NEUROLEPTIC-INDUCED MOVEMENT DISORDERS

T0312108

Neuroleptics, one of the most widely prescribed groups of psychotropic drugs, are indispensable in the management of the majority of patients with schizophrenia, as well as patients with other psychoses. But neuroleptic treatment has not proved to be an unmixed blessing. Neuroleptics are associated with troublesome adverse side effects, of which movement disorders are the most serious in terms of frequency, persistence, and overall impact on the well-being of patients and caregivers. Medication-induced movement disorders have now been recognized as a separate category in DSM-IV.

This book was compiled with the aim of improving our understanding and clinical management of these iatrogenic conditions. It deals with the historical, clinical, and neurobiological aspects of tardive dyskinesia and related movement disorders, such as parkinsonism, dystonia, and akathisia. There are also chapters devoted to the measurement of tardive dyskinesia, its geographic and ethnic differences, and its management with novel neuroleptic agents and biofeedback.

With authoritative contributions and an international perspective, this book will be valuable to clinicians and researchers alike in psychiatry, neurology, and related disciplines.

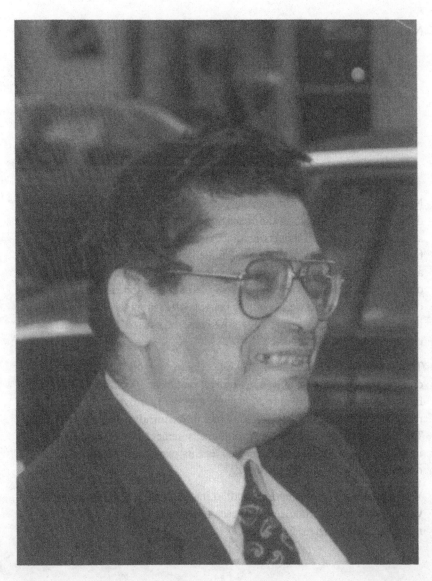

Ramzy Yassa, M.D.

NEUROLEPTIC-INDUCED MOVEMENT DISORDERS

Edited by

RAMZY YASSA, M.D.
Douglas Hospital, Quebec

N. P. V. NAIR, M.D.
Douglas Hospital, Quebec

DILIP V. JESTE, M.D.
University of California, San Diego

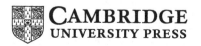

CAMBRIDGE
UNIVERSITY PRESS

CAMBRIDGE UNIVERSITY PRESS
Cambridge, New York, Melbourne, Madrid, Cape Town, Singapore, São Paulo

Cambridge University Press
The Edinburgh Building, Cambridge CB2 2RU, UK

Published in the United States of America by Cambridge University Press, New York

www.cambridge.org
Information on this title: www.cambridge.org/9780521433648

© Cambridge University Press 1997

First published 1997
This digitally printed first paperback version 2006

A catalogue record for this publication is available from the British Library

Library of Congress Cataloguing in Publication data
Neuroleptic-induced movement disorders/[edited by] Ramzy Yassa,
   N.P.V. Nair, Dilip V. Jeste.
      p.   cm.
   Includes bibliographical references.
   ISBN 0-521-43364-9 (hc)
   1. Tardive dyskinesia – Etiology.   2. Antipsychotic drugs – Side
effects.   3. Movement disorders – Etiology.   I. Yassa, Ramzy.
II. Nair, N.P.V.   III. Jeste, Dilip V.
   RC394.T37N48   1996
616.8'3 – dc20   95-50009

ISBN-13   978-0-521-43364-8 hardback
ISBN-10   0-521-43364-9 hardback

ISBN-13   978-0-521-03352-7 paperback
ISBN-10   0-521-03352-7 paperback

Contents

Contributors

Margot Albus, M.D., Ph.D.
State Mental Hospital Haar, Vockestrasse 72, D-85529 Haar, Germany

José Ma. J. Alvir, Dr. P.H.
Department of Psychiatry, Hillside Hospital, Long Island Jewish Medical Center, Glen Oaks, New York 11004, and Albert Einstein College of Medicine, Bronx, New York 10461

Jeffrey S. Aronowitz, M.D.
Mercy Center for Health Services, Watertown, New York 13601

Peter Buckley, M.R.C.Psych.
St. John of God Psychiatric Service, Dublin, Ireland

Robert E. Burke, M.D.
Department of Neurology, College of Physicians and Surgeons, Columbia University, New York, New York 10032

Michael P. Caligiuri, Ph.D.
Department of Psychiatry, School of Medicine, University of California, San Diego, San Diego, California 92093, and Veterans Affairs Medical Center, San Diego, California 92161

Shawn L. Cassady, M.D.
Maryland Psychiatric Research Center, University of Maryland School of Medicine, Baltimore, Maryland 21228

Jonathan O. Cole, M.D.
McLean Hospital, Belmont, Massachusetts 02178

Alan S. DeWolfe, Ph.D.
Department of Psychology, Loyola University, Chicago, Illinois

John Doucette, M.Phil.
Department of Epidemiology and Public Health, Yale University School of Medicine, New Haven, Connecticut 06520

Cheryl Flynn, Ph.D.
The Nathan S. Kline Institute for Psychiatric Research, State of New York Office of Mental Health, Orangeburg, New York 10962

Ronald C. Fudge, Ph.D.
Department of Veterans Affairs, Franklin Delano Roosevelt Hospital, Montrose, New York 10548

Linda Ganzini, M.D.
Department of Psychiatry, School of Medicine, Oregon Health Sciences University, Portland, Oregon 97201-3098, and Consultation-Liaison Section, Psychiatry Section Service, Portland Veterans Affairs Medical Center, Portland, Oregon

George Gardos, M.D.
McLean Hospital, Belmont, Massachusetts 02178

Jes Gerlach, M.D.
Saint Hans Hospital, DK-4000 Roskilde, Denmark

William M. Glazer, M.D.
Associate Clinical Professor of Psychiatry, Harvard School of Medicine, Massachusetts General Hospital, P.O. Box 121, Beach Plum Lane, Menemsha, MA 02552

Paul Greene, M.D.
The Neurological Institute, Columbia-Presbyterian Medical Center, 710 West 168th Street, New York, New York 10032-3784

Thomas E. Hansen, M.D.
Psychiatry Service, Department of Veterans Affairs Medical Center, Portland, Oregon, and Department of Psychiatry, Oregon Health Sciences University, Portland, Oregon 97201-3098

Teruo Hayashi, M.D., Ph.D.
Department of Psychiatry and Neurosciences, Hiroshima University School of Medicine, Kasumi 1-2-3, Minami-ku, Hiroshima 734, Japan

William F. Hoffman, Ph.D., M.D.
Psychiatry Service, Department of Veterans Affairs Medical Center, Portland, Oregon, and Department of Psychiatry, Oregon Health Sciences University, Portland, Oregon 97201-3098

Dilip V. Jeste, M.D.
Department of Psychiatry, University of California, San Diego, San Diego, California 92093, and Geriatric Psychiatry Clinical Research Center, San Diego Veterans Affairs Medical Center, San Diego, California 92161

John M. Kane, M.D.
Department of Psychiatry, Hillsdale Hospital, Long Island Jewish Medical Center, Glen Oaks, New York 11004, and Albert Einstein College of Medicine, Bronx, New York 10461

George A. Keepers, M.D.
Department of Psychiatry, School of Medicine, Oregon Health Sciences University, Portland, Oregon 97201-3098

T. A. Kerr, M.D.
Newcastle Mental Health N.H.S. Trust, St. Nicholas Hospital, Newcastle upon Tyne, United Kingdom

Bruce J. Kinon, M.D.
Department of Psychiatry, Hillside Hospital, Long Island Jewish Medical Center, Glen Oaks, New York 11004

Anthony Kinsella, M.Sc.
Department of Mathematics, Dublin Institute of Technology, Dublin 8, Ireland

Jonathan P. Lacro, Pharm.D.
Department of Psychiatry, University of California, San Diego, San Diego, California 92093, and San Diego Veterans Affairs Medical Center, San Diego, California 92161

Conall Larkin, F.R.C.Psych.
St. John of God Psychiatric Service, Dublin, Ireland

Jeffrey A. Lieberman, M.D.
Department of Psychiatry, Hillside Hospital, Long Island Jewish Medical Center, Glen Oaks, New York 11004, and Albert Einstein College of Medicine, Bronx, New York 10461

Pierre-Michel Llorca, M.D.
Douglas Hospital Research Centre, Verdun, Quebec H4H 1R3, Canada

H. A. McClelland, M.D.
Newcastle Mental Health N.H.S. Trust, St. Nicholas Hospital, Newcastle upon Tyne NE4 9BE, United Kingdom

Cathy Madigan, M.A.
St. John of God Psychiatric Service, Dublin, Ireland

Mark Magulac, M.D.
Department of Psychiatry, School of Medicine, University of California, San Diego, San Diego, California 92093, and Children's Hospital and Health Center, Children's Way, San Diego, California 92123

Sahebarao P. Mahadik, Ph.D.
Department of Psychiatry, Medical College of Georgia, Augusta, Georgia 30912-3800

Hal Morgenstern, Ph.D.
Department of Epidemiology, UCLA School of Public Health, University of California, Los Angeles, Los Angeles, California

Aron D. Mosnaim, Ph.D.
Department of Pharmacology and Molecular Biology, Finch University of Health Sciences, The Chicago Medical School, 3333 Green Bay Road, North Chicago, Illinois 60064-3095

Driss Moussaoui, M.D.
Centre Psychiatrique University Ibn Rochd, Rue Tarik Ibn Ziad, Casablanca, Morocco

Sukdeb Mukherjee, M.D.
Medical College of Georgia, Augusta, Georgia 30912

Ikuo Nagaoka, M.D.
Department of Psychiatry and Neurosciences, Hiroshima University School of Medicine, Kasumi 1-2-3, Minami-ku, Hiroshima 734, Japan

N. P. V. Nair, M.D.
6875 Boul. Lasalle, Douglas Hospital Research Centre, Verdun, Quebec H4H 1R3, Canada

Eadbhard O'Callaghan, F.R.C.P.I.
St. John of God Psychiatric Service, Dublin, Ireland

Linda Peacock, M.D.
Saint Hans Hospital, DK-4000 Roskilde, Denmark

Laura Read, Ph.D.
The Nathan S. Kline Institute for Psychiatric Research, State of New York Office of Mental Health, Orangeburg, New York 10962

Margaret Reilly, Ph.D.
The Nathan S. Kline Institute for Psychiatric Research, State of New York Office of Mental Health, Orangeburg, New York 10962

Mary Ann Richardson, Ph.D.
The Nathan S. Kline Institute for Psychiatric Research, State of New York Office of Mental Health, Orangeburg, New York 10962

Allan Z. Safferman, M.D.
Pfizer, Inc., New York, New York 10021

Hiroshi Saitoh, M.D., Ph.D.
Department of Psychiatry and Neurosciences, Hiroshima University School of Medicine, Kasumi 1-2-3, Minami-ku, Hiroshima 734, Japan

Bruce L. Saltz, M.D.
Department of Psychiatry, Hillside Hospital, Long Island Jewish Medical Center, Glen Oaks, New York 11004, and Albert Einstein College of Medicine, Bronx, New York 10461

Christian L. Shriqui, M.D., M.Sc., F.R.C.P.C.
Assistant Professor of Psychiatry, Laval University, and Clinical Research Psychiatrist and Clinical Research Scientist, Fonds de la Recherche en Santé du Québec (FRSQ), Centre de Recherche Université Laval Robert Giffard and Centre Hospitalier Robert-Giffard, Beauport, Québec G1J 2G3, Canada

Cecile E. Sison, Ph.D.
Franklin Delano Roosevelt Department of Veterans Affairs Medical Center, Montrose, New York 10548

Raymond Suckow, Ph.D.
The Nathan S. Kline Institute for Psychiatric Research, State of New York Office of Mental Health, Orangeburg, New York 10962

Carol A. Tamminga, M.D.
Maryland Psychiatric Research Center, University of Maryland School of Medicine, Baltimore, Maryland 21228

Gunvant K. Thaker, M.D.
Maryland Psychiatric Research Center, University of Maryland School of Medicine, Baltimore, Maryland 21228

Yosuke Uchitomi, M.D., Ph.D.
Department of Psychiatry and Neurosciences, Hiroshima University School of Medicine, Kasumi 1-2-3, Minami-ku, Hiroshima 734, Japan

Daniel Umbricht, M.D.
Department of Psychiatry, Hillside Hospital, Long Island Jewish Medical Center, Glen Oaks, New York 11004

John L. Waddington, D.Sc.
Department of Clinical Pharmacology, Royal College of Surgeons in Ireland, Dublin 2, Ireland

Donna Raye Wagner, M.A.
Department of Epidemiology and Public Health, Yale University School of Medicine, New Haven, Connecticut 06520

T. E. G. West, Ph.D.
Douglas Hospital Research Centre, Verdun, Quebec H4H 1R3, Canada

Margaret G. Woerner, Ph.D.
Department of Psychiatry, Hillside Hospital, Long Island Jewish Medical Center, Glen Oaks, New York 11004

Marc-Alain Wolf, M.D.
Douglas Hospital Research Centre, Verdun, Quebec H4H 1R3, Canada

Marion E. Wolf, M.D.
Department of Psychiatry, Stritch School of Medicine, Loyola University, Chicago, Illinois, and Veterans Affairs Medical Center, North Chicago, Illinois 60064

Shigeto Yamawaki, M.D., Ph.D.
Department of Psychiatry and Neurosciences, Hiroshima University School of Medicine, Kasumi 1-2-3, Minami-ku, Hiroshima 734, Japan

Ramzy Yassa, M.D.
Douglas Hospital Research Centre, Verdun, Quebec H4H 1R3, Canada

Norio Yokota, M.D., Ph.D.
Department of Psychiatry and Neurosciences, Hiroshima University School
of Medicine, Kasumi 1-2-3, Minami-ku, Hiroshima 734, Japan

Preface

It is interesting to note that the three classes of psychotropic drugs that were introduced into psychiatry within the span of a few years around 1950 have had greater impact in the treatment of the major psychiatric disorders than have any other forms of treatment in this century. These include the antipsychotic drugs or neuroleptics, the tricyclic antidepressants, and lithium. Of the three groups, neuroleptics are easily the most widely prescribed agents worldwide. They are being used – and sometimes overused and misused – to treat not only schizophrenia and other psychoses but also a host of additional behavioral disorders. Although neuroleptics continue to be indispensable in the management of a majority of schizophrenic patients, as well as some other psychotic individuals, they have not proved to be an unmixed blessing. In terms of frequency, persistence, and overall impact on the quality of well-being for patients and caregivers, movement disorders are the most serious adverse side effects of neuroleptics.

The importance of iatrogenic movement disorders in psychiatry can be deduced from the fact that the *Diagnostic and Statistical Manual of Mental Disorders,* fourth edition (DSM-IV), recently published by the American Psychiatric Association, includes a separate category of "medication-induced movement disorders." This newly delineated group of conditions primarily includes neuroleptic-induced movement disorders such as parkinsonism, dystonia, akathisia, and, especially, tardive dyskinesia. The American Psychiatric Association had previously appointed two task forces on tardive dyskinesia, and those groups published reports in 1980 and 1992.

In the past few years, there have been exciting advances in psychopharmacology. Dopamine and serotonin antagonists, including clozapine, risperidone, and olanzapine, are being used to treat increasing numbers of patients. In contrast to the traditional dopamine-blocking antipsychotic agents, it has been shown that these newer drugs significantly reduce the negative symptoms of schizophrenia and produce fewer extrapyramidal side effects. Nonetheless, they are not free of the risk of inducing movement disorders. In all probability, the neuroleptic-associated movement disorders will be with us for at least the immediate future. Until the emergence of a new generation of antipsychotic agents that can act highly selectively, with no risk of causing movement disorders, we need to study these iatrogenic conditions in depth so as to understand them better and improve the management of our patients. We hope that this book will be of value to those interested in understanding the clinical uses of neuroleptic agents and the research into their adverse effects.

This book is divided into seven parts. Part I has a chapter that provides the historical perspective on neuroleptic-induced movement disorders. Part II deals with the clinical aspects of tardive dyskinesia – the most serious of the iatrogenic movement disorders. The nine chapters in Part II discuss studies of the epidemiology of tardive dyskinesia, the various predisposing risk factors such as aging, gender, primary psychiatric disorders (e.g., schizophrenia, affective disorder), and physical co-morbidity (especially diabetes mellitus), other patient-related factors such as family medical history and smoking, and treatment-related factors (principally neuroleptic and anticholinergic medications). Part III focuses on the neurobiological mechanisms likely involved in tardive dyskinesia. Its seven chapters consider the possible neurochemical abnormalities (involving mainly the neurotransmitters in the basal ganglia, with particular emphasis on dopamine and phenylalanine) and the neuroendocrine, cognitive, and structural brain abnormalities related to tardive dyskinesia. There is also a discussion of animal models pertaining to the disorder. Part IV presents a chapter on clinical and instrumental measurements of the severity of tardive dyskinesia. Part V focuses on the manifestations of tardive dyskinesia in different patient populations. Its five chapters summarize numerous studies of tardive dyskinesia in Asia, North Africa, the Middle East, and Europe, as well as studies of patients from diverse racial/ethnic groups and studies involving children and adolescents. Part VI deals with other movement disorders induced by neuroleptics – parkinsonism, acute and tardive dystonia, and tardive akathisia. The chapters in Part VII discuss the management of tardive dyskinesia using novel neuroleptic agents, GABA-ergic drugs, and biofeedback. Although this book may not contain a chapter on every single aspect of neuroleptic-induced movement disorders, we have attempted to cover all the critical issues in the clinical and research arenas pertaining to this topic.

We find it indescribably sad that this preface is being written by only two of the original three editors. Ramzy Yassa, M.D., died unexpectedly at the age of 52 on October 3, 1992, while working on this volume. We consider ourselves blessed to have worked with Dr. Yassa on this and many other projects.

Dr. Yassa was born in Cairo, Egypt. After completing his medical training in Cairo, he earned M.B. and B.Ch. degrees before moving to Montreal, Canada, where he completed his residency in psychiatry at the Douglas Hospital, Montreal, subsequently becoming a Fellow of the Royal College of Physicians and Surgeons (Canada) and a Diplomate of the American Board of Psychiatry and Neurology. Dr. Yassa joined the staff of the Douglas Hospital and the faculty of McGill University, where he became a professor of psychiatry. He published more than a hundred papers and book chapters on various topics, mainly in the area of psychopharmacology.

Dr. Yassa was truly a remarkable man. A gentleman and a scholar, he was also an outstanding scientist. He set a role model for others, conducting high-quality clinical research without the benefit of external grant support and without laboratories and other such resources. He was a gifted phenomenological researcher, with exquisite powers of observation. Many clinical observations first reported by Dr. Yassa have subsequently been replicated by other investigators with much greater resources at hand. Dr. Yassa was an inspirational teacher and mentor for a large number of young investigators. As caring and compassionate with his junior and senior colleagues as he was with his patients, he touched forever the lives of those fortunate enough to know him. He will be sorely missed by his patients, colleagues, and friends. We dedicate this book to the achievements of Ramzy Yassa, M.D.

N. P. V. Nair, M.D.
Dilip V. Jeste, M.D.

Part I

Historical Perspective

1

Neuroleptic-Induced Movement Disorders: Historical Perspective

MARC-ALAIN WOLF, M.D., RAMZY YASSA, M.D.,
and PIERRE-MICHEL LLORCA, M.D.

In February 1952, Laborit, Huguenard, and Alluaume published an article concerning the anesthetic properties of a new medication, chlorpromazine, mentioning therein the induction of a "psychic disinterest." That same year, Delay, Deniker, and Harl (1952a,b), Delay et al. (1952c), and Hamon, Paraire, and Velluz (1952) first reported the effects of chlorpromazine in patients with various psychiatric conditions. A few months later, the effectiveness of the first neuroleptic was considered to have been demonstrated.

Initial Descriptions

The first description of an extrapyramidal syndrome during the course of neuroleptic treatment dates back to the 1953 Swiss symposium on chlorpromazine. The next year, Labhardt (1954) and Staehelin (1954) reported certain extrapyramidal complications caused by neuroleptics. It was Steck (1954, 1956), however, who vividly described such symptoms in a convincing manner. (Not until 1961 did Lambert and Broussolle note that it was not surprising that the Swiss authors had reported good results from their use of neuroleptics, given the high dosages used, which of course entailed a greater likelihood of developing extrapyramidal side effects.) Steck (1954) stated that "since the summer of 1953, we were impressed by the appearance of a well-developed parkinsonian syndrome in a chronic, cyclically agitated patient who also manifested schizophrenic symptomatology. This patient presented the well-known picture of post-encephalitic parkinsonism with psychomotor rigidity, tremors, facial seborrhea, marked salivation and akathisia." Steck (1954) also reported the presence of extrapyramidal symptoms in 78 of 232 (34%) women and 33 of 77 (43%) men treated with neuroleptics. He claimed, as well, that this syndrome was completely reversible and that its occurrence depended on the dosage used. Comparing the symptoms of this syndrome

with those of encephalitis lethargica, Steck identified both an initial phase of
somnolence, akin to the lethargic period of the encephalitis, and a parkinsonian syndrome similar to postencephalitic parkinsonism. That analogy
prompted him to postulate an extrapyramidal and diencephalic localization for
the actions of the neuroleptics.

A symposium on neuroleptic medications was held in Paris in October
1955; 5 of the 150 presentations discussed neuroleptic-induced extrapyramidal symptoms. Investigators reported that the "pseudoparkinsonian signs" of
neurolepticized patients, which presented rarely as a typical parkinsonian
syndrome, were more often seen as a forme fruste (Letailleur, Morin, &
Monnerie 1956). Others reported that when compared with parkinsonian
patients, the neurolepticized patients had more frequent tremors and different
characteristic electromyographic tracings (Deniker, Bourguignon, & Lempérière, 1956). The positive effects of anticholinergic drugs were also noted
(Letailleur et al., 1956).

In that same year, 1955, Delay and Deniker, on observing the similarities
in therapeutic efficacy and extrapyramidal activity of two such seemingly
different compounds as chlorpromazine and reserpine, used the term "neuroleptic" to characterize their combination of properties (Deniker, 1989).

In the following year, Flügel (1956) was the first to hypothesize the apparent necessity of inducing a parkinsonian state to obtain a therapeutic effect in
the psychiatric condition. As concern with the extrapyramidal side effects
grew, an international symposium on the subject was scheduled for Montreal
in 1960, and there the questions regarding the efficacy of neuroleptics and
their relationship to parkinsonism were fully discussed. Delay and Deniker
(1961) reported that the percentage of patients who had experienced improvement when taking certain neuroleptics (perphenazine, trifluoperazine) seemed
to be directly related to the appearance of extrapyramidal symptoms. Haase
(1961) reported that it was only when extrapyramidal manifestations appeared
that the neuroleptics led to improvements in the underlying psychiatric conditions. On the other hand, Lambert and Broussolle (1961) stated that some
psychiatric patients had shown improvement without exhibiting extrapyramidal side effects, that others had exhibited extrapyramidal side effects without
showing improvement, and that the addition of an anticholinergic did not
affect the therapeutic outcome. Cole and Clyde (1961), in an efficacy comparison of thioridazine (which causes relatively fewer extrapyramidal side
effects) and fluphenazine (which causes relatively more), found the two products equally effective.

Somewhat earlier, Delay and Deniker (1957) had outlined five characteristics by way of defining the new class of neuroleptics. Neuroleptics, they said,

produced psychomotor indifference, a sedative effect, an antipsychotic effect, and vegetative and extrapyramidal effects and had a dominantly subcortical site of action. Those authors were criticized, however, by their American counterparts, as recounted by Deniker: "Naturally, this definition did not please everybody. In fact, Americans were horrified. It was a matter of defining a group of drugs by their adverse effects, and they preferred such terms as tranquilizers, later on using the expression 'major tranquilizers', and finally, using the expression 'antipsychotic'. In 1970, Stille and Hippius announced that clozapine was a powerful antipsychotic without extrapyramidal effects: our theory was therefore seriously attacked. In reality, this was the exception which proved the rule" (Deniker, 1989).

By 1960, the sequence of appearance of neuroleptic-induced extrapyramidal side effects had been precisely described (Goldman, 1961; Lambert & Broussolle, 1961), as follows: For the first few days, dyskinetic or dystonic excitomotor crises occur; the next few weeks bring about an akinetohypertonic parkinsonian syndrome; during the following weeks, a tardive excitomotor syndrome with akathisia occurs; and finally, after several months of neuroleptic treatment, continuous oral or choreiform movements appear. At the Montreal symposium, Lambert and Broussolle (1961) proposed a classification of the neuroleptics based on their therapeutic efficacy and extrapyramidal side effects. Those researchers distinguished a sedative group, with levomepromazine as its main referent, and an antipsychotic group, with thioproperazine and piperazine derivatives as examples of its products. It was that latter group, they said, that produced higher rates of extrapyramidal side effects. Goldman (1961), who stated that anticholinergic drugs could prevent the development of extrapyramidal side effects, also noted that parkinsonian manifestations could spontaneously disappear and that akathisia was difficult to treat. At that same symposium, epidemiologic (Ayd, 1961) and psychoanalytic (Sarwer-Foner, 1961) studies of neuroleptic-induced extrapyramidal side effects were presented.

Tardive Dyskinesia

The tardive complications of neuroleptic treatment were not mentioned in the literature until the late 1950s. Moreover, they were referred to only anecdotally at the Montreal symposium (Goldman, 1961; Lambert & Broussolle, 1961). In 1983, Tarsy reconstructed the early history of tardive dyskinesia as follows:

• In 1957, Matthias Schonecker, in Germany, reported on 3 women, ages 60 years and older, who presented with bucco-oral movements a few weeks after beginning chlorpromazine treatment. Although the neuroleptic dosage was decreased for one patient and the drug was discontinued for the other two, the symptoms continued. Those patients suffered from depressive or anxiety symptoms, with cerebral arteriosclerosis. Schonecker concluded that those manifestations differed from acute extrapyramidal side effects.

- In 1959, a French group (Sigwald et al., 1959) described 4 women, ages 54 years and older, in whom involuntary movements of the tongue, lips, and facial muscles had appeared after several years of phenothiazine treatment. Calling those movements "facio-bucco-linguo-masticatory dyskinesias," the group proposed a first classification of the dyskinesias into acute and chronic types.

- In 1960, the Danish authors Uhrbrand and Faurbye described 29 patients who exhibited buccolinguomasticatory movements, sometimes associated with trunk and foot movements, that still persisted in 50% of the patients after discontinuation of the neuroleptics. Those authors noted that whereas discontinuation of the neuroleptics aggravated the syndrome in some patients, it unmasked the condition in others. They also noted that the movements were more frequent for aged patients suffering from organic abnormalities. Faurbye et al. (1964) proposed the term "tardive dyskinesia" for this condition.

- The first North American observations date to 1960. First, Kruse (1960) reported on 3 women, ages 50 years and older, who developed akathisia accompanied by abnormal movements of the legs, arms, and mouth that continued for several months after neuroleptics were discontinued. Then Druckman, Seelinger, and Thulin (1962) described severe dystonia of the neck and trunk in a 46-year-old man whose manifestations had not changed during 20 months following discontinuation of neuroleptics. It was Keegan and Rajput (1973) who first used the term "tardive dystonia."

- The first British observations were reported by Hunter, Earl, and Janz (1964a) and Hunter, Earl, and Thornicroft (1964b), who described the different manifestations of tardive dyskinesia as bucco-oral, choreiform movements of the limbs, along with respiratory dyskinesia. Comparing that condition to encephalitis lethargica, with its viral origin, they suggested the presence of a chemical encephalitis.

As shown by those historical vignettes, the patients described in the early literature were mainly of advanced age, a time when organic involvement is common. It was not until the late 1960s that serious epidemiologic studies were undertaken, showing prevalences varying between 0.5% and 65% (Wolf & Gautier, 1987). Indeed, most of the predisposing factors suspected in the early studies (cerebral lesions, lobotomy, electroconvulsive treatment) have never been decisively confirmed by more recent studies, whereas such factors as older age and female gender were confirmed only later (Tarsy, 1983).

Deniker (1989) showed that interest in tardive dyskinesia varied widely from one country to another. French researchers, for example, were less concerned about this side effect than were their American counterparts. Perhaps dyskinesia was a more severe problem in the United States because of the Americans' more liberal use of neuroleptics, at higher dosages, and because fewer such medications had been approved for use in the United States (Deniker, 1989). Medicolegal concerns in the United States had also increased the apprehension of American physicians (Wolf, Grunberg, & Garneau, 1988). Periodically the American College of Neuropsychopharmacology (1973) and the American Psychiatric Association (1980, 1992) have published reports by various "task forces" synthesizing the current knowledge concerning tardive dyskinesia. Yassa and Jeste (1988) have speculated that the new antipsychotic molecules that are devoid of neurological side effects may lead to the disappearance of tardive dyskinesia.

Conclusion

Tardive dyskinesia remains an enigmatic phenomenon, not only because of its paradoxical clinical aspects but also from a scientific viewpoint. It will constitute a challenge for basic and clinical researchers for generations to come.

Acknowledgment

The authors thank Dr. D. Bloom for his help in editing the manuscript.

References

American College of Neuropsychopharmacology/Food and Drug Administration Task Force (1973). Neurologic syndromes associated with antipsychotic drug use. *Arch. Gen. Psychiatry* 28:463–6.

American Psychiatric Association Task Force on Late Neurological Effects of Antipsychotic Drugs (1980). Tardive dyskinesia. *Am. J. Psychiatry* 137:1163–72.

American Psychiatric Association (1992). *Tardive dyskinesia. A Task Force Report.* Washington, D.C.: American Psychiatric Association.

Ayd, F. (1961). Neuroleptics and extrapyramidal reactions in psychiatric patients. In *Extrapyramidal System and Neuroleptics,* ed. J. M. Bordeleau, pp. 355–63. International symposium, Montreal, November 1960. Montreal: Editions Psychiatriques.

Cole, J., & Clyde, D. (1961). Extrapyramidal side effects and clinical response to the phenothiazines. In *Extrapyramidal System and Neuroleptics,* ed. J. M.

Bordeleau, pp. 469–78. International symposium, Montreal, November 1960. Montreal: Editions Psychiatriques.

Delay, J., & Deniker, P. (1957). Caracteristiques psychophysiologiques des médicaments neuroleptiques. Rapport au Symposium International sur les médicaments psychotropiques, Milan, 9–11 mai 1957. In *Psychotropic Drugs*, pp. 485–501. Amsterdam: Elsevier.

Delay, J., & Deniker, P. (1961). Apport de la clinique à la connaissance de l'action des neuroleptiques. In *Extrapyramidal System and Neuroleptics*, ed. J. M. Bordeleau, pp. 301–27. International symposium, Montreal, November 1960. Montreal: Editions Psychiatriques.

Delay, J., Deniker, P., & Harl, J. M. (1952a). Utilisation en thérapeutique psychiatrique d'une phénothiazine d'action centrale élective. *Ann. Med. Psychol. (Paris)* 110:112–17.

Delay, J., Deniker, P., & Harl, J. M. (1952b). Traitement des états d'excitation et d'agitation par une méthode médicamenteuse dérivée de l'hibernothérapie. *Ann. Med. Psychol. (Paris)* 110:267–73.

Delay, J., Deniker, P., Harl, J. M., & Grasset, A. (1952c). Traitement d'états confusionnels par le 4560 RP. *Ann. Med. Psychol. (Paris)* 110:398–403.

Deniker, P. (1989). From chlorpromazine to tardive dyskinesia (brief history of the neuroleptics). *Psychiatr. J. Univ. Ottawa* 14:253–9.

Deniker, P., Bourguignon, A., & Lempérière, T. (1956). Complications d'allure extrapyramidale au cours des traitements par la chlorpromazine et la réserpine. (Etude clinique et électromyographique). In *Colloque international sur la chlorpromazine et les médicaments neuroleptiques en thérapeutique psychiatrique (Paris, octobre 1955). Encephale (Paris), Numéro spécial*, pp. 793–8.

Druckman, R., Seelinger, D., & Thulin, B. (1962). Chronic involuntary movements induced by phenothiazines. *J. Nerv. Ment. Dis.* 135:69–76.

Faurbye, A., Rasch, P. J., Petersen, P. B., Brandborg, G., & Pakkenberg, H. (1964). Neurological symptoms in pharmacotherapy of psychoses. *Acta Psychiatr. Scand.* 40:10–27.

Flügel, F. (1956). Thérapeutique par médication neuroleptique obtenue en réalisant systématiquement des états parkinsoniformes. In *Colloque international sur la chlorpromazine et les médicaments neuroleptiques en thérapeutique psychiatrique (Paris, octobre 1955). Encephale (Paris), Numéro spécial*, pp. 790–2.

Goldman, D. (1961). Parkinsonism and related phenomena from administration of drugs: their production and control under clinical conditions and possible relation to therapeutic effect. In *Extrapyramidal System and Neuroleptics*, ed. J. M. Bordeleau, pp. 453–64. International symposium, Montreal, November 1960. Montreal: Editions Psychiatriques.

Haase, H. (1961). Extrapyramidal modification of fine movements – a "conditio sine qua non" of the fundamental therapeutic action of neuroleptic drugs. In *Extrapyramidal System and Neuroleptics*, ed. J. M. Bordeleau, pp. 329–53. International symposium, Montreal, November 1960. Montreal: Editions Psychiatriques.

Hamon, J., Paraire, J., & Velluz, J. (1952). Remarques sur l'action du 4560 RP sur l'agitation maniaque. *Ann. Med. Psychol. (Paris)* 110:331–5.

Hunter, R., Earl, C. J., & Janz, D. (1964a). A syndrome of abnormal movements and dementia in leucotomized patients treated with phenothiazines. *J. Neurol. Neurosurg. Psychiatry* 27:219–23.

Hunter, R., Earl, C. J., & Thornicroft, S. (1964b). An apparently irreversible syndrome of abnormal movements following phenothiazine medication. *Proc. R. Soc. Med.* 57:758–62.

Keegan, D. L., & Rajput, A. H. (1973). Drug-induced dystonia tarda: treatment with L-dopa. *Dis. Nerv. Syst.* 38:167–9.

Kruse, W. (1960). Persistent muscular restlessness after phenothiazine treatment: report of 3 cases. *Am. J. Psychiatry* 117:152–3.

Labhardt, F. (1954). Technik, Nebeuerscheinungen und Komplikationen der Largactiltherapie (Largactil-Symposium Basel, Nov. 28, 1953). *Schweiz. Arch. Neurol. Psychiatr.* 73:338–45.

Laborit, H., Huguenard, P., & Alluaume, R. (1952). Un nouveau stabilisateur végétatif (le 4560 RP). *Presse Med.* 60:206–8.

Lambert, P. A., & Broussolle, P. (1961). Activité thérapeutique et incidence neurologique de divers neuroleptiques: comparaisons et réflexions. In *Extrapyramidal System and Neuroleptics*, ed. J. M. Bordeleau, pp. 405–26. International symposium, Montreal, November 1960. Montreal: Editions Psychiatriques.

Letailleur, M., Morin, J., & Monnerie, R. (1956). Syndromes transitoires pseudo-parkinsoniens provoqués par la chlorpromazine. In *Colloque international sur la chlorpromazine et les médicaments neuroleptiques en thérapeutique psychiatrique (Paris, Octobre 1955). Encephale (Paris), Numéro spécial*, pp. 806–9.

Sarwer-Foner, G. (1961). Some comments on the psychodynamic aspects of the extrapyramidal reactions. In *Extrapyramidal System and Neuroleptics*, ed. J. M. Bordeleau, pp. 527–33. International symposium, Montreal, November 1960. Montreal: Editions Psychiatriques.

Schonecker, M. (1957). Beitrag zu der Mitteilung von Kulenkampff und Tarnow. Ein eigentumliches Syndrom im oralen Bereich bei Megaphenapplikation. *Nervenarzt* 28:35.

Sigwald, J., Bouttier, D., Raymondeaud, C., & Piot, C. (1959). Quatre cas de dyskinésie facio-bucco-linguo-masticatrice à l'évolution prolongée secondaire à un traitement par les neuroleptiques. *Rev. Neurol. (Paris)* 100:751–5.

Staehelin, J. E. (1954). Largactil-Symposion in der psychiatrischen Universitätsklinik Basel. *Schweiz. Arch. Neurol. Psychiatr.* 73:288–91.

Steck, H. (1954). Le syndrome extrapyramidal et diencéphalique au cours des traitements au largactil et au serpasil. *Ann. Med. Psychol. (Paris)* 112:737–44.

Steck, H. (1956). Le syndrome extrapyramidal dans les cures de chlorpromazine et serpasil. Sa symptomatologie clinique et son rôle thérapeutique. In *Colloque international sur la chlorpromazine et les médicaments neuroleptiques en thérapeutique psychiatrique (Paris, Octobre 1955). Encephale (Paris), Numéro spécial*, pp. 783–9.

Tarsy, D. (1983). History and definition of tardive dyskinesia. *Clin. Neuropharmacol.* 6:91–9.

Uhrbrand, L., & Faurbye, A. (1960). Reversible and irreversible dyskinesia after treatment with perphenazine, chlorpromazine, reserpine and electroconvulsive therapy. *Psychopharmacologia* 1:408–18.

Wolf, M. A., & Gautier, J. (1987). Tardive dyskinesia: a clinical update. *Mod. Med. Can.* 42:143–50.

Wolf, M. A., Grunberg, F., & Garneau, Y. (1988). Aspects médico-légaux des dyskinésies tardives aux États-unis. *Encephale (Paris)* 24:133–8.

Yassa, R., & Jeste, D. V. (1988). Tardive dyskinesia 1988: 31 years later. *J. Clin. Psychopharmacol. (Suppl. 4)* 8:1.

Part II
Clinical Aspects of Tardive Dyskinesia

2

Aging and Tardive Dyskinesia

BRUCE L. SALTZ, M.D., JOHN M. KANE, M.D.,
MARGARET G. WOERNER, Ph.D., JEFFREY A.
LIEBERMAN, M.D., and JOSÉ MA. J. ALVIR, Dr. P.H.

Tardive dyskinesia, a syndrome of abnormal, involuntary body movements, is produced by administration of antipsychotic drugs. The movements can involve the face, lips, jaw, tongue, neck, trunk, upper extremities, and lower extremities. Less obvious internal body regions can also be
involved, such as the muscles of respiration. "Dyskinesia" is a generic
term, referring to excessive or abnormal movements of any etiology or
character. Historically, it has been used predominantly to refer to
choreoathetoid-type movements; more recently it has also been used to
include tics, dystonia, akathisia, myoclonus, and ballismus. Although
tremors are also, by definition, abnormal movements, they have traditionally been recorded as a separate form of movement disorder. When an
antipsychotic drug is believed to be the cause of the dyskinesia, the term
"tardive" is employed. When an antipsychotic drug is implicated in the
appearance of tremors, the term "drug-induced parkinsonism" is used. In
general, it has been the rule that at least 3 months of neuroleptic treatment
should precede any attribution of these drugs as causative agents in the
development of tardive dyskinesia (Schooler & Kane, 1982), although
recent work with older individuals suggests that shorter exposure times
may be sufficient. The abnormal movements themselves can be distinguished phenomenologically by their rhythmicity, speed, and repetition, as
well as by the presence or absence of sustained postures at the termination
of the movement. Combinations of different movements are frequently
seen, with parkinsonism, choreiform dyskinesia, and akathisia being
among the most common in elderly patients. Generally, the movements do
not occur during sleep, and frequently they are exacerbated by anxiety and
stress.

Many different rating systems have been used to document the location and
character of abnormal involuntary movements; none, however, can be diagnostic without a family history and concurrent medical, neurological, physi-

cal, and laboratory information. The Abnormal Involuntary Movement Scale (AIMS) (Guy, 1976) is one of the most widely used instruments for recording the severity and location of dyskinetic activity.

Relationship Between Spontaneous Dyskinesia and Tardive Dyskinesia

Many studies of tardive dyskinesia have shown that abnormal movements resembling those of tardive dyskinesia can occur in individuals who have not been treated with neuroleptics, either young or old. The reported prevalence rates have varied, depending on the diagnostic method used (Kane & Smith, 1982). It has been estimated, for instance, that 1% of elderly people living outside of institutions have spontaneous dyskinesia. Yet patients in institutions have an average dyskinesia prevalence of 5%, with some groups exhibiting much higher rates. It is possible that many institutional cases are in fact instances of "occult dyskinesia," related to past use of neuroleptics. One survey of an institutional sample of elderly patients (Ticehurst, 1990) revealed a much higher rate of past exposure to antipsychotics (86%) than of current use (26%) among organically impaired patients. Despite a high prevalence of dyskinesia, no cases were found without past exposure to antipsychotics.

Khot and Wyatt (1991) reviewed nine studies of dyskinesia prevalence that, apart from revealing a history of neuroleptic treatment, indicated that prevalence was related to age. Dyskinesias were characterized as neuroleptic-associated if the patients had taken neuroleptics for longer than 3 months. All other dyskinesias were considered spontaneous. The prevalence of tardive dyskinesia was defined as the rate of neuroleptic-associated dyskinesia minus the rate of spontaneous dyskinesia. Those investigators found a true rate of tardive dyskinesia below 20% for all age groups except the 70–79-year-olds. They noted a low correlation between the rate of neuroleptic-associated dyskinesia and the rate of spontaneous dyskinesia. Those authors concluded that after age 40, the prevalence of tardive dyskinesia was sufficiently high to say that the abnormal movements in many patients with diagnoses of tardive dyskinesia were attributable to causes other than neuroleptics. They acknowledged that the likelihood of developing abnormal movements during treatment increased with increasing age. They also acknowledged that although it was possible that the movements of tardive dyskinesia were physiologically the same as spontaneous movements, the neuroleptics had induced their appearance earlier than might have been the case if the patients had never taken neuroleptics. Nevertheless, the assumption that the dyskinesias in individuals with less than 3 months of exposure to neuroleptics are spontaneous dyskinesias remains somewhat controversial, in view of recent incidence data on the development of tardive dyskinesia in the elderly.

One commonly prescribed drug that may be overlooked as a neuroleptic – it is not usually prescribed for antipsychotic properties – is metoclopramide (Reglan). An antagonist to the dopamine-2 (D_2) receptor, it is used for various gastrointestinal disorders and as an antiemetic in cancer chemotherapy. In one study of metoclopramide (Miller & Jankovic, 1989), 16 patients were evaluated, ranging in age from 24 to 85 years (average 63), with a female:male ratio of 3:1. The average duration of metoclopramide exposure prior to onset of abnormal movements was 12 months (range 1 day to 4 years). Those authors advised against long-term use of metoclopramide.

Other drugs that are more clearly nonneuroleptic have also been implicated as causative agents. Some cases of antihistamine- and benzodiazepine-associated dyskinesias and dystonias have been reported. One cannot, however, rule out other causes, such as local oral abnormalities and toxic, metabolic, infectious, and other neuromedical conditions and agents that are not affecting the central nervous system (CNS) (Thach, Chase, & Bosma, 1976; Kaplan & Murkofsky, 1978).

Prevalence of Tardive Dyskinesia

Kane and Smith (1982) reviewed 56 prevalence studies of dyskinesia in neuroleptic-treated psychiatric populations and compared those data with the data from 19 samples of individuals not treated with neuroleptics. They found average rates of 20% and 5%, respectively. Their data support the notion that exposure to neuroleptics plays a highly significant role in producing abnormal movements in susceptible patients. However, care must be taken when comparing rates directly, as differences possibly could be due to so many other variables, such as age, sex, diagnosis, and history of other extrapyramidal signs. Although spontaneous dyskinesias may occur in individuals not treated with neuroleptics, and though tardive dyskinesia may occur in neuroleptic-treated individuals, many studies have shown increasing age to be the most consistently associated risk factor for the development of tardive dyskinesia.

In a prevalence survey of 2,250 individuals from psychiatric and geriatric medical settings, Woerner et al. (1991) found the rates of abnormal movements among neuroleptic-treated individuals to range widely – from 13.3% in a voluntary-admission psychiatric-hospital sample to 36.1% among subjects in a state-hospital sample. There was a steady increase in the prevalence of tardive dyskinesia with increasing age and increasing duration of neuroleptic exposure. In the geriatric-hospital sample, 85% of patients had orofacial movements. Preliminary analysis of the data from a neuroleptic-discontinuation study of 70 patients from the psychiatric sample indicates that false-negative (masked dyskinesia) rates increased with age, as well as with longer duration of neuroleptic exposure, and that they were highest in the state-hospital population. Those findings suggest that the prevalence of tardive dyskinesia may be particularly underestimated among older patients with longer treatment histories who are examined while taking neuroleptics. The role of dentures was also examined in that study. Those who used dentures were subdivided into two groups: those who were and those who were not wearing dentures at the time of the examination. Neuroleptic users not wearing dentures were found to be more likely to be rated as having tardive dyskinesia, especially those between the ages of 35 and 55 years. Moreover, once regression analysis had been used to adjust for the effects of age, gender, site, and duration of treatment, it was found that individuals who had dentures but did not wear them were 3.5 times more likely to be rated as having tardive dyskinesia than were those without dentures.

Incidence of Tardive Dyskinesia

In a prospective study of more than 600 individuals (mean age 29 years), Kane et al. (1986) found a 40% cumulative incidence of tardive dyskinesia after 8 years of neuroleptic exposure. They noted that for any given length of exposure, there was a higher incidence rate among older patients. In fact, after only 4 years of treatment, the rate was already 30% for individuals 50 years of age and older.

Saltz et al. (1991), in another prospective study that examined 160 elderly individuals undergoing treatment with antipsychotic drugs for the first time, showed a cumulative incidence (95% confidence intervals) of dyskinesia of $31 \pm 11\%$ after only 43 weeks of neuroleptic treatment (Figure 2.1). Those movements appeared predominantly, but not exclusively, in the orofacial region and were mild in severity. Although the incidence of tardive dyskinesia was not significantly related to neuroleptic class or dosage, nor to patient gender, it decreased significantly with increasing age. That relationship was not affected by stratification by gender. However, diagnosis was a factor. Patients given a nonorganic (psychiatric) diagnosis (mainly affective disorder) showed greater vulnerability to tardive dyskinesia than did those with diagnoses of "organic mental syndrome." Also, the subjects with psychiatric diagnoses were significantly younger than those with diagnoses of organic mental syndrome. When the effect of diagnosis was statistically controlled, the relationship of age to the incidence of tardive dyskinesia was no longer

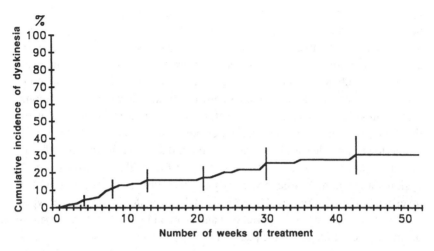

Figure 2.1.

significant. However, patients who had had parkinsonian signs during the first 4 weeks of neuroleptic treatment developed tardive dyskinesia at a faster rate than did those without such signs. The spontaneous dyskinesia rate, moreover, was only 5%. Thus, one can infer that when abnormal movements occur during the course of neuroleptic treatment, the movements may not result solely from a preexisting neurological condition. It is also possible that short-term neuroleptic treatment alone, although perhaps insufficient to induce tardive dyskinesia, may provoke abnormal movements in neurologically predisposed individuals. That study highlights the importance of conducting a careful examination for abnormal involuntary movements prior to initiating a course of neuroleptic treatment.

Relationships Between Other Neuromedical Disorders and Tardive Dyskinesia

Because disorders involving intellectual impairment are also prevalent at high rates among the elderly, and because the presence of such CNS disorders has been implicated as a risk factor in certain studies of tardive dyskinesia, several investigators have examined the relationship between cognitive deficits and tardive dyskinesia more closely. In the interest of assessing the roles of both intellectual dysfunction and negative symptoms as vulnerability factors in the development of tardive dyskinesia, Karson et al. (1990) assessed the presence or absence of tardive dyskinesia, cognitive impairment, and negative symptoms in a group of elderly male neuropsychiatric patients ($N = 49$) in a nursing-home setting. For the 25 patients found to have tardive dyskinesia, the presence of tardive dyskinesia was associated with greater degrees of cognitive impairment and more severe negative symptoms. That finding was not related to obvious macroscopic organic abnormalities; indeed, such pathologic conditions were less common among the dyskinetic patients than among those without tardive dyskinesia. In fact, patients with frontal lesions (primarily lobotomies) had a significantly lower prevalence of tardive dyskinesia.

The lower prevalence of macroscopic brain disease in the group with tardive dyskinesia is consistent with the findings in the incidence study of tardive dyskinesia mentioned earlier and clearly warrants further investigation. Other investigators (Mukherjee et al., 1985; Sandyk & Bamford, 1988) have hypothesized that impairments of peripheral and central glucose and insulin metabolism may be significant in the pathophysiology of tardive dyskinesia. This is a particularly interesting area in view of the high prevalence of diabetes among the elderly. Ganzini et al. (1991), in a comparison of the prevalence of tardive dyskinesia among 38 neuroleptic-treated diabetics and 38 nondiabetic controls (matched for age, sex, diagnosis, and dosage and duration of neuroleptic treatment), found significantly higher prevalence rates and degrees of severity of tardive dyskinesia among the neuroleptic-treated diabetic group. No differences between the groups were found for other risk factors, however, including parkinsonism, anticholinergic drug treatment, and cognitive dysfunction. These data suggest that diabetes should be investigated further as a risk factor for tardive dyskinesia.

The effects of alloxan-induced hyperglycemia on the incidence and severity of haloperidol-induced perioral movements in rats were studied by Sandyk (1990). The hyperglycemic rats showed a significantly higher incidence and greater severity of abnormal perioral movements than did the control rats. Moreover, the severity ratings for abnormal movements were significantly related to blood glucose levels in the hyperglycemic rats. Those findings suggest that hyperglycemia may increase the severity of neuroleptic-induced perioral movements; they also support the possibility that glucose intolerance may increase the risk for tardive dyskinesia.

Other work on the epidemiology of tardive dyskinesia suggests that increasing age is a factor associated with both the persistence and severity of this condition. From their review of the literature, Smith and Baldessarini (1980) concluded that the rate of improvement was 83% for patients younger than the median age of 54.4 years, versus 46% for older patients. Kane et al. (1986) and other investigators have suggested that the duration of neuroleptic exposure prior to and following the development of tardive dyskinesia is an important predictor of remission. However, certain forms of tardive dyskinesia, such as tardive dystonia, can be both severe and persistent, even after discontinuation of neuroleptics; furthermore, those at risk are not readily identifiable (Burke, Fahn, & Jankovic, 1982). Interestingly, acute dystonia seems to be less prevalent in older patient samples (Moleman et al., 1986). There is some evidence that tardive dyskinesia becomes more severe with increasing age, particularly between the ages of 40 and 69 years (Smith & Baldessarini, 1980). Perhaps the overall mild severity of tardive dyskinesia seen in the prospective incidence study of Saltz et al. (1991) was a function of both the relatively low dosages used and the brief duration of follow-up. Nevertheless, both young and old patients undergoing standard neuroleptic treatment can develop severe symptoms of tardive dyskinesia. These symptoms can cause distress and lead to disability, and in some cases severe complications can develop, such as dysphagia, respiratory distress, and renal failure from dehydration or rhabdomyolysis – witness the case of severe life-threatening tardive dyskinesia that resulted in esophageal and respiratory difficulties in a 66-year-old man with clear-cell carcinoma of the biliary duct who had undergone treatment with metoclopramide; despite discontinuation of the offending drug, a gastrostomy tube had to be placed to maintain nutritional support because of persistent severe dyskinesia (Samie, Dannenhoffer, & Rozek, 1987).

Lieberman and Reife (1989) reported a case of choreoathetoid dyskinesia and spastic dysphonia associated with clinical and electromyographic signs of muscle denervation, suggesting that the neurological syndrome originated within the basal-ganglia nuclei, but also may have extended to the peripheral neuromuscular system. Although that occurred in a young man, the possibility of such presentations of tardive dyskinesia must be considered, particularly in elderly patients who present with neuromuscular symptoms of any kind and a prior history of neuroleptic exposure.

To be diagnosed as having tardive dyskinesia, a patient must exhibit involuntary abnormal movements and have a history of neuroleptic treatment, in the absence of other known causes of dyskinesia, such as Wilson's disease, Huntington's disease, or L-dopa administration (as might be used to treat Parkinson's disease). The conditions that might produce abnormal movements in the absence of neuroleptic treatment presumably can contribute to the development of such movements during neuroleptic treatment. Recognition of non-motor signs that can coexist with disorders of movement is also important for the diagnostic formulation. For example, the combination of

Table 2.1. *Conditions and agents associated with adventitious movements*

Congenital or hereditary conditions
Acanthocytosis, acute intermittent porphyria, ataxia, telangiectasia, olivoponto-
cerebellar atrophy, benign familial chorea, cerebral palsy, dystonia musculorum
deformans, glutaric acidemia, Hallervorde-Spatz syndrome, hereditary lipidoses,
Huntington's disease, Lesch-Nyhan syndrome, perinatal injury (e.g., anoxia, ker-
nicterus), Wilson's disease
Inflammatory or infectious conditions
Brain tumors, diphtheria, Henoch-Schönlein purpura, Jakob-Creutzfeldt disease,
Lyme disease, multiple sclerosis, periarteritis nodosa, pertussis, rheumatoid
arthritis, serum sickness, subactue sclerosing panencephalitis, Sydenham's chorea,
syphilis, systemic lupus erythematosus, varicella, other encephalitides
Toxic/metabolic agents
Amphetamines, carbon monoxide, phenytoin, hypernatremia, hepatic encephalopa-
thy, hypocalcemia, hypoglycemia, hypokalemia, L-dopa, lithium, manganese, mer-
cury, methyl bromide, methylphenidate, neuroleptics, oral contraceptives, para-
thyroid disease, strychnine, thyroid disease
Psychogenic conditions
Mannerisms associated with illnesses such as schizophrenia
Posttraumatic syndromes
Subdural hematoma
Miscellaneous conditions
Alzheimer's disease, Brueghel's syndrome, cerebrovascular accidents, edentulous
dyskinesia, epilepsy, idiopathic torsion dystonia, Meige's syndrome, Parkinson's
disease, Pick's disease, polycythemia, progressive supranuclear palsy, senile chorea,
Tourette's syndrome, transient facial myokymia

Source: Adapted from Saltz and Lieberman (1992).

intellectual impairment, chorea, and a family history of dyskinesia may be
suggestive of Huntington's disease. Table 2.1 lists conditions and agents that
can be associated with abnormal movements (Saltz & Lieberman, 1992).

Motor phenomena can be principal features of a primary movement disorder (e.g., Sydenham's chorea, Huntington's disease). They can also occur as a
primary association (as in Alzheimer's disease) or as an uncommon association (as in polycythemia vera).

Many different lesions in the basal ganglia, cerebellum, and cerebral cortex
have been associated with spontaneous movement disorders. Despite a number of case reports dealing with such clinical and pathological correlates, no
large controlled studies have been done on this topic.

Edentulousness and Tardive Dyskinesia

Edentulousness is a particularly relevant condition for investigation, not only
because the condition is highly prevalent in the elderly and has been linked to

abnormal orofacial movements but also because the site of this condition is one of the parts of the body most commonly affected by tardive dyskinesia. If the trigeminal proprioceptive input from the oral cavity to the basal ganglia is disrupted, the risk for neuroleptic-induced orofacial dyskinesia may be increased (Sutcher et al., 1971). Because lesions of the globus pallidus will alter the trigeminal, sensory-induced reflexive activity of neck muscles in rats, and because the putamen-caudate complex regulates vestibular and proprioceptive mechanisms, edentulousness can also facilitate expression of neuroleptic-induced neck and trunk movements. In a sample of 131 chronic schizophrenic patients being treated with neuroleptics, Sandyk and Kay (1990) found that edentulous patients exhibited significantly more neck and trunk dyskinesias than did nonedentulous patients. In contrast, the two groups did not differ in regard to dyskinesias of the face, tongue, and extremities. Those findings imply that edentulousness may increase the risk for neck and trunk dyskinesias; they also highlight the importance of the dental status for patients with tardive dyskinesia.

Cerebrovascular Disease, Imaging, and Dyskinesias in Older Adults

Cerebrovascular disease, which can be a risk factor for the development of abnormal involuntary motor activity, is of interest because cerebrovascular accidents (strokes) are more common in the elderly. Appenzeller and Biehl (1968) reported a series of 11 cases of elderly (ages 55–95 years; 9 males, 2 females) edentulous individuals with "mouthing" and a variety of neuromedical/psychiatric presentations, but no known history of neuroleptic exposure. The relative contributions of subdural hematomas, recurrent seizures, and cerebrovascular accidents could not, however, be determined. Other investigators have reported decreased cell sizes and cell counts in the basal ganglia in individuals with no known disease of the cerebral cortex or cerebral vasculature (Alcock, 1936).

Modern imaging techniques have been used to detect the structural brain changes associated with disorders of movement (Saris, 1983; Tabaton, Mancardi, & Loeb, 1985; Biller et al., 1986). Most of those studies used computed tomography (CT) to show evidence of basal-ganglia hemorrhage, atrophy, or infarction. There is evidence that magnetic-resonance imaging (MRI) may be superior to CT scanning for identification of such lesions, whether or not other manifestations of brain disease exist. Biller et al. (1986), for example, described 2 patients with hemiballismus who had MRI evidence of lacunar infarction in the subthalamic nucleus, not seen on cranial CT scans. Tabaton et al. (1985) reported a case of generalized chorea due to MRI-documented bilateral lacunar infarcts in the caudate nucleus, putamen, and deep frontal white matter.

Pathophysiological Considerations

Long-term treatment of schizophrenic patients with neuroleptics is associated with neuroleptic accumulation in neuromelanin-containing cells, with ensuing nigral-cell damage (Seeman, 1988). This process has been postulated as a pathophysiological mechanism underlying the development of tardive dyskinesia. Thus, in addition to early or short-term up-regulation of D_2 dopamine receptors, the late-stage denervation supersensitivity may result in a further proliferation of D_2 dopamine receptors in those parts of the human striatum controlling the motions of mouth, lips, and tongue. Young individuals, on reduction or withdrawal of neuroleptics, may have neural sprouting, with subsequent D_2 down-regulation and reversal of their dyskinesia. Older individuals do not readily exhibit sprouting and D_2 down-regulation, possibly thereby accounting for a more persistent form of dyskinesia.

Conclusion

Abnormal involuntary body movements can develop in many different internal and external body regions, and in association with many different neuromedical conditions. Many of these neuromedical conditions are found more commonly in older adults than in younger individuals. When these adventitious movements develop as a consequence of neuroleptic treatment, they are known as tardive dyskinesia. Increasing age is one of the most consistently identified risk factors for the development of tardive dyskinesia.

The relationships between specific neurological, medical, and psychiatric disorders and tardive dyskinesia will require further investigation, but affective disorders appear to increase the risk for tardive dyskinesia in both young and old individuals who undergo neuroleptic treatment. It is still controversial whether those disorders that produce intellectual deficits increase or decrease the rate of development of tardive dyskinesia and its severity in the elderly, and this issue clearly requires further investigation. The finding that diabetes mellitus is associated with higher rates of tardive dyskinesia is particularly interesting, because diabetes is common in older adults and is associated with higher rates of cerebrovascular disease. Further investigation of this relationship may reveal important information about the pathophysiology of the development of tardive dyskinesia in both older and younger individuals. Edentulousness is another type of medical condition associated with dyskinesias in the elderly. Individuals who need dentures may appear to have abnormal involuntary oral movements even in the absence of neuroleptic treatment. Also, the presence of dentures during a physical examination may mask abnormal movements that occur in the absence of the dentures. On the other hand, the presence of loose-fitting dentures may produce abnormal movements in the orofacial region that would not otherwise be present if the dentures were not in place or were better fitted. The proprioceptive changes that are associated with edentulousness have not been well characterized and may be etiologically related to the increased rates of dyskinesia seen in older adults, either with or without neuroleptic treatment.

There are as yet no unifying theories of the pathogenic and pathophysiological mechanisms involved in dyskinetic disorders. It would be difficult to hypothesize similar mechanisms for chorea associated with proprioceptive abnormalities (such as might occur with stroke) and chorea associated with neurodegenerative processes (such as might occur with Alzheimer's disease). In the absence of additional pathophysiological data on dyskinesias, whether neuroleptic-related or not, treatment strategies must employ an empirical approach based on earlier work done with younger populations. Mention of certain applicable principles, however, may be helpful. First, neuroleptics should not be prescribed for elderly patients in circumstances where less toxic treatments might be efficacious. For example, nonpsychotic individuals with Alzheimer's disease and nighttime agitation may benefit from environmental changes, such as improved lighting, or improved sleep hygiene, in conjunction with increased daytime activity and low-dosage benzodiazepines at night. Second, the indications for antipsychotic drugs should be reviewed at regular intervals. For example, for depressed individuals who have had delusions, but who have responded to a combination of tricyclic antidepressant and low-dosage neuroleptic, later maintenance treatment consisting of only a tricyclic antidepressant may be adequate. Third, individuals with multiple risk factors for tardive dyskinesia, such as drug-induced parkinsonism early in treatment and affective illness, may benefit from a change to a less toxic treatment, such as electroconvulsive treatment (acute) and follow-up antidepressant treatment consisting of maintenance tricyclics, without needing further exposure to neuroleptics.

References

Alcock, N. S. (1936). A note on the pathology of senile chorea (non-hereditary). *Brain* 59:376–87.

Appenzeller, O., & Biehl, J. P. (1968). Mouthing in the elderly: a cerebellar sign. *J. Neurol. Sci.* 6:249–60.

Berkovic, S. F., Karpati, G., Carpenter, S., & Lang, A. E. (1987). Progressive dystonia with bilateral putaminal hypodensities. *Arch. Neurol.* 44:1184–7.

Biller, J., Graff-Radford, N. R., Smoker, W. R., Adams, H. P., and Johnston, P. (1986). MR imaging in "lacunar" hemiballismus. *J. Conput. Assist. Tomogr.* 10:793–7.

Burke, R. E., Fahn, S., & Jankovic, J. (1982). Tardive dystonia: late onset and persistent dystonia caused by antipsychotic drugs. *Neurology* 32:1335–46.

Ganzini, L., Heintz, R. T., Hoffman, W. F., & Casey, D. E. (1991). The prevalence of tardive dyskinesia in neuroleptic-treated diabetics. A controlled study. *Arch. Gen. Psychiatry* 48:259–63.

Guy, W. (ed.) (1976). *ECDEU Assessment Manual for Psychopharmacology,* rev. ed. Publication ADM 76-338. Washington, DC: U.S. Department of Health, Education, and Welfare.

Kane, J. M., & Smith, J. M. (1982). Tardive dyskinesia: prevalence and risk factors. *Arch. Gen. Psychiatry* 39:473–81.

Kane, J. M., Woerner, M., Lieberman, J. A., & Kinon, B. J. (1986). Tardive dyskinesia and drugs. In *Drug Development Research,* ed. M. L. Cornfelot & G. M. Shutske, pp. 41–51. New York: Alan R. Liss Inc.

Kaplan, S. R., & Murkofsky, C. (1978). Oral-buccal dyskinesia symptoms associated with low dose benzodiazepine treatment. *Am. J. Psychiatry* 135:1558–9.

Karson, C. N., Bracha, H. S., Powell, A., & Adams, L. (1990). Dyskinetic movements, cognitive impairment, and negative symptoms in elderly neuropsychiatric patients. *Am. J. Psychiatry* 147:1646–9.

Khot, V., & Wyatt, R. J. (1991). Not all that moves is tardive dyskinesia. *Am. J. Psychiatry* 148:661–6.

Lieberman, J. A., & Reife, R. (1989). Spastic dysphonia and denervation signs in a young man with tardive dyskinesia. *Br. J. Psychiatry* 154:105–9.

Miller, L. G., & Jankovic, J. (1989). Metoclopramide induced movement disorders. Clinical findings with a review of the literature. *Arch. Intern. Med.* 149:2486–92.

Moleman, P., Janzen, G., von Bargen, B. A., Kappers, E. J., Pepplinkhuizen, L., & Schmitz, P. I. (1986). Relationship between age and incidence of parkinsonism in psychiatric patients treated with haloperidol. *Am. J. Psychiatry* 143:232–4.

Mukherjee, S., Wisniewski, A., Bilder, R., and Sackeim, H. A. (1985). Possible association between tardive dyskinesia and altered carbohydrate metabolism. *Arch. Gen. Psychiatry* 42:205.

Saltz, B. L., & Lieberman, J. A. (1992). Spontaneous and drug induced disorders of movement in the elderly. In *Disorders of Movement in Psychiatry and Neurology,* ed. R. Young & A. B. Joseph, pp. 155–63. Oxford: Blackwell Scientific Publications.

Saltz, B. L., Woerner, M. G., Kane, J. M., Lieberman, J. A., Alvir, J. M., Bergmann, K. J., Blank, K., Koblenzer, J., & Kahaner, K. (1991). Prospective study of tardive dyskinesia incidence in the elderly. *JAMA* 266:2401–6.

Samie, M. R., Dannenhoffer, M. A., & Rozek, S. (1987). Life-threatening tardive dyskinesia caused by metoclopramide. *Mov. Disord.* 2:125–9.

Sandyk, R. (1990). Increased incidence of neuroleptic-induced perioral movements in the rat by hyperglycemia. *Int. J. Neurosci.* 50:227–32.

Sandyk, R., & Bamford, C. R. (1988). Neuroleptic mediated hypothalamic deregulation of central insulin and peripheral glucose metabolism in tardive dyskinesia: a hypothesis. *Int. J. Neurosci.* 40:213–16.

Sandyk, R., & Kay, S. R. (1990). Edentulousness and neuroleptic induced neck and trunk dyskinesia. *Funct. Neurol.* 5:361–3.

Saris, S. (1983). Chorea caused by caudate infarction. *Arch. Neurol.* 40:590–1.

Schooler, N. R., & Kane, J. M. (1982). Research diagnoses for tardive dyskinesia. *Arch. Gen. Psychiatry* 39:486–7.

Seeman, P. (1988). Tardive dyskinesia, dopamine receptors, and neuroleptic damage to cell membranes. *J. Clin. Psychopharmacol.* 8:3s–9s.

Smith, J. M., & Baldessarini, R. J. (1980). Changes in prevalence, severity, and recovery in tardive dyskinesia with age. *Arch. Gen. Psychiatry* 37:1368–71.

Sutcher, H. D., Underwood, R. B., Beatty, R. A., & Sugar, O. (1971). Orofacial dyskinesia. A dental dimension. *JAMA* 216:1459–63.

Tabaton, M., Mancardi, G., & Loeb, C. (1985). Generalized chorea due to bilateral small, deep cerebral infarcts. *Neurology* 35:588–9.

Thach, B. T., Chase, T. N., & Bosma, J. F. (1976). Oral facial dyskinesia associated with prolonged use of antihistaminic decongestants. *N. Engl. J. Med.* 293:486–7.

Ticehurst, S. B. (1990). Is spontaneous orofacial dyskinesia an artifact due to incomplete drug history? *J. Geriatr. Psychiatry Neurol.* 3:208–11.

Woerner, M. G., Kane, J. M., Lieberman, J. A., Alvir, J., Bergmann, K. J., Borenstein, M., Schooler, N. R., Mukherjee, S., Rotrosen, J., Rubinstein, M., & Basavarju, N. (1991). The prevalence of tardive dyskinesia. *J. Clin. Psychopharmacol.* 11:34–42.

3

Gender as a Factor in the Development of Tardive Dyskinesia

RAMZY YASSA, M.D., and DILIP V. JESTE, M.D.

Ever since the syndrome of tardive dyskinesia was introduced into the literature more than 30 years ago, older age has been the only consistent risk factor confirmed by most authors (Smith & Baldessarini, 1980). However, several other factors, detailed elsewhere in this volume, have now been implicated.

Gender has been suggested to be an important factor in the development of tardive dyskinesia, and whereas some authors have concluded that women have a higher prevalence of tardive dyskinesia than do men, others have found no gender difference (Jeste & Wyatt, 1981). Elsewhere, we have reviewed, in detail, the studies that discussed and compared the prevalences of tardive dyskinesia for the two genders (Yassa & Jeste, 1992). Only articles published in English or French (or in other languages, if a detailed summary was provided in English or French) were reviewed. We found 93 English or French prevalence studies published prior to the end of 1989. To be included in our review, a study had to meet the following criteria:

- report on 50 patients or more. The study by Crane and Smeets (1974), a study of 39 patients, was therefore excluded.
- include both genders in its sample. We excluded three women-only studies (Uhrbrand & Faurbye, 1960; Pryce & Edwards, 1966; Edwards, 1970) and two studies of men only (Dynes, 1970; Goldberg et al., 1982).
- include the numbers of men and women affected by tardive dyskinesia. Eleven studies were excluded (Paulson, 1968; Yagi et al., 1976; Bell & Smith, 1978; Alexopoulos, 1979; Gardos et al., 1980; McCreadie, Barron, & Winslow, 1982; Cunningham-Owens, Johnstone, & Frith, 1982; Holden, Sandler, & Myslobodsky, 1984; Lieberman et al., 1984; Kane, Woerner, & Lieberman, 1985; Waddington & Youssef, 1986). For the final analysis, we reviewed a total of 76 prevalence studies comprising 39,187 patients (Table 3.1). The sample sizes ranged from 50 patients (Famujiwa et al., 1979) to

Table 3.1. *Prevalence studies and gender differences for tardive dyskinesia (TD)*

Author/year	Overall total prevalence		Men		Women		χ² (p)	Odds ratio	95% confidence interval	
	N	% with TD	Total n	% with TD	Total n	% with TD			Lower	Upper
Hunter et al. (1964)	450	3.3	200	0	250	5.2	<0.005	10.92[a]	1.4	84.2
Demars (1966)	371	7.0	166	4.8	205	8.8	NS	1.90	0.8	4.5
Dincman (1966)	1,700	3.4	850	1.6	850	5.2	<0.001	3.26	1.8	6.0
Crane & Paulson (1967)	182	14.8	66	15.2	116	14.7	NS	0.96	0.4	2.2
Turunen & Achte (1967)	480	5.4	207	3.4	273	7.3	NS	2.14	0.9	5.2
Degkwitz & Wenzel (1967)	766	17.0	303	10.9	463	21.0	<0.001	2.17	1.4	3.3
	499	22.8	193	20.7	306	24.2	NS	1.22	0.8	1.9
Siede & Muller (1967)	404	11.4	109	7.0	295	13.0	NS	1.87	0.8	4.1
Heinrich et al. (1968)	554	17.0	228	12.3	326	20.2	<0.025	1.81	1.1	2.9
Crane (1968)	379	27.4	207	31.0	172	23.3	NS	0.68	0.4	1.1
Villeneuve et al. (1969)	3,280	2.1	1,929	1.3	1,351	3.2	<0.001	2.50	1.5	4.1
Jones & Hunter (1969)	82	30.5	13	7.7	69	34.8	<0.05[b]	6.40	0.8	52.2
Lehmann et al. (1970)	350	6.6	168	4.2	182	8.8	NS	2.22	0.9	5.5
Crane (1970)	127	26.8	62	27.4	65	26.1	NS	0.94	0.4	2.1
Hippius & Lange (1970)	531	34.4	244	34.4	287	34.1	NS	0.99	0.7	1.4
Kennedy et al. (1971)	63	62.0	32	53.0	31	71.0	NS	2.16	0.8	6.1
Brandon et al. (1971)	625	25.1	264	17.0	361	31.0	<0.001	2.19	1.5	3.2
Fann et al. (1972)	193	34.7	138	31.1	55	43.6	NS	1.71	0.9	3.3
Ogita (1972)	454	17.9	70	17.1	53	18.9	NS	1.12	0.4	2.8
Lehmann & Ban (1974)	123	6.8	199	5.5	255	7.8	NS	1.45	0.7	3.1
Jus et al. (1976)	332	56.0	142	53.5	190	58.0	NS	1.19	0.8	1.9
Bourgeois et al. (1976)	1,660	7.2	737	4.9	923	9.1	<0.001	1.95	1.3	2.9

(*continues*)

Table 3.1. (*cont.*)

Author/year	Overall total prevalence		Men		Women		χ^2 (p)	Odds ratio	95% confidence interval	
	N	% with TD	Total n	% with TD	Total n	% with TD			Lower	Upper
Asnis et al. (1977)	69	43.4	16	31.0	53	47.0	NS	1.96	0.6	6.4
Simpson et al. (1978)	3,319	11.0	1,577	7.5	1,742	13.8	<0.001	1.97	1.6	2.5
Smith et al. (1978)	293	45.7	150	39.0	143	52.4	<0.025	1.70	1.1	2.7
Smith et al. (1979)	213	41.3	96	36.4	117	45.3	NS	1.44	0.8	2.5
Perris et al. (1966)	347	17.0	213	9.4	134	29.8	<0.001	4.11	2.3	7.4
Famujiwa et al. (1979)	50	34.0	26	26.9	24	41.7	NS	1.94	0.6	6.4
Wojcik et al. (1980)	208	18.0	92	16	116	19.0	NS	1.20	0.6	2.5
Perenyi & Arato (1980)	200	23.5	100	31	100	16.0	<0.02	0.42	0.2	0.8
Jeste & Wyatt (1981)	95	31.6	25	24	70	34.3	NS	1.65	0.6	4.7
Ezrin-Waters et al. (1981)	94	43.6	58	39.6	36	50.0	NS	1.52	0.7	3.5
Rey et al. (1981)	66	43.9	39	39	27	52.0	NS	1.72	0.6	4.7
Yesavage et al. (1982)	3,140	8.2	1,568	5.8	1,572	10.6	<0.001	1.93	1.5	2.5
Ananth & Yassa (1982)	223	20.6	116	16.3	107	25.2	NS	1.72	0.9	3.3
Mukherjee et al. (1982)	152	30.7	41	34.1	112	29.1	NS	0.81	0.4	1.7
Doongaji et al. (1982)	1,801	9.6	1,141	9.5	660	9.8	NS	1.04	0.8	1.4
Kane & Smith (1982)	328	15.8	193	13.5	135	19.2	NS	1.53	0.8	2.8
Yassa et al. (1983)	180	27.0	83	22	97	32.0	NS	1.70	0.9	3.3
Kulhanek et al. (1984)	861	15.0	398	14.8	463	15.3	NS	1.04	0.7	1.5
Yassa et al. (1984)	108	7.4	55	5.5	53	9.4	NS[b]	1.81	0.4	8.0
Itoh et al. (1984)	2,274	19.0	969	19.6	1,305	18.8	NS	0.95	0.8	1.2
Branchey & Branchen (1984)	57	24.6	43	25.6	14	21.4	NS	0.79	0.2	3.4
Richardson et al. (1984)	167	61.7	87	50.6	80	73.8	<0.005	2.75	1.4	5.3
Kane et al. (1984)	554	12.4	288	12.8	266	12.0	NS	0.93	0.6	1.5
Fleischhauer et al. (1985)	608	31.6	255	29.8	353	32.9	NS	1.15	0.8	1.6

Study										
Kok & Christopher (1985)	211	9.9	100	7.0	111	12.6	NS	1.92	0.7	5.0
Guy et al. (1985)	768	11.0	430	11.0	338	11.0	NS	1.00	0.6	1.6
Waddington & Youssef (1985)	68	41.0	22	36.4	46	43.4	NS	1.35	0.5	3.8
Ramsay & Millard (1986)	426	11.5	92	7.6	334	12.6	NS	1.75	0.8	4.0
Yassa et al. (1986)	76	25.0	32	22.0	44	40.9	NS	2.47	0.9	6.9
Rittmannsberger & Schony (1986)	76	25.0	46	19.6	30	33.3	NS	2.06	0.7	5.9
Fanget et al. (1986)	52	4.0	22	0	30	6.7	NS[b]	1.50[a]	0.1	17.7
Chouinard et al. (1986)	224	45.0	113	45.0	111	44.0	NS	0.96	0.6	1.6
Williams & Dalby (1986)	196	34.2	106	34.0	90	34.4	NS	1.02	0.6	1.8
Kolakowska et al. (1986)	91	25.0	59	27.0	32	22.0	NS	0.75	0.3	2.1
Richardson et al. (1986)	211	30.0	139	23.0	72	43.0	<0.005	2.53	1.4	4.7
Holden (1987)	100	39.0	50	26.0	50	52.0	<0.01	3.08	1.3	7.1
Morgenstern et al. (1987)	180	33.0	89	37.0	91	30.0	NS	0.72	0.4	1.3
Gurge (1987)	70	37.0	54	39.0	16	31.0	NS	0.94	0.3	3.0
Binder et al. (1987)	126	35.0	66	41.0	60	28.3	NS	0.57	0.3	1.2
Yassa et al. (1988)	135	45.0	58	45.5	77	44.8	NS	0.97	0.5	1.9
Yassa & Nair (1988)	315	32.4	150	6.0	165	38.1	<0.025	1076.00	1.1	2.8
Ahrens et al. (1988)	385	19.7	256	17.0	129	26.0	<0.05	1.66	1.0	2.8
Delance (in Bourgeois, 1988)	262	39.0	126	37.3	136	40.7	NS	1.14	0.7	1.9
Moussaoui et al. (1988)	1,070	12.1	272	16.7	798	10.7	<0.05	0.60	0.4	0.9
Youssef & Waddington (1988)	77	19.5	51	19.6	26	19.2	NS	0.98	0.3	3.2
Arisco & Holden (1989)	90	5.5	50	2.0	40	10.0	NS[b]	5.44	0.6	50.8
Ko et al. (1989)	866	8.4	641	10.0	225	6.6	NS	0.65	0.4	1.2
Muscettola et al. (1989)	1,651	19.0	991	15.7	660	24.2	<0.001	1.73	1.3	2.2
Stone et al. (1989)	1,227	48.0	638	45.0	589	52.0	<0.05	1.33	1.1	1.7
Gurge (1989)	137	27.0	101	27.7	36	25.0	NS	0.87	0.4	2.1
Total	39,187	24.2	19,337	21.6	19,850	26.6		1.34	1.3	1.4

[a] A significantly *lower* odds ratio.
[b] Used Fisher's exact probability test, rather than χ^2.

29

Table 3.2. *Study characteristics*

Characteristics	Number of studies
Inpatient setting, psychiatric hospital	45
Outpatient setting, psychiatric hospital	12
General-hospital psychiatric department	11
Private hospital	1
Multicenter institution	1
Setting not known	5
Rating scales not used	8
Mean ages of men and women indicated	20
Patients older than 65 years	9
Only psychogeriatric patients included	2
Mentally retarded patients only	3

3,319 patients (Simpson et al., 1978), with a mean of 530 patients per study.

The study characteristics are outlined in Table 3.2. Most of those studies emerged from psychiatric institutions.

Prevalences of Tardive Dyskinesia

We estimated the overall prevalence of tardive dyskinesia to be 24.2% (range 3.3–62%), with a prevalence of 21.6% (range 0–50%) among men and 26.6% (range 3.2–73.8%) among women. After the findings were combined from all studies (Table 3.1), we calculated the mean odds ratio (OR) as 1.34 (93% CI: 1.3–1.4). Of the 76 studies, 18 reported significantly higher women/men relative risks for tardive dyskinesia ($p < .05$; lower boundary of 95% CI > 1.0). Only two studies (Perényi & Arato, 1980; Moussaoui et al., 1988) found significantly higher men/women relative risks ($p < .05$; upper boundary of 95% CI < 1.0).

When the prevalences of tardive dyskinesia were reanalyzed into occurrences by decade (1960–69, 1970–79, 1980–89), we found the mean prevalences to be 13.5%, 28.6%, and 25.1%, respectively. When the material was reanalyzed by gender, we found the prevalences of tardive dyskinesia to be 9.6% for men and 15.6% for women (M:W = 1:1.6) during 1960–69, as compared with 25.0% for men and 33.1% for women (M:W = 1:1.3) during 1970–79, and 23.5% for men and 27.1% for women (M:W = 1:1.2) during 1980–89. Of the 12 studies during the first decade, 6 (50%) reported that women had significantly more tardive dyskinesia than men, as compared with 5 of 18 studies (28%) in the second decade, and 10 of 46 studies (19.6%) in the third decade.

Age and Gender Interaction

We found 6 studies (Degkwitz & Wenzel, 1967; Villeneuve, Lavallée, & Lemieux, 1969; Brandon, McClelland, & Protheroe, 1971; Smith et al., 1978, 1979; Yassa & Nair, 1988) that presented the prevalences of tardive dyskinesia according to age group and gender. They showed that although the prevalence increased with age (Table 3.3), in women, it did not do so in men. Also, whereas tardive dyskinesia was significantly more prevalent among women than among men 51–70 years and over 70 years, it was equally distributed in the lower age groups. The increase in the prevalence of tardive dyskinesia was particularly apparent in the over-70 age group.

Gender and Severity of Tardive Dyskinesia

Eight studies (Degkwitz & Wenzel, 1967; Villeneuve et al., 1969; Brandon et al., 1971; Simpson et al., 1978; Smith et al., 1978; Perényi & Arato, 1980; Yesavage et al., 1982; Richardson et al., 1984), covering 7,964 patients, discussed severe tardive dyskinesia. The mean reported prevalence of severe tardive dyskinesia was 2.2% (1.3% among men, 3.1% among women, $\chi^2 = 31$, df $= 1$, $p < .001$). Whereas in 6 studies the women had more severe tardive dyskinesia than the men (Degkwitz & Wenzel, 1967; Brandon et al., 1971; Simpson et al., 1978; Smith et al., 1978; Yesavage et al., 1982; Richardson et al., 1984), in 2 other studies the two genders were equally affected (Villeneuve et al., 1969; Perényi & Arato, 1980).

Differences in Manifestations of Tardive Dyskinesia

No consensus emerged regarding the manifestations of tardive dyskinesia by gender. Two studies found that whereas men had more bucco-oral manifestations of tardive dyskinesia (Perris et al., 1966; Binder et al., 1987), women had more generalized movement manifestations of tardive dyskinesia (Perris et al., 1966). Smith et al. (1979) found that women with tardive dyskinesia had more lip-movement difficulties than men, whereas Ezrin-Waters, Seeman, and Seeman (1981) found that men in the over-40 population with tardive dyskinesia had more total-body afflictions than did women.

Table 3.3. *Studies comparing age and gender prevalence*

| | Patients <50 years old | | | | Patients 51–70 years old | | | | Patients >70 years old | | | |
| | Men | | Women | | Men | | Women | | Men | | Women | |
Author/year	n	% TD	n	% TD	n	% TD	n	% TD	n	% TD	n	% TD
Degkwitz & Wenzel (1967)	216	6.9	187	7.0	79	20.2	231	29.9	8	25.0	45	33.3
Villeneuve et al. (1969)	137	8.8	65	1.5	136	8.1	133	17.3	85	2.0	68	27.9
Brandon et al. (1971)	124	4.0	86	15.1	158	27.2	120	50.0	79	22.8	130	57.7
Smith et al. (1978, 1979)	90	26.7	61	19.7	90	48.9	131	54.2	66	39.4	68	66.2
Yassa et al. (1988)	60	6.7	37	10.8	62	41.9	60	30.0	28	32.1	68	60.3
Total	627	10.6	436	10.8	525	29.3[a]	675	36.1[a]	266	24.3[b]	379	49.1[b]

[a] $\chi^2 = 10.7$; $p < 0.001$.
[b] $\chi^2 = 58.8$; $p < 0.001$.

32

Discussion

Our review of the prevalence studies of tardive dyskinesia indicates that this condition occurs in an estimated 24% of the neuroleptic-treated population, some 40,000 patients in all. The prevalence of tardive dyskinesia apparently increased from 13.5% during the 1960s to 28.6% during the 1970s, stabilizing at 25.0% during the 1980s. One possible explanation for that increase may be that many of the 1960 studies did not use standardized scales to measure tardive dyskinesia; also, some included only patients with bucco-oral movements, thus omitting patients that today might be diagnosed as exhibiting tardive dyskinesia. Other changes that have occurred over the past three decades – such as improvements in study designs, narrowing concepts of schizophrenia, and increasing awareness of tardive dyskinesia – may also have contributed to the observed differences in the prevalence of tardive dyskinesia. Nonetheless, it is notable that the reported mean prevalence of tardive dyskinesia did not change appreciably from the 1970s to the 1980s. Indeed, we found that the mean odds ratio for tardive dyskinesia among women/men was 1.34 (CI_{95} = 1.3–1.4). Of the studies reviewed, 15 showed significantly higher women/men odds ratios for tardive dyskinesia, whereas only 2 studies (Perényi & Arato, 1980; Moussaoui et al., 1988) found significantly higher men/women odds ratios. However, when the studies are categorized into the three decades, the M/W odds ratio seems to narrow in the latter decades (from 1:1.6 during the first decade to 1:1.2 in the third decade), despite the fact that many studies reported that the women assessed were older than the men. Although the explanation for that finding is not clear, it is conceivable that the narrowing of the concept of schizophrenia following publication of the *Diagnostic and Statistical Manual of Mental Disorders,* third edition (DSM-III), with its more stringent criteria, may have had differential effects on diagnoses in men and women. In other words, it is possible that more women (than men) with affective disorders (affective disorder being a risk factor for tardive dyskinesia), who in previous decades would have been diagnosed as suffering from schizophrenia, are no longer receiving such diagnoses and therefore are not being treated with neuroleptics.

Table 3.3 suggests that only women continue to show an increasing prevalence of tardive dyskinesia with age. In fact, that increase is fivefold when women over 70 are compared with those less than 50 years of age. Among men, that increase is only twofold.

To date, the controversial issues of tardive dyskinesia severity and assessment have not been adequately addressed (Yassa et al., 1990). At present, severe tardive dyskinesia is rather arbitrarily classified according to various criteria: the investigators' experience (Brandon et al., 1971; Bourgeois, Graux, & Arretche-Berthelot, 1976); selection of an item on a scale, for example, an AIMS rating of 4 (severe) (Smith et al., 1978; Simpson et al., 1979; Richardson et al., 1984; Yassa et al., 1990); the degree of the patient's incapacitation resulting from tardive dyskinesia (Gardos et al., 1987). Thus, one can expect large variations in the definitions of severe tardive dyskinesia. In our review, women were reported to have more severe tardive dyskinesia than men (3.1% vs. 1.3%).

Several hypotheses have been put forward to explain the discrepancy in the prevalences of tardive dyskinesia between men and women. Certain investigators have reported that women tend to have more chronic illnesses and longer hospitalizations than men (Kennedy, Hershon, & McGuire, 1971). Several reports have indicated that women tend to receive larger doses of neuroleptics (Degkwitz & Wenzel, 1967; Kane & Smith, 1982) or to experience longer periods of neuroleptic treatment than men (Doongaji et al., 1982). However, evidence has accumulated in studies conducted on schizophrenic patients (most prevalence studies have dealt mainly with schizophrenic populations) to the effect that women have better prognoses vis-à-vis tardive dyskinesia than do men (Huber et al., 1980; Seeman, 1983; Goldstein, 1988; Yassa, Uhr, & Jeste, 1991). Thus, it is difficult to attribute the higher prevalence of tardive dyskinesia among women to a poorer prognosis regarding their schizophrenia.

Another possible explanation is that, in some studies, the women were older than the men. Women have longer life spans than men and therefore tend to be overrepresented in surveys of older patients (Yesavage et al., 1982). Also, aging is accompanied by a tendency to develop more severe tardive dyskinesia (Smith & Baldessarini, 1980; Yassa, Nair, & Schwartz, 1986) – witness those studies that failed to include older women in their samples and reported an absence of severe tardive dyskinesia (Gardos et al., 1980; Mukherjee et al., 1982). All in all, age does not seem to increase the prevalence of tardive dyskinesia among men to the same degree as among women. Thus, older women may be more vulnerable to tardive dyskinesia, especially the severe forms.

A third possibility is that psychosis may tend to develop later in life among women than among men (Harris & Jeste, 1988) – witness the studies that showed tardive dyskinesia to have developed after shorter periods of neuroleptic treatment, and in more severe forms, when neuroleptic treatment was initiated later rather than earlier in life (Jeste & Wyatt, 1982; Yassa et al., 1986). Perhaps, too, women are simply protected by estrogens earlier in life. Estrogens have an antidopaminergic activity (Raymond, Beaulieu, & Labrie,

1978), thus possibly protecting premenopausal women from developing tardive dyskinesia. Premenopausal women, therefore, may need lower neuroleptic dosages than do men of the same age (Seeman, 1983). In fact, one study has reported improvement among patients with tardive dyskinesia following estrogen administration, for both men and women (Villeneuve, Cazejust, & Coté, 1980); that finding, however, has not been replicated (Jeste et al., 1988).

Finally, it is possible that the catecholaminergic changes that accompany aging may play a role in the development of tardive dyskinesia in older patients (Smith & Baldessarini, 1980; Jeste & Wyatt, 1987). The role of those changes in the pathophysiology of tardive dyskinesia needs further study.

References

Ahrens, T. N., Sramek, J. J., Herrera, J. M., Jewett, C. M., & Alcorn, V. E. (1988). Pharmacy-based screening program for tardive dyskinesia. *Drug Intell. Clin. Pharm.* 22:205–8.

Alexopoulos, G. (1979). Lack of complaints in schizophrenics with tardive dyskinesia. *J. Nerv. Ment. Dis.* 167:125–6.

Ananth, J., & Yassa, R. (1982). Tardive dyskinesia and skin pigmentation. *Psychiatry* 141:94–5.

Arisco, J. P., & Holden, L. D. (1989). Prevalence of tardive dyskinesia in private psychiatric inpatients. *Tex. Med.* 85:25–8.

Asnis, G., Leopold, M. A., Duvoisin, R. C., & Shwartz, A. H. (1977). A survey of tardive dyskinesia in psychiatric outpatients. *Psychiatry* 134:1367–70.

Bell, R. C. H., & Smith, R. C. (1978). Tardive dyskinesia: characterization and prevalence in a state-wide system. *Psychiatry* 39:39–47.

Binder, R., Kazamatsuri, H., Nishimura, T., & McNiel, D. E. (1987). Tardive dyskinesia and neuroleptic-induced parkinsonism in Japan. *Psychiatry* 144:1494–6.

Bourgeois, M. (1988). Les dyskinésies tardives des neuroleptiques en France. *Encephale* 14:195–201.

Bourgeois, M., Graux, C., & Arretche-Berthelot, N. (1976). Les dyskinésies tardives des neuroleptiques: enquête sur 1660 malades d'hôpital psychiatrique. *Ann. Med. Psychol. (Paris)* 134:737–46.

Branchey, M., & Branchen, L. (1984). Patterns of psychotropic drug use and tardive dyskinesia. *Clin. Psychopharmacol.* 4:41–5.

Brandon, S., McClelland, H. A., & Protheroe, C. (1971). A study of facial dyskinesia in a mental hospital population. *Br. J. Psychiatry* 118:171–84.

Chouinard, G., Annable, L., & Ross-Chouinard, A. (1986). Supersensitivity psychosis and tardive dyskinesia: a survey of schizophrenic outpatients. *Psychopharmacol. Bull.* 22:891–6.

Crane, G. E. (1968). Tardive dyskinesia in schizophrenic patients treated with psychotropic drugs. *Agressologie* 9:209–18.

Crane, G. E. (1970). High doses of trifluoperazine and tardive dyskinesia. *Arch. Neurol.* 22:176–80.

Crane, G. E., & Paulson, G. (1967). Involuntary movements in a sample of chronic mental patients and their relation to the treatment with neuroleptics. *Int. Neuropsychiatry* 3:286–91.

Crane, G. E., & Smeets, R. A. (1974). Tardive dyskinesia and drug therapy in geriatric patients. *Arch. Gen. Psychiatry* 30:341–3.

Cunningham-Owens, D. G., Johnstone, E. C., & Frith, C. D. (1982). Spontaneous involuntary disorders of movements. *Arch. Gen. Psychiatry* 39:452–61.

Degkwitz, R., & Wenzel, W. (1967). Persistent extrapyramidal side effects after long-term application of neuroleptics. In *Neuropsychopharmacology*, ed. J. Amsterdam & H. Brill, pp. 608–15. Amsterdam: Excerpta Medica.

Demars, J.-P. C. A. (1966). Neuromuscular effects of long-term phenothiazine medication, electroconvulsive therapy and leucotomy. *J. Nerv. Ment. Dis.* 143:73–9.

Dincmen, K. (1966). Chronic psychotic choreoathetosis. *Dis. Nerv. Syst.* 27:399–402.

Doongaji, D. R., Jeste, D. V., Jape, N. M., Sheth, A. S., Apte, J. S., Vahia, V. N., Desai, A. B., Vahora, A., Thatte, S., Vevaina, T., & Bharadwaj, J. (1982). Tardive dyskinesia in India: a prevalence study. *J. Clin. Psychopharmacol.* 2:341–4.

Dynes, J. B. (1970). Oral dyskinesias – occurrence and treatment. *Dis. Nerv. Syst.* 31:854–9.

Edwards, H. (1970). The significance of brain damage in persistent oral dyskinesia. *Br. J. Psychiatry* 116:271–5.

Ezrin-Waters, C., Seeman, M. V., & Seeman, P. (1981). Tardive dyskinesia in schizophrenic outpatients: prevalence and significant variables. *Clin. Psychiatry* 42:16–22.

Famujiwa, O. O., Eccleston, D., Donaldson, A. A., & Garside, R. F. (1979). Tardive dyskinesia and dementia. *Br. J. Psychiatry* 135:500–4.

Fanget, F., Henry, E., & Aimard, G. (1986). Incidence des dyskinésies tardives sous traitement neuroleptique. *Presse Med.* 15:2147–50.

Fann, W. E., Davis, J. M., & Janowsky, D. S. (1972). The prevalence of tardive dyskinesias in mental hospital patients. *Dis. Nerv. Syst.* 33:182–6.

Fleischhauer, J., Kocher, J., Hobi, V. F., & Gilsdorf, U. (1985). Prevalence of tardive dyskinesia in a clinic population. Dyskinesia – research and treatment. *Psychopharmacology (Suppl.)* 2:162–72.

Gardos, G., Cole, J. O., Salomon, M., & Schniebolk, S. (1987). Clinical forms of severe tardive dyskinesia. *Am. J. Psychiatry* 144:895–902.

Gardos, G., Samu, I., Kallos, M., & Cole, J. O. (1980). Absence of severe tardive dyskinesia in Hungarian schizophrenic outpatients. *Psychopharmacology* 71:29–34.

Goldberg, S., Shenoy, R. S., Julius, D., Hamer, R. M., Ross, B., Minten, T., & Spiro, M. (1982). Do long-acting injectable neuroleptics protect against tardive dyskinesia? *Psychopharmacol. Bull.* 18:177–9.

Goldstein, J. M. (1988). Gender differences in the course of schizophrenia. *Am. J. Psychiatry* 145:684–9.

Gurge, O. (1987). Tardive dyskinesia in schizophrenics. *Acta Psychiatr. Scand.* 76:523–8.

Gurge, O. (1989). The significance of subtyping tardive dyskinesia: a study of prevalence and associated factors. *Psychol. Med.* 19:121–8.

Guy, W. (ed.) (1979). *ECDEU Assessment Manual for Psychopharmacology.* Publication ADH 76-338, pp. 534–7. Washington, DC: U.S. Department of Health, Education, and Welfare.

Guy, W., Ban, T. A., & Wilson, W. H. (1985). An international survey of tardive dyskinesia. *Prog. Neuropsychopharmacol. Biol. Psychiatry* 9:401–5.

Harris, M. J., & Jeste, D. V. (1988). Late-onset schizophrenia: an overview. *Schizophrenia Bull.* 14:39–55.

Heinrich, K., Wagener, I., & Bender, H-J. (1968). Spate extrapyramidal Hyperkinesen bei neuroleptischer Langzeittherapie. *Pharmakopsychiatr. Neuropsychopharmakol.* 1:169–95.

Hippius, V., & Lange, J. (1970). Zur Problematik der spaten extrapyramidalen Hyperkinesen nach langfristiger neuroleptischer Therapie. *Arzneimittelforschung* 20:888–90.

Holden, T. J. (1987). Tardive dyskinesia in long-term hospitalized Zulu psychiatric patients. *S. Afr. Med. J.* 71:88–90.

Holden, T. J., Sandler, R., & Myslobodsky, M. (1984). Tardive dyskinesia prevalence and subtypes at Valkenberg Hospital, Cape Town. *S. Afr. Med. J.* 66:132–4.

Huber, G., Cross, G., Schuttler, R., & Linz, M. (1980). Longitudinal studies of schizophrenic patients. *Schizophrenia Bull.* 6:592–605.

Hunter, R., Earl, C. J., & Thornicroft, S. (1964). An apparently irreversible syndrome of abnormal movements following phenothiazine medication. *Proc. R. Soc. Med.* 57:758–62.

Itoh, M., Fuju, Y., Kamisada, M., & Kamishima, K. (1984). Recent trend on the prevalence of tardive dyskinesia in Japan. *Prog. Neuropsychopharmacol. Biol. Psychiatry* 8:39–49.

Jeste, D. V., Kleinman, J. E., Potkin, S. G., Luchins, D. J., & Weinberger, D. R. (1986). Ex uno multi: subtyping the schizophrenia syndrome. *Biol. Psychiatry* 17:199–222.

Jeste, D. V., Lohr, J. B., Clark, K., & Wyatt, R. J. (1988). Pharmacological treatment of tardive dyskinesia in the 1980s. *J. Clin. Psychopharmacol. (Suppl).* 84:38S–48S.

Jeste, D. V., & Wyatt, R. J. (1981). Changing epidemiology of tardive dyskinesia. *Am. J. Psychiatry* 138:297–309.

Jeste, D. V., & Wyatt, R. J. (1982). *Understanding and Treating Tardive Dyskinesia.* New York: Guilford Press.

Jeste, D. V., & Wyatt, R. J. (1987). Aging and tardive dyskinesia. In *Schizophrenia and Aging: Schizophrenia, Paranoid and Schizophreniform Disorders in Later Life,* ed. N. E. Miller & G. D. Cohen, pp. 275–86. New York: Guilford Press.

Jones, M., & Hunter, R. (1969). Abnormal movements in patients with chronic psychiatric illness. In *Psychotropic Drugs and Dysfunctions of the Basal Ganglia,* Public Health Service Publication no. 1938, pp. 53–65. Washington, DC: U.S. Public Health Service.

Jus, A., Pineau, R., Lachance, R., Pelchat, G., Jus, K., Pires, P., & Villeneuve, R. (1976). Epidemiology of tardive dyskinesia, Part I. *Dis. Nerv. Syst.* 20:387–9.

Kane, J. M., & Smith, J. M. (1982). Tardive dyskinesia: prevalence and risk factors, 1959 to 1979. *Arch. Gen. Psychiatry* 39:473–81.

Kane, J. M., Woerner, M., & Lieberman, J. (1985). The prevalence of tardive dyskinesia. *Psychopharmacol. Bull.* 21:136–9.

Kane, J. M., Woerner, M., Weinhold, P., & Lieberman, J. (1984). Incidence of tardive dyskinesia: five-year data from a prospective study. *Psychopharmacol. Bull.* 20:387–9.

Kane, J. M., Woerner, M., Weinhold, P., Wegner, J., & Kinon, B. (1986). A prospective study oof tardive dyskinesia development: preliminary results. *J. Clin. Psychopharmacol.* 2:345–59.

Kennedy, P. F., Hershon, H. I., & McGuire, R. J. (1971). Extrapyramidal disorders after prolonged phenothiazine therapy. *Br. J. Psychiatry* 118:509–18.

Ko, G. N., Zhang, L. D., Yan, W. W., Zhang, M. D., Buchner, D., Xia, Z. Y., Wyatt, R. J., & Jeste, D. V. (1989). The Shanghai 800: prevalence of tardive dyskinesia in a Chinese psychiatric hospital. *Ann. J. Psychiatry* 146:387–9.

Kok, L. P., & Christopher, Y. S. (1985). Tardive dyskinesia in schizophrenic outpatients. *Ann. Acad. Med. Singapore* 14:87–90.

Kolakowska, T., Williams, A. O., & Ardern, M. (1986). Tardive dyskinesia and current dose of neuroleptic drugs. *Arch. Gen. Psychiatry* 43:614.

Kulhanek, F., Schwitzer, J., Hebenstreit, G., Hinterhuber, H., & Schubert, H. (1984). Tardive dyskinesia and correlating factors in a mental hospital in Austria. *Neuropsychiatric Clin.* 3:281–7.

Lehmann, H. E., & Ban, T. A. (1974). Sex differences in long-term adverse effects of phenothiazines. In *The Phenothiazines and Structurally Related Drugs*, ed. I. S. Forrest, C. J. Carr, & E. Usdin, pp. 249–54. New York: Raven Press.

Lehmann, H. E., Ban, T. A., & Saxena, S. M. (1970). A survey of extrapyramidal manifestations in the inpatient population of a psychiatric hospital. *Laval Med.* 41:909–16.

Lieberman, J., Kan, J. M., Woerner, M., & Weinhold, P. (1984). Prevalence of tardive dyskinesia in elderly samples. *Psychopharmacol. Bull.* 20:22–6.

McCreadie, R. G., Barron, E. T., & Winslow, G. S. (1982). The Nithsdale schizophrenia survey. II: Abnormal movements. *Br. J. Psychiatry* 40:587–90.

Morgenstern, H., Glazer, W. M., Gibowski, L. D., & Holmbey, S. (1987). Predictors of tardive dyskinesia: results of a cross-sectional study in an outpatient population. *J. Chronic Dis.* 40:319–27.

Moussaoui, D., Douki, S., Bentounsi, B., Otarid, A., Chorfi, M., Mamou, A., & Benamor, L. (1988). Épidémiologie des dyskinésies tardives au Maghreb. *Encephale* 14:203–8.

Mukherjee, S., Rosen, A. M., Cardinas, C., Varia, V., & Olarte, S. (1982). Tardive dyskinesia in schizophrenic outpatients. *Arch. Gen. Psychiatry* 39:466–9.

Muscettola, G., Pampollona, S., Barbato, G., Casillo, M., & Bollini, P. (1989). Tardive dyskinesia in Italy: preliminary findings. *Arch. Gen. Psychiatry* 46:754–5.

Ogita, K. (1972). A study of tardive dyskinesia following prolonged administration of neuroleptics. *Keio J. Med.* 50:297–310.

Paulson, G. (1968). Permanent or complex dyskinesias in the aged. *Geriatrics* 25:105–10.

Perényi, A., & Arato, M. (1980). Tardive dyskinesia in Hungarian psychiatric wards. *Psychosomatics* 21:904–9.

Perris, C., Dimitrijevic, P., Jacobsson, L., Paulson, P., Rapp, W., & Froberg, H. (1966). Tardive dyskinesia in psychiatric patients treated with neuroleptics. *Br. J. Psychiatry* 112:983–7.

Pryce, I. G., & Edwards, H. (1966). Persistent oral dyskinesia in female mental hospital patients. *Br. J. Psychiatry* 112:983–7.

Ramsay, F. M., & Millar, P. H. (1986). Tardive dyskinesia in the elderly. *Age Ageing* 15:145–50.

Raymond, V., Beaulieu, M., & Labrie, F. (1978). Potent antidopaminergic activity of oestradiol at the pituitary level on prolactin release. *Science* 200:1173–5.

Rey, J. M., Hunt, G. E., & Johnson, G. F. S. (1981). Assessment of tardive dyskinesia in psychiatric outpatients using a standardized rating scale. *Aust. N.Z. J. Psychiatry* 15:33–7.

Richardson, M. A., Hangland, G., Pass, R., & Craig, T. J. (1986). The prevalence of tardive dyskinesia in a mentally retarded population. *Psychopharmacol. Bull.* 22:245–9.

Richardson, M., Pass, R., Craig, T. J., & Vickers, E. (1984). Factors influencing the prevalence and severity of tardive dyskinesia. *Psychopharmacol. Bull.* 30:33–8.

Rittmannsberger, H., & Schony, W. (1986). Prevalenz tardiven Dyskinesie bei langzeit-hospitalisierten schizophrenen Patienten. *Nervenarzt* 57:116–18.

Seeman, M. V. (1983). Interaction of sex, age and neuroleptic dose. *Compr. Psychiatry* 24:125–8.

Siede, H., & Muller, H. F. (1967). Choreiform movements as side effects of phenothiazine medication in geriatric patients. *J. Am. Geriatr. Soc.* 15:517–22.

Simpson, G. M., Lee, J. H., Zoubok, B., & Gardos, G. (1979). A rating scale for tardive dyskinesia. *Psychopharmacology* 64:171–9.

Simpson, G. M., Varga, E., Lee, J. H., & Zoubok, B. (1978). Tardive dyskinesia and psychotropic drug history. *Psychopharmacology* 58:117–24.

Smith, J. M., & Baldessarini, R. J. (1980). Changes in prevalence, severity and recovery in tardive dyskinesia with age. *Arch. Gen. Psychiatry* 37:1368–73.

Smith, J. M., Kucharski, L. T., Eblen, C., Knutsen, E., & Linn, C. (1978). An assessment of tardive dyskinesia in schizophrenic outpatients. *Psychopharmacology* 64:99–104.

Smith, J. M., Oswald, W. T., Kucharski, L. T., & Walterman, L. J. (1979). Tardive dyskinesia: age and sex differences in hospitalized schizophrenics. *Psychopharmacology* 58:207–11.

Stone, R. K., Msy, J. E., Alvarez, W. F., & Ellman, G. (1989). Prevalence of dyskinesia and related movement disorders in a developmentally disabled population. *J. Mental Def. Res.* 33:41–53.

Turunen, S., & Achte, K. A. (1967). The buccolinguomasticatory syndrome as a side effect of neuroleptic therapy. *Psychiatr. Q.* 41:268–79.

Uhrbrand, L., & Faurbye, A. (1960). Reversible and irreversible dyskinesia after treatment with perphenazine, chlorpromazine, reserpine and ECT. *Psychopharmacologia* 1:408–18.

Villeneuve, A., Cazejust, T., & Coté, M. (1980). Estrogens in tardive dyskinesia in male psychiatric patients. *Neuropsychobiology* 6:145–51.

Villeneuve, A., Lavallée, J.-C., & Lemieux, L.-H. (1969). Dyskinésie tardive postneuroleptique. *Laval Med.* 40:832–7.

Waddington, J. L., & Youssef, H. A. (1985). Late onset involuntary movements in chronic schizophrenia: age-related vulnerability to "tardive" dyskinesia independent of extent of neuroleptic medication. *Irish Med. J.* 78:143–6.

Waddington, J. L., & Youssef, H. A. (1986). Involuntary movements and cognitive dysfunction in late onset schizophrenic outpatients. *Irish Med. J.* 79:347–50.

Williams, R., & Dalby, J. T. (1986). Tardive dyskinesia in outpatient schizophrenics treated with depot phenothiazines. *J. Clin. Psychopharmacol.* 6:318–19.

Wojcik, J. D., Gelenberg, A. J., LaBrie, R., & Mieske, M. (1980). Prevalence of tardive dyskinesia in an outpatient population. *Compr. Psychiatry* 21:370–80.

Yagi, G., Ogita, K., Ohtsuka, N., Itoh, H. B., & Miura, S. (1976). Persistent dyskinesia after long-term treatment with neuroleptics in Japan. *Keio J. Med.* 25:25–7.

Yassa, R., Ananth, J., Cordozo, S., & Ally, J. (1983). Tardive dyskinesia in an outpatient population: prevalence and predisposing factors. *Can. J. Psychiatry* 28:391–4.

Yassa, R., & Jeste, D. V. (1992). Gender differences in tardive dyskinesia: a critical review of the literature. *Schiz. Bull.* 18:701–15.

Yassa, R., & Nair, V. (1988). The association of tardive dyskinesia and pseudoparkinsonism. *Prog. Neuropsychopharmacol. Biol. Psychiatry* 12:909–14.

Yassa, R., Nair, V., Iskandar, H., & Schwartz, G. (1990). Factors in the development of severe forms of tardive dyskinesia. *Am. J. Psychiatry* 147:1156–63.

Yassa, R., Nair, V., & Schwartz, G. (1984). Tardive dyskinesia and the primary psychiatric diagnosis. *Psychosomatics* 25:135–8.

Yassa, R., Nair, V., & Schwartz, G. (1986). Early versus late onset psychosis and tardive dyskinesia. *Biol. Psychiatry* 21:1291–7.

Yassa, R., Nastase, C., Camille, Y., & Belzile, L. (1988). Tardive dyskinesia in a psychogeriatric population. In *Tardive Dyskinesia: Biological Mechanisms and Clinical Aspects*, ed. M. E. Wolf & A. D. Mosnaim, pp. 123–33. Washington, DC: American Psychiatric Press.

Yassa, R., Uhr, S., & Jeste, D. V. (1991). Gender differences in chronic schizophrenia: need for further research. In *The Elderly with Chronic Mental Illness*, ed. E. Light & B. D. Lebowitz, pp. 16–30. Berlin: Springer-Verlag.

Yesavage, J. A., Bourgeois, M., Kraemer, M., Csernansky, J. G., & Berger, P. A. (1982). Prevalence of tardive dyskinesia in 3140 French inpatients. *J. Nerv. Ment. Dis.* 170:111–12.

Youssef, H. A., & Waddington, J. L. (1988). Involuntary orofacial movements in hospitalized patients with mental handicaps or epilepsy: relationship to development/intellectual deficit and presence or absence of long-term exposure to neuroleptics. *J. Neurol. Neurosurg. Psychiatry* 51:863–5.

4

The Yale Tardive Dyskinesia Study: A Prospective Incidence Study Among Long-Term Outpatients

WILLIAM M. GLAZER, M.D., HAL MORGENSTERN, Ph.D., DONNA RAYE WAGNER, M.A., and JOHN DOUCETTE, M.Phil.

Tardive dyskinesia is now relatively common among psychiatric patients maintained on neuroleptics. A study of young patients newly exposed to neuroleptic medication (Kane, Woerner, & Weinhold, 1982) suggested an average tardive dyskinesia occurrence rate of 0.039/year during a 7-year follow-up period. The frequency of occurrence of tardive dyskinesia and its associated risk factors in older, chronically treated patients are not clearly understood, however. Without such an understanding, those who treat schizophrenia and other disorders requiring maintenance neuroleptic medication do not have adequate means to prevent and control this condition and its sequelae (Gardos & Cole, 1983). To improve this situation, we have been conducting a prospective follow-up study of new tardive dyskinesia occurrences among long-term outpatients, the goal being to identify risk factors for this disorder. The purpose of this chapter is to describe the design and methods of this study and to summarize the effects of variables on the incidence of tardive dyskinesia in this population (Morgenstern and Glazer, 1993; Glazer, Morgenstern, & Doucette, 1993, 1994).

Most epidemiologic investigations of tardive dyskinesia have been limited by several factors. First, because they have been cross-sectional (Jeste & Wyatt, 1981; Kane & Smith, 1982; Morgenstern et al., 1987; Waddington, 1987), that has not permitted a clear distinction between *risk factors* (those that affect disease development) and *prognostic factors* (those that affect the course of disease once it is present). Furthermore, cross-sectional studies of patient populations are particularly vulnerable to selection biases and temporal ambiguities of cause and effect. Second, the statistical analyses used in most published studies of tardive dyskinesia often have been too simplistic, ignoring the influences of other variables (i.e., confounders, modifiers, and mediating variables). Third, methodologic problems abound concerning the diagnosis and classification of tardive dyskinesia cases (Glazer, Morgenstern, & Niedzwiecki, 1988). For example, whereas diagnoses of new tardive dyskinesia occurrences (incidence) are best generated from longitudinal data (Jeste & Wyatt, 1981; Schooler & Kane, 1982), most studies to date have relied on a single examination to identify cases. The prospective design employed in the study reported here attempts to address these limitations.

Our earlier investigations had found limited published data pertaining to *the incidence of tardive dyskinesia among specific populations at risk* (Gibson, 1981; Kane et al., 1982; Yassa & Nair, 1984; Chouinard et al., 1986; Gardos et al., 1988; Waddington, Youssef, & Kinsella, 1990; Saltz et al., 1991; APA Task Force, 1992; Glazer et al., 1993, 1994). To compare those studies (excluding the study by Saltz et al., 1991, because it had focused only on geriatric patients), we (Glazer et al., 1993) estimated average tardive dyskinesia incidence rates from the published reports for all those studies and found that they ranged from 0.0385/year (Yassa & Nair, 1984) to 0.1093/year (Waddington et al., 1990). We then concluded that the sources of such variability had been differences in population characteristics and differences in the diagnostic criteria used for tardive dyskinesia.

Design and Methods

For this ongoing prospective study, we have established the major outcome variable as the rate of new occurrences (incidence) of tardive dyskinesia, as diagnosed at semiannual examinations. Nearly 400 study subjects at risk for tardive dyskinesia have been followed since the fall of 1985. The data that follow cover the 1985–90 time period.

Subject Selection

Our source population comes from the outpatient clinic at the Connecticut Mental Health Center (CMHC), which at the time of the study's initiation served a population of about 450,000 people in the greater New Haven area and carried an average daily census of 1,278 patients distributed among five units: emergency and evaluation; individuals; groups; couples and families; and "coffee and . . ." groups. Most of the patients being followed in this study were being treated by full-time staff members via low-contact modalities, with contacts ranging from biweekly to monthly. The patients were receiving maintenance neuroleptic medications, prescribed on a refillable basis over 3–6-month periods.

To be eligible for participation in the study, an individual had to meet three criteria: (1) be actively enrolled as a CMHC outpatient at any time between

July 1, 1985, and June 30, 1987; (2) be currently on neuroleptic medication, as evidence by at least a 3-month prescription in the pharmacy; and (3) be free of persistent tardive dyskinesia at the time of study intake, with no history of persistent involuntary abnormal movements.

In order to verify study eligibility, all patients whose names were selected from the pharmacy records were cross-checked against the list of patients previously diagnosed with tardive dyskinesia in the Yale tardive dyskinesia clinic (Glazer & Moore, 1981). Clinic patients previously diagnosed as having persistent tardive dyskinesia were ineligible for study inclusion. If the patients had no history of persistent tardive dyskinesia but met the criteria described for this study's baseline examination, they were considered to be in the category of *probable cases* of tardive dyskinesia and were reexamined in 6 months. If, at the 6-month follow-up, they again met the diagnostic criteria, they were considered to be in the category of *prevalent cases* of tardive dyskinesia; such patients were dropped from the incidence study and were followed in the tardive dyskinesia clinic. Conversely, if they failed to meet the criteria at the 6-month follow-up, they were considered to be in the category of *transient cases* of tardive dyskinesia; such patients were kept in the incidence study and considered to be at risk.

Data and Variables

Data for this study come from three sources: baseline interviews of 60–80 minutes with all subjects, medical records, and regularly scheduled follow-up visits every 6 months, starting on the day of the baseline interview. Baseline data include a wide variety of demographic, medical, psychosocial, and behavioral variables collected from patient interviews and medical records. Medical records are used as additional sources of information on past use of any psychiatric medications, any history of certain medical conditions, and any history of psychiatric hospitalization and use of certain treatments (electroshock, insulin coma, and lobotomy). Patients' charts are abstracted by a research assistant who did not conduct the baseline interview, thereby ensuring independent assessment of this important information. Demographic data include age, gender, race, marital status, employment status, and occupational status (using the Hollingshead coding system) (Hollingshead, 1975).

Follow-up data are collected at regularly scheduled visits (every 6 months) by a research assistant. Each visit involves two examinations using the Abnormal Involuntary Movement Scale (AIMS) (Guy, 1976) (at the beginning and end of the visit), one modified Webster examination to measure neuroleptic-induced involuntary movements (Webster, 1968), and patients' reports on the

Table 4.1. *Measures used in tardive dyskinesia incidence study schedule*

Variable	Baseline	6 months	12 months	18 months
Demographic/treatment-history data				
Sociodemographic data	×			
Medication history	×	×	×	×
Rehospitalization history		×	×	×
Diagnostic/symptom scales				
SADS-L/RDC	×			
SANS/SAPS	×			
SCL-90		×	×	×
Premorbid adjustment			×	
Movement-disorder scales				
AIMS	×	×	×	×
Webster	×	×	×	×
Cognitive functioning scales				
Mini Mental State Examination		×		×
Trail Making Test			×	
Verbal-fluency test			×	
Handedness			×	

types and dosages of all current medications, which are then confirmed via medical records. Patients are asked to describe their psychiatric symptoms during the preceding week and any hospitalizations since they were interviewed 6 months earlier. In addition, there are assessments of psychopathology, development, and neuropsychological status at various times during the study (Table 4.1).

Diagnosis and Detection. Each patient's tardive dyskinesia status is determined via the AIMS, a clinical instrument that includes 10 items (each coded 0–4). Seven items assess the severity of abnormal movements in different anatomic areas; three global items assess general severity, incapacitation, and the patient's awareness of the condition. The AIMS exam, conducted by a research assistant twice each visit, generally takes about 5 minutes per patient and has been shown to be reliable for detecting tardive dyskinesia (Lane, Glazer, & Hansen, 1985; Glazer, 1992).

Our definition of tardive dyskinesia, derived from our previous research (Glazer & Moore, 1981; Glazer et al., 1984; Glazer, Moore, & Bowers, 1985), is based on a modification of the definition by Schooler and Kane (1982). To be placed in the category of probable tardive dyskinesia at a given visit, a patient must have a total AIMS score (item 13) or 3 or more on both AIMS exams and at least one anatomic score of 2 (mild) or more on both exams. Patients meeting these criteria are reexamined by the principal investigator to confirm the diagnosis.

These criteria, because they are broader (less conservative) than the criteria proposed by Schooler and Kane (1982), have the potential disadvantage of increasing the proportion of false-positive diagnoses. Because this is an incidence study, however, we want to identify true cases of tardive dyskinesia as early as possible. To examine this issue, we have reviewed data from another earlier study (Glazer et al., 1988) in which 238 probable cases of tardive dyskinesia had been diagnosed in the Yale tardive dyskinesia clinic using the Glazer-Morgenstern criteria (i.e., the previously described criteria, but with only one AIMS exam). Among the 118 patients who had been examined at least four times (at quarterly visits), 28 (24%) met the Glazer-Morgenstern criteria but did not meet the Schooler-Kane criteria for tardive dyskinesia at baseline. However, of those 28 discrepant diagnoses, 23 (82%) had become "probable" cases within three visits, according to the Schooler-Kane criteria. From that unpublished analysis, we concluded that the Glazer-Morgenstern criteria are more sensitive for detecting tardive dyskinesia cases early. For this study, therefore, and in order to minimize the problem of additional false positives that would be created by setting the symptom threshold lower, we conduct the AIMS exam twice at every visit. A diagnosis of tardive dyskinesia will then be made only if both sets of AIMS scores meet our criteria described earlier. Our reasoning is that despite the adequate interrater reliability among experienced examiners, there can be much intrapersonal variability in the assessed levels of severity of tardive dyskinesia, variability that may, to some extent, reflect true biological changes in the condition or measurement error. Hence, we believe that our two AIMS exams per visit not only will enhance diagnostic reliability but also will permit a quantitative analysis of the intrapersonal variability. This approach is similar to the procedures customarily employed to measure blood pressure in epidemiologic studies.

A *new persistent case* of tardive dyskinesia is declared when any patient, after a negative baseline evaluation, meets the previously described criteria for two consecutive visits. Thus, on the second visit, if these criteria are met, the patient is diagnosed as having *persistent* tardive dyskinesia and is dropped from the incidence study and followed in the tardive dyskinesia clinic.

Determination of History of Neuroleptic Exposure. Any history of neuroleptic exposure was determined at the time of the baseline interview by patient interview and chart review, the latter including reports sent from other facilities. When questioning patients about their use of neuroleptics, the interviewer used the brand names of the neuroleptic medications and showed the actual tablets or capsules in their different dosages. For all positive responses, the patients were asked to identify the dosages and the time periods during which they had taken those medications. Another reviewer examined each patient's medical chart and recorded the medications and dosages prescribed by CMHC physicians, as well as those prescribed earlier at other institutions. If the reviewer learned from the patient or from the chart review of undocumented episodes of neuroleptic treatment, that fact was recorded. As long as there were no undocumented periods during which there might have been unrecorded use of neuroleptics, we relied on chart information exclusively for our determination of the total duration of neuroleptic use. If there were undocumented periods, we supplemented the chart information with patients' reports that coincided with the undocumented periods. Actual neuroleptic dosages were determined from medical records alone, because most outpatients at CMHC were unable to recall their dosages reliably. Thus, the total durations of neuroleptic use and the dosages were determined from both patients' self-reports and records reviews, with heavy reliance on chart information. To compare dosage levels for different drugs, we used the values of Baldessarini (1985) for chlorpromazine-equivalent dosages.

Other Clinical Measures. Patients' psychiatric diagnoses, via the Research Diagnostic Criteria (RDC) (Spitzer & Endicott, 1978a), and their psychopathologic conditions were determined at baseline. For that we used the Schedule for Affective Disorder and Schizophrenia, Lifetime Version (SADS-L) (Endicott & Spitzer, 1978; Spitzer & Endicott, 1978a). At all follow-up visits, patients are examined for certain symptoms from the Symptom Checklist (SCL-90) (Derogatis, 1983).

Psychological status and developmental level were evaluated with the Premorbid Asocial Adjustment Scale (PAAS) at month 12 (Gittelman-Klein & Klein, 1969), the Scale for Assessment of Negative Symptoms (SANS) at baseline and at 24 months (Andreasen, 1984a), and the Scale for Assessment of Positive Symptoms (SAPS) at baseline and at 24 months (Andreasen, 1984b).

Cognitive functioning is measured annually with the Mini Mental State Examination (MMSE) (Folstein, Folstein, & McHugh, 1975), beginning at the 6-month examination, with the Trail Making Test (TMT) (Reitan, 1958; Reitan & Davison, 1976), at months 12 and 24, and with a test of verbal fluency (Goodglass & Kaplan, 1972), at months 12 and 24. Handedness was measured at the 12-month visit by the Raczkowski, Kalat, and Nebes (1974) modification of the Edinburgh questionnaire (Oldfield, 1971).

Raters. Each research assistant participating in this project has had at least 3 years of clinical experience with psychiatric patients. In an initial training phase, they were given relevant journal articles and one-on-one instruction in the use of the various rating scales used in the study. In order to ensure reliability of ratings, weekly interrater meetings were held for a year; since then, monthly sessions have been held on an ongoing basis. In these sessions, ratings of patients are completed independently, and then discussed. The intraclass correlation coefficients (Shrout & Fleiss, 1979) for agreement on total AIMS scores for groups of two to four raters have ranged from 0.71 to 0.88.

Statistical Methods

The average incidence rate (per unit time) of persistent tardive dyskinesia in the study population is estimated as a ratio: the number of new cases detected at follow-up visits divided by the number of person-years for the population at risk during the study – that is, from the baseline period to either the time of initial disease detection or the time of withdrawal from the study. This person-time or "survival" approach takes into consideration the different durations of follow-up among the subjects. Estimates of the *risk* (cumulative incidence) for tardive dyskinesia during the follow-up period are based on a life-table procedure using Rothman's method for deriving confidence limits (Rothman, 1978).

Crude effects of the categorical variables on the incidence of tardive dyskinesia are measured by the rate ratio, which is the average incidence rate in a certain group divided by the corresponding rate in a reference group. By means of a standard asymptotic method (Kleinbaum, Kupper, & Morgenstern, 1982), 95% confidence intervals are computed for each rate ratio. To examine the nature of possible dosage–response relationships, most predictor variables are categorized into three or four groups, where one group is designated as the referent. The *p* values for testing the effects of ordinal variables are based on two-sided Mantel-Haenszel tests for linear trend (Kleinbaum et al., 1982). Where possible, the weighted mean value of the underlying continuous variable within each group is used as the exposure score for that group when computing the test statistic.

After performing crude (i.e., unadjusted) analyses, we conduct multivariable analyses, using stratification methods and model fitting to adjust for confounding effects and to consider possible interaction effects. In all cases, the results of stratified analyses have been consistent with those obtained from model fitting; thus, only the modeling results are presented here. The determination of modeling rates is made with Cox's proportional-hazards analysis (i.e., life-table regression), using maximization of the partial-likelihood function to estimate the multiplicative regression coefficients (Cox, 1972; Breslow, 1974). Rate-ratio estimates and confidence intervals for each predictor are derived from the model coefficients and their standard errors (Kelsey, Thompson, & Evans, 1986).

Results

The mean baseline age for the entire cohort of 398 patients at risk was 42 years (range 19–73); 52% were women, and 26% were nonwhite (23% African-American). Eighty-three percent of the patients were single, separated, divorced, or widowed. Forty-seven percent of the patients were Catholic, 38% protestant, and 5% Jewish. Thirty-four percent had received less than 12 years of education, 38% had received 12 years, and 28% had received more than 12 years. Seventy percent of the patients were unemployed at baseline.

At the baseline interview, the mean duration of previous neuroleptic use was 8 years (range 3 months to 33 years). The mean age at first neuroleptic exposure was 29 years (range 4–72). The mean age at first outpatient treatment was 25 years (range 1–72), and the mean age at first hospitalization was 26 years (range 8–65). Six percent of the patients had never been hospitalized, 53% had been hospitalized fewer than five times, and 41% had been hospitalized five or more times.

The 398 patients were divided into five mutually exclusive RDC diagnostic groups, called the "primary-diagnosis" groups. Equal weights were given to definite and probable diagnoses and to present, past, and lifetime designations. The numbers of patients in the five groups were as follows: 167 (41%) schizophrenics; 67 (16%) schizoaffectives; 60 (15%) with affective disorders (i.e., manic, hypomanic, bipolar with mania, and major depressive disorder); 40 with (10%) "mixed" diagnoses (i.e., combinations of the first three categories); 64 (16%) with other diagnoses (i.e., minor depressive disorder, alcoholism, drug-use disorder, other psychotic disorder, and schizotypal features). In addition, 90 (23%) of the patients in the total cohort were diagnosed with alcohol-abuse or drug-abuse disorders – 42 (25%) of the schizophrenics, 22

(33%) of the schizoaffectives, 8 (13%) of the affectives, 10 (25%) with mixed diagnoses, and 8 (13%) with other diagnoses.

Incidence Rates

There were 62 new persistent cases of tardive dyskinesia detected during 1,167 person-years of follow-up (1985–90), yielding an average incidence rate of 0.053/year. When considering individual follow-up intervals between successive visits, we found that the average incidence rates were relatively high (6.6–8.2 per 100 per year) during the first three follow-up intervals, covering an average of 2.1 years; the rates then dropped over the next six intervals (0.0–4.8 per 100 per year), covering another 3.1 years of follow-up time.

Risk (Cumulative Incidence)

To address the important question of the probability of developing tardive dyskinesia over long periods of exposure to neuroleptics, we combined data (Glazer et al., 1993) from patients who had had different durations of neuroleptic exposure at baseline; we are thus able to estimate the *risk,* that is, the probability of developing tardive dyskinesia, for exposure periods that greatly exceed the observed durations of follow-up (about 5 years). Thus, for example, if the baseline histories of previous neuroleptic exposure for patients with no history of tardive dyskinesia range from nearly zero to more than 20 years, we can estimate the risk for tardive dyskinesia for periods as long as 20 + 5 = 25 years of neuroleptic treatment. The major assumption required for these long-term risk estimates is that the tardive dyskinesia incidence *rate* (i.e., new cases per person-year of follow-up experience at risk) for a given duration of previous neuroleptic exposure will remain approximately constant over (calender) time in the source population of neuroleptic users. We thus find that the estimated risk of a newly exposed patient developing tardive dyskinesia is 0.318 after 5 years of exposure, 0.494 after 10 years, 0.567 after 15 years, 0.647 after 20 years, and 0.684 after 25 years of neuroleptic exposure.

Risk Factors

A modified stepwise procedure, incorporating our a priori knowledge, was used to identify a core (best) set of predictors for tardive dyskinesia: age, race, years of previous neuroleptic use at baseline, and average neuroleptic dosage. The results of the core prediction model are summarized in Figure 4.1, which

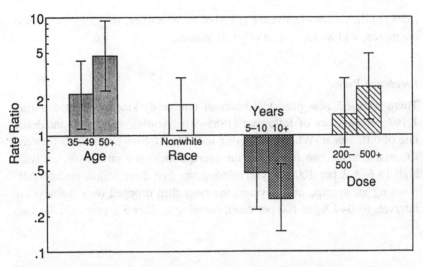

Figure 4.1. Adjusted rate ratios for the effects of age at baseline, race, years of previous neuroleptic use at baseline, and average dosage (CPZE) during follow-up, by nonreference category of each predictor – results of a multiple-proportional-hazards analysis ($n = 362$). The reference categories are as follows: <35 years (age); white (race); <5 years (previous neuroleptic use); CPZE at <200 mg/day (average dosage).

shows adjusted rate ratios and 95% confidence intervals (vertical bands) for the effects of these four core predictors in a multiple-proportional-hazards analysis. Note that the estimated rate ratio for each nonreference category is a comparison of the tardive dyskinesia incidence rate for that category with the rate for the reference category, adjusting for all other predictors in the core model.

We found that on the basis of adjusted results, the incidence rate for tardive dyskinesia is positively affected by *age*. Compared with patients less than 35 years of age, patients between ages 35 and 49 years have a rate ratio of 2.2, and those over 50 years of age have a rate ratio of 4.7 (p for trend <.001).

Another notable predictor is *race*. The rate ratio for nonwhites to whites is 1.8 ($p = .026$).

The third predictor, *years of previous neuroleptic use at baseline*, inversely affects the incidence of tardive dyskinesia. Compared with patients exposed to neuroleptics for less than 5 years at baseline, the rate ratio for patients with 5–10 years of exposure was 0.5 (confidence interval, CI, 0.2–0.9); the rate ratio comparing patients with 10 or more years to those with less than 5 years was 0.3 (CI, 0.2–0.6; p for trend <.001). Thus, the tardive dyskinesia rate is greatest during the first 5 years of neuroleptic treatment, although new persistent cases continue to occur many years after first exposure.

The final core predictor is the *average neuroleptic dosage* during follow-up. The rate ratio comparing patients receiving an average of 200–499 mg/day to those patients receiving less than 200 mg/day (chlorpromazine equivalents, CPZE) was 1.5 (CI, 0.8–2.9); the rate ratio for those receiving more than 500 mg/day compared to the low-dosage group was 2.5 (CI, 1.3–4.8). The *p* for the trend in this tripartite comparison was 0.006.

Although other variables of interest were added to this model, one at a time, in an effort to estimate their (adjusted) effects, controlling for the core predictors as confounders, no other variable added to this core model appreciably altered the effects estimated for the four predictors just outlined. Gender, education, occupation, employment status, and marital status were among the variables tried. Furthermore, when we estimated the effects of other neuroleptic variables on this core model, including the effects of chemical type, relative potency, age at first exposure to neuroleptics, and depot route of administration, no appreciable effects were observed (Morgenstern & Glazer, 1993). Finally, we found that other psychiatric medications and/or psychiatric diagnoses had no substantial effect on the core model.

Discussion

The major findings of this study are that the incidence rate for tardive dyskinesia in a long-term outpatient cohort is positively affected by increased age, nonwhite status, and higher neuroleptic dosages and is inversely affected by net years of previous neuroleptic use at baseline. Additionally, the estimated long-term risk for developing tardive dyskinesia as a function of previous neuroleptic treatment is high; that is, 2 of every 3 patients maintained on neuroleptics can be expected to develop persistent tardive dyskinesia within 25 years if there is continuing exposure. Furthermore, the risk for tardive dyskinesia is not uniform over the course of treatment; it is substantially greater in the first 5 years of exposure.

Several points should be considered apropos the finding that the incidence risk for tardive dyskinesia is highest in the first 5 years of neuroleptic exposure, as compared with subsequent 5-year periods. First, perhaps not all the cases detected in this study represent first-time occurrences of tardive dyskinesia. Indeed, some subjects may have had tardive dyskinesia before the study, even though it was not clinically detectable at baseline. Assuming that possibility to be true, one would expect these recurrent cases to reappear during the first 1–2 years of follow-up. However, because we were careful to review medical records and ask patients for signs of previous movement disorders, we doubt that that explanation can account for the observed trend.

Second, in another study of the same source population, we found that 80% of all prevalent cases of tardive dyskinesia had previously been diagnosed at the Yale tardive dyskinesia clinic (Morgenstern et al., 1987), our primary source for determining prevalence in the incidence study. Third, perhaps the secular trends in treatment practices within the source population can account for the decrease in tardive dyskinesia risk after long-term neuroleptic exposure. However, we found no obvious indication that practice patterns had changed at the CMHC between 1985 and 1990 (when the inverse effect was *directly* observed via rate estimates) in a manner that could explain the reduction in rates.

Of the four predictors of the incidence of tardive dyskinesia, the least expected was that of race. Despite extensive analysis of the data, we are still unclear as to what this finding represents (W. Glazer, unpublished data). It seems that although African-American patients in this study population were more likely than their white counterparts to be diagnosed as schizophrenic, to receive higher dosages of neuroleptics, and to be placed on the depot route, none of these variables actually accounts for the race effect. In the absence of an explanation, these data should stimulate more attention to race effects in studies of tardive dyskinesia, schizophrenia, and neuroleptic medication effects.

One concern raised about the design of this study is that at the start of the follow-up, many subjects had already been exposed to neuroleptics, and for many years. But such a criticism actually reflects a basic lack of appreciation for the cohort (incidence) study design. Proponents of this critical view maintain that the only way to identify risk factors for tardive dyskinesia is to follow a group of patients from the very start of (first) neuroleptic treatment. However, although we would agree that the ideal study of risk factors for tardive dyskinesia would follow newly exposed cases throughout the entire course of treatment, and setting aside the practical problems that would preclude such a study, it is important to note that because our subjects were initially free of dyskinetic movements and had no history of persistent dyskinesia, they were still only *at risk* of developing tardive dyskinesia. It is therefore appropriate and, we believe, informative to examine possible risk factors in this population. Indeed, it is quite possible that predictors of "early" tardive dyskinesia (e.g., in the first few years of neuroleptic treatment) are not predictors of "late" tardive dyskinesia (Kane et al., 1982). In addition, the variability in the durations of previous neuroleptic use at baseline was considerable, ranging from 3 months to 33 years. Thus, we can, with this design, compare the tardive dyskinesia rates for different periods of neuroleptic treatment, in addition to estimating the effects of other factors on tardive dyskinesia for different durations of neuroleptic use. One last point: If the foregoing criticism were valid, and if it were generalized to other areas of epidemiologic research, it would be pointless to conduct incidence studies of chronic diseases in the elderly. Yet we know that examining the possible effects of high serum concentrations of cholesterol in terms of the risk for coronary heart disease among 65–79-year-olds, for example, has important etiologic, clinical, and policy implications – even though such individuals may have been "exposed" to high (or low) cholesterol levels for many decades. As pointed out by numerous researchers over the past 10–15 years, the findings from such aging studies complement the findings from analogous studies conducted in younger populations.

Conclusion

This chapter, a further ramification of the original Yale study of tardive dyskinesia, presents our initial findings concerning the effects of demographic and clinical variables on the incidence of tardive dyskinesia. Our findings contradict several commonly held beliefs about the cases of tardive dyskinesia, in that we found no overall effect due to gender, type of neuroleptic, depot route, or affective diagnosis. Perhaps, however, these factors influence the course of tardive dyskinesia once it develops. In any event, we are following the incidence cases and will address this possibility in future analyses. Future analyses will also address other possible risk factors. We hope that these data will contribute to an understanding of the causes of tardive dyskinesia and to the development of methods to prevent, manage and treat this condition.

References

Andreasen, N. C. (1984a). *Scale for the Assessment of Negative Symptoms (SANS)*. Iowa City: University of Iowa.

Andreasen, N. C. (1984b). *Scale for the Assessment of Positive Symptoms (SAPS)*. Iowa City: University of Iowa.

APA Task Force (1992). *Task Force Report of the American Psychiatric Association: Tardive Dyskinesia*. Washington, DC: American Psychiatric Association.

Baldessarini, R. J. (1985). Antipsychotic agents. In *Chemotherapy in Psychiatry: Principles and Practice*, pp. 14–92. Cambridge, MA: Harvard University Press.

Breslow, N. (1974). Covariance analysis of censored survival data. *Biometrics* 30:89–97.

Chouinard, G., Annable, L., Mercier, P., & Ross-Chouinard, A. (1986). A five-year follow-up study of tardive dyskinesia. *Psychopharmacol. Bull.* 22:259–63.

Cox, D. (1972). Regression models and life-tables. *J. Roy. Statist. Soc. (Series B)* 34:187–202.

Derogatis, L. R. (1983). *SCL-90-R. Administration, Scoring & Procedures Manual, II, for the Revised Version*. Towson, MD: Clinical Psychometric Research.

Endicott, J., & Spitzer, R. L. (1978). A diagnostic interview: the schedule for affective disorders and schizophrenia. *Arch. Gen. Psychiatry* 35:837–44.

Folstein, M., Folstein, S., & McHugh, P. (1975). Mini-mental state: a practical method for grading the cognitive state of patients for the clinician. *Psychiatr. Res.* 12:189–98.

Gardos, G., & Cole, J. O. (1983). Tardive dyskinesia and anticholinergic drugs. *Am. J. Psychiatry* 140:210–22.

Gardos, G., Perenyi, A., Cole, J., Samu, I., Kocsis, E., & Casey, D. E. (1988). Seven-year follow-up of tardive dyskinesia in Hungarian outpatients. *Neuropsychopharmacology* 1:169–72.

Gibson, A. C. (1981). Incidence of tardive dyskinesia in patients receiving depot neuroleptic injection. *Acta Psychiatr. Scand.* 63:111–16.

Gittelman-Klein, R., & Klein, D. F. (1969). Premorbid asocial adjustment and prognosis in schizophrenia. *J. Psychiatr. Res.* 7:35–54.

Glazer, W. (1992). Doctors' response to managed care. *Med. Interface* 5:14–16.

Glazer, W., & Moore, D. C. (1981). A tardive dyskinesia clinic in a mental health center. *Hosp. Community Psychiatry* 32:572–4.

Glazer, W. M., Moore, D., & Bowers, M. (1985). The treatment of tardive dyskinesia with Baclofen. *Psychopharmacology* 87:480–3.

Glazer, W. M., Moore, D., Schooler, N., Brenner, L., & Morgenstern, H. (1984). Tardive dyskinesia: a discontinuation study. *Arch. Gen. Psychiatry* 41:623–7.

Glazer, W. M., Morgenstern, H., & Doucette, J. (1993). Predicting the long-term risk of tardive dyskinesia in outpatients maintained on neuroleptic medications. *J. Clin. Psychiatry* 54:133–9.

Glazer, W., Morgenstern, H., & Doucette, J. (1994). Race and tardive dyskinesia in a community health center outpatient population. *Hosp. Community Psychiatry* 45:38–42.

Glazer, W., Morgenstern, H., & Niedzwiecki, D. (1988). Heterogeneity of tardive dyskinesia: a multivariate analysis. *Br. J. Psychiatry* 152:253–9.

Goodglass, H., & Kaplan, E. (1972). *The Assessment of Aphasia and Related Disorders*. Philadelphia: Lea & Febiger.

Guy, W. (1976). Abnormal involuntary movement scale (AIMS). In *ECDEU Assessment Manual for Psychopharmacology*, rev. ed. DHEW publication (ADM) 76-338, pp. 534–7. Rockville, MD: U.S. Department of Health, Education, and Welfare.

Hollingshead, A. (1975). *A Two-Factored Index of Social Position*. New Haven: Yale University Press.

Jeste, D., & Wyatt, R. (1981). Changing epidemiology of tardive dyskinesia. *Am. J. Psychiatry* 138:297–309.

Kane, J. M., & Smith, J. M. (1982). Tardive dyskinesia. *Arch. Gen. Psychiatry* 39:473–81.

Kane, J. M., Woerner, M., & Weinhold, P. (1982). A prospective study of tardive dyskinesia development: preliminary results. *J. Clin. Psychopharmacol.* 2:345–9.

Kelsey, J. L., Thompson, W. D., & Evans, A. S. (1986). Methods. In *Observational Epidemiology*, p. 141. Oxford University Press.

Kleinbaum, D., Kupper, L., & Morgenstern, H. (1982). *Epidemiologic Research: Principles and Quantitative Methods*. Belmont, CA: Lifetime Learning.

Lane, R., Glazer, W., & Hansen, T. (1985). Assessment of tardive dyskinesia using the abnormal involuntary movement scale. *J. Nerv. Ment. Dis.* 173:353–7.

Morgenstern, H., & Glazer, W. (1993). Identifying risk factors for tardive dyskinesia among chronic outpatients maintained on neuroleptic medications: results of the Yale Tardive Dyskinesia Study. *Arch. Gen. Psychiatry*, 50:723–33.

Morgenstern, H., Glazer, W., Gibowski, L., & Holmberg, S. (1987). Predictors of tardive dyskinesia: results of a cross-sectional study in an outpatient population. *J. Chronic Dis.* 40:319–27.

Oldfield, R. C. (1971). The assessment and analysis of handedness: the Edinburgh Inventory. *Neuropsychologia* 9:97–113.

Raczkowski, D., Kalat, J. W., & Nebes, R. (1974). Reliability and validity of some handedness questionnaire items. *Neuropsychologia* 12:43–7.

Reitan, R. M. (1958). Validity of the Trail Making Test as an indicator of organic brain damage. *Percept. Mot. Skills* 8:271–6.

Reitan, R. M., & Davison, L. A. (1976). *Current Status and Applications. Clinical Neuropsychology*. New York: Winston/Wiley.

Rothman, K. J. (1978). Estimation of confidence limits for the cumulative probability of survival in life table analysis. *J. Chronic Dis.* 31:557–60.

Saltz, B. L., Woerner, M. G., Kane, J. M., Leiberman, J. A., Alvir, J. M. J., Bergmann, K. J., Blank, K., Koblenzer, J., & Kahaner, K. (1991). Prospective study of tardive dyskinesia in the elderly. *JAMA* 266:2402–6.

Schooler, N., & Kane, J. (1982). Research diagnoses for tardive dyskinesia. *Arch. Gen. Psychiatry* 39:486–7.

Shrout, P. E., & Fleiss, J. L. (1979). Intraclass correlations: uses in assessing rater reliability. *Psychol. Bull.* 86:420–8.

Spitzer, R., & Endicott, J. (1978a). *Research Diagnostic Criteria*, 3rd. ed., no. 59. New York: New York State Psychiatric Institute.

Spitzer, R., & Endicott, J. (1978b). *Schedule for Affective Disorders and Schizophrenia – Lifetime Version (SADS-L)*, 3rd ed. New York: New York State Psychiatric Institute.

Waddington, J. L. (1987). Tardive dyskinesia in schizophrenia and other disorders: associations with ageing, cognitive dysfunction and structural brain pathology in relation of neuroleptic exposure. *Hum. Psychopharmacol.* 2:11–22.

Waddington, J. L., Youssef, H. A., & Kinsella, A. (1990). Cognitive dysfunction in schizophrenia followed up over 5 years, and its longitudinal relationship to the emergence of tardive dyskinesia. *Psychol. Med.* 20:835–42.

Webster, D. (1968). Critical analysis of the disability in Parkinson's disease. *Mod. Treat.* 5:257–82.

Yassa, R., & Nair, V. (1984). Incidence of tardive dyskinesia in an outpatient population. *Psychosomatics* 25:479–81.

5

Vulnerability to Tardive Dyskinesia in Schizophrenia: An Exploration of Individual Patient Factors

JOHN L. WADDINGTON, Ph.D., EADBHARD
O'CALLAGHAN, F.R.C.P.I., PETER BUCKLEY,
M.R.C.Psych., CATHY MADIGAN, M.A., CONALL
LARKIN, F.R.C.Psych., and ANTHONY KINSELLA,
M.Sc.

After almost 40 years of research, we still do not know why some patients, but not others, develop late-onset involuntary movements – that is, tardive dyskinesia – when they are prescribed neuroleptics on a long-term basis. Although neuroleptics are the primary offending medications in the general sense (but see the conclusion to this chapter), there is little evidence to indicate that patients with tardive dyskinesia may simply have received neuroleptics (or other drugs) for longer periods or at higher dosages than have otherwise similar patients who remain unaffected (Kane & Smith, 1982; Waddington, 1989; Chapter 9, this volume). Much interest centers, therefore, on vulnerability factors *within* the individual patient.

One of the more consistent findings in research on tardive dyskinesia is a general association with increasing age. It is evident, however, that the syndrome is by no means restricted to the middle-aged or elderly, for it can constitute a substantial clinical problem in younger patients (Kane & Smith, 1982; Waddington, 1989; Chapter 2, this volume), whose fundamental vulnerability apparently resides elsewhere. Similarly, it is often asserted that tardive dyskinesia is more likely to emerge in women than in men, although the evidence to support such an assertion is complex and is far from robust statistically. In fact, among both men and women, an important but often overlooked interaction has emerged between age and severity of the involuntary movements of tardive dyskinesia (Kane & Smith, 1982; Waddington, 1989; Chapter 3, this volume). Another factor possibly associated with the varying risks for tardive dyskinesia is the diagnosis itself. Although patients with affective or "organic" disorders may be somewhat more likely to develop the syndrome (Kane & Smith, 1982; Waddington, 1989; Chapter 6, this volume), reports indicate that it has emerged in every diagnostic group for which neuroleptics have been prescribed, with most of the affected individuals carrying a diagnosis of schizophrenia. Such evidence, together with the other issues reviewed in Part II of this volume, would suggest that a family of factors may exist, each of which can exert a general, modulatory influence on the likelihood of developing tardive dyskinesia and on its severity, but none of which, alone, is sufficient to predispose to the emergence of the syndrome. The question remains: Does the notion of individual vulnerability in some way integrate these general risk factors? Alternatively, perhaps the operation of some other, more fundamental process or processes still needs clarification.

This issue can most readily be addressed by comparing groups of patients with and without tardive dyskinesia who are well matched for multiple variables such as age, gender distribution, and diagnostic composition. Indeed, studies comparing schizophrenic patients with tardive dyskinesia and similar patients without the disorder have shown cognitive impairment as the most consistently (though not invariably) reported measure. This association, particularly with an orofacial site of the involuntary movements (Waddington, 1995; Waddington et al., 1987, 1993; DeWolfe, Ryan, & Wolfe, 1988), has been reported after testing a wide variety of patients (in terms of age range and chronicity) using a broad range of neuropsychological procedures. Although such findings usually have been interpreted as consonant with the organic-vulnerability hypothesis, other interpretations are possible (Waddington, 1989, 1995; Waddington et al., 1993; Chapter 1, this volume), as considered later. A further question is then raised: What are the antecedents of this apparent association? That is, what are the cerebral processes that might result in only some schizophrenic patients showing cognitive impairment and the emergence of tardive dyskinesia? And what might be the origins of such processes? Current theory and much of the available evidence suggest that schizophrenia is a neurodevelopmental disorder whereby environmental and/or genetically programmed events in utero disrupt the establishment of certain fundamental aspects of brain structure and function. Although such early cerebral disturbances might then give rise to typical diagnostic symptoms some two decades later, perhaps that occurs only on the subsequent functional maturation or completion of other associated cerebral systems or processes (Weinberger, 1987; Murray & Lewis, 1987; Waddington, 1993a,b).

The extent and form of the structural and functional consequences of any such neuronal "maldevelopment" might be elements in one's vulnerability to tardive dyskinesia. But how could this be indexed? Obstetric complications, perhaps uncommonly frequent in the early history of patients with schizophrenia, suggest one potential source of early cerebral insult (Lewis, 1989; O'Callaghan et al., 1992b), and a family history of schizophrenia might reflect the operation of genetic factors as well. Although both of those aspects have been considered as potential risk factors for tardive dyskinesia, a consistent picture has yet to emerge (O'Callaghan et al., 1990; McCreadie et al., 1992). An additional factor might be that patients with schizophrenia have an excess of peripheral markers of neurodevelopmental perturbation reflected in minor physical anomalies (those slight anatomic, though clinically insignificant, malformations of the head or body and limbs that reflect early disturbances of ectodermally derived structures, including the brain) (Green et al., 1989; O'Callaghan et al., 1991; Lohr & Flynn, 1993).

The purpose of this chapter is to elaborate these issues by way of an account of a recent study of tardive dyskinesia (Waddington et al., 1995). In this analysis, we compared a variety of cognitive, symptomatological, biological, and other measures in diagnostically homogeneous and demographically comparable patients, with and without tardive dyskinesia, who shared a number of putative neurodevelopmental factors.

The Study

Subjects and Procedures

We studied 47 subjects who attended a day center or outpatient clinic (ages 21–65 years) and who met DSM-III criteria (American Psychiatric Association, 1980) for schizophrenia. We examined each subject using the Abnormal Involuntary Movement Scale (Guy, 1976) and determined the presence or absence of tardive dyskinesia by applying the criteria of Schooler and Kane (1982). From case notes, the following demographic variables were transcribed: age at first presentation to a psychiatric service; duration of illness; current neuroleptic dosage in chlorpromazine (CPZ) equivalents (Davis, 1976); current exposure to anticholinergics. For those patients whose biological mothers were living, we ascertained any history of obstetric complications related to the patient and any family history of schizophrenia in a first-degree relative (O'Callaghan et al., 1990). Each patient was examined for, inter alia, the following: (1) minor physical anomalies (MPAs), using the Waldrop scale (O'Callaghan et al., 1991), which gave a total MPA score (MPAT), separate scores for the head (MPAH) and periphery (MPAP), and an anomalies-distribution index [(MPAH − MPAP)/MPAT]; (2) handedness, as left-handed (exclusive or ambidextrous) or non-left-handed; (3) current psychopathology using the Scale for Assessment of Positive Symptoms

(SAPS) and the Scale for Assessment of Negative Symptoms (SANS) (Andreasen, 1990); (4) premorbid intelligence, using the National Adult Reading Test (NART); (5) current cognitive function, using Trail Making Tests A and B (O'Callaghan et al., 1991) and the Wisconsin Card Sorting Test (Nelson, 1976); (6) cerebral structure, using magnetic-resonance imaging (MRI), which gave the total volume of the lateral ventricles (TVV), the volumes of the left (LVV) and right (RVV) ventricles separately, and a ventricular asymmetry index [(LVV − RVV)/TVV] and revealed the presence or absence of cortical atrophy (Waddington et al., 1990a; O'Callaghan et al., 1992a).

Results

As shown in Table 5.1, 18 (38%) of 47 patients satisfied the criteria of Schooler and Kane (1982) for tardive dyskinesia; the orofacial (buccal-lingual-masticatory) region was affected in each instance, with or without additional involvement of the limbs or trunk. We found that patients with and without tardive dyskinesia were indistinguishable in terms of mean age, gender distribution, age at first illness, duration of illness, mean current neuroleptic dosage, and current exposure to anticholinergics.

In terms of current psychopathologic manifestations, patients with and without tardive dyskinesia showed indistinguishable severities of positive and negative symptoms. Regarding cognitive function, it was found that the two groups could not be distinguished either on the basis of premorbid IQ or by their performances on Trail Making Tests A and B. The patients with tardive dyskinesia, however, made 48% more perseverative errors and sorted 35% fewer categories ($p = .04$) on the Wisconsin Card Sorting Test than did patients without such movement disorder.

At the level of putative neurodevelopmental factors, patients with tardive dyskinesia were no more or less likely than those without such movement disorder to have experienced obstetric complications, to have a family history of schizophrenia, or to show anomalous handedness. Neither were the patients with tardive dyskinesia distinguishable by total scores for MPAs, a finding that held for separate scores for the head and periphery, although the nonsignificant trend was toward more anomalies of the head and fewer of the periphery in the dyskinetic group. In this regard, among patients with MPAs, those with tardive dyskinesia showed a higher ($p = 0.02$) distribution index, indicating that dyskinetic patients had a greater relative likelihood that their anomalies would be of the head rather than the periphery.

Table 5.1. *Characteristics of schizophrenic patients with and without tardive dyskinesia*

	Tardive dyskinesia[a]	
Characteristic	Absent	Present
Number (male/female)	29 [15M, 14F]	18 [11M, 7F]
Age (years)	34.7 ± 10.8	37.7 ± 14.5
Age at first illness (years)	22.7 ± 6.2	24.5 ± 7.4
Duration of illness (years)	12.0 ± 9.2	13.1 ± 9.5
Current neuroleptic dose (mg CPZ)	453 ± 527	611 ± 463
Current anticholinergic exposure	15/29 [52%]	10/18 [56%]
Positive symptom score[b]	8.2 ± 2.9	9.6 ± 3.5
	(28)	(18)
Negative symptom score[b]	8.4 ± 5.0	10.2 ± 4.5
	(28)	(18)
Premorbid IQ	109.8 ± 12.4	107.3 ± 10.3
	(27)	(16)
Trail Making Test		
Form A (seconds)	64.6 ± 44.3	75.2 ± 4.6
Form B (seconds)	124.5 ± 60.1	139.7 ± 68.0
	(23)	(14)
Wisconsin Card Sorting Test		
Perseverative errors	0.27 ± 0.33	0.41 ± 0.37
Categories	3.9 ± 2.1	2.5 ± 2.0[c]
	(28)	(17)
Obstetric complication(s)	8/24 [33%]	3/12 [25%]
Family history	6/28 [21%]	4/15 [27%]
Left-handedness	7/27 [26%]	2/18 [11%]
Minor physical anomalies		
Total score	4.3 ± 3.8	4.1 ± 4.5
Head score	3.3 ± 3.0	3.5 ± 3.5
Periphery score	1.0 ± 1.1	0.6 ± 1.1
	(29)	(17)
Anomalies distribution index[d]	0.49 ± 0.44	0.85 ± 0.19[e]
	(24)	(13)
Magnetic-resonance imaging		
TVV (ml)[f]	13.9 ± 11.3	14.7 ± 7.3
LVV (ml)	7.6 ± 6.0	7.6 ± 3.9
RVV (ml)	6.7 ± 5.5	7.1 ± 3.6
Ventricular asymmetry index	0.06 ± 0.15	0.03 ± 0.15
	(28)	(17)
Cortical atrophy	5/29 [17%]	5/18 [28%]

[a]Not all measures available on each patient; numbers in parentheses below values indicate relevant group size.
[b]As mean total of *global* ratings for each subscale.
[c]$p < 0.05$ versus patients without tardive dyskinesia (Student's *t* test).
[d]Excludes patients in whom minor physical anomalies were absent.
[e]$p < 0.02$.
[f]TVV, total ventricular volume; LVV, left ventricular volume; RVV, right ventricular volume.

As for the MRI examination, patients with and without tardive dyskinesia were again indistinguishable; that is, they could not be distinguished on the basis of total, left, or right ventricular volumes, ventricular asymmetry, or cortical atrophy.

Discussion

That greater exposure to neuroleptics did not distinguish the schizophrenic patients with tardive dyskinesia from those without such movement disorder is in keeping with the majority of studies on this issue (Waddington, 1989; Chapter 9, this volume). Our failure to distinguish the dyskinetic group in terms of either positive or negative psychopathologic symptoms is also in accordance with a number of studies in similar patient populations (Waddington, 1989, 1995; Gureje, 1989; Gold et al., 1991; Perenyi, Norman, & Burrows, 1992). In fact, those studies in which a positive association with negative symptoms was reported not only generally involved older, chronically ill patients (Waddington, 1989; 1995; Manschreck et al., 1990; Brown & White, 1991a; Davis, Borde, & Sharma, 1992) but also demonstrated the primary association to be with orofacial (Waddington et al., 1987) or a limb-truncal (Brown & White, 1991a) topography of involuntary movements. There is, however, a single report of a negative association based on electro-mechanical quantification, rather than observer ratings of such movement disorder (Bartzokis et al., 1989). In relation to positive symptoms, recent studies have reported tardive dyskinesia to be associated positively with formal thought disorder (Manschreck et al., 1990; Davis et al., 1992) or negatively with total positive-symptom scores (White, Brown, & Woods, 1991). On the basis of such disparate findings and the potential confounding effects of current neuroleptic treatment, it is difficult to elaborate any explanatory model involving positive or negative symptoms, other than to note that there is perhaps an overall excess of negative symptoms in older, chronically ill patients with tardive dyskinesia (Waddington, 1995). This might suggest a delayed association, between the emergence of such a movement disorder and the presence of signs of poor outcome, that may be considerably less evident in the earlier phases of the illness.

In terms of cognitive function, patients with and without tardive dyskinesia were distinguishable using the Wisconsin Card Sorting Test, but not with Trail Making Tests A or B. That patients with this movement disorder showed greater cognitive impairment is in keeping with a now substantial (though by no means entirely consistent) body of evidence (Waddington, 1989, 1995; Waddington et al., 1993; Chapter 15, this volume). Indeed, the most recent studies have reported positive (Brown & White, 1991a) and essentially negative (Gold et al., 1991) findings. In contrast to our recent report in a less severely ill population (O'Callaghan et al., 1990), we could not, in this study, distinguish the dyskinetic patients from the nondyskinetic patients using the Trail Making Tests, although the nonsignificant trends were in the expected direction. The distinction effected using the Wisconsin Card Sorting Test, however, is consistent with a recent report by Brown, White, and Palmer (1992b), who found such a distinction to be most easily made in patients with prominent negative symptoms (Brown & White, 1991b). This finding might, in fact, indicate a particular association between tardive dyskinesia and frontal-lobe dysfunction. Nevertheless, we should not overlook the apparent association, especially in older, chronically ill inpatient populations, between tardive dyskinesia and more global cognitive dysfunction (Waddington, 1989, 1995; Waddington et al., 1993), an association that may relate primarily to involuntary movements with an orofacial (Waddington et al., 1987; De-Wolfe et al., 1988; Waddington, Youssef, & Kinsella, 1990b) or limb-truncal (Brown & White, 1991a) topography.

How should such associations be interpreted in the long term? Brown et al. (1992b) have argued that in patients with schizophrenia, tardive dyskinesia "produces" a frontal-lobe deficit in addition to that derived from the disease process of schizophrenia. The basis of this presumed direction of cause and effect, however, is unclear; it could equally be argued that patients with the greater frontal-lobe dysfunction are in some way more vulnerable to tardive dyskinesia. The organic-vulnerability hypothesis, with its long history based essentially on cross-sectional studies, predicts that indices of organicity should already be present to excess in such patients *before* they go on to develop tardive dyskinesia. Although the findings in one *prospective* neuro-psychological study of a young, mixed patient population are consistent with this notion (Wegner et al., 1985), our own prospective study, in a much older and more chronically ill patient population, showed that measures of more global cognitive function actually declined over the same time period during which tardive orofacial (but not limb-truncal) dyskinesia emerged. This would suggest that these phenomena may be distinct manifestations of a common process, with cognitive dysfunction constituting a "state marker" for tardive dyskinesia, rather than them being sequential events in a cause–effect cascade (Waddington et al., 1990b; Waddington & Youssef, in press). Current research in schizophrenia posits "core" abnormalities of structure and function in frontotemporal and corticostriatopallidothalamic networks (Waddington, 1993a), the extent of which may be associated with vulnerability to, or indeed an integral part of, the development of tardive dyskinesia. Such a process may also accommodate certain symptomatological correlates of such movement disorder, as it relates to the course of illness in schizophrenia.

In the study population reported here (Waddington et al., 1995), we were unable to fully replicate our previous findings (O'Callaghan et al., 1990) of an *underrepresentation* of obstetric complications and an *overrepresentation* of a positive family history of schizophrenia in patients with tardive dyskinesia, as compared with patients without tardive dyskinesia; in each instance, although they tended to be in the same direction, our findings reported here failed to attain statistical significance. Similar trends have recently been reported by McCreadie et al. (1992). It is curious, as well, that involuntary movements appear to be more prominent both in lithium-treated patients with major affective disorders who have a family history of dementia (though not of other mental disorders) (Axelsson & Nilsson, 1991) and in child/adolescent psychiatric patients who have been treated with neuroleptics and have a family history of psychiatric hospitalization (Richardson, Haughland, & Craig, 1991). Furthermore, we reported a positive family history of psychiatric disorder to be predictive of de novo emergence of tardive dyskinesia in a longitudinal study of older, more chronically ill inpatients with schizophrenia (Waddington et al., 1990b). The foregoing findings, together with earlier findings regarding family-history variables (Waddington, 1989), suggest the possible operation of a subtle "genetic-vulnerability" factor, the basis of which cannot yet be specified.

It has been argued that patterns of manual dominance (and, by inference, of cerebral dominance) may be associated with vulnerability to tardive dyskinesia. The data are in conflict, however, as to directionality. Because excesses of both left-handedness (McCreadie et al., 1982; Joseph, 1990) and right-handedness (Barr et al., 1989; Kern et al., 1991; Brown et al., 1992a) have been reported in (predominantly schizophrenic) patients with tardive dyskinesia, the nonsignificant trend we have found in the direction of an overrepresentation of "normal" dominance would suggest that any role for anomalous cerebral dominance is relatively minor.

We were able to detect no significant relationship between tardive dyskinesia and any of the scores for MPAs (total, head, or peripheral) and thus were unable to replicate the findings of Lohr & Flynn (1993). There was, however, a significant increase in the anomalies-distribution index in patients with tardive dyskinesia, as compared with patients without tardive dyskinesia. Although this latter exploratory analysis was of necessity confined to patients exhibiting such anomalies, it suggests that those individuals with tardive (orofacial) dyskinesia show a predominance of head anomalies, as compared with peripheral anomalies. Indeed, they may have experienced developmental disturbances that were particularly selective for regions of the head.

In the study reported here, we could not distinguish patients with and those without tardive dyskinesia on the basis of several indices of cerebral structure demonstrated by MRI: total, left, and right ventricular volumes, ventricular asymmetry index, and cortical atrophy. As for the literature reports that have examined whether or not patients with tardive dyskinesia show greater evidence of structural brain abnormalities, particularly ventricular enlargement or cortical atrophy, when examined with computed tomography or MRI, they are far from consistent. In fact, positive associations have tended to be more common among older, chronically ill inpatient populations (Waddington, 1989, 1995; Hoffman & Casey, 1991; McClelland et al., 1991), except for one report of decreased ventricular size in younger patients (Gold et al., 1991). The greater anatomic resolution afforded by MRI, however, now allows individual brain regions to be examined. Also of interest is a preliminary report of reduced caudate volume in the presence of tardive dyskinesia (Mion et al., 1991), which may indicate the way forward in addressing these issues.

Conclusion

Perhaps the principal message of the study reported here is our difficulty in distinguishing patients with and those without tardive dyskinesia when they are drawn from a nonelderly population that is diagnostically homogeneous, at least for schizophrenia, as well as from a common clinical service encompassing patients with similar courses of illness. Our patients could not be distinguished on the basis of a large number of demographic, medication, symptomatological, clinical, and neuroimaging variables.

Of the two measures that did distinguish our patients with from those without such movement disorder, the dyskinesia group's poorer performance on the Wisconsin Card Sorting Test suggests an association between involuntary movements and frontal-lobe dysfunction. This notion is in keeping with, and elaborative of, the present body of evidence indicating that neuropsychological deficits are more common in patients with tardive dyskinesia (Waddington, 1995). However, the longitudinal relationship between this movement disorder and such neuropsychological impairment over the course of schizophrenic illness, and its treatment with neuroleptics, remains to be determined. For example, it is less clear how the apparent predominance of MPAs of the head, relative to those of the periphery, in patients with tardive dyskinesia can be conceptualized in any simple manner. Indeed, in view of the large number of exploratory comparisons made, we cannot exclude a chance association. However, all of our patients with tardive dyskinesia showed involuntary movements that either included or were confined to the orofacial region. Thus, the topography of early developmental disturbances in patients with schizophrenia, for which MPAs provide an index, may in some way be associated with a topographic vulnerability to tardive dyskinesia when neuroleptics are ultimately prescribed. It may also be that the extent to which the totality of "tardive" dyskinesia can include instances of spontaneous involuntary movements as overt expressions of vulnerability, in the absence of any requirement for neuroleptic treatment, has actually been underestimated (Waddington & Crow, 1988; Waddington, 1989, 1995; Khot & Wyatt, 1991).

These data highlight the complexity of seeking simple, unitary vulnerability factors for tardive dyskinesia, at least in patients with schizophrenia. They also focus renewed attention on the interaction between neuroleptic drugs and features of the illness for which neuroleptic treatment is prescribed.

Acknowledgment

The authors' studies are supported by the Health Research Board.

References

American Psychiatric Association (1980). *Diagnostic and Statistical Manual of Mental Disorders,* 3rd ed. Washington, DC: American Psychiatric Association.

Andreasen, N. C. (1990). *Schizophrenia: Positive and Negative Symptoms and Syndromes.* Basel: Karger.

Axelsson, R., & Nilsson, A. (1991). On the pathogenesis of abnormal involuntary movements in lithium-treated patients with major affective disorder. *Eur. Arch. Psychiatry Clin. Neurosci.* 241:1–7.

Barr, W. B., Mukherjee, S., Degreef, G., & Caracci, G. (1989). Anomalous dominance and persistent tardive dyskinesia. *Biol. Psychiatry* 25:826–34.

Bartzokis, G., Hill, M. A., Altshuler, L., Cummings, J. L., Wirshing, W., & May, P. R. A. (1989). Tardive dyskinesia in schizophrenic patients: correlation with negative symptoms. *Biol. Psychiatry* 28:145–51.

Brown, K. W., & White, T. (1991a). The psychological consequences of tardive dyskinesia: the effects of drug-induced parkinsonism and the topography of the dyskinetic movements. *Br. J. Psychiatry* 159:399–403.

Brown, K. W., & White, T. (1991b). The association among negative symptoms, movement disorders, and frontal lobe psychological deficits in schizophrenic patients. *Biol. Psychiatry* 30:1182–90.

Brown, K. W., White, T., Anderson, F., & McGilp, R. (1992a). Handedness as a risk factor for neuroleptic-induced movement disorders. *Biol. Psychiatry* 31:746–8.

Brown, K. W., White, T., & Palmer, D. (1992b). Movement disorders and psychological tests of frontal lobe function in schizophrenic patients. *Psychol. Med.* 22:69–77.

Davis, E. J. B., Borde, M., & Sharma, L. N. (1992). Tardive dyskinesia and type II schizophrenia. *Br. J. Psychiatry* 160:253–6.

Davis, J. M. (1976). Comparative doses and costs of antipsychotic medication. *Arch. Gen. Psychiatry* 33:858–61.

DeWolfe, A. S., Ryan, J. J., & Wolfe, M. E. (1988). Cognitive sequelae of tardive dyskinesia. *J. Nerv. Ment. Dis.* 176:270–4.

Gold, J. M., Egan, M. F., Kirch, D. G., Goldberg, T. E., Daniel, D. E., Bigelow, L. B., & Wyatt, R. J. (1991). Tardive dyskinesia: neuropsychological, computerized tomographic and psychiatric symptom findings. *Biol. Psychiatry* 30:587–99.

Green, M. F., Satz, P., Gaier, D. J., Ganzell, S., & Kharabi, F. (1989). Minor physical anomalies in schizophrenia. *Schizophr. Bull.* 15:91–9.

Gureje, O. (1989). Correlates of positive and negative schizophrenic syndromes in Nigerian patients. *Br. J. Psychiatry* 155:628–32.

Guy, W. (1976). Abnormal involuntary movement scale. In *Early Clinical Drug Evaluation Unit Assessment Manual*, ed. W. Guy, pp. 534–7. Rockville, MD: U.S. Department of Health and Human Services.

Hoffman, W. F., & Casey, D. E. (1991). Computed tomographic evaluation of patients with tardive dyskinesia. *Schizophr. Res.* 5:1–12.

Joseph, A. B. (1990). Non-right-handedness and maleness correlate with tardive dyskinesia among patients taking neuroleptics. *Acta Psychiatr. Scand.* 81:530–3.

Kane, J. M., & Smith, J. M. (1982). Tardive dyskinesia: prevalence and risk factors, 1959–1979. *Arch. Gen. Psychiatry* 39:473–81.

Kern, R. S., Green, M. F., Satz, P., & Wirsching, W. C. (1991). Patterns of manual dominance in patients with neuroleptic-induced movement disorders. *Biol. Psychiatry* 30:483–92.

Khot, V., & Wyatt, R. J. (1991). Not all that moves is tardive dyskinesia. *Am. J. Psychiatry* 148:661–6.

Lewis, S. W. (1989). Congenital risk factors for schizophrenia. *Psychol. Med.* 19:5–13.

Lohr, J. B., & Flynn, K. (1993). Minor physical anomalies in schizophrenia and mood disorders. *Schizophr. Bull.* 19:551–6.

McClelland, H. A., Metcalfe, A. V., Kerr, T. A., Dutta, D., & Watson, P. (1991). Facial dyskinesia: a 16-year follow-up study. *Br. J. Psychiatry* 158:691–6.

McCreadie, R. G., Crone, J., Barron, E. T., & Winslow, G. S. (1982). The Nithsdale schizophrenia survey. III. Handedness and tardive dyskinesia. *Br. J. Psychiatry* 140:591–4.

McCreadie, R. G., Hall, D. J., Berry, I. J., Robertson, L. J., Ewing, J. I., & Geals, M. F. (1992). The Nithsdale schizophrenia surveys. X. Obstetric complications, family history and abnormal movements. *Br. J. Psychiatry* 161:799–805.

Manschreck, T. C., Keuthen, N. J., Schneyer, M. L., Caleda, M. T., Laughery, J., & Collins, P. (1990). Abnormal involuntary movements and chronic schizophrenic disorders. *Biol. Psychiatry* 27:150–8.

Mion, C. C., Andreasen, N. C., Arndt, S., Swayze, V. W., & Cohen, G. A. (1991). MRI abnormalities in tardive dyskinesia. *Psychiatry Res.* 40:157–66.

Murray, R. M., & Lewis, S. W. (1987). Is schizophrenia a neurodevelopmental disorder? *Br. Med. J.* 295:681–2.

Nelson, H. E. (1976). A modified card sorting test sensitive to frontal lobe deficits. *Cortex* 12:313–24.

O'Callaghan, E., Buckley, P., Redmond, O., Stack, J., Ennis, J. T., Larkin, C., & Waddington, J. L. (1992a). Abnormalities of cerebral structure in schizophrenia on magnetic resonance imaging: interpretation in relation to the neurodevelopmental hypothesis. *J. R. Soc. Med.* 85:227–31.

O'Callaghan, E., Gibson, T., Colohan, H. A., Buckley, P., Walshe, D. G., Larkin, C., & Waddington, J. L. (1992b). Risk of schizophrenia in adults born after obstetric complications and their association with early onset of illness: a controlled study. *Br. Med. J.* 305:1256–9.

O'Callaghan, E., Larkin, C., Kinsella, A., & Waddington, J. L. (1990). Obstetric complications, the putative familial–sporadic distinction and tardive dyskinesia in schizophrenia. *Br. J. Psychiatry* 157:578–84.

O'Callaghan, E., Larkin, C., Kinsella, A., & Waddington, J. L. (1991). Familial, obstetric and other clinical correlates of minor physical anomalies in schizophrenia. *Am. J. Psychiatry* 148:479–83.

Perenyi, A., Norman, T., & Burrows, G. D. (1992). Relationship of symptomatology of schizophrenia and tardive dyskinesia. *Eur. Neuropsychopharmacol.* 2:51–5.

Richardson, M. A., Haughland, G., & Craig, T. J. (1991). Neuroleptic use, parkinsonian symptoms, tardive dyskinesia, and associated factors in child and adolescent psychiatric patients. *Am. J. Psychiatry* 148:1322–8.

Schooler, N. R., & Kane, J. M. (1982). Research diagnoses for tardive dyskinesia. *Arch. Gen. Psychiatry* 39:486–7.

Waddington, J. L. (1989). Schizophrenia, affective psychoses and other disorders treated with neuroleptic drugs: the enigma of tardive dyskinesia, its neurobiological determinants, and the conflict of paradigms. *Int. Rev. Neurobiol.* 31:297–353.

Waddington, J. L. (1993a). The neurodynamics of abnormalities in cerebral metabolism and structure in schizophrenia. *Schizophr. Bull.* 19:55–69.

Waddington, J. L. (1993b). Schizophrenia: developmental neuroscience and pathobiology. *Lancet* 341:531–6.

Waddington, J. L. (1995). Psychopathological and cognitive correlates of tardive dyskinesia in schizophrenia and other disorders treated with neuroleptic drugs. In *Behavioral Neurology of Movement Disorders,* ed. W. J. Weiner & A. E. Lang, pp. 211–29. New York: Raven Press.

Waddington, J. L., & Crow, T. J. (1988). Abnormal involuntary movements and psychosis in the preneuroleptic era and in unmedicated patients: implications for the concept of tardive dyskinesia. In *Tardive Dyskinesia: Biological Mechanisms and Clinical Aspects,* ed. M. E. Wolf & A. D. Mosnaim, pp. 51–66. Washington, DC: American Psychiatric Press.

Waddington, J. L., O'Callaghan, E., Buckley, P., Madigan, C., Redmond, O., Stack, J. P., Kinsella, A., Larkin, C., & Ennis, J. T. (1995). Tardive dyskinesia in schizophrenia: relationship to minor physical anomalies, frontal lobe dysfunction and cerebral structure on magnetic resonance imaging. *Br. J. Psychiatry* 167:41–4.

Waddington, J. L., O'Callaghan, E., Larkin, C., & Kinsella, A. (1993). Cognitive dysfunction in schizophrenia: organic vulnerability factor or state marker for tardive dyskinesia? *Brain Cogn.* 23:56–70.

Waddington, J. L., O'Callaghan, E., Larkin, C., Redmond, O., Stack, J., & Ennis, J. T. (1990a). Magnetic resonance imaging and spectroscopy in schizophrenia. *Br. J. Psychiatry (Suppl. 9)* 157:56–65.

Waddington, J. L., & Youssef, H. A. (in press). Cognitive dysfunction in chronic schizophrenia followed prospectively over 10 years, and its longitudinal relationship to the emergence of tardive dyskinesia. *Psychol. Med.* (in press).

Waddington, J. L., Youssef, H. A., Dolphin, C., & Kinsella, A. (1987). Cognitive dysfunction, negative symptoms and tardive dyskinesia in schizophrenia: their association in relation to topography of involuntary movements and criterion of their abnormality. *Arch. Gen. Psychiatry* 44:907–12.

Waddington, J. L., Youssef, H. A., & Kinsella, A. (1990b). Cognitive dysfunction in schizophrenia followed up over 5 years, and its longitudinal relationship to the emergence of tardive dyskinesia. *Psychol. Med.* 20:835–42.

Wegner, J. T., Kane, J. M., Weinhold, P., Woerner, M., Kinon, B., & Lieberman, J. (1985). Cognitive impairment in tardive dyskinesia. *Psychiatry Res.* 16:331–7.

Weinberger, D. R. (1987). Implications of normal brain development for the pathogenesis of schizophrenia. *Arch. Gen. Psychiatry* 44:660–9.

White, T., Brown, K. W., & Woods, J. P. (1991). Tardive dyskinesia and positive symptoms of schizophrenia. *Acta Psychiatr. Scand.* 83:377–9.

6

Tardive Dyskinesia and Affective Disorder

GEORGE GARDOS, M.D.,
and JONATHAN O. COLE, M.D.

Neuroleptic antipsychotic drugs are used in the treatment of a variety of psychiatric conditions, including affective disorder. This chapter concerns the association between tardive dyskinesia and affective disorder, inasmuch as affective illness has been established as a risk factor in the development of tardive dyskinesia (Gardos & Casey, 1984; Casey, 1988). The evidence for this association will be reviewed, and possible mechanisms will be considered. Because the somatic treatments used for bipolar and unipolar patients may influence the development and manifestations of tardive dyskinesia, we shall briefly review the effects on tardive dyskinesia of antidepressants, electroconvulsive treatment (ECT), lithium carbonate, and anticonvulsants.

Epidemiology

The earliest relevant studies grew out of clinical observations that some tardive dyskinesia patients were experiencing concurrent depression or had been depressed in the past (Rosenbaum et al., 1977). Other studies suggested that many patients with tardive dyskinesia had been improperly diagnosed as schizophrenic and that the more appropriate psychiatric diagnosis would have been affective disorder (Davis, Berger, & Hollister, 1976; Rush, Diamond, & Alpert, 1982; Casey & Toenniessen, 1983). Several studies compared tardive dyskinesia patients with non-dyskinetic control subjects and found affective disorder to be more common in the tardive dyskinesia groups (Hamra et al., 1983b; Alpert & Rush, 1984; Wolf et al., 1985). In a recent study, Yassa et al. (1992) showed that major depression among tardive dyskinesia patients was significantly more frequent (12 of 20, or 60%) than was primary degenerative dementia (42 of 49, or 24.5%) among a cohort of psychogeriatric inpatients. In all of the studies cited earlier, the rate of tardive dyskinesia among patients with affective disorder exceeded the rate among non-affective-

69

disorder (usually schizophrenic) patients, as well as the 15–20% base rate for the prevalence of tardive dyskinesia reported in the relevant literature (Casey, 1987). Nasrallah, Churchill, and Hamdan-Allan (1988) found that a significantly higher proportion of manic patients (26.1%) than of schizophrenic patients (5.9%) developed acute dystonia, which they interpreted as supporting a greater vulnerability of affective-disorder patients to acute extrapyramidal symptoms (EPS), as well as to tardive dyskinesia. Glazer et al. (1988) found a statistically significant association between orofacial dyskinesia and schizoaffective and affective disorders in 228 outpatients with tardive dyskinesia. Our group of investigators (Cole et al., 1992), using the Structured Clinical Interview for DSM-III-R Diagnosis (SCID-P) to arrive at psychiatric diagnoses for 100 patients with recently developed dyskinesia, found that both unipolar and bipolar patients were more vulnerable to tardive dyskinesia (in terms of both developing dyskinesia after shorter durations of neuroleptic treatment and needing lesser total amounts of neuroleptics) than were schizophrenic and schizoaffective patients. However, no difference in the incidence of tardive dyskinesia between affective-disorder patients and schizophrenics has been seen in the early data (11–13 months) from an ongoing prospective longitudinal study in Japan (Inada & Yagi, 1992).

Slightly different methods were employed in a few studies involving only patients with affective disorder. With 58 outpatients and 25 inpatients, Yassa, Ghadirian, and Schwartz (1983) found a prevalence rate of 41% (35 of 83) for tardive dyskinesia in a clinic for affective disorder, using as their criterion at least one "mild" score (2) on the Abnormal Involuntary Movement Scale (AIMS) (Guy, 1976). The diagnoses, based on the *Diagnostic and Statistical Manual of Mental Disorders,* third edition (DSM-III), yielded 69 bipolar patients and 14 patients who had "schizophrenia with a superimposed atypical affective disorder." Mukherjee et al. (1986) reported a 35.4% prevalence of persistent tardive dyskinesia among 131 bipolar outpatients. Longer durations of maintenance neuroleptic treatment and shorter durations of previous lithium carbonate treatment characterized the tardive dyskinesia patients, as compared with the bipolar patients without persistent tardive dyskinesia. No instance of persistent tardive dyskinesia was noted in the subgroup of 35 bipolar patients without neuroleptic exposure. A slightly higher tardive dyskinesia prevalence rate was reported by Parepally et al. (1989), who found that 22 (44%) of 50 bipolar inpatients satisfied the research criteria for tardive dyskinesia, a rate not significantly different from the 43% rate for tardive dyskinesia found in their schizophrenic patients.

The most compelling evidence for affective disorder as a risk factor for tardive dyskinesia comes from a prospective longitudinal study of tardive dyskinesia development in a large cohort (Kane et al., 1984). In that study, preliminary analysis of 5-year dyskinesia rates showed 23.3% for schizophrenics, 26.9% for schizoaffectives, and 37.9% for patients with affective disorder (including both unipolar and bipolar patients). The relationship between affective illness and tardive dyskinesia remains statistically significant even after controlling for other risk factors such as age, gender, lithium treatment, and ECT (M. Woerner, personal communication, 1992).

Unipolar versus Bipolar Depression

Although the foregoing data are impressive regarding the overall impact of affective illness on the development of tardive dyskinesia, the relative risks for tardive dyskinesia among bipolar versus unipolar patients or among affective versus schizoaffective patients remain unclear. Several studies, for example, have noted an association between tardive dyskinesia and depression (Davis et al., 1976; Rosenbaum et al., 1977; Rush et al., 1982), whereas Mukherjee et al. (1986) found no cases of persistent tardive dyskinesia among their patients with unipolar mania. In a recently completed study of the course of dyskinesia (Cole et al., 1992) in which unipolar patients showed vulnerability comparable to that for bipolar patients, both sets of patients developed tardive dyskinesia after significantly shorter neuroleptic exposures than did schizophrenic patients or schizoaffective patients (Table 6.1).

Observations of mood-dependent dyskinesia have suggested that the state of depression may induce and/or aggravate dyskinesia. Indeed, patients who tend to be rapid-cycling bipolars, responding poorly to conventional pharmacotherapy, have shown increased dyskinesia during depression and decreased dyskinesia during mania (Cutler et al., 1981; Cutler & Post, 1982;

Table 6.1. *Months of antipsychotic treatment prior to dyskinesia onset*

Diagnosis	Mean	SD	n
Schizophrenia	70.1[a]	±70.6	77
Schizoaffective	78.1	±68.7	57
Bipolar	33.1	±33.0	30
Unipolar	38.0	±61.2	40

[a]$F = 4.29$, $p = .0023$.

Applebaum, 1982; Weiner & Werner, 1982; DePotter, Linkowski, & Mendlewicz, 1983; Linnoila et al., 1983). The validity of those observations notwithstanding, mood-dependent dyskinesia has not been observed in the vast majority of bipolar patients (Casey, 1988).

In summary, the evidence to date has not conclusively demonstrated increased vulnerability to tardive dyskinesia among unipolar patients as compared with bipolar patients as had been suggested by some of the research data.

Possible Mechanisms

Because neither the pathogenesis of tardive dyskinesia nor that of affective disorder has been clearly established, it is no surprise that explanations of their association remain speculative. Perhaps decreased aminergic activity – whether the indoleamine serotonin or the catecholamines norepinephrine and dopamine – is the fundamental neurotransmitter abnormality in patients with depression (Casey, 1984). Such decreased neurotransmitter activity could lead to "chemical denervation" and consequent supersensitivity. Similarly, neuroleptic treatment could lead to a state of chemical denervation by antagonizing the relevant neurotransmitters and producing receptor supersensitivity. This oversimplified hypothesis is compatible with the notion that depression increases the risk for tardive dyskinesia. Manic states, however, as well as antidepressant drugs, are believed to involve opposite changes, that is, increased activities of norepinephrine, serotonin, and dopamine, which could in turn induce subsensitivity of receptors. Patients with affective disorder have been shown to have increased noradrenergic activity, as reflected by low platelet concentrations of monoamine oxidase (MAO) and higher serum concentrations of dopamine β-hydroxylase (DBH) (Jeste et al., 1981). Evidence to implicate defective serotonergic functions in patients with tardive dyskinesia (Sandyk & Fisher, 1988), as well as in those with affective disorder, has been accumulating. Recent data suggest that abnormalities of phenylalanine metabolism may affect the development of tardive dyskinesia (Richardson, 1990; Rosenberg et al., 1992). However, these biochemical abnormalities will need confirmation before they can be advanced as common pathogenetic links between tardive dyskinesia and affective disorder. Also, simplistic explanations probably should be abandoned, inasmuch as neuroleptics and antidepressants, for instance, are often administered simultaneously, and depressive and manic symptoms may coexist or change in rapid succession. It will be of interest to consider the effects of the usual somatic treatments for affective disorder on patients with tardive dyskinesia.

Antidepressants

In a review of the literature on dyskinesia associated with antidepressants, Yassa, Camille, and Belzile (1987) found 24 cases, 15 of which involved patients more than 60 years old. Amoxapine was implicated in 6 patients, amitriptyline in 7, imipramine in 3, doxepin in 2, tranylcypromine in 2, nomifensine in 2, and clomipramine and trazodone in 1 each. The dyskinesia usually developed within 2 months of initiation of antidepressant treatment and tended to disappear once the drug was reduced or discontinued. The prevalence of persistent dyskinesia was extremely low, especially given the large number of antidepressant-exposed patients. The same authors (Yassa et al., 1992) studied 50 psychogeriatric patients on antidepressants and found 3 new cases of dyskinesia (for a prevalence of 6%): 2 patients with buccolingual tardive dyskinesia, and a third patient with dyskinesia of the limbs and trunk. In 2 of the 3 patients, the dyskinetic manifestations decreased after withdrawal of an antidepressant drug. In our recently completed study of early dyskinesia, the number of months on antidepressants correlated negatively ($r = .26$, $p < .01$) with the total amount of neuroleptic administered before development of tardive dyskinesia, suggesting that antidepressants enhanced the vulnerability to tardive dyskinesia (Cole et al., 1992). Although the pathophysiology of these antidepressant-induced dyskinesias is not understood, their largely reversible courses suggest similarities to withdrawal dyskinesias, and they may have been associated with functional overactivity of biogenic amines (dopamine, norepinephrine, and/or serotonin). In addition, therapeutic effects of tricyclic antidepressants in combination with lithium have been reported by Rosenbaum (1984) for patients with treatment-resistant depression and tardive dyskinesia. Also, antidepressants have been employed for indications other than affective disorder. For example, occasional patients with tics related to Tourette's syndrome and myoclonus have improved when given antidepressants (Riley, 1992).

Lithium and Tardive Dyskinesia

Because of the growing evidence that affective disorder is a risk factor in the development of tardive dyskinesia, and because neuroleptics remain the primary causes of tardive dyskinesia, or at the very least the main precipitating factors, it stands to reason that a great deal of attention has been focused on the use of lithium carbonate both to prevent and to treat tardive dyskinesia.

That focused effort was prompted by case reports in the early 1970s that described the effects of lithium on movement disorders. First, Dalen (1973) described a 65-year-old woman with severe tardive dyskinesia who responded very well "as soon as adequate blood level of lithium was reached." He also reported striking reductions in hyperkinetic movements in 3 of 6 patients with Huntington's chorea who were treated with lithium (0.7–1.5 mEq/L). Then Simpson (1973) reported disappearance of tardive dyskinesia when 3 manic patients were switched from neuroleptics to lithium treatment. Improvement was seen in nonmanic patients with tardive dyskinesia as well, once they were switched to lithium. Prange et al. (1973) and Pickar and Davis (1978) also reported positive results from lithium treatment in tardive dyskinesia patients.

Lithium has been tried for neurological conditions as well. Aminoff and Marshall (1974), in a study of 9 patients with Huntington's chorea, found lithium (0.6–1.5 mEq/L) to be ineffective. Leonard et al. (1974) reported only negative findings in a double-blind study of lithium for treatment of Huntington's chorea. Hamra, Dunner, and Larson (1983a) described a patient with cyclothymia whose chronic tics, when treated with lithium, gradually disappeared over 2 months. Although improvement has been reported in individual cases of spasmodic torticollis or segmental dystonia, Riley (1992) concluded that only a minority of patients with various types of dystonia treated with lithium have actually benefited.

Systematic studies of the effects of lithium in patients with tardive dyskinesia began to be reported in the mid-1970s. Reda, Escobar, and Scanlen (1975) reported an open trial of lithium in 6 tardive dyskinesia patients, with alternating 2-week lithium/no-lithium periods added to previous medications. At lithium concentrations of 0.7–1.0 mEq/L, they found a statistically significant improvement, but only in the 15–20% range. In a double-blind trial in which Gerlach, Thorsen, and Munkvad (1975) compared lithium treatment with placebo in 15 tardive dyskinesia patients, dyskinesia was found to have diminished by an average of 25% after lithium treatment, with the best responses occurring at a serum concentration of 0.8 mEq/L. At higher concentrations, there were lesser degrees of improvement. Jus, Villeneuve, and Gautier (1978), in a double-blind crossover study comparing deanol, lithium, and placebo in patients with chronic schizophrenia and tardive dyskinesia, low lithium doses yielding serum concentrations between 0.7 and 0.9 mEq/L were employed. For the 5 patients who showed improvement (2 became worse), the decreases in dyskinetic manifestations persisted for 1–2 months after discontinuation of lithium. However, Simpson, Branchey, and Lee (1976), who carried out a double-blind crossover study in which lithium (0.6–1.0 mEq/L) or a placebo was given to 16 patients following neuroleptic withdrawal, found no significant improvement regarding dyskinetic movements in the 10 patients who completed the 6-week drug trial. Mackay et al.

(1980) also came up with negative results in a placebo-controlled double-blind study of 11 neuroleptic-maintained tardive dyskinesia patients. They found no consistent changes in tardive dyskinesia or psychiatric states associated with lithium treatment (0.8–1.3 mEq/L).

A few patients have shown worsening of their dyskinetic movements when given lithium. Beitman (1978) described a 56-year-old woman whose tardive dyskinesia was reinduced by lithium and suppressed by trihexyphenidyl, suggesting a pharmacologically atypical dyskinesia. Other cases of lithium-induced tardive dyskinesia have been associated with toxic serum concentrations of the drug (Cohen and Cohen, 1974; Crews & Carpenter, 1977; Prakash, Keluvla, & Ban, 1982; Reed, Wise, & Timmerman, 1989). Sternbach and Jordan (1990) reported on a 63-year-old woman with bipolar disorder without neuroleptic exposure who developed oral dyskinesia, as well as gastrointestinal complaints and confusion, at serum lithium concentrations of 0.9–1.0 mEq/L. Those problems lasted for 2 years, but subsequently remitted when her dosage was reduced to 600 g/d (serum concentration 0.57 mEq/L). Severe abnormal involuntary movements in women more than 50 years of age have been associated with high, 12-hour lithium concentrations in a longitudinal study of lithium treatment for major affective disorder (Axelsson & Nilsson, 1991). In our own double-blind 8-week study of lithium versus placebo added to the usual antipsychotics in 18 schizophrenics with tardive dyskinesia, we found statistically significant differences favoring lithium on AIMS score for face, lips, jaw, and tongue and on the choreoathetosis cluster of the Simpson dyskinesia scale (Cole et al., 1984). An extension of that study involving neuroleptic withdrawal, to test the feasibility of maintaining patients on lithium alone, was deemed a failure in all but 2 lithium patients (the majority of patients relapsed or dropped out of the study). Meanwhile, the early lithium-related improvements regarding dyskinetic manifestations dissipated as well. The previously described heterogeneous group of studies suggest (1) that occasional tardive dyskinesia patients may show improvement on lithium whether or not antipsychotics are administered concurrently and (2) that toxic serum concentrations can precipitate dyskinesia, with the lower (<0.8 mEq/L) lithium concentrations possibly being more likely to reduce tardive dyskinesia than the higher (>0.8 mEq/L) concentrations.

The absence of clear therapeutic effects still leaves open the question whether or not lithium carbonate can actually prevent the development of tardive dyskinesia. Evidence that lithium blocks neuroleptic-induced proliferation of dopamine receptors (Klawans, Weiner, & Nausieda, 1977; Pert et al., 1978; Gallagher, Pert, & Bunney, 1978; Goodnick & Meltzer, 1983) might suggest that in neuroleptic-treated patients, lithium not only could prevent the development of dopamine supersensitivity but also might delay or prevent the onset of tardive dyskinesia. However, our data from a recently completed study of the course of early dyskinesia did not support that hypothesis (Cole et al., 1992): Our patients who received lithium showed a weak trend toward developing dyskinesia more readily. As for Kane and associates' longitudinal study of the development of tardive dyskinesia, the incidence of tardive dyskinesia was lower among patients with affective disorder who had a history of lithium exposure than the incidence among those without lithium treatment (Kane, Woerner, & Borenstein, 1986); among non-affective-disorder patients, however, no relationship between tardive dyskinesia and lithium use was found (M. Woerner, personal communication, 1992).

Carbamazepine and Valproic Acid

The two anticonvulsants carbamazepine and valproic acid have become established as effective alternatives to lithium carbonate treatment for patients with bipolar disorder. Thus, many bipolar patients at risk of developing tardive dyskinesia because of neuroleptic exposure may already have been treated with carbamazepine or valproic acid.

Because carbamazepine is structurally related to the phenothiazines, it can be expected to produce extrapyramidal symptoms. However, carbamazepine does not have a biochemical profile typical of neuroleptics and does not exert its antimanic effects by blocking dopamine receptors (Post et al., 1986). Several reports have implicated carbamazepine in cases of chorea or choreoathetoid dyskinesia (Jacome, 1979; Joyce & Gunverson, 1980; Bimpong-Buta & Froescher, 1982; Schwartzman & Leppik, 1990). Such dyskinesia, which usually appears after chronic treatment, tends to resolve with decreasing carbamazepine concentrations (Lang, 1992). Carbamazepine has also been reported to cause tics in occasional patients, both children (Neglia, Glazer, & Zion, 1984) and adults (Kurlan et al., 1989). Also, a single case of carbamazepine-induced akathisia has been reported (Schwarcz et al., 1986). Cutler and Post (1982) described a mood-dependent dyskinesia in a rapid-cycling bipolar patient who experienced substantial improvement during carbamazepine treatment. Carbamazepine induces hepatic microsomal enzymes and therefore may decrease the blood concentrations and efficacies of compounds used in the treatment of bipolar disorders, such as clonazepam and neuroleptics (Post & Uhde, 1986). For example, carbamazepine has been reported to decrease the concentrations of haloperidol by 40–60% (Post & Uhde, 1986).

Valproate is finding increasing acceptance in the treatment of bipolar disorder, alone or in combination with lithium, and, less frequently, with carbamazepine. However, some 20–25% of patients on chronic valproate treatment develop tremors (Karas et al., 1982). The tremors, which usually begin 3–14 months after initiation of treatment, are most commonly seen in the arms. In general, they will be of the postural or action type, although occasional resting tremors or involvement of the head, neck, or trunk may occur (Karas et al., 1982). Valproate tremors typically occur when patients are at therapeutic blood concentrations and are at dosages of more than 750 mg daily (Lang, 1992). Reductions of the valproate dosages or treatment with propranolol usually have improved such tremors (Karas et al., 1982). The pharmacologic mechanism underlying valproate-induced tremor is unknown, however. Recently, a syndrome of valproate-induced parkinsonism–dementia was reported (Armon et al., 1991); it is awaiting confirmation. Thus far, no clear effects on tardive dyskinesia have been demonstrated.

Electroconvulsive Treatment

There is conflicting information concerning the nature of the effect of ECT on tardive dyskinesia. According to one report, ECT exacerbated tardive dyskinesia in a patient with parkinsonism and depression (Holcomb, Sternberg, & Heninger, 1983). Other depressed patients with tardive dyskinesia, however, have shown improvement with ECT (Rosenbaum et al., 1980; Chacko & Root, 1983; Gosek & Weller, 1988; Webb, 1988). Epidemiologic studies have yielded conflicting results as well, with some studies showing weak positive associations between ECT and the presence or severity of dyskinesia (Jeste & Wyatt, 1982). Simpson et al. (1978), on the other hand, found that patients without tardive dyskinesia were more likely to have been given ECT than were patients with tardive dyskinesia. We have recently reported that patients who have been exposed to ECT seem to be less vulnerable to the development of dyskinesia (Cole et al., 1992).

Conclusion

Our review of the association between tardive dyskinesia and affective disorder, and the effects of its somatic treatments, has yielded several points. Affective disorder is now established as a risk factor for development of tardive dyskinesia. Unipolar depressed patients may be more vulnerable to tardive dyskinesia than are bipolar patients. Antidepressants sometimes induce dyskinesia, which tends to be reversible. Lithium treatment occasionally leads to a decrease in the severity of the dyskinesia, although in a few patients, high or toxic lithium concentrations can induce or aggravate dyskinesia. Attempts to substitute lithium for neuroleptics in treating patients with affective disorder have been disappointing. Carbamazepine will induce choreiform dyskinesia in a few bipolar patients. Finally, valproic acid tends to be associated with tremors.

References

Alpert, M., & Rush, M. (1984). Early depressive signs in patients with tardive dyskinesia. In *Tardive Dyskinesia and Affective Disorders,* ed. G. Gardos & D. E. Casey, pp. 29–36. Washington, DC: American Psychiatric Press.

Aminoff, M. J., & Marshall, J. (1974). Treatment of Huntington's chorea with lithium carbonate. *Lancet* 1:107–9.

Applebaum, P. S. (1982). Dyskinesia and unipolar depression. *Am. J. Psychiatry* 139:140–1.

Armon, C., Miller, P., Carwile, S., Brown, E., Edinger, J. D., Paul, R. G., & Shin, C. (1991). Valproate-induced parkinsonism–dementia syndrome: clinical features. *Mov. Disord.* 6:269.

Axelsson, R., & Nilsson, A. (1991). On the pathogenesis of abnormal involuntary movements in lithium-treated patients with major affective disorder. *Eur. Arch. Psychiatry Clin. Neurosci.* 24:1–7.

Beitman, B. D. (1978). Tardive dyskinesia reinduced by lithium carbonate. *Am. J. Psychiatry* 135:1229–30.

Bimpong-Buta, K., & Froescher, W. (1982). Carbamazepine-induced choreoathetotic dyskinesias. *J. Neurol. Neurosurg. Psychiatry* 45:560–7.

Casey, D. E. (1984). Tardive dyskinesia and affective disorders. In *Tardive Dyskinesia and Affective Disorders,* ed. G. Gardos & D. E. Casey, pp. 1–20. Washington, DC: American Psychiatric Press.

Casey, D. E. (1987). Tardive dyskinesia. In *Psychopharmacology. The Third Generation of Progress,* ed. H. Y. Meltzer, pp. 1411–19. New York: Raven Press.

Casey, D. E. (1988). Affective disorders and tardive dyskinesia. *Encephale* 14:221–6.

Casey, D. E., & Toenniessen, L. M. (1983). Neuroleptic treatment in tardive dyskinesia: Can it be developed into a clinical strategy for long-term treatment? In *New Directions in Tardive Dyskinesia Research,* ed. J. Bannet & R. H. Belmaker, pp. 65–79. Basel: S. Karger.

Chacko, R. C., & Root, L. (1983). ECT and tardive dyskinesia: two cases and a review. *J. Clin. Psychiatry* 44:265–6.

Cohen, W. J., & Cohen, N. H. (1974). Lithium carbonate, haloperidol and irreversible brain damage. *JAMA* 230:1283–7.

Cole, J. O., Gardos, G., Boling, L. A., Marby, D., Haskell, D., & Moore, P. (1992). Early dyskinesia – vulnerability. *Psychopharmacology* 107:503–10.

Cole, J. O., Gardos, G., Rapkin, R. M., Gelernter, J., Haskell, D., Moore, P., Schniebolk, S., & Bird, M. (1984). Lithium carbonate in tardive dyskinesia and schizophrenia. In *Tardive Dyskinesia and Affective Disorders,* ed. G. Gardos & D. E. Casey, pp. 49–73. Washington, DC: American Psychiatric Press.

Crews, E. L., & Carpenter, A. E. (1977). Lithium-induced aggravation of tardive dyskinesia. *Am. J. Psychiatry* 134:933.

Cutler, N. R., & Post, R. M. (1982). State-related cyclical dyskinesias in manic–depressive illness. *J. Clin. Psychopharmacol.* 2:350–4.

Cutler, N. R., Post, R. M., Rey, A., & Bunney, W. E., Jr. (1981). Depression-dependent dyskinesias in two cases of manic–depressive illness. *New Engl. J. Med.* 304:1088–9.

Dalen, P. (1973). Lithium therapy in Huntington's chorea and tardive dyskinesia. *Lancet* 1:107–8.

Davis, K. L., Berger, P. A., & Hollister, L. E. (1976). Tardive dyskinesia and depressive illness. *Psychopharmacol. Com.* 2:125–30.

DePotter, R. W., Linkowski, P., & Mendlewicz, J. (1983). State-dependent tardive dyskinesia in manic–depressive illness. *J. Neurol. Neurosurg. Psychiatry* 46:666–8.

Gallagher, D. W., Pert, A., & Bunney, W. E. (1978). Haloperidol-induced presynaptic dopamine supersensitivity is blocked by chronic lithium. *Nature* 273:309–12.

Gardos, G., & Casey, D. E. (eds.) (1984). *Tardive Dyskinesia and Affective Disorders*. Washington, DC: American Psychiatric Press.

Gerlach, J., Thorsen, K., & Munkvad, I. (1975). Effect of lithium on neuroleptic-induced tardive dyskinesia compared with placebo in a double-blind crossover trial. *Pharmakopsychiatr. Neuropsychopharmakol.* 8:51–6.

Glazer, W. M., Morgenstern, H., Niedzwieckie, D., & Hughes, J. (1988). Heterogeneity of tardive dyskinesia. *Br. J. Psychiatry* 152:253–9.

Goodnick, P. J., & Meltzer, H. Y. (1983). Effect of subchronic lithium treatment on apomorphine-induced change in prolactin and growth hormone secretion. *J. Clin. Psychopharmacol.* 3:239–43.

Gosek, E., & Weller, R. E. (1988). Improvement of tardive dyskinesia associated with electroconvulsive therapy. *J. Nerv. Ment. Dis.* 176:120–2.

Guy, W. (ed). (1976). *ECDEU Assessment Manual for Psychopharmacology*, pp. 534–7. Washington, DC: U.S. Department of Health, Education, and Welfare.

Hamra, B. J., Dunner, F., & Larson, C. (1983a). Remission of tics with lithium therapy. *J. Clin. Psychiatry* 44:73–4.

Hamra, B. J., Nasrallah, H. A., Clancy, J., & Finn, R. (1983b). Psychiatric diagnosis and risk for tardive dyskinesia. *Arch. Gen. Psychiatry* 40:346–7.

Holcomb, H. H., Sternberg, D. E., & Heninger, G. (1983). Efficacy of electroconvulsive therapy on mood, parkinsonism and tardive dyskinesia in a depressed patient: ECT and dopamine system. *Biol. Psychiatry* 18:865–73.

Inada, T., & Yagi, G. (1992). Incidence of tardive dyskinesia in affective disorder patients. *J. Clin. Psychopharmacol.* 12:301–2.

Jacome, D. (1979). Carbamazepine-induced dystonia. *JAMA* 241:2263.

Jeste, D. V., Delisi, L. E., Zalcman, S., Wise, D. C., Phelps, B. H., Rosenblatt, J. E., Potkin, S. G., Bridge, T. P., & Wyatt, R. J. (1981). A biochemical study of tardive dyskinesia in young male patients. *Psychiatry Res.* 4:327–31.

Jeste, D. V., & Wyatt, R. J. (1982). *Understanding and Treating Tardive Dyskinesia*. New York: Guilford Press.

Joyce, R. P., & Gunverson, C. H. (1980). Carbamazepine-induced orofacial dyskinesia. *Neurology* 30:1333–4.

Jus, A., Villeneuve, A., & Gautier, J. (1978). Deanol, lithium and placebo in the treatment of tardive dyskinesia. *Neuropsychobiology* 4:140–9.

Kane, J. M., Woerner, M., & Borenstein, M. (1986). Integrating incidence and prevalence of tardive dyskinesia. *Psychopharmacol. Bull.* 22:254–8.

Kane, J. M., Woerner, M., Weinhold, P., Kinon, B., Lieberman, J., & Borenstein, M. (1984). Incidence and severity of tardive dyskinesia in affective illness. In *Tardive Dyskinesia and Affective Disorders,* ed. G. Gardos & D. E. Casey, pp. 21–8. Washington, DC: American Psychiatric Press.

Karas, B. J., Widder, B. J., Hammond, E. J., & Bauman, A. W. (1982). Valproate tremors. *Neurology* 32:1380–2.

Klawans, H. L., Weiner, W. J., & Nausieda, P. A. (1977). The effect of lithium on animal models of tardive dyskinesia. *Prog. Neuropsychopharmacol.* 1:53–60.

Kurlan, R., Kersun, J., Behr, J., Leborici, A., Tarid, P., Lichter, D., & Shoulson, I. (1989). Carbamazepine-induced tics. *Clin. Neuropharmacol.* 12:298–302.

Lang, A. E. (1992). Miscellaneous drug-induced movement disorders. In *Drug-induced Movement Disorders,* ed. A. E. Lang & W. J. Weiner, pp. 339–81. Mount Kisko, NY : Futura Publishing.

Leonard, D. P., Kidson, M. A., Shannon, P. J., & Brown, J. (1974). Double-blind trial of lithium carbonate and haloperidol in Huntington's chorea. *Lancet* 2:1208–9.

Linnoila, M., Karoum, F., Cutler, N. R., & Potter, W. Z. (1983). Temporal association between depression-dependent dyskinesias and high urinary phenylethylamine output. *Biol. Psychiatry* 18:513–16.

Mackay, A., Sheppard, G. P., Saha, B. K., Motley, B., Johnson, A. L., & Marsden, C. D. (1980). Failure of lithium treatment in established tardive dyskinesia. *Psychol. Med.* 10:583–7.

Mukherjee, S., Rosen, A. M., Caracci, G., & Shukla, S. (1986). Persistent tardive dyskinesia in bipolar patients. *Arch. Gen. Psychiatry* 43:342–6.

Nasrallah, H. A., Churchill, C. M., & Hamdan-Allan, G. A. (1988). Higher frequency of neuroleptic-induced dystonia in mania than in schizophrenia. *Am. J. Psychiatry* 145:1455–5.

Neglia, J. P., Glazer, D. G., & Zion, T. E. (1984). Tics and vocalizations in children treated with carbamazepine. *Pediatrics* 73:841–4.

Parepally, H., Mukherjee, S., Schnur, B. B., & Caracci, G. (1989). Tardive dyskinesia in bipolar patients. *Biol. Psychiatry* 25:163A.

Pert, A., Rosenblatt, J. E., Sivit, C., Pert, C. B., & Bunney, W. E., Jr. (1978). Long-term treatment with lithium prevents the development of dopamine receptor supersensitivity. *Science* 201:171–3.

Pickar, D., & Davis, R. K. (1978). Tardive dyskinesia in younger patients. *Am. J. Psychiatry* 135:385–6.

Post, R. M., Rubinow, D. R., Uhde, T. W., Ballenger, J. C., & Linnoila, M. (1986). Dopaminergic effects of carbamazepine: relationship to clinical response and affective illness. *Arch. Gen. Psychiatry* 43:392–6.

Post, R. M., & Uhde, T. W. (1986). Anticonvulsants in nonepileptic psychosis. In *Epilepsy in Psychiatry,* ed. T. G. Bolurg & M. R. Trimble, pp. 177–212. New York: Wiley.

Prakash, R., Keluvla, S., & Ban, T. A. (1982). Neurotoxicity in patients with schizophrenia during lithium therapy. *Compr. Psychiatry* 23:271–3.

Prange, A. J., Wilson, I. C., Morris, C. E., & Hall, C. D. (1973). Preliminary experience with tryptophan and lithium in the treatment of tardive dyskinesia. *Psychopharmacol. Bull.* 9:36–7.

Reda, F. A., Escobar, I. L., & Scanlen, J. M. (1975). Lithium carbonate in the treatment of tardive dyskinesia. *Am. J. Psychiatry* 132:560–2.

Reed, S. M., Wise, M. G., & Timmerman, I. (1989). Choreoathetosis: a sign of lithium toxicity. *J. Neuropsychiatry* 1:57–60.

Richardson, M. A. (1990). *Amino Acids in Psychiatric Disease.* Progress in Psychiatry series no. 22. Washington, DC: American Psychiatric Press.

Riley, D. E. (1992). Antidepressant therapy and movement disorders. In *Drug-induced Movement Disorders,* ed. A. E. Lang & W. J. Weiner, pp. 231–56. Mount Kisco, NY: Futura Publishing.

Rosenbaum, A. (1984). Biological markers and treatment of affective disorder patients with tardive dyskinesia. In *Tardive Dyskinesia and Affective Disorders,* ed. G. Gardos & D. E. Casey, pp. 37–48. Washington, DC: American Psychiatric Press.

Rosenbaum, A. H., Niven, R. G., Hanson, N. P., & Swanson, D. W. (1977). Tardive dyskinesia: relationship with a primary affective disorder. *Dis. Nerv. Syst.* 38:423–7.

Rosenbaum, A. H., O'Connor, M. K., Duane, D. D., & Auger, R. G. (1980). Treatment of tardive dyskinesia in an agitated, depressed patient. *Psychosomatics* 21:765–6.

Rosenberg, P. B., Gardos, G., Cole, J. O., Lindley, C., Wycoff, W., Nierenberg, A., Matthews, J. D., & Dugan, S. J. (1992). Acute effects of oral phenylalanine in patients with or without tardive dyskinesia. Presented at the 31st annual meeting of American College of Neuropsychopharmacology, San Juan, Puerto Rico, December 15, 1992.

Rush, M., Diamond, F., & Alpert, M. (1982). Depression as a risk factor in tardive dyskinesia. *Biol. Psychiatry* 17:387–92.

Sandyk, R., & Fisher, H. (1988). Serotonin in involuntary movement disorders. *Int. J. Neurosci.* 42:185–205.

Schwarcz, G., Gosenfeld, L., Gilderman, A., Jiwesh, J., & Ripple, R. E. (1986). Akathisia associated with carbamazepine therapy. *Am. J. Psychiatry* 143:1190–1.

Schwartzman, M. J., & Leppik, I. E. (1990). Carbamazepine-induced dyskinesia and ophthalmoplegia. *Cleveland Clin. T. Med.* 57:367–72.

Simpson, G. M. (1973). Tardive dyskinesia. *Br. J. Psychiatry* 122:618.

Simpson, G. M., Branchey, M. H., & Lee, J. H. (1976). Lithium in tardive dyskinesia. *Pharmakopsychiatr. Neuropsychopharmakol.* 9:76–80.

Simpson, G. M., Varga, E., Lee, J. H., & Zoubok, B. (1978). Tardive dyskinesia and psychotropic drug history. *Psychopharmacology* 58:117–24.

Sternbach, H., & Jordan, S. (1990). Lithium associated tardive dyskinesia. *J. Clin. Psychopharmacol.* 10:143–4.

Webb, M. (1988). Effects of electroconvulsive therapy and depression on tardive dyskinesia. *Ann. Neurol.* 23:181.

Weiner, W. J., & Werner, T. R. (1982). Mania-induced remission of tardive dyskinesia in manic–depressive illness. *Ann. Neurol.* 12:229–30.

Wolf, M. E., DeWolfe, A. S., Ryan, J. J., Lips, O., & Mosnaim, A. D. (1985). Vulnerability to tardive dyskinesia. *J. Clin. Psychiatry* 46:367–8.

Yassa, R., Camille, Y., & Belzile, L. (1987). Tardive dyskinesia in the course of antidepressant therapy: a prevalence study and review of the literature. *J. Clin. Psychopharmacol* 7:243–6.

Yassa, R., Ghadirian, A. M., & Schwartz, G. (1983). Prevalence of tardive dyskinesia in affective disorder patients. *J. Clin. Psychiatry* 44:410–12.

Yassa, R., Nastase, C., Dupont, D., & Thibeau, S. C. (1992). Tardive dyskinesia in elderly psychiatric patients: a 5-year study. *Am. J. Psychiatry* 149:1206–11.

7

Diabetes Mellitus and Tardive Dyskinesia

SUKDEB MUKHERJEE, M.D., and SAHEBARAO P.
MAHADIK, Ph.D.

In spite of considerable research, tardive dyskinesia remains an enigmatic
syndrome: Its pathologic basis is not understood, the role of neuroleptic
treatment in its pathogenesis remains controversial insofar as chronic schizophrenic patients are concerned, and it is not clear why, with comparable
exposures to neuroleptics, some patients develop the syndrome and others do
not. It seems unlikely that this differential risk pattern can be explained by
pharmacokinetic considerations alone. Also, the search for patient characteristics associated with greater risk for developing tardive dyskinesia has
yielded largely disparate findings. Indeed, increasing age is the one factor that
has consistently been associated with higher incidences and prevalences,
increased severity, and stubborn persistence of tardive dyskinesia.

Diabetes Mellitus and Tardive Dyskinesia

On the basis of incidental observations and findings from pilot studies, we
earlier hypothesized that impaired glucose metabolism is associated with
increased risk for tardive dyskinesia (Mukherjee et al., 1985; Mukherjee,
Bilder, & Sackeim 1986). That view was based on the following observations: (1) In two separate studies, the proportion of tardive dyskinesia patients
also diagnosed as having non-insulin-dependent diabetes mellitus (NIDDM)
was considerably higher than would have been expected on the basis of the
known rates of NIDDM in the general population (Mukherjee et al., 1985,
1986). (2) On average, fasting blood glucose concentrations were found to be
significantly higher in patients with tardive dyskinesia than in patients without
tardive dyskinesia, an effect that remained significant after controlling for
variance due to age and gender (Mukherjee et al., 1985). (3) A disproportionately large number of nondiabetic tardive dyskinesia patients had a positive family history of NIDDM (Mukherjee et al., 1986). (4) In a survey of 20

82

elderly, neuroleptic-treated, diabetic schizophrenic patients, 15 (75%) were found to have tardive dyskinesia, a considerably higher rate than had previously been reported for any group (Mukherjee et al., 1986).

Subsequently, using a within-subject, repeated-measures design, we found differential effects of neuroleptic treatment on glucose tolerance in schizophrenic patients as a function of their tardive dyskinesia status. Specifically, haloperidol treatment was associated with decreased glucose tolerance in tardive dyskinesia patients, but increased glucose tolerance in patients without tardive dyskinesia. Also, independent of neuroleptic effects on glucose tolerance, a family history of NIDDM was significantly associated with the presence of tardive dyskinesia (Mukherjee et al., 1989a). When both factors (family history of NIDDM and neuroleptic-associated decrease in glucose tolerance) were considered together to classify the patients, tardive dyskinesia was present in 8 of the 10 patients who met this criterion, and in none of the 5 patients who did not ($\chi^2 = 5.7$, df = 1, $p = .02$, with continuity correction). Unfortunately, we could not determine from that study whether neuroleptic effects on glucose tolerance influenced the subsequent development of tardive dyskinesia or whether neurometabolic changes associated with tardive dyskinesia accounted for the differential peripheral effects of haloperidol on glucose tolerance. Muscle is the tissue primarily involved in peripheral glucose utilization, and it is rather difficult to imagine how impaired glucose utilization in this peripheral tissue might account for an increased risk for a specific brain abnormality.

Our initial hypothesis recently received support from an independent group of investigators (Ganzini et al., 1991) who found a significantly higher prevalence of tardive dyskinesia among neuroleptic-treated diabetic patients than among a nondiabetic control group whose members were matched for age, gender, duration of neuroleptic treatment, psychiatric diagnosis, and neuroleptic dosage. The diabetic and nondiabetic groups did not differ in regard to severity of parkinsonism or exposure to anticholinergic drugs. Interestingly, those investigators found 79% of the neuroleptic-treated diabetic patients to have tardive dyskinesia, similar to the 75% we had earlier observed. Because a non-neuroleptic-treated diabetic group showed a higher-than-expected prevalence (23%) of dyskinesia that except for the treatment condition would have met the criteria for tardive dyskinesia, those authors suggested that diabetes mellitus may contribute to an increased prevalence of tardive dyskinesia through an additive effect. The same investigators subsequently found a high prevalence and greater severity of tardive dyskinesia in metoclopramide-treated, nonpsychiatric, diabetic patients than in similarly treated nondiabetic controls, thereby extending to a nonpsychiatric population the possibility that diabetes mellitus may be associated with increased risk for tardive dyskinesia (Ganzini et al., 1992).

These findings are at best suggestive and leave unresolved the nature of the relationship between tardive dyskinesia and diabetes mellitus. Any two variables may be associated because of chance (thus confounding any association of a third variable with both the risk factor and the disease) or because they are linked in a causal pathway. It would be difficult to establish retrospectively that diabetes mellitus was an antecedent to the emergence of tardive dyskinesia, although the late age at initiation of neuroleptic treatment in the study by Ganzini et al. (1991) suggests that such may well have been the case. Regardless, the hypothesis that NIDDM is associated with increased risk for tardive dyskinesia gains credibility from the finding in a prospective study that NIDDM at initiation of neuroleptic treatment was associated with a significantly higher incidence of subsequent tardive dyskinesia, even after controlling for the variance due to age and gender (Woerner et al., 1993). Specifically, the incidence of tardive dyskinesia was more than 50% among the diabetic patients and approximately 25% among the nondiabetic patients.

Although the studies of Ganzini et al. (1991) and Woerner et al. (1993) provide strong support for our original hypothesis, their findings must be interpreted with caution, for in neither study were patients systematically screened for diabetes mellitus by a glucose-tolerance test. On the basis of evidence from population surveys (Harris et al., 1987; Wingard et al., 1990), it seems likely that many patients in those studies were falsely classified as nondiabetic. Indeed, a more precise classification of patients based on diabetes status might have increased the proportion of variance in the prevalence (or incidence) of tardive dyskinesia accounted for by diabetes mellitus; the converse might also have been observed. Obviously, this is an issue that merits further systematic study.

Contributing environmental factors notwithstanding, NIDDM has a strong genetic basis (O'Rahilly, Wainscoat, & Turner, 1988): For instance, concordance for NIDDM approaches 100% for identical twins (Barnett et al., 1981). In longitudinal studies, a family history of NIDDM has been a robust predictor of subsequent NIDDM (Zimmet, 1982). An increased incidence of impaired glucose tolerance has been found among the offspring of conjugal diabetic (NIDDM) parents (Viswanathan et al., 1988). We therefore decided to ascertain the family histories of NIDDM for young, nondiabetic patients admitted to the Creedmoor Research Division. In an initial report, after drawing attention to the unexpectedly high rate of a positive family history of NIDDM among schizophrenic patients, we proposed that a genetic risk for NIDDM plays a permissive role by interfering with the brain's developmental and maturational events (Mukherjee, Schnur, & Reddy 1989b). That hypothesis remains to be examined. In a subsequent study, we found that a family history of NIDDM was significantly associated with tardive dyskinesia among both schizophrenic and bipolar patients, all of whom were nondiabetic and none of whom had entered the risk age for NIDDM (S. Mukherjee & D. B. Schnur, unpublished data). It is interesting in this regard that the data provided by Ganzini et al. (1991) show that 34.2% of their neuroleptic-treated diabetic patients had a family history of diabetes, in contrast to 13.2% of the nondiabetic controls (our analysis: $\chi^2 = 4.7$, df = 1, $p = .03$). However, those investigators did not examine the relationship between a family history of diabetes and the presence of tardive dyskinesia.

The studies of Ganzini et al. (1991, 1992) and Woerner et al. (1993) suggest that the presence of NIDDM at the initiation of neuroleptic treatment increases the risk for subsequent development of tardive dyskinesia. Critical to the subject at issue is whether hyperglycemia per se or some other factor underlying the diabetic disease process is responsible for the increased risk for tardive dyskinesia. Furthermore, the majority of patients receiving long-term neuroleptic treatment suffer from schizophrenia, and in such patients the onset of psychosis, its treatment with neuroleptics, and, in most cases, the emergence of tardive dyskinesia all long antedate the onset of NIDDM, which typically becomes manifest at or after the fifth decade. Clearly, in such patients diabetes (hyperglycemia) cannot be a risk factor. Nevertheless, it was in such young, nondiabetic patients that we observed an association between a family history of NIDDM and the presence of tardive dyskinesia (Mukherjee et al., 1986, 1989a; S. Mukherjee & D. B. Schnur, unpublished data). This association suggests that a genetic factor that antedates, or is independent of, the development of overt diabetes is responsible for the increased risk for tardive dyskinesia in patients with a family history of NIDDM. We have proposed insulin resistance in the brain as the critical factor (Mukherjee, Reddy, & Schnur, 1991).

Insulin Resistance and NIDDM

Kahn (1978) has defined insulin resistance as a condition in which normal concentrations of insulin produce a less-than-normal biological response. This varies from the earlier and commonly used definition of insulin resistance as "a state in which greater than normal amounts of insulin are required to elicit a quantitatively normal response" (Berson & Yalow, 1970). A major difference between the two definitions is the latter's implication that a normal biological response is possible; the former makes no such assumption. It is interesting in this regard that one study found that low doses of insulin, which conceivably could compensate for the deleterious effects of insulin resistance, ameliorated the severity of tardive dyskinesia (Mouret et al., 1991).

Several lines of evidence suggest the primacy of insulin resistance in the pathogenesis of NIDDM. Numerous longitudinal and cross-sectional studies have conclusively documented that hyperinsulinemia (reflecting insulin resistance) antedates the development of NIDDM. Normal glucose-tolerant offspring of conjugal diabetic (NIDDM) parents show a high prevalence of insulin resistance before entering the risk age for NIDDM (Ho et al., 1990; Ramachandran et al., 1990). In Pima Indians, who have a high familial incidence of NIDDM, it has been demonstrated prospectively that the transition from normal to impaired glucose tolerance is associated with insulin resistance, whereas insulin secretory failure is observed only after the onset of overt diabetes (Lillioja et al., 1988). Not only is impairment of the post-binding action of insulin in these subjects, as well as in other groups, a familial characteristic (Lillioja et al., 1987; Martin et al., 1992), but also there is evidence suggesting that insulin sensitivity is determined by a single gene with a co-dominant mode of inheritance (Bogardus et al., 1989). In prospective studies, insulin resistance during the early years of life has been shown to be a robust predictor of subsequent NIDDM (Warram et al., 1990; Zimmet et al., 1992), and in prospective and longitudinal studies of events leading to the development of spontaneous NIDDM in rhesus monkeys, insulin resistance has been found to be the first identifiable metabolic abnormality (Hansen & Bodkin, 1986).

Thus, it is likely that the observed relationship between a family history of NIDDM and tardive dyskinesia may be due to the confounding effect of insulin resistance. Because insulin resistance is a characteristic of NIDDM patients, the possibility exists that in the studies of Ganzini et al. (1991) and Woerner et al. (1993) the increased risk for tardive dyskinesia among NIDDM patients is also attributable to the underlying insulin resistance. Perhaps, then, tardive dyskinesia does not develop in some diabetic patients because of an insulin-non-resistant variant of NIDDM (Banerjee & Lebovitz, 1989). Perhaps an underlying insulin resistance can also explain the occurrence of tardive dyskinesia in nondiabetic subjects. Regardless of genetic considerations, it is well established that both increased body weight, especially central obesity, and a sedentary existence contribute to insulin resistance. Both of these factors are common in psychiatric patients. Furthermore, a wide range of insulin sensitivity is seen in normoglycemic individuals (Hollenbeck & Reaven, 1987), indicating that insulin resistance occurs in nondiabetic subjects and can exist without progressing to NIDDM if adequate compensatory mechanisms, such as hyperinsulinemia, are maintained. Clearly, we need to examine whether or not the diabetic state has an additive effect that increases the risk beyond that attributable to insulin resistance.

It is becoming increasingly apparent that complications commonly associated with diabetes mellitus, such as hypertension, coronary artery disease, and hyperlipidemia, are independent consequences of insulin resistance. Reaven (1988) has named this cluster "syndrome X." Our hypothesis extends syndrome X to include a decreased threshold for the pathogenesis of specific movement disorders. Reaven (1988) implicated the compensatory hyperinsulinemia that accompanies insulin resistance in nondiabetic individuals as the pathogenic factor in syndrome X. DeFronzo and Ferrannini (1991) have suggested a more complicated paradigm in which insulin resistance (or hyperinsulinemia) has a permissive or facilitory effect on the genetic determination of specific complications. The alternative possibility, that the pathogenesis of the complications involves altered cellular events as a direct consequence of insulin resistance, has received less attention.

Insulin Resistance and the Brain

Because studies of insulin resistance are limited to peripheral insulin actions, our hypothesis that insulin resistance is associated with increased risk for tardive dyskinesia (Mukherjee et al., 1991) requires evidence that peripheral insulin resistance is also associated with resistance of insulin receptors in the brain. The presence of insulin receptors in the brain is well established (Havrankova & Roth, 1978; Adamo, Raizada, & LeRoith, 1989; Unger, Livingston, & Moss 1991). Although there are structural differences between the brain's insulin receptors and peripheral insulin receptors (Heidenreich et al., 1983), both are coupled to tyrosine kinase activity (Rees-Jones et al., 1984), which is integrally involved in the action of insulin (Kahn & White, 1988). In an animal model of NIDDM, we found markedly decreased insulin-stimulated tyrosine kinase activity in both brain and peripheral tissue, even in the absence of hyperglycemia, thereby demonstrating that peripheral insulin resistance is associated with brain insulin resistance (Mukherjee, Mahadik, & Makar, 1992). It deserves mention that the cellular actions of insulin involve many discrete cascades (Marshall, Garvey, & Traxinger, 1991), only some of which are involved in glucose utilization, and that tyrosine kinase activity is not involved in all of those cascades. This is a critical consideration, for it raises the possibility that the cascade of events following the binding of insulin to its receptor, so critical for the pathogenesis of tardive dyskinesia, may not be the same as that involved in glucose utilization. In fact, it is known that the regulation of glucose utilization is not a major function of insulin where neurons are concerned. Insofar as insulin resistance affects peripheral sites of glucose utilization as well as the brain, one may observe an association between peripheral insulin resistance or diabetes mellitus and tardive dyskinesia. But that should not lead to the conclusion that abnormal glucose regulation is the factor responsible for this association – an error we made in formulating our initial hypothesis (Mukherjee et al., 1985, 1986).

Although the role of insulin in the brain is yet to be fully elucidated, the emerging evidence suggests that insulin plays critical metabolic, trophic, and neuromodulatory roles in the brain (Adamo et al., 1989; Unger et al., 1991). Central to our research in this area is the view that a generalized abnormality (such as insulin resistance) may have differential pathologic consequences in the brain and peripheral tissues and that differential effects may also occur across various brain regions. This view of differential risk is supported by the finding that insulin corrects diabetes-associated chromatin changes in peripheral tissues, but not in brain tissues (Hartnell, Storrie, & Mooradian, 1990). It has been suggested that this pattern of differential effects may be a function of the replicative potential of tissues (Mooradian, 1988a). From a theoretical perspective, selective insulin resistance (Houslay, 1989) might result in abnormal insulin actions in the brain while peripheral glucose utilization remained normal. At this point, little is known of the effects of brain insulin resistance on functions presumed to be affected in neuropsychiatric diseases. Direct investigation of the cellular and molecular effects of brain insulin resistance cannot be conducted in humans in vivo and will require studies in animal models and primary neuronal cultures.

How Does Insulin Resistance Influence the Pathogenesis of Tardive Dyskinesia?

The fact that the pathophysiology of tardive dyskinesia is poorly understood makes it difficult to answer this question. The adequacy of the dopamine-supersensitivity hypothesis to explain tardive dyskinesia, especially its persistent form, has been questioned (Jeste & Wyatt, 1981; Fibiger & Lloyd, 1984; Gerlach & Casey, 1988); moreover, it is not supported by findings from postmortem studies (Cross, Crow, & Owen, 1981; Kornhuber et al., 1989). Dopamine supersensitivity is a compensatory phenomenon that attempts to restore normal nigrostriatal dopaminergic function in the face of loss, as occurs in Parkinson's disease. Both in vivo positron-emission tomography and postmortem brain studies have found D_2 dopamine supersensitivity in early-onset untreated patients with Parkinson's disease (Rinne et al., 1990). This may not necessarily exclude a role for dopamine supersensitivity in the pathogenesis of tardive dyskinesia. Neuroleptic-induced parkinsonism has been shown to predict the development of tardive dyskinesia in prospective studies, and neuroleptics (e.g., clozapine) that do not cause parkinsonism as an adverse effect also appear to be associated with low risk for tardive dyskinesia. Thus, parkinsonism may be an initial event in the cascade of pathologic change leading ultimately to tardive dyskinesia. Thus, even if it is a necessary factor, dopamine-receptor supersensitivity would not qualify as a sufficient factor. Other possibilities, such as GABAergic deficiency (Fibiger & Lloyd, 1984; Gunne, Häggström, & Sjöquist, 1984) and abnormal noradrenergic activity (Jeste & Wyatt, 1981), remain largely conjectural at this stage. To explain the topographic heterogeneity of tardive dyskinesia, Lohr, Wisniewski, and Jeste (1986) have suggested that orofacial dyskinesia may be the consequence of loss of neostriatal cholinergic neurons, with limb-axial dyskinesias being due to the loss of neostriatal GABAergic neurons. There is no evidence that the increased risk for tardive dyskinesia among diabetic patients has differential effects on the topography of tardive dyskinesia.

Numerous studies in rodents have examined the effects of overt diabetes on the brain. They have shown that diabetes is associated with abnormal functioning of various brain neurotransmitter systems, such as decreased dopaminergic activity with dopamine-receptor supersensitivity, decreased noradrenergic activity, decreased GABAergic activity, and abnormal serotonergic activity (Mooradian, 1988b). Those studies all involved induction of diabetes with alloxan or streptozotocin. This acute-onset diabetes due to pancreatic dysfunction is not a model of NIDDM, which has a relatively insidious onset and generally does not result from marked pancreatic hypofunction. Thus, although it may be tempting to extrapolate the findings from those studies to propose an explanation for the increased risk for tardive dyskinesia among diabetic patients (e.g., dopamine supersensitivity, decreased GABAergic functions), such an approach would be questionable, because there are no animal or human data to suggest that insulin resistance or NIDDM is associated with brain changes similar to those that occur following acute induction of experimental diabetes.

Recently, the emphasis has shifted from neurotransmitter hypotheses to consideration of cellular events in the pathogenesis of tardive dyskinesia. The view best supported by evidence is that of an oxyradical-mediated abnormality (Cadet, Lohr, & Jeste, 1986). This does not conflict with neurotransmitter hypotheses, but rather, at a different explanatory level, attempts to define a final, common pathway leading to cell abnormalities that may manifest as tardive dyskinesia. This hypothesis is supported by the findings that tardive dyskinesia is associated with increased concentrations of lipid-peroxidation products in the cerebrospinal fluid (Lohr et al., 1990) and that α-tocopherol, an antioxidant, ameliorates the manifestations of tardive dyskinesia (Lohr et al., 1987; Elkashef et al., 1990; Scapicchio et al., 1991). Further, increased lipid peroxidation results in decreased membrane fluidity (Watanabe et al., 1990), and tardive dyskinesia has been reported to be associated with decreased membrane fluidity (Zubenko & Cohen, 1986).

We propose that insulin resistance or NIDDM or both can increase the risk for tardive dyskinesia by impairing the capacity of the antioxidant defense system to cope with the increased oxidative stress that can result from the schizophrenic disease process or from neuroleptic treatment, or from both. Most studies that have examined the activities of the antioxidant enzymes in patients with schizophrenia have reported abnormal findings. Superoxide dismutase activity has been found to be increased (Lohr, 1991; Reddy et al., 1991), suggesting increased oxidative tone. In contrast, catalase activity has been found to be reduced (Glazov & Mamzev, 1976; Reddy et al., 1991), suggesting a failure to limit production of highly toxic hydroxyl ions from H_2O_2 formed by the dismutation of superoxide. None of those studies examined whether or not abnormal activities of these enzymes were associated with membrane lipid peroxidation. One study (Pall et al., 1987) found high levels of lipid-peroxidation products in the cerebrospinal fluid in phenothiazine-treated patients, especially those with neuroleptic-induced parkinsonism. This is noteworthy, considering that neuroleptic-induced parkinsonism may be a predictor for subsequent development of tardive dyskinesia.

Diabetes mellitus also has been associated with increased lipid peroxidation and decreased membrane fluidity (Sato et al., 1979; Bryszewska & Leko, 1983; Jain et al., 1989; Abdella et al., 1990; Winocour et al., 1990; Rajeswari et al., 1991), especially in patients with complications (Mooradian, 1991), and it is also associated with reduced Na^+-K^+ ATPase activity in red blood cells (RBCs) (Baldini et al., 1989; Rajeswari et al., 1991), all of which are consistent with cell membrane dysfunction. The RBC activities of superoxide dismutase, plasma thiol (a free-radical scavenger), and the glutathione-dependent antioxidant system have been found to be reduced in NIDDM patients (Fujiwara et al., 1989; Collier et al., 1990). Increased lipid-peroxidation products (conjugated dienes) have been found in the brains of diabetic rats (Mooradian, Dickerson, & Smith, 1990), and in an animal model of NIDDM we found that brain insulin resistance was associated with reduced brain catalase activity prior to the onset of manifest diabetes (Mahadik et al., 1992). It has been suggested that oxyradical-mediated damage underlies the complications of NIDDM, especially microvascular abnormalities (Gillery et al., 1989; Mullarkey, Edelstein, & Brownlee, 1990; Baynes, 1991; Mooradian, 1991). Thus, consideration of microvascular abnormalities to explain the risk for tardive dyskinesia among diabetic patients (Ganzini et al., 1991) may not be in conflict with the oxyradical hypothesis of tardive dyskinesia. Further, high insulin concentrations have been found to increase lipid-peroxidation products in erythrocytes in vitro (Salnikova & Musatova, 1990), suggesting that oxyradical-mediated membrane damage can occur as a consequence of the hyperinsulinemia associated with insulin resistance prior to the development of frank hyperglycemia. No study, however, has yet examined blood insulin concentrations in patients with tardive dyskinesia.

There may be pathways other than impairment of antioxidant defenses through which insulin resistance can increase oxidative damage to membranes. Relative to normal controls, patients with NIDDM have higher blood lactate concentrations both during the fasting state and after a glucose load (Reaven et al., 1988); schizophrenic patients also have been reported to have higher blood lactate concentrations after a glucose load (Henneman, Altschule, & Goncz, 1954) and to show increased conversion of glucose to lactate in the brain (Sacks, 1961). These findings suggest that in diabetic and schizophrenic patients, pyruvate formed during glycolysis is preferentially metabolized to lactate, rather than converted to acetyl coenzyme A (acetyl-CoA) by the pyruvate dehydrogenase complex (PDHC) for oxidation through the citric acid cycle. That would decrease cellular energy production, because glucose metabolism through glycolytic pathways yields only 12 molecules of adenosine triphosphate (ATP), in contrast to the 36 molecules of ATP when glucose is metabolized through the oxidative pathway. The reduced availability of ATP can limit the capability for membrane repair by phospholipid replacement. Increased lactate production will also result in a decrease in intracellular pH, making the intracellular milieu more suitable for lipid peroxidation, and bring about increased intracytosolic free Ca^{2+}. Both low pH and increased availability of free Ca^{2+} can activate phospholipase A_2 (PLA_2) and further increase oxyradical production via the arachidonic acid cascade. It is noteworthy in this regard that increased PLA_2 activity has been reported in schizophrenic patients (Gattaz et al., 1987, 1990), although its relation to insulin resistance or tardive dyskinesia has not yet been examined. It has been demonstrated that both insulin resistance and NIDDM are associated with decreased responsiveness of PDHC to insulin (Buffington, Givens, &

Kitabchi, 1990). Alternatively, because PDHC is located on the mitochondrial membrane, its function can be impaired by lipid-peroxidation damage to mitochondrial membranes.

Concluding Remarks

Our fundamental position is that insulin resistance plays a *permissive* role in
the pathogenesis of specific neurological disorders, especially those in which
oxidative damage is involved, by impairing the ability of the antioxidant
defense system to cope with oxidative stress. A corollary of this view is that
insulin resistance per se is not a sufficient factor for the pathogenesis of a
neurological syndrome, which requires the presence of additional pathogenic
factors that are discrete for, and thereby define the nature of, the particular
syndrome (e.g., neuroleptic treatment and/or the schizophrenic disease process, where tardive dyskinesia is concerned). This brief overview does not
address the functional organization of the basal ganglia or the differential
vulnerability of specific striatal neuronal populations to explain how insulin
resistance or NIDDM could lower the threshold for development of tardive
dyskinesia. This is primarily because of the prevailing uncertainty as to which
basal-ganglia systems are critical for the pathogenesis of tardive dyskinesia.
Instead, a hypothesis has been proposed that may be but a small step forward
in our understanding of the pathologic basis of the tardive dyskinesia syndrome. It is, nevertheless, a testable proposition.

Traditionally, the brain has not been regarded as a target organ for the
complications of insulin resistance or NIDDM, except when severe derange-
ments of glucose homeostasis occur. Recent evidence indicates that that view
should be revised. In addition to the evidence presented earlier, patients with
NIDDM have been found to have greater cognitive impairments than matched
nondiabetic controls (Perlmutter et al., 1984; Mooradian et al., 1986; Reaven
et al., 1990) and a much higher prevalence of major depression than would be
expected on the basis of known population base rates (Lustman et al., 1986).
Interestingly, tardive dyskinesia has been reported to be associated with
greater cognitive impairment, and depression may be a risk factor for tardive
dyskinesia (Waddington, 1989; American Psychiatric Association, 1990). It
is also noteworthy that more than two decades ago, an association of Parkinson's disease to insulin resistance and impaired glucose tolerance was suggested (Barbeau, Giguere, & Hardy, 1961; van Woert and Mueller, 1971); it
was never pursued, however, despite the absence of any negative report. As
mentioned earlier, parkinsonism is recognized as a risk factor for tardive
dyskinesia. More recently, it has been suggested that impaired insulin actions

in the brain may be critical for the pathogenesis of Alzheimer's disease (Hoyer, Osterreich, & Wagner, 1988), a disorder in which dyskinetic movements often occur and bode a more malignant course. It may be more than mere coincidence that oxyradical-mediated damage has been implicated in the pathogenesis of both disorders.

In 1899, Sir Henry Maudsley wrote in *The Pathology of Mind* that "diabetes is a disease which often shows itself in families in which insanity prevails: whether one disease predisposes in any way to the other or not, or whether they are independent outcomes of a common neurosis, they are certainly found to run side by side, or alternately with one another more often than can be accounted for by accidental coincidence or sequence." That prescient remark appears to have had little impact on the past three decades of biological research into the bases of neuropsychiatric disorders. This is all the more surprising considering the large body of literature spanning many decades that provides evidence of high rates of diabetes mellitus, impaired glucose tolerance, and insulin resistance among patients with a variety of neuropsychiatric disorders, including schizophrenia and major mood disorders. Nevertheless, efforts to elucidate the implications of this co-morbidity for an understanding of neuropsychiatric disease processes are conspicuous by their virtual absence. It is hoped that this overview will encourage more systematic research in this area.

References

Abdella, N., Awadi, F., Salman, A., & Armstrong, D. (1990). Thiobarbituric acid test as a measure of lipid peroxidation in Arab patients with NIDDM. *Diabetes Res.* 15:173–7.

Adamo, M., Raizada, M. K., & LeRoith, D. (1989). Insulin and insulin-like growth factor receptors in the nervous system. *Mol. Neurobiol.* 3:71–100.

Alexander, G. E., & Crutcher, M. D. (1990). Functional architecture of basal ganglia circuits: neural substrates of parallel processing. *Trends Neurosci.* 13:266–71.

American Psychiatric Association (1990). *Task Force Report on Tardive Dyskinesia.* Washington, DC: American Psychiatric Press.

Baldini, P., Incerpi, S., Lambert-Gardini, S., Spinedi, A., & Luly, P. (1989). Membrane lipid alterations and Na^+-pumping activity in erythrocytes from IDDM and NIDDM subjects. *Diabetes* 38:825–31.

Banerjee, M. A., & Lebovitz, H. E. (1989). Insulin-sensitive and insulin-resistant variants in NIDDM. *Diabetes* 38:784–92.

Barbeau, A., Giguere, R., & Hardy, J. (1961). Expérience clinique avec le tolbutamide dans la maladie de Parkinson. *Union Med. Can.* 90:147–51.

Barnett, A. H., Eff, C., Leslie, R. D. G., & Pyke, D. A. (1981). Diabetes in identical twins. A study of 200 pairs. *Diabetologia* 20:87–93.

Baskin, D. G., Wilcox, B. J., Figlewicz, D. P., & Dorsa, D. M. (1988). Insulin and insulin-like growth factors in the CNS. *Trends Neurosci.* 11:107–11.

Baynes, J. W. (1991). Role of oxidative stress in development of complications in diabetes. *Diabetes* 40:405–12.

Berson, S. A., & Yalow, R. S. (1970). Insulin "antagonists" and insulin resistance. In *Diabetes Mellitus: Theory and Practice*, ed. M. Ellenberg & H. Rifkin, pp. 388–423. New York: McGraw-Hill.

Bogardus, C., Lillioja, S., Nyomba, B. L., Zurlo, F., Swinburn, B., Esposito-del Puente, A., Knowler, W. C., Ravussin, E., Mott, D. M., & Bennett, P. H. (1989). Distributions of in vivo insulin action in Pima Indians as a mixture of three normal distributions. *Diabetes* 38:1423–32.

Bryszewska, M., & Leko, W. (1983). Effect of insulin on human erythrocyte membrane fluidity in diabetes mellitus. *Diabetes* 24:311–31.

Buffington, C. K., Givens, J. R., & Kitabchi, A. E. (1990). Sensitivity of pyruvate dehydrogenase to insulin in activated T lymphocytes. *Diabetes* 39:361–8.

Cadet, J. L., Lohr, J. B., & Jeste, D. V. (1986). Free radicals and tardive dyskinesia. *Trends Neurosci.* 9:107–8.

Collier, A., Wilson, R., Bradley, H., Thomson, J. A., & Small, M. (1990). Free radical activity in type 2 diabetes. *Diabetic Med.* 7:27–30.

Cross, A. J., Crow, T. J., & Owen, F. (1981). ^{3}H-flupenthixol binding in postmortem brains of schizophrenics. *Psychopharmacology* 74:122–4.

DeFronzo, R. A., & Ferrannini, E. (1991). Insulin resistance: a multifaceted syndrome responsible for NIDDM, obesity, hypertension, dyslipidemia, and atherosclerotic cardiovascular disease. *Diabetes Care* 14:173–94.

Dexter, D. T., Carter, C. J., Wells, F. R., Javoy-Agid, F., Agid, Y., Lees, A., Jenner, P., & Marsden, C. D. (1989). Basal lipid peroxidation in substantia nigra is increased in Parkinson's disease. *J. Neurochem.* 52:381–9.

Elkashef, A. M., Ruskin, P. E., Bacher, N., & Barrett, D. (1990). Vitamin E in the treatment of tardive dyskinesia. *Am. J. Psychiatry* 147:505–6.

Fibiger, H. C., & Lloyd, K. G. (1984). Neurobiological substrates of tardive dyskinesia: the GABA hypothesis. *Trends Neurosci.* 7:462–4.

Fujiwara, Y., Kondo, T., Murakami, K., & Kawakami, Y. (1989). Decrease of inhibition of lipid peroxidation by glutathione-dependent system in erythrocytes of non-insulin dependent diabetics. *Klin Wochenschr.* 67:336–41.

Ganzini, L., Casey, D. E., Hoffman, W. F., & McCall, A. (1992). Metoclopramide-induced movement disorders. *Biol. Psychiatry (Suppl.)* 29:156A.

Ganzini, L., Heintz, R. T., Hoffman, W. F., & Casey, D. E. (1991). The prevalence of tardive dyskinesia in neuroleptic treated diabetics. *Arch. Gen. Psychiatry* 48:259–63.

Gattaz, W. F., Hubner, C. K., Nevalainen, T. J., Thuren, T., & Kinnunen, P. K. J. (1990). Increased serum phospholipase A_2 activity in schizophrenia: a replication study. *Biol. Psychiatry* 28:495–501.

Gattaz, W. F., Köllisch, M., Thuren, T., Virtanen, J. A., & Kinnunen, P. J. (1987). Increased plasma phospholipase A_2 activity in schizophrenic patients: reduction after neuroleptic therapy. *Biol. Psychiatry* 22:421–6.

Gerlach, J., & Casey, D. E. (1988) Tardive dyskinesia. *Acta Psychiatr. Scand.* 77:369–78.

Gillery, P., Monboissa, J.-C., Maquart, F. X., & Borel, J. P. (1989). Does oxygen free radical increased formation explain long term complications of diabetes mellitus? *Med. Hypotheses* 29:47–50.

Glazov, V. A., & Mamzev, V. P. (1976). Catalase in the blood and leucocytes in patients with nuclear schizophrenia. *Zh. Nevropatol. Psikhiatr.* 4:549–52.

Gunne, L.-M., Häggström, J.-E., & Sjöquist, B. (1984). Association with persistent neuroleptic-induced dyskinesia of regional changes in brain GABA synthesis. *Nature* 309:347–9.

Halliwell, B., & Gutteridge, J. M. C. (1989). *Free Radical in Biology and Medicine*, 2nd ed. Oxford: Clarendon Press.

Hansen, B. C., & Bodkin, N. L. (1986). Heterogeneity of insulin responses: phases leading to the type 2 (non-insulin-dependent) diabetes mellitus in the rhesus monkey. *Diabetologia* 29:713–19.

Harris, M. I., Hadden, W. C., Knowler, W. C., & Bennett, P. H. (1987). Prevalence of diabetes and impaired glucose tolerance and plasma glucose levels in U.S. population aged 20–74 yr. *Diabetes* 36:523–34.

Hartnell, J. M., Storrie, M. C., & Mooradian, A. D. (1990). Diabetes-related changes in chromatin structure of brain, liver, and intestinal epithelium. *Diabetes* 39:348–53.

Havrankova, J., & Roth, J. (1978). Insulin receptors are widely distributed in the central nervous system of the rat. *Nature* 272:827–9.

Heidenreich, K. A., Zahniser, N. R., Berhanu, P., Brandenburg, D., & Olefsky, J. M. (1983). Structural differences between insulin receptors in the brain and peripheral tissues. *J. Biol. Chem.* 258:8527–30.

Henneman, D. H., Altschule, M. D., & Goncz, R. M. (1954). Carbohydrate metabolism in brain disease. II. Glucose metabolism in schizophrenic, manic-depressive, and involutional psychoses. *Arch. Intern. Med.* 94:402–16.

Ho, L. T., Chang, Z. Y., Wang, J. T., Li, S. H., Liu, Y. F., Chen, Y.-D. I., & Reaven, G. M. (1990). Insulin insensitivity in offspring of parents with type 2 diabetes mellitus. *Diabetic Med.* 7:31–4.

Hollenbeck, C., & Reaven, G. M. (1987). Variations in insulin-stimulated glucose uptake in healthy individuals with normal glucose tolerance. *J. Clin. Endocrinol. Metab.* 64:1169–73.

Houslay, M. D. (1989). Distinct functional domains on the insulin receptor β-subunit: Do they provide a molecular basis for "selective" insulin resistance? *Trends Endocrinol. Metab.* 1:83–9.

Hoyer, S., Osterreich, K., & Wagner, O. (1988). Glucose metabolism as the site of the primary abnormality in early-onset dementia of Alzheimer type? *J. Neurol.* 235:143–8.

Jain, S. K., McVie, R., Duett, J., & Herbst, J. J. (1989). Erythrocyte membrane lipid peroxidation and glycosylated hemoglobin in diabetes. *Diabetes* 38:1539–43.

Jeste, D. V., & Wyatt, R. J. (1981). Dogma disputed: Is tardive dyskinesia due to postsynaptic dopamine receptor supersensitivity? *J. Clin. Psychiatry* 42:455–7.

Kahn, C. R. (1978). Insulin resistance, insulin sensitivity, and insulin unresponsiveness: a necessary distinction. *Metabolism (Suppl. 2)* 27:1893–902.

Kahn, C. R., & White, M. F. (1988). The insulin receptor and the molecular mechanism of insulin action. *J. Clin. Invest.* 82:1151–6.

Kane, J., Woerner, M., & Lieberman, J. (1988). Tardive dyskinesia: prevalence, incidence and risk factors. *J. Clin. Psychopharmacol. (Suppl.)* 8:52–6.

Kish, S. J., Morito, C., & Hornykiewicz, O. (1985). Glutathione peroxidase activity in Parkinson's disease brain. *Neurosci. Lett.* 58:343–6.

Kornhuber, J., Riederer, P., Reynolds, G. P., Beckmann, H., Jellinger, K., & Gabriel, E. (1989). ^{3}H-spiperone binding sites in post-mortem brains from schizophrenic patients: relationship to neuroleptic drug treatment, abnormal movements and positive symptoms. *J. Neural Transm.* 75:1–10.

Lillioja, S., Mott, D. M., Howard, B. V., Bennett, P. H., Yki-Järvinen, H., Frey-
mond, D., Nyomba, B. L., Zurlo, F., Swinburn, B., & Bogardus, C. (1988).
Impaired glucose tolerance as a disorder of insulin action: longitudinal and
cross-sectional studies in Pima Indians. *N. Engl. J. Med.* 318:1217–25.
Lillioja, S., Mott, D. M., Zawadzki, J. K., Young, A. A., Abbott, W. G. H.,
Knowler, W. C., Bennett, P. H., Moll, P., & Bogardus, C. (1987). In vivo
insulin action is a familial characteristic in nondiabetic Pima Indians. *Diabetes*
36:1329–35.
Lohr, J. B. (1991). Oxygen radicals and neuropsychiatric illness. *Arch. Gen. Psy-
chiatry* 48:1097–106.
Lohr, J. B., Cadet, J. L., Lohr, M. A., Jeste, D. V., & Wyatt, R. J. (1987).
Alpha-tocopherol in tardive dyskinesia. *Lancet* 1:913–14.
Lohr, J. B., Kuczenski, R., Bracha, H. S., Moir, M., & Jeste, D. V. (1990).
Increased indices of free radical activity in the cerebrospinal fluid of patients
with tardive dyskinesia. *Biol. Psychiatry* 28:535–9.
Lohr, J. B., Wisniewski, A., & Jeste, D. V. (1986). Neurological aspects of tar-
dive dyskinesia. In *Handbook of Schizophrenia. Vol. 1: Neurology of Schizo-
phrenia*, ed. H. Nasrallah & D. R. Weinberger, pp. 97–119. Amsterdam:
Elsevier.
Lustman, P. J., Griffith, L. S., Clouse, R. E., & Cryer, P. E. (1986). Psychiatric
illnesses in diabetes mellitus: relationship to symptoms and glucose control. *J.
Nerv. Ment. Dis.* 174:736–42.
Mahadik, S. P., Mukherjee, S., Reddy, R., Korenovsky, A., & Makar, T. (1992).
Brain insulin resistance and deregulation of antioxidant enzymes in an animal
model of NIDDM. *Biol. Psychiatry (Suppl)* 31:219A.
Marshall, S., Garvey, W. T., & Traxinger, R. R. (1991). New insights into the
metabolic regulation of insulin action and insulin resistance: role of glucose
and amino acids. *FASEB J.* 5:3031–6.
Martin, B. C., Warram, J. H., Rosner, B., Rich, S. S., Soeldner, J. S., &
Krolewski, A. S. (1992) Familial clustering of insulin sensitivity. *Diabetes*
41:850–4.
Marttila, B. J., Lorentz, H., & Rinne, U. K. (1988). Oxygen toxicity protecting
enzymes in Parkinson's disease: increase of superoxide dismutase-like activity
in the substantia nigra and basal nucleus. *J. Neurol. Sci.* 86:321–31.
Maudsley, H. (1899). *The Pathology of Mind*, 3rd ed., p. 113. New York:
Appleton.
Mooradian, A. D. (1988a). Tissue specificity of premature aging in diabetes mellitus:
the role of cellular replicative capacity. *J. Am. Geriatr. Soc.* 36:831–8.
Mooradian, A. D. (1988b). Diabetic complications of the central nervous system.
Endocr. Rev. 9:346–56.
Mooradian, A. D. (1991). Increased serum conjugated dienes in elderly diabetic
patients. *J. Am. Geriatr. Soc.* 39:571–4.
Mooradian, A. D., Dickerson, F., & Smith, T. L. (1990). Lipid order and compo-
sition of synaptic membranes in experimental diabetes mellitus. *Neurochem.
Res.* 15:981–5.
Mooradian, A. D., Perryman, K., Fitten, J., Kavonian, G. D., & Morley, J. E.
(1986). Cortical functions in elderly non-insulin-dependent diabetic patients:
behavioral and electrophysiologic studies. *Arch. Intern. Med.* 148:2369–72.
Mouret, J., Khomais, M., Lemoine, P., & Sebert, P. (1991). Low doses of insulin
as a treatment of tardive dyskinesia: conjuncture or conjecture? *Eur. Neurol.*
31:199–203.

Mukherjee, S., Bilder, R. M., & Sackeim, H. A. (1986). Tardive dyskinesia and glucose metabolism. *Arch. Gen. Psychiatry* 43:192–3.

Mukherjee, S., Mahadik, S. P., & Makar, T. (1992). Insulin sensitivity in brain and periphery. *Biol. Psychiatry (Suppl)* 31:219A.

Mukherjee, S., Reddy, R., & Schnur, D. B. (1991). Diabetes mellitus and tardive dyskinesia. In *Biological Psychiatry*, vol. 2, ed. G. Racagni, N. Brunello, & T. Fukuda, pp. 624–7. Amsterdam: Elsevier.

Mukherjee, S., Roth, S. D., Sandyk, R., & Schnur, D. B. (1989a). Persistent tardive dyskinesia and neuroleptic effects on glucose tolerance. *Psychiatry Res.* 29:17–27.

Mukherjee, S., Schnur, D. B., & Reddy, R. (1989b). Family history of type 2 diabetes in schizophrenic patients. *Lancet* 1:495.

Mukherjee, S., Wisniewski, A., Bilder, R. M., & Sackeim, H. A. (1985). Possible association between tardive dyskinesia and altered carbohydrate metabolism. *Arch. Gen. Psychiatry* 42:205.

Mullarkey, C. J., Edelstein, D., & Brownlee, M. (1990). Free radical generation by early glycation products: a mechanism for accelerated atherogenesis in diabetes. *Biochem. Biophys. Res. Comm.* 173:932–9.

O'Rahilly, S., Wainscoat, J. S., & Turner, R. C. (1988). Type 2 (non-insulin-dependent) diabetes mellitus: new genetics for old nightmares. *Diabetologia* 31:407–14.

Pall, H. S., Williams, A. C., Blake, D. R., & Lunec, J. (1987). Evidence of enhanced lipid peroxidation in the cerebrospinal fluid of patients taking phenothiazines. *Lancet* 2:596–9.

Perlmutter, L. C., Hakami, M. K., Hodgson-Harrington, C., Ginsberg, J., Katz, J., Singer, D. E., & Nathan, D. M. (1984). Decreased cognitive function in aging non-insulin-dependent diabetic patients. *Am. J. Med.* 77:1043–8.

Rajeswari, P., Natarajan, R., Nadler, J. L., Kumar, D., & Kalra, V. K. (1991). Glucose induces lipid peroxidation and inactivation of membrane-associated ion-transport enzymes in human erythrocytes in vivo and in vitro. *J. Cell. Physiol.* 149:100–9.

Ramachandran, A., Snehalatha, C., Mohan, V., Bhattacharyya, P. K., & Viswanathan, M. (1990). Decreased insulin sensitivity in offspring whose parents both have type 2 diabetes. *Diabetic Med.* 7:331–4.

Reaven, G. M. (1988). Role of insulin resistance in human disease. *Diabetes* 37:1595–607.

Reaven, G. M., Hollenbeck, C., Jeng, C.-Y., Wu, M. S., & Chen, Y.-D. I. (1988). Measurement of plasma glucose, free fatty acid, lactate, and insulin for 24 h in patients with NIDDM. *Diabetes* 37:1020–4.

Reaven, G. M., Thompson, L. W., Nahum, D., & Haskins, E. (1990). Relationship between hyperglycemia and cognitive functions in older NIDDM patients. *Diabetes Care* 13:16–21.

Reddy, R., Mahadik, S. P., Mukherjee, S., & Murthy, J. N. (1991). Enzymes of the antioxidant defence system in chronic schizophrenic patients. *Biol. Psychiatry* 30:409–12.

Rees-Jones, R. W., Hendricks, A., Quarum, M., & Roth, J. (1984). The insulin receptor of rat brain is coupled to tyrosine kinase activity. *J. Biol. Chem.* 259:3470–4.

Rinne, U. K., Laihinen, A., Rinne, J. O., Någren, K., Bergman, J., & Ruotsalainen, U. (1990). Positron emission tomography demonstrates dopamine D_2

receptor supersensitivity in the striatum of patients with early Parkinson's disease. *Mov. Disord.* 5:55–9.

Sacks, W. (1961). Cerebral metabolism of glucose-3-C^{14}, pyruvate-1-C^{14}, and lactate-1-C^{14} in mental disease. *J. Appl. Physiol.* 16:175–80.

Salnikova, L. A., & Musatova, N. V. (1990). The action of insulin on the antioxidative enzymes and lipid peroxidation in the erythrocytes. *Probl. Endokrinol. (Mosk)* 36:32–4.

Sato, Y., Hotta, N., Sakamoto, N., Matsuoka, S., Ohishi, N., & Yagi, K. (1979). Lipid peroxide levels in plasma of diabetic patients. *Biochem. Med.* 21:104–7.

Scapicchio, P. L., Decina, P., Mukherjee, S., & Caracci, G. (1991). Effects of α-tocopherol on persistent tardive dyskinesia in elderly schizophrenic patients. *Ital. J. Psychiatry* 1:111–14.

Unger, J. W., Livingston, J. N., & Moss, A. M. (1991). Insulin receptors in the central nervous system: localization, signalling mechanisms, and functional aspects. *Prog. Neurobiol.* 36:343–62.

van Woert, M. H., & Mueller, P. S. (1971). Glucose, insulin, and free fatty acid metabolism in Parkinson's disease treated with levodopa. *Clin. Pharmacol. Ther.* 12:360–7.

Viswanathan, M., Mohan, V., Snehalatha, C., & Ramachandran, A. (1988). High prevalence of type 2 (non-insulin-dependent) diabetes among the offspring of conjugal type 2 diabetic parents in India. *Diabetologia* 28:907–10.

Waddington, J. L. (1989). Schizophrenia, affective psychoses, and other disorders treated with neuroleptic drugs: the enigma of tardive dyskinesia, its neurobiological determinants, and the conflict of paradigms, *Int. Rev. Neurobiol.* 31:297–353.

Warram, J. H., Martin, B. C., Krolewski, A. S., Soeldner, J. S., & Kahn, C. R. (1990). Slow glucose removal rate and hyperinsulinemia precede the development of type II diabetes in the offspring of diabetic parents. *Ann. Intern. Med.* 113:909–15.

Watanabe, H., Kobayashi, A., Yamamoto, T., Suzuki, S., Hayashi, H., & Yamazaki, N. (1990). Alterations of human erythrocyte membrane fluidity by oxygen-derived free radicals and calcium. *Free Radic. Biol. Med.* 9:507–14.

Wingard, D. L., Sinsheimer, P., Barrett-Connor, E., & McPhillips, J. B. (1990). A community-based study of NIDDM in older adults. *Diabetes Care (Suppl. 2)* 13:3–8.

Winocour, P. D., Bryszewska, M., Watala, C., Rand, M. L., Epand, R. M., Kinlough-Rathbone, R. L., Pacham, M. A., & Mustard, J. F. (1990). Reduced membrane fluidity in platelets from diabetic patients. *Diabetes* 39:241–4.

Woerner, M. G., Saltz, B. L., Kane, J. M., Lieberman, J. A., & Alvir, J. (1993). Diabetes and the development of tardive dyskinesia. *Am. J. Psychiatry* 150:966–8.

Zimmet, P. (1982). Type 2 (non-insulin-dependent) diabetes: an epidemiological overview. *Diabetologia* 22:399–411.

Zimmet, P. Z., Collins, V. R., Dowse, G. K., & Knight, L. T. (1992). Hyperinsulinemia in youth is a predictor of type 2 (non-insulin-dependent) diabetes mellitus. *Diabetologia* 35:534–41.

Zubenko, G. S., & Cohen, B. M. (1986). A cell membrane correlate of tardive dyskinesia in patients treated with phenothiazines. *Psychopharmacology* 88:230–6.

8

Other Factors in the Development of Tardive Dyskinesia

RAMZY YASSA, M.D.

Although tardive dyskinesia is defined as a movement disorder that develops after 3 months of drug treatment (Jeste & Wyatt, 1982), the fact that some patients develop this side effect earlier means that they may have a greater predisposition to the condition. Various authors have speculated as to the different mechanisms for this vulnerability; in this chapter we shall look at genetic factors and smoking.

Genetic Factors

Recently, hereditary susceptibility to tardive dyskinesia has been the subject of much discussion. Brandon, McClelland, and Protheroe (1971), for example, have suggested that blue-eyed men are more prone to develop tardive dyskinesia than brown-eyed men, although Gardos, Sokol, and Coel (1976) could not confirm that finding, nor could it be confirmed in women. In a study of six pairs of twin patients (four monozygotic and two dizygotic) treated with high-dosage neuroleptics, Jacob Brody found that the specific type of neurological side effect was *not* determined genetically, inasmuch as the identical twins showed distinctly different reaction patterns (Jeste & Wyatt, 1982). Moreover, Jeste, Phelps, and Wyatt (1982), in a study of 50-year-old female schizophrenic quadruplets on neuroleptic treatment, found that only one of the four had definite tardive dyskinesia. Weinhold, Wegner, and Kane (1981), however, reported the presence of tardive dyskinesia in two schizophrenic brothers treated with neuroleptics. Yassa and Ananth (1981) found that of eight pairs of family members, two were concordant for tardive dyskinesia, and six for the absence of tardive dyskinesia. Pair 4 (two male twins) subsequently developed TD – interestingly, in the same body areas, as evidenced by their buccolingual masticatory movements.

In a series of studies, Waddington and colleagues (Waddington & Youssef,

1987; Waddington, 1989) reported concordance for buccolingual masticatory dyskinesia, as well as cognitive dysfunction, in each of 4 schizophrenic siblings. Subsequently, O'Callaghan et al. (1990) determined that schizophrenic patients without family histories of psychiatric disorders as well as those with an earlier onset of their illness were more likely to have obstetric complications than were the patients with positive family histories and those with later onset of illness, respectively. However, those investigators also found that tardive dyskinesia patients, as compared with patients without tardive dyskinesia, were more likely to have had family histories of psychiatric disorders and less likely to have experienced obstetric complications; they also found greater cognitive deficits in the tardive dyskinesia patients than in patients without tardive dyskinesia.

Thus, at present, vulnerability to tardive dyskinesia seems to run in families. The mechanism of this vulnerability, however, has yet to be explored. As suggested by Waddington and colleagues, perhaps the greater cognitive and neurological impairments evident in tardive dyskinesia patients may be related, in part, to some familial component of their illness (Waddington, 1989).

Smoking

Nicotine affects several neurotransmitters, particularly those of the dopaminergic system. It increases the turnover of dopamine in the nigrostriatal and mesolimbic systems (Anderson, Fuxe, & Agnati, 1981). Enhancement of the dopamine function by nicotine in the nigrostriatal pathway might therefore be expected to foster the development of tardive dyskinesia (Yassa et al., 1987). In addition to its central dopaminergic effects, smoking is believed to induce hepatic microsomal enzymes and accelerate the metabolism of neuroleptics. Thus, tardive dyskinesia patients who smoke may need more neuroleptic intake than nonsmokers (Swett, 1974; Stimmel & Falloon, 1983; Vinarova, Vinar, & Kalvach, 1984). As well, Jann et al. (1986) found that smokers, compared with nonsmokers, had significantly lower plasma concentrations of haloperidol and reduced haloperidol. Several investigations on the prevalence of movement disorders among smokers have resulted from these findings.

Smoking and Parkinson's Disease

Nicotine causes significant releases of dopamine (Chesselet, 1984). Parkinsonism, moreover, is believed to be secondary to dopamine depletion in the substantia nigra (Miller, 1989). The current epidemiologic data suggest that smokers have a lower risk for developing Parkinson's disease than do nonsmokers (Nefzger, Quadfasel, & Karl, 1968; Kessler & Diamond, 1971; Kessler, 1972; Miller, 1989), though not all authors agree (Haack et al., 1981). In fact, nicotine has been found to induce tremors in normal individuals (Shiffman et al., 1983) and to exacerbate essential tremors (Marshall & Schnieden, 1966). Nevertheless, cessation of smoking has been reported to relieve the "restless-leg syndrome," albeit in only 1 patient (Mountifield, 1985).

Neuroleptic-induced parkinsonism has recently been studied in relation to smoking. Decina et al. (1990) found that smokers presented with significantly lower prevalence and severity of neuroleptic-induced parkinsonism than did nonsmokers. However, two other studies found no relation between smoking and neuroleptic-induced parkinsonism (Yassa et al., 1987; Menza et al., 1991).

Smoking and Tardive Dyskinesia

The relationship between tardive dyskinesia and smoking has been a topic of much debate. Both Binder et al. (1987) and Yassa et al. (1987) found a higher prevalence of tardive dyskinesia among smokers than among nonsmokers. But Yassa et al. (1987) noted that smokers were receiving higher neuroleptic dosages than nonsmokers, whereas Binder et al. (1987) found no difference in current neuroleptic dosages for smokers and nonsmokers. Kirch, Alho, and Wyatt (1988) showed not only that patients with tardive dyskinesia were more likely to be smokers but also that smokers with tardive dyskinesia had higher blood concentrations of nicotine and its metabolite, cotinine, than did smokers without tardive dyskinesia. On the other hand, two studies (Youssef & Waddington, 1987; Menza et al., 1991) found no relationship between smoking and tardive dyskinesia. However, Menza et al. (1991) found that akathisia was more prevalent among female smokers than among nonsmokers.

Clearly, the question of smoking as a factor in the development of movement disorders, particularly tardive dyskinesia, has not yet been settled.

References

Anderson, K., Fuxe, K., & Agnati, L. F. (1981). Effects of single injection of nicotine on the ascending dopamine pathways in the rat: evidence for increase of dopamine turnover in the mesostriatal and mesolimbic dopamine neurons. *Acta Physiol. Scand.* 112:345–7.

Binder, R. L., Kazamatsuri, H., Nishimura, T., & McNiel, D. E. (1987). Smoking and tardive dyskinesia. *Biol. Psychiatry* 22:1280–2.

Brandon, S., McClelland, H. A., & Protheroe, C. (1971). A study of facial dyskinesia in a mental hospital. *Br. J. Psychiatry* 118:171–84.

Chesselet, M. F. (1984). Presynaptic regulation of neurotransmitter release in the brain: facts and hypothesis. *Neuroscience* 12:347–75.

Decina, P., Caracci, G., Snadik, R., Berman, W., Mukherjee, S., & Scapicchio, P. (1990). Cigarette smoking and neuroleptic-induced parkinsonism. *Biol. Psychiatry* 28:502–8.

Gardos, G., Sokol, M., & Coel, J. O. (1976). Eye color and tardive dyskinesia. *Psychopharmacol. Bull.* 22:7–9.

Haack, D. G., Baumann, R. J., McKean, H. E., Jameson, H. D., & Turbek, J. A. (1981). Nicotine exposure and Parkinson disease. *Am. J. Epidemiol* 114:191–200.

Jann, M. W., Saklad, S. R., Ereshefsky, L., Richards, A. L., Harington, C. A., & Davis, C. M. (1986). Effects of smoking on haloperidol and reduced haloperidol plasma concentrations and haloperidol clearance. *Psychopharmacology* 90:468–70.

Jeste, D. V., Phelps, B. H., & Wyatt, R. J. (1982). Enzyme studies in tardive dyskinesia. II. Familial aspects. *J. Clin. Psychopharmacol.* 2:315–17.

Jeste, D. V., & Wyatt, R. J. (1982). *Understanding and Treating Tardive Dyskinesia.* New York: Guilford Press.

Kessler, I. I. (1972). Epidemiologic studies of Parkinson's disease: a community band survey. *Am. J. Epidemiol.* 96:242–54.

Kessler, I. I., & Diamond, K. L. (1971). Epidemiologic studies of Parkinson's disease. I. Smoking and Parkinson's disease. *Am. J. Epidemiol.* 94:16–25.

Kirch, D. G., Alho, A.-M., & Wyatt, R. J. (1988). Hypothesis: a nicotine–dopamine interaction linking smoking with Parkinson's disease and tardive dyskinesia. *Cell. Mol. Neurobiol.* 8:285–91.

Marshall, J., & Schnieden, H. (1966). Effect of adrenaline, noradrenaline, atropine and nicotine on some types of human tremor. *J. Neurol. Neurosurg. Psychiatry* 29:214–18.

Menza, M. A., Grossman, N., Van Horn, M., Cody, R., & Forman, N. (1991). Smoking and movement disorders in psychiatric patients. *Biol. Psychiatry* 30:109–15.

Miller, L. C. (1989). Recent developments in the study of the effects of cigarette smoking on clinical pharmacokinetics and clinical pharmaco-dynamics. *Clin. Pharmacokinet.* 17:90–108.

Mountifield, J. A. (1985). Restless leg syndrome relieved by cessation of smoking. *Can. Med. Assoc. J.* 133:426–7.

Nefzger, M. D., Quadfasel, F. A., & Karl, V. C. (1968). A retrospective study of smoking and Parkinson's disease. *Am. J. Epidemiol.* 88:149–58.

O'Callaghan, E., Larkin, C., Kinsella, A., & Waddington, J. L. (1990). Obstetric complications, the putative familial–sporadic distinction and tardive dyskinesia in schizophrenia. *Br. J. Psychiatry* 157:578–84.

Shiffman, S. M., Gritz, E. R., Maltese, J., Lee, M. A., Schnieder, N. G., & Jarvik, M. E. (1983). Effects of cigarette smoking and oral nicotine on hand tremor. *Clin. Pharmacol. Ther.* 33:800–5.

Stimmel, G. L., & Falloon, I. R. H. (1983). Chlorpromazine plasma levels, adverse effects, and tobacco smoking: case report. *J. Clin. Psychiatry* 44:420–2.

Swett, C. (1974). Drowsiness due to chlorpromazine in relation to cigarette smoking. *Arch. Gen. Psychiatry* 31:211–13.

Vinarova, E., Vinar, O., & Kalvach, Z. (1984). Smokers need higher doses of neuroleptic drugs. *Biol. Psychiatry* 19:1265–8.

Waddington, J. L. (1989). Schizophrenia, affective psychoses and other disorders treated with neuroleptic drugs: the enigma of tardive dyskinesia, its neurobiological determinants and the conflict of paradigms. *Int. Rev. Neurobiol.* 31:297–353.

Waddington, J. L., & Youssef, H. A. (1987). Familial predisposition both to tardive dyskinesia and to cognitive dysfunction in a large psychotic sibship. *Psychopharmacol. Bull.* 23:505–7.

Weinhold, P., Wegner, J. T., & Kane, J. M. (1981). Familial occurrence of tardive dyskinesia. *J. Clin. Psychiatry* 42:165–6.

Yassa, R., & Ananth, J. (1981). Familial tardive dyskinesia. *Am. J. Psychiatry* 138:1618–19.

Yassa, R., Lal, S., Korpassy, A., & Ally, J. (1987). Nicotine exposure and tardive dyskinesia. *Biol. Psychiatry* 22:67–72.

Youssef, H. A., & Waddington, J. L. (1987). Morbidity and mortality in tardive dyskinesia: associations in chronic schizophrenia. *Acta Psychiatr. Scand.* 75:74–7.

9

Neuroleptic Treatment and Tardive Dyskinesia

GEORGE GARDOS, M.D.,
and JONATHAN O. COLE, M.D.

Any reasonable, informed clinician will accept the overwhelming epidemiologic evidence implicating neuroleptic drugs in the causation of tardive dyskinesia, with the caveat that not every case that looks like tardive dyskinesia is neuroleptic-related. Spontaneous dyskinesia (Marsden, 1985; Casey, 1987) and dyskinesias induced by drugs other than neuroleptics, such as antihistamines, antidepressants, and metoclopramide, often are indistinguishable from tardive dyskinesia. As Marsden (1985) pointed out, the causative relationship implies either that neuroleptics induce tardive dyskinesia in individuals who otherwise would not develop it or that neuroleptics precipitate tardive dyskinesia in patients who already carry the substrate for development of tardive dyskinesia.

Patients exposed to neuroleptics differ regarding variables such as age at first neuroleptic exposure, time since the start of neuroleptic treatment, duration of neuroleptic treatment (i.e., actual time on neuroleptics), number and duration of neuroleptic-free intervals, number of neuroleptics used, amount of neuroleptic (i.e., total quantity delivered), average neuroleptic dosage, and maximum neuroleptic dosage. Other areas of interest include comparisons of exposures to high- and low-potency neuroleptics, the number of neuroleptics simultaneously prescribed, the route of administration (depot vs. oral), and different schedules, such as a dose once daily versus twice daily (BID), or doses as needed (PRN) (oral and/or intramuscular). Only adequate knowledge of the pathogenesis of tardive dyskinesia will enable us to decide which of these drug variables are of particular relevance to tardive dyskinesia. In the 15 years since we first addressed the issue of the relative importance of neuroleptic variables (Gardos, Cole, & LaBrie, 1977), although extensive research has been conducted, few definitive answers have emerged. We are far from being able to delineate precisely those features of neuroleptic treatment that pose the greatest risk for development of tardive dyskinesia.

In this chapter we shall review the available information concerning the commonly investigated neuroleptic variables.

Type of Neuroleptic

A common question raised by clinicians is whether or not one neuroleptic is less likely than another to induce tardive dyskinesia. ("Does thioridazine cause less tardive dyskinesia than haloperidol?"). A related issue is whether or not tardive dyskinesia in an individual patient is attributable to a particular neuroleptic ("Was Mrs. B's tardive dyskinesia caused by chlorpromazine?"). This problem is of great interest to patients and their families (not to mention attorneys) and has been previously discussed elsewhere (Cole, Gardos, & Schniebolk, 1986).

If a patient who has been exposed to only one neuroleptic develops tardive dyskinesia while on the drug, or within 1–2 months of drug discontinuation, the best clinical opinion will be that the drug has caused the tardive dyskinesia in that patient. Surprisingly, published reports have cited few such instances. In the early literature on tardive dyskinesia, reserpine was reported to have caused tardive dyskinesia in a few patients (Uhrbrand & Faurbye, 1960; Degkwitz, 1969; Wolf, 1973). Crane and Smeets (1974) mentioned 6 elderly patients treated only with thioridazine (3 patients), perphenazine (2 patients), or chlorpromazine (1 patient). Yassa and Dmitry (1983) added cases concerning only chlorpromazine (1 patient) and thioridazine (1 patient). However, Yassa et al. (1992), in a study of 58 patients in a geriatric psychiatry unit each treated with a single neuroleptic, reported that among 47 haloperidol patients, 14 (29.8%) developed tardive dyskinesia, and among 4 pimozide patients, 2 developed tardive dyskinesia, whereas no tardive dyskinesia developed among patients taking perphenazine (3 patients), chlorpromazine (2 patients), fluphenazine (1 patient), or thioridazine (1 patient). Information provided by one of the authors of the Borison et al. (1983) study allows us to infer that in their sample of 122 British geriatric patients each exposed to only a single neuroleptic, roughly 11 of 25 haloperidol patients developed tardive dyskinesia, as did 4 of 17 patients on promazine, 4 of 27 patients on chlorpromazine, 2 of 18 patients on prochlorperazine, 3 of 10 patients on trifluoperazine, and 3 of 10 patients on perphenazine-amitriptyline; however, none of the 13 patients on thioridazine developed tardive dyskinesia. In our own study of the course of dyskinesia (Cole et al., 1992), 11 of 104 patients were each exposed to only a single neuroleptic (2 to thioridazine, 2 to thiothixene, 2 to haloperidol, 2 to chlorpromazine, and 2 to trifluoperazine, with 1 patient on perphenazine only). One tardive dyskinesia patient was exposed only to amoxapine, an antidepressant with neuroleptic properties.

The Food and Drug Administration (FDA) receives reports of drug side effects from individual physicians and from drug companies, which obtain them from individual physicians. The numbers of cases of tardive dyskinesia reported for 1984 and their associated drugs were as follows: haloperidol (18 cases), trifluoperazine (11), thioridazine (9), amoxapine (6), molindone (4), fluphenazine (3), chlorpromazine (2), perphenazine-amitriptyline (2), metoclopramide (2), thiothixene (1), and loxapine (1). The FDA reports of tardive dyskinesia cases are of limited use (Cole et al., 1986), however, because accurate information regarding physicians' relative frequencies of prescribing the specific neuroleptics is not known, nor is it known why doctors would report particular cases of tardive dyskinesia to the FDA. Perhaps the primary value of reports of single cases of neuroleptic-associated tardive dyskinesia is to document that tardive dyskinesia can be induced by most, if not all, neuroleptic drugs.

Attempts have been made to correlate the specific pharmacologic activities of neuroleptics with the potential to induce movement disorders (Anden et al., 1970; Borison et al., 1983; Hyttel et al., 1985). Nevertheless, although differential affinities for dopamine-receptor subtypes, as well as for norepinephrine and β-adrenergic, muscarinic, and other receptors, may explain certain neuroleptic side effects (e.g., hypotension), they have not helped in predicting movement disorders (Miller & Jankovic, 1992).

A statistical approach has been taken by some investigators to demonstrate greater or lesser degrees of "tardive dyskinesia–inducing propensity" for specific neuroleptics. Smith, Strizich, and Klass (1978) found a negative correlation between the amount of thioridazine received over the preceding 9-year period and scores for dyskinesia among 103 chronic inpatients; a comparable positive correlation was found between the amount of fluphenazine received over the same period and the incidence of dyskinesia. Mukherjee et al. (1982), who studied 155 outpatients given neuroleptics for 1 year or longer, found positive correlations between measures of tardive dyskinesia and exposure to thiothixene, haloperidol, and fluphenazine, and negative correlations between low-potency neuroleptics and Abnormal Involuntary Movement Scale (AIMS) scores. We found that the degree of exposure to low-potency neuroleptics was positively correlated to the severity of dyskinesia, as was exposure to fluphenazine (Gardos et al., 1977). An apparently higher prevalence of tardive dyskinesia among depot-fluphenazine-treated patients was found by Klawans, Tanner, and Goetz (1988). Gibson (1981) found the risk for developing tardive dyskinesia among patients on depot fluphenazine to be

5% at 1 year and 40% after 11 years. On the other hand, Yassa, Iskandan, and Alley (1988) did not find a significantly greater prevalence of tardive dyskinesia among depot-fluphenazine-treated patients.

The data regarding thioridazine are also conflicting, compared with those for patients taking other oral neuroleptics. For example, in a comparison of mild and severe forms of tardive dyskinesia, we found that patients with severe cases were much less likely ever to have been exposed to thioridazine (Gardos et al., 1987). And yet, in a series of 125 patients, thioridazine was responsible for 15 cases of tardive dyskinesia, second only to haloperidol among the drugs causing movement disorders (Miller & Jankovic, 1990). In our study of the course of dyskinesia (Cole et al., 1992), we recorded the "primary" antipsychotic as that given at least 80% of the time. Trifluoperazine, thioridazine, haloperidol, thiothixene, chlorpromazine, and fluphenazine accounted for the majority of "primary" neuroleptics. Inasmuch as these six neuroleptics were likely to be those most frequently employed in the Boston area, our data failed to identify any single neuroleptic associated with a higher prevalence of tardive dyskinesia. These six were also the neuroleptics that patients were receiving at the time dyskinesia emerged (Cole et al., 1992). Unfortunately, therefore, these findings simply reflect prescription practices and probably shed little light on the relative vulnerability to tardive dyskinesia.

Gerlach and Casey (1988) discussed the hypothesis that the neuroleptics that produce parkinsonian symptoms and suppress tardive dyskinesia also induce greater rebound exacerbation of tardive dyskinesia and carry greater risk for the development of tardive dyskinesia. According to that hypothesis, higher potency neuroleptics with more potent antidopaminergic effects would be more likely to cause tardive dyskinesia than would low-potency neuroleptics. Gunne and Barany (1979) studied *Cebus* monkeys with tardive dyskinesia and found that haloperidol (0.05 mg/kg/d) chlorpromazine (1 mg/kg/d) caused more initial dystonia, greater initial suppression of tardive dyskinesia, and longer rebound aggravation of tardive dyskinesia than did either thioridazine (1 mg/kg/d) or clozapine (1 mg/kg/d). Also supporting that hypothesis was a 4-week clinical study in which haloperidol (5.25 mg/d) evoked more parkinsonism and more withdrawal dyskinesia than did thioridazine (225 mg/d) (Gerlach & Simmelsgaard, 1978). In a second study by Gerlach and Simmelsgaard (1986), neither haloperidol nor perphenazine produced greater rebound dyskinesia than did comparable dosages of the low-potency neuroleptic chlorprothixene.

The strongest claims for a reduced propensity to induce tardive dyskinesia have been made for the newer, atypical neuroleptics: sulpiride and clozapine.

Uncontrolled studies and worldwide observations have revealed only a small number of patients receiving sulpiride who have developed tardive dyskinesia (Alberts, François, & Josserand, 1985). The case is even stronger for clozapine. Of the more than 15,000 patients treated with clozapine in the United States, the rate of development of tardive dyskinesia has been negligible. Occasional patients in Europe (Doepp & Buddeberg, 1975) and the United States have apparently developed tardive dyskinesia attributable to clozapine, but the incidence is still extremely low (Kane et al., 1992). Patients with preexisting tardive dyskinesia who are switched to clozapine often continue to show tardive dyskinesia (Bajulaiye & Addonizio, 1992), though many others manifest remission (Lieberman et al., 1989). Risperidone is a recently introduced atypical neuroleptic that may reduce the severity of already existing tardive dyskinesia and may possibly be less likely to lead to the development of tardive dyskinesia (Chouinard et al., 1993).

The foregoing review suggests that the more widely used neuroleptics appear to cause tardive dyskinesia more often – no great discovery. Although depot fluphenazine seemed to involve greater risk, the relevant studies did not control for compliance, plasma concentrations of neuroleptics, or population differences. Also, certain drugs marketed as antidepressants, such as amoxapine and perphenazine-amitriptyline, and such antiemetics as metoclopramide or prochlorperazine have neuroleptic properties and may induce tardive dyskinesia.

The only tentative answer to the basic clinical questions raised earlier is that clozapine almost certainly (and sulpiride and risperidone possibly) causes less tardive dyskinesia than other neuroleptics. As far as the classic neuroleptics are concerned, we cannot state that any single neuroleptic has a lesser or greater propensity to cause tardive dyskinesia.

Dosage and Duration of Treatment

Common sense would suggest that if neuroleptics are "bad" in terms of causing tardive dyskinesia, then more neuroleptic treatment is worse, and less is better. One might therefore predict a positive correlation between neuroleptic dosage and the incidence of tardive dyskinesia. But the duration of neuroleptic treatment must also be a key variable, for, by definition, tardive dyskinesia occurs late in neuroleptic treatment. Although the earliest-onset case of tardive dyskinesia was reported after only 3 months of neuroleptic treatment (Chouinard & Jones, 1979; Fleischhauer et al., 1985), tardive dyskinesia typically is recognized after 2 years or more of neuroleptic treatment (Crane, 1973). In our long-term study of the course of dyskinesia, for instance, the onset of tardive dyskinesia occurred after an average of 59 months of neuroleptic treatment (Cole et al., 1992). Just how the different patterns of neuroleptic use alter the risk for development of tardive dyskinesia is still unknown. Additional factors that increase the unpredictability of the relationship between neuroleptic exposure and tardive dyskinesia include the following: (1) neuroleptic dosage at the time of tardive dyskinesia assessment, which may correlate negatively with ratings, because of the neuroleptic's effect of suppressing tardive dyskinesia; (2) medication noncompliance, which is likely to exert at least a short-term effect on the severity of tardive dyskinesia; (3) interindividual variability in the pharmacokinetic parameters of neuroleptics, as demonstrated by large variances in the plasma concentrations of neuroleptics for the same dosages, which is bound to dilute whatever may be the true relationship between neuroleptic dosage and tardive dyskinesia.

The relevant literature bears out what the foregoing discussion would predict: the difficulty of demonstrating a powerful effect of neuroleptic exposure on the prevalence of tardive dyskinesia. For example, Kane and Smith (1982) reviewed the prevalences and risk factors for tardive dyskinesia and found 18 studies that had explored the relationship between the cumulative dose and the prevalence of tardive dyskinesia. Only 4 of the 18 studies reported a significant positive association.

A few controlled studies have compared different neuroleptic dosages. For example, Kane et al. (1986b), in a prospective double-blind study, compared the usual doses (12.5–50 mg) and low doses (1.25–5.0 mg) of depot fluphenazine given every 2 weeks. After 52 weeks, the low-dose group showed significantly fewer early signs of tardive dyskinesia. Marder, Van Putten, and Mintz (1987) evaluated the effectiveness and side effects of conventional doses (25 mg) and low doses (5 mg) of fluphenazine every 2 weeks, using a double-blind comparison. Although at 3 and 6 months the rates of akathisia were significantly higher among the conventional-dose group, the degrees of dyskinesia did not differ significantly for the two groups at any time during the 2 years of observations. Hogarty et al. (1988), in a comparison of standard doses (average 25 mg) and minimal doses (average 3–8 mg) of fluphenazine every 2 weeks, found significant differences in the first year for extrapyramidal symptoms (less severe on minimal doses), but no significant differences regarding dyskinesia.

Innovative treatment strategies devised to reduce neuroleptic exposure without substantially increasing psychotic relapse rates have been expected to reduce the rate of development of tardive dyskinesia. To date, studies of intermittent or targeted neuroleptic treatment have yielded short-term findings of fewer early signs of tardive dyskinesia among the groups given intermittent or targeted neuroleptic treatment, as compared with those receiving continuous neuroleptic treatment (Carpenter, Heinrichs, & Hanlan, 1987; Herz & Glazer, 1988; Jolley et al., 1989). However, longer follow-up will be needed to establish the validity of those early differences.

Drug holidays that involve interruption of neuroleptic treatment, though usually for only brief periods of days or weeks, have lost favor. It was discovered that they might increase the risk for development of tardive dyskinesia, as well as for psychotic relapse (Jeste et al., 1979; Goldman & Luchins, 1984).

Other than total (cumulative) neuroleptic exposure, the dosage variables that may have a bearing on the development of tardive dyskinesia and/or the appearance of tardive dyskinesia include the maximum neuroleptic dosage and the dosage at the time of assessment. The maximum neuroleptic dosage (usually expressed in chlorpromazine equivalents and given for at least 1 month) was found in some studies to be correlated with the development of tardive dyskinesia (Crane, 1974; Smith et al., 1978), whereas in other studies no significant association was found (Jus et al., 1976b; Gardos et al., 1977; Perényi, Norman, & Burrows, 1992). The negative correlation between current neuroleptic dosage and tardive dyskinesia, expected on the basis of tardive dyskinesia suppression, was found in only a few studies (Richardson et al., 1984); meanwhile, relevant review articles have concluded that no clear association can be found between current neuroleptic dosages and tardive dyskinesia (Kane & Smith, 1982; Kane et al., 1992).

It has been suggested that measurements of plasma concentrations of neuroleptics, inasmuch as they circumvent the variance due to individual differences in absorption and metabolism of the drugs, may bring us one step closer to the true association between neuroleptic dosage and tardive dyskinesia. However, a recent American Psychiatric Association survey (Kane et al., 1992) found that whereas only two studies had reported a significant positive association between plasma concentrations of neuroleptics and the presence of tardive dyskinesia, five relevant studies had shown no significant correlation. At the present time, it is reasonable to conclude that higher plasma concentrations of neuroleptics do not appear to pose a major risk factor for development of tardive dyskinesia.

In summary, the literature reveals a weak positive association between neuroleptic exposure and development of tardive dyskinesia, insofar as a meta-analysis shows more studies with a positive, rather than negative, correlation, with a sizable proportion of studies showing no association at all. Yet the patterns of neuroleptic treatment in individual patients that would reveal how neuroleptics are distributed over time have never been studied systematically. Moreover, it remains unclear whether or not there is a dosage threshold below which tardive dyskinesia does not develop, no matter how long the exposure continues. For instance, is thioridazine at 50 mg/d sufficient to produce tardive dyskinesia if prescribed long enough? At the other end of the spectrum, we do not know if brief exposures to very high dosages pose greater risks for tardive dyskinesia than do moderate dosages over longer periods.

Age and Diagnosis

Before concluding our discussion of neuroleptics and the development of tardive dyskinesia, we must consider the interactions of neuroleptics with two other factors: age and diagnosis.

Age

Advanced age is the most consistently reported risk factor for the development of tardive dyskinesia (Kane & Smith, 1982; Saltz et al., 1989). Older patients, for example, tend to develop tardive dyskinesia after shorter neuroleptic exposures than do younger patients (Jus et al., 1976a; Jeste, Jeste, & Wyatt, 1983; Kane, Woerner, & Borenstein, 1986a). Barnes and colleagues (Kidger et al., 1980; Barnes, Rossor, & Tremer, 1983) suggested that neuroleptic-treated patients in their sixth decade are at the highest risk for developing orofacial dyskinesia. Toenniessen, Casey, and McFarland (1985) found that in elderly patients the maximal risk for development of tardive dyskinesia was seen during the first 2 years of neuroleptic treatment. Interactions between age and neuroleptic treatment partly account for the large variability in the reported prevalences of tardive dyskinesia when statistical comparisons are not controlled for age.

Diagnosis

Patients suffering from affective disorder appear to be more vulnerable to the development of tardive dyskinesia (Kane et al., 1986a; Gardos & Casey, 1984). That increased vulnerability seems to hold for both bipolar patients (Mukherjee et al., 1986) and unipolar patients (Cole et al., 1992). Gardos and Cole (1986), who reviewed prevalence studies in which (1) tardive dyskinesia was assessed separately for different diagnostic groups and (2) tardive dyskinesia patients were matched with controls who did not have tardive dyskinesia, found that affective disorder, organic mental disorder, and mental retardation posed greater risks than did schizophrenia for development of tardive dyskinesia. Among patients with schizophrenia, tardive dyskinesia has been found to be more common among patients with negative symptoms (Jeste et al., 1984; Waddington et al., 1987), although that finding is not unanimous and may be weakened by confounding variables such as depression or bradykinesia (Kane et al., 1992). As for alcohol abuse, a recent study implicated it as an independent risk factor for development of tardive dyskinesia (Dixon et al., 1992).

Because neuroleptic treatment strategies differ greatly for patients with different diagnoses (Gardos & Cole, 1986), the relationship between the diagnosis and the development of tardive dyskinesia is not a simple one. Schizophrenics tend to be given higher neuroleptic dosages for longer periods, and more nearly continuously, than are patients with affective disorder (Cole et al., 1992). The use of neuroleptics for patients with organic mental disorders and mental retardation has been decreasing (Gardos & Cole, 1986). Indeed, it appears to be very much lower than the rate of neuroleptic use for schizophrenia. The more extensive use of neuroleptics for schizophrenic patients than for those in other diagnostic groups suggests that schizophrenia may confer resistance to the development of tardive dyskinesia. It is conceivable that such resistance may apply to only a minority of schizophrenic patients: those resistant to antipsychotic drugs as well as to the development of tardive dyskinesia. Whether or not differential sensitivity to neuroleptics across diagnostic groups can be demonstrated in future studies, it seems possible that an interaction between psychiatric diagnosis and exposure to neuroleptics is involved in determining the risk for tardive dyskinesia.

Interactions

The foregoing data suggest that the risk for development of tardive dyskinesia during neuroleptic treatment is affected by both age and diagnosis. Triple or higher-order interactions involving neuroleptics and other risk factors may, nevertheless, be involved. For instance, patients with affective disorder tend to be older and predominantly female, usually being started on neuroleptics at more advanced ages and receiving neuroleptic treatment with more interruptions and at lower dosages, as compared with schizophrenics. The relevant epidemiologic studies have rarely, if ever, controlled for all these variables. Therefore, the indications that patients with affective disorder tend to develop tardive dyskinesia more readily than do schizophrenic patients, as suggested by the studies of Yassa, Ghadirian, and Schwartz (1983), Yassa et al. (1992), and our own group (Cole et al., 1992), may need to be interpreted as showing the interplay of several risk factors, particularly age, diagnosis, and neuroleptic exposure, and possibly female gender as well.

Conclusion

Somewhat like happiness – which is readily understood until one is asked to define it – the apparently straightforward, causative relationship between neuroleptic treatment and development of tardive dyskinesia unravels under scrutiny. The foregoing literature review has yielded few clear answers and raised many new questions. The thrust of this presentation is not to view neuroleptic treatment as a univariate risk factor producing tardive dyskinesia in proportion to age and neuroleptic type, dosage, and duration, but to consider the impact of neuroleptic treatment in a multivariate interactive system, where its propensity to cause tardive dyskinesia can be modified by patient variables.

References

Alberts, J. L. François, F., & Josserand, F. (1985). Etude des effets secondaires rapportés à l'occasion de traitements par dogmatil. *Sem. Hop. Paris* 61:1352–7.

Anden, N. E., Butcher, S. G., Corrodi, H., Fuxe, K., & Ungerstedt, U. (1970). Receptor activity and turnover of dopamine and noradrenaline after neuroleptics. *Eur. J. Pharmacol.* 11:303–14.

Bajulaiye, R., & Addonizio, G. (1992). Clozapine in the treatment of psychosis in an 82-year-old woman with tardive dyskinesia (letter to the editor). *J. Clin. Pharmacol.* 12:364–5.

Barnes, T. R. E., Rossor, M., & Tremer, T. (1983). A comparison of purposeless movements in psychiatric patients treated with antipsychotic drugs and normal individuals. *J. Neurol. Neurosurg. Psychiatry* 46:540–6.

Borison, R., Mitri, A., Blowers, A., & Diamond, B. I. (1983). Antipsychotic drug actions: clinical, biochemical and pharmacological evidence for site specificity of action. *Clin. Neuropharmacol.* 6:137–49.

Carpenter, W. T., Heinrichs, D. W., & Hanlan, T. E. (1987). A comparative trial of pharmacologic strategies in schizophrenia. *Am. J. Psychiatry* 144:1466–70.

Casey, D. E. (1987). Tardive dyskinesia. In *Psychopharmacology. The Third Generation of Progress,* ed. H. Y. Meltzer, pp. 1411–19. New York: Raven Press.

Chouinard, G., & Jones, B. D. (1979). Early onset of tardive dyskinesia: case report. *Am. J. Psychiatry* 136:1323–4.

Chouinard, G., Jones, B., Remington, G., Bloom, D., Addington, D., MacEwan, G. W., Labelle, A., Beauclair, L., & Arnett, W. (1993). A Canadian multicenter placebo-controlled study of fixed doses of risperidone and haloperidol in the treatment of chronic schizophrenic patients. *S. J. Clin. Psychopharmacology* 13:25–40.

Cole, J. O., Gardos, G., Boling, L. A., Marbey, D., Haskell, D., & Moore, P. (1992). Early dyskinesia – vulnerability. *Psychopharmacology* 107:503–10.

Cole, J. O., Gardos, G., & Schniebolk, S. (1986). Differences in incidence of tardive dyskinesia with different neuroleptics. In *Tardive Dyskinesia and Neuroleptics: From Dogma to Reason,* ed. D. E. Casey & G. Gardos, pp. 34–54. Washington, DC: American Psychiatric Press.

Crane, G. E. (1973). Persistent dyskinesia. *Br. J. Psychiatry* 122:395–405.

Crane, G. E. (1974). Factors predisposing to drug-induced neurologic effects. In *The Phenothiazines and Structurally Related Drugs,* ed. I. S. Forest, C. J. Carr, & E. Usdin, pp. 269–79. New York: Raven Press.

Crane, G. E., & Smeets, R. (1974). Tardive dyskinesia and drug therapy in geriatric patients. *Arch. Gen. Psychiatry* 30:341–8.

Degkwitz, R. (1969). Extrapyramidal motor disorders following long-term treatment with neuroleptic drugs. In *Psychotropic Drugs and Dysfunction of the Basal Ganglia,* ed. G. E. Crane & R. Gardner, Jr. U.S. Public Health Service publication no. 1938. Washington, DC: U.S. Government Printing Office.

Dixon, L., Weiden, P. J., Haas, G., Sweeney, J., & Frances, R. J. (1992). Increased tardive dyskinesia in alcohol-abusing schizophrenic patients. *Compr. Psychiatry* 33:121–2.

Doepp, S., & Buddeberg, C. (1975). Extrapyramidale Symptome unter Clozapine. *Nervenarzt* 46:589–90.

Fleischhauer, J., Kocher, R. Hobi, V., & Gilsdorf, U. (1985). Prevalence of tardive dyskinesia in a chronic population. In *Dyskinesia – Research and Treatment (Psychopharmacology Suppl. 2),* ed. D. E. Casey, T. N. Chase, A. V. Christensen, & J. Gerlach, pp. 162–72. Berlin: Springer-Verlag.

Gardos, G., & Casey, D. E. (eds.) (1984). *Tardive Dyskinesia and Affective Disorders.* Washington, DC: American Psychiatric Press.

Gardos, G., & Cole, J. O. (1986). Neuroleptics and tardive dyskinesia in nonschizophrenic patients. In *Tardive Dyskinesia and Neuroleptics: From Dogma to Reason,* ed. D. E. Casey & G. Gardos, pp. 56–74. Washington, DC: American Psychiatric Press.

Gardos, G., Cole, J. O., & LaBrie, R. (1977). Drug variables in the etiology of tardive dyskinesia: application of discriminant function analysis. *Prog. Neuropsychopharmacol.* 1:147–55.

Gardos, G., Cole, J. O., Schniebolk, S., & Salomon, M. (1987). Comparison of severe and mild tardive dyskinesia: implications for etiology. *J. Clin. Psychiatry* 48:359–62.

Gerlach, J., & Casey, D. C. (1988). Tardive dyskinesia. *Acta Psychiatr. Scand.* 77:369–78.

Gerlach, J., & Simmelsgaard, H. (1978). Tardive dyskinesia during and following treatment with haloperidol, haloperidol and biperiden, thioridazine, and clozapine. *Psychopharmacology* 59:105–12.

Gerlach, J., & Simmelsgaard, H. (1986). Effect of chlorprothixene, haloperidol, and perphenazine in tardive dyskinesia and parkinsonism. *Psychopharmacology* 90:423–9.

Gibson, A. C. (1981). Incidence of tardive dyskinesia in patients receiving depot neuroleptic injections. *Acta Psychiatr. Scand. (Suppl.)* 63:111–16.

Goldman, M. B., & Luchins, D. J. (1984). Intermittent neuroleptic therapy and tardive dyskinesia: a literature review. *Hosp. Community Psychiatry* 35:1215–19.

Gunne, L.-M., & Barany, S. (1979). A monitoring test for the liability of neuroleptic drugs to induce tardive dyskinesia. *Psychopharmacology* 63:195–8.

Herz, M. I., & Glazer, W. (1988). Intermittent medication in schizophrenia – preliminary results. *Schizophr. Res.* 1:224–5.

Hogarty, G. B., McEvoy, J. P., Munetz, M., DiBarry, A. L., Barone, P., Cather, R., Cooley, S. J., Ulrich, R. F., Carter, M., & Madonia, M. J. (1988). Dose of fluphenazine, familial expressed emotion, and outcome in schizophrenia. *Arch. Gen. Psychiatry* 45:797–805.

Hyttel, J., Larsen, J.-J., Christensen, A. V., & Arnt, J. (1985). Receptor binding profile of neuroleptics. In *Dyskinesia – Research and Treatment (Psychopharmacology Suppl. 2)*, ed. D. E. Casey, T. N. Chase, A. V. Christensen, & J. Gerlach, pp. 9–18. Berlin: Springer-Verlag.

Jeste, D. V., Jeste, S. D., & Wyatt, R. J. (1983). Reversible tardive dyskinesia: implications for therapeutic strategy and prevention of tardive dyskinesia. In *New Directions in Tardive Dyskinesia Research*, ed. J. Bannet & R. H. Belmaker, pp. 34–48. Basel: S. Karger.

Jeste, D. V., Karson, C. M., Iager, A. C., Bigelow, L. B., & Wyatt, R. J. (1984). Association of abnormal involuntary movements and negative symptoms. *Psychopharmacol. Bull.* 20:380–1.

Jeste, D. V., Potkin, S. G., Sinha, S., Feder, S., & Wyatt, R. J. (1979). Tardive dyskinesia, reversible and persistent. *Arch. Gen. Psychiatry* 36:585–90.

Jolley, A. G., Hirsh, S. R., McRink, A., & Mauchauda, R. (1989). Trial of brief intermittent neuroleptic prophylaxis for selected schizophrenic outpatients: clinical outcome at one year follow-up. *Br. Med. J.* 298:985–90.

Jus, A., Pineau, R., Lachance, R., Pelchat, G., Jus, K., Pires, P., & Villeneuve, R. (1976a) Epidemiology of tardive dyskinesia. Part I. *Dis. Nerv. Syst.* 37:210–14.

Jus, A., Pineau, R., Lachance, R., Pelchat, G., Jus, K., Pires, P., & Villeneuve, R., (1976b). Epidemiology of tardive dyskinesia. Part II. *Dis. Nerv. Syst.* 37:257–61.

Kane, J. M., Jeste, D. V., Barnes, T. R. E., Casey, D. E., Cole, J. O., Davis, J. M., & Gualteri, C. T. (1992). *Tardive Dyskinesia: A Task Force Report of the American Psychiatric Association*, pp. 61–102. Washington, DC: American Psychiatric Association.

Kane, J. M., & Smith, J. M. (1982). Tardive dyskinesia: prevalence and risk factors 1959 to 1979. *Arch. Gen. Psychiatry* 39:473–81.

Kane, J. M., Woerner, M., & Borenstein, M. (1986a). Integrating incidence and prevalence of tardive dyskinesia. *Psychopharmacol. Bull.* 22:254–8.

Kane, J. M., Woerner, M., Sarantakos, S., Kinon, B., & Lieberman, J. (1986b). Do low dose neuroleptics prevent or ameliorate tardive dyskinesia? In *Tardive Dyskinesia and Neuroleptics: From Dogma to Reason*, ed. D. E. Casey & G. Gardos, pp. 100–7. Washington, DC: American Psychiatric Press.

Kidger, T., Barnes, T. R. E., Rossor, M., & Tremer, T. (1980). Subsyndromes of tardive dyskinesia. *Psychol. Med.* 10:513–20.

Klawans, H. L., Tanner, C. M., & Goetz, C. G. (1988). Epidemiology and pathophysiology of tardive dyskinesia. In *Advances in Neurology*, vol. 49, ed. J. Jankovic & E. Tolosa, pp. 185–97. New York: Raven Press.

Lieberman, J. A., Saltz, B. L., Johns, C. A., Pollack, S., & Kane, J. M. (1989). Clozapine effects on tardive dyskinesia. *Psychopharmacol. Bull.* 25:57–62.

Marder, S. R., Van Putten, T., & Mintz, J. (1987). Low- and conventional-dose maintenance therapy with fluphenazine decanoate: two-year outcome. *Arch. Gen. Psychiatry* 44:518–21.

Marsden, C. M. (1985). Is tardive dyskinesia a unique disorder? In *Dyskinesia: Research and Treatment*, ed. D. E. Casey, T. N. Chase, & J. Gerlach, pp. 64–71. Berlin: Springer-Verlag.

Miller, L. G., & Jankovic, J. (1990). Neurologic approach to drug-induced movement disorders in 125 patients. *South Med. J.* 83:525–32.

Miller, L. G., & Jankovic, J. (1992). Drug-induced movement disorders: an overview. In *Movement Disorders in Neurology and Neuropsychiatry,* ed. A. B. Joseph & R. R. Young, pp. 5–32. Boston: Blackwell Scientific.

Mukherjee, S., Rosen, A. M., Caracci, G., & Shukla, S. (1986). Persistent tardive dyskinesia in bipolar patients. *Arch. Gen. Psychiatry* 43:342–6.

Mukherjee, S., Rosen, A., Cardenas, C., Varva, V., & Olarte, S., (1982). Tardive dyskinesia in psychiatric outpatients. *Arch. Gen. Psychiatry* 39:466–9.

Perenyi, A., Norman, T., & Burrows, G. D. (1992). Relationship of symptomatology of schizophrenia and tardive dyskinesia. *Eur. Neuropsychopharmacol.* 2:51–5.

Richardson, M. A., Pass, R., Craig, T. J., & Vickers, E. (1984). Factors influencing the prevalence and severity of tardive dyskinesia. *Psychopharmacol. Bull.* 20:33–8.

Saltz, B. L., Kane, J. M., Woerner, M. G., Lieberman, J. A., Aliro, J. M. J., Blank, K., Kahaner, K., & Foley, K. (1989). Prospective study of tardive dyskinesia in the elderly. *Psychopharmacol. Bull.* 25:52–6.

Smith, R., Strizich, M., & Klass, D. (1978). Drug history in tardive dyskinesia. *Am. J. Psychiatry* 135:1402–3.

Toenniessen, L. M., Casey, D. E., & McFarland, B. H. (1985). Tardive dyskinesia in the aged. *Arch. Gen. Psychiatry* 42:278–84.

Uhrbrand, L., & Faurbye, A. (1960). Reversible and irreversible dyskinesia after treatment with perphenazine, chlorpromazine, reserpine and electroconvulsive therapy. *Psychopharmacology* 1:408–18.

Waddington, J. L., Youssef, H. A., Dolphin, C., & Kinsella, A. (1987). Cognitive dysfunction, negative symptoms and tardive dyskinesia in schizophrenia. *Arch. Gen. Psychiatry* 44:907–12.

Wolf, S. M. (1973). Reserpine: cause and treatment of oral-facial dyskinesia. *Bull. Los Angeles Neurol. Soc.* 38:80–4.

Yassa, R., & Dmitry, R. (1983). Single phenothiazines and tardive dyskinesia. *J. Clin. Psychiatry* 44:223–4.

Yassa, R., Ghadirian, A. M., & Schwartz, G. (1983). Prevalence of tardive dyskinesia in affective disorder patients. *J. Clin. Psychiatry* 44:410–12.

Yassa, R., Iskandan, H., & Alley, R. (1988). The prevalence of tardive dyskinesia in fluphenazine-treated patients. *J. Clin. Psychopharmacology* 8:17S–19S.

Yassa, R., Nastase, C., Dupont, D., & Thibeau, M. K. (1992). Tardive dyskinesia in elderly psychiatry patients: a 5-year study. *Am. J. Psychiatry* 149:1206–11.

10

Anticholinergic Drugs as Factors in the Development of Tardive Dyskinesia

RAMZY YASSA, M.D., and N. P. V. NAIR, M.D.

As discussed elsewhere in this book, several neurotransmitter systems have been implicated in the development of tardive dyskinesia. The most consistently cited abnormality is a disturbance in the dopaminergic–cholinergic balance at the nigrostriatal level (Klawans, 1973; Berger & Dunner, 1985). According to that hypothesis, dopaminergic overactivity can lead to an imbalance between dopamine and acetylcholine in the nigrostriatum and consequently can lead to the development of tardive dyskinesia (Klawans, 1973).

Since the early descriptions of tardive dyskinesia, anticholinergic drugs have been reported to be ineffective for treatment of this condition (Jeste & Wyatt, 1982). Indeed, that lack of efficacy has been considered an important diagnostic aspect of the condition (Jeste & Wyatt, 1982). In the ensuing years, two claims relating to increasing use of antiparkinsonian medications vis-à-vis tardive dyskinesia have been made:

- Antiparkinsonian medications increase the risk for development of tardive dyskinesia (Klawans, 1973).
- Antiparkinsonian medications may aggravate existing tardive dyskinesia (Chouinard, DeMontigny, & Annable, 1979).

To test those claims, we have reviewed the pertinent literature, seeking to discern the importance of prescribing antiparkinsonian medications for patients with tardive dyskinesia and the effects of such drugs on tardive dyskinesia. This review does not deal with animal models.

Do Anticholinergic Drugs Increase the Risk for Tardive Dyskinesia?

Klawans, Goetz, and Perlik (1980) recommended avoidance of anticholinergic drugs, because those medications potentiate anew the development of tardive dyskinesia. Klawans (1973) had suggested that the incidence of tardive dyskinesia would be greater among patients receiving both neuroleptics and anticholinergics than among patients receiving neuroleptics alone.

The most convincing evidence for a higher incidence of tardive dyskinesia would be direct observation of this side effect during the course of anticholinergic treatments. Such drugs have been part of the treatment for Parkinson's disease since the 1940s (Nomoto, Thompson, & Sheehy, 1987).

Birket-Smith (1974) described 6 elderly women who had never received neuroleptics but who developed buccolingual and choreoathetoid movements while receiving benztropine for treatment of their parkinsonism. The movements disappeared after discontinuation of benztropine. Warne and Gubbay (1979) and Nomoto et al. (1987) described the development of tardive dyskinesia in patients treated with anticholinergic drugs alone. The related movements disappeared after the anticholinergic drugs were discontinued, only to reappear upon provocation (Warne & Gubbay, 1979).

In addition, some antihistaminic drugs with anticholinergic properties (Smith & Domino, 1980) have been reported to cause sporadic tardive dyskinesia of the orofacial type (Davis, 1975; Thacht, Chase, & Basma, 1975); subsequent withdrawal of those medications led to disappearance of the movement disorders.

The literature also contains reports on the anticholinergic activities of certain antidepressants (Yassa, Camille, & Belzile, 1987). The rule has been that the movement disorder will disappear after discontinuation of the antidepressant (Yassa et al., 1987). Although some patients have developed tardive dyskinesia after using a medication with anticholinergic properties, such cases have been sporadic, occurring mainly in older patients, and the tardive dyskinesia usually has disappeared once the offending agent has been discontinued. On the other hand, 30–80% of patients treated with L-dopa, a dopamine agonist, can develop movement disorders (Bédard et al., 1992).

Another way of testing whether or not anticholinergic drugs increase the incidence of tardive dyskinesia is to measure total anticholinergic intake for patients with and without the condition. Theoretically, tardive dyskinesia patients should have received more anticholinergic drugs than patients without tardive dyskinesia. However, as shown in Table 10.1, more studies have shown negative (11) rather than positive (5) results. Some authors (Mallya, Jose, & Brig, 1977) found tardive dyskinesia patients to have had longer durations of exposure to anticholinergic drugs than patients without tardive dyskinesia, although Perris, Dimitrijevic, and Jacobsson (1979) found a significant positive correlation between patients' total tardive dyskinesia scores and their total amounts of anticholinergic drugs.

Table 10.1. *Discussions of how anticholinergics affect the development of tardive dyskinesia (TD)*

Total anticholinergic intake	
Increased risk for TD (n = 5)	No increased risk for TD (n = 11)
Mallya et al. (1977)	Jus et al. (1976)
Perris et al. (1979)	Gardos et al. (1977, 1980)
Chien et al. (1980)	Simpson et al. (1978)
Itil et al. (1981)	Doongaji et al. (1982)
Yassa et al. (1992)	Branchey & Branchey (1984)
	Yassa (1985, 1988)
	Waddington & Youssef (1986)
	Rao et al. (1987)
Current anticholinergic intake	
Higher drug concentrations in TD patients (n = 12)	Drug concentrations unchanged (n = 21)
Perris et al. (1979)	Kennedy et al. (1971)
Crane (1980)	Asnis et al. (1977)
Perenyi & Arato (1980)	Gardos et al. (1977)
Ezrin-Waters et al. (1981)	Bell & Smith (1978)
Itil et al. (1981)	Simpson et al. (1978)
Barnes et al. (1983)	Chouinard et al. (1979)
Yassa et al. (1983)	Wojeik et al. (1980)
Greil et al. (1984)	Rey et al. (1981)
Holden et al. (1984)	McCreadie et al. (1982)
Kulhanek et al. (1984)	Branchey & Branchey (1984)
Fleishhauer et al. (1985)	Chacko et al. (1985)
Kolakowska et al. (1985)	Kok & Christopher (1985)
	Ramsay & Millard (1985)
	Waddington & Youssef (1986)
	Williams et al. (1986)
	Holden (1987)
	Morgenstern et al. (1987)
	Rao et al. (1987)
	Yassa & Nair (1988)
	Altamura et al. (1990)
	Sramek et al. (1991)

A third avenue for testing the hypothesis that the incidence of tardive dyskinesia is increased by the use of anticholinergic drugs would involve finding higher rates of use of these medications in prospective studies. Indeed, all prospective studies published to date (Kane et al., 1984; Chouinard et al., 1986; Imada et al., 1991; Saltz et al., 1991) have found that patients who develop parkinsonian side effects are more prone to subsequent development

of tardive dyskinesia. However, their conclusions as to the use of anticholinergic drugs differ. For example, Kane et al. (1984) found a high rate of
use of anticholinergics among patients with tardive dyskinesia, as compared
with patients without tardive dyskinesia. Chouinard et al. (1986) found the
use of anticholinergic medications particularly important in brain-damaged
patients, whereas Imada et al. (1991) and Saltz et al. (1991) found no difference between patients with and those without tardive dyskinesia.

Thus, at present, the evidence is unconvincing that anticholinergic drugs
increase the incidence of tardive dyskinesia.

Do Anticholinergic Drugs Uncover or Aggravate Tardive Dyskinesia?

Some authors have said that the use of anticholinergic drugs may uncover
tardive dyskinesia in neuroleptic-treated patients with no prior clinical evidence of tardive dyskinesia. Kiloh, Smith, and Williams (1973) described
3 patients who presented with tardive dyskinesia manifestations that were
subsequently suppressed by neuroleptics; when an antiparkinsonian medication was added, tardive dyskinesia reappeared, only to disappear again
after discontinuation of the anticholinergic drug. West and Newgreen
(1979) described a patient who experienced marked choreiform symptoms
after a mix-up in medication; benztropine had accidentally been substituted
for haloperidol.

Fifteen challenge studies that tested the dopaminergic–cholinergic paradigm (examining 123 patients) have been reviewed elsewhere (Yassa, 1988).
For 104 patients (81.4%), anticholinergic medication was found to increase
the severity of tardive dyskinesia, whereas 17 patients (13.9%) responded
paradoxically, and in 2 patients (1.6%) the severity of tardive dyskinesia
remained unchanged. Perhaps some patients who responded in a paradoxical
manner had dystonic symptoms that really did respond better to anticholinergic drugs (Burke, Fahn, & Jankovic, 1982). Perhaps, too, investigators should be examining whether or not anticholinergic drugs uncover or
aggravate tardive dyskinesia, by withdrawing those medications and measuring the reductions in tardive dyskinesia symptoms. Five studies (Burnett,
Prange, & Wilson, 1980; Good, 1981; Reunanen, Kaartinen, & Varsanen,
1982; Greil, Haag, & Rossangl, 1984; Yassa, 1985), including two double-
blind studies (Burnett et al., 1980; Greil et al., 1984), showed that withdrawing antiparkinsonian medication led to reductions of tardive dyskinesia symptoms in 34 of 37 patients (91.9%). Those improvements were not related to
increases in parkinsonian symptoms nor to changes in plasma concentrations
of neuroleptics (Greil et al., 1984).

Finally, the question whether or not anticholinergic drugs uncover tardive dyskinesia has been examined by comparing current dosages of anticholinergic drugs in patients with and those without tardive dyskinesia. Twenty-one studies (Table 10.1) found no differences in current dosages of anticholinergic drugs between patients with and those without tardive dyskinesia. On the other hand, 12 studies reported that tardive dyskinesia patients received more anticholinergic drugs than did patients without tardive dyskinesia. Whereas several studies found a positive relationship between the severity of tardive dyskinesia and the amount of antiparkinsonian medication taken (Crane, 1980; Perényi & Arato, 1980; Barnes, Kidger, & Gore, 1983; Fleischhauer, Kocher, & Hobi, 1985), other studies found a positive relationship between total tardive dyskinesia score and amount of antiparkinsonian medication taken (Ezrin-Waters, Seeman, & Seeman, 1981). Some studies also showed that tardive dyskinesia patients had received less anticholinergic drugs than had patients without tardive dyskinesia (Gardos, Samm, & Kollos, 1980; Itoh, Fugui, & Kanusada, 1984).

Thus, we can conclude that anticholinergic drugs tend to uncover and/or aggravate preexisting tardive dyskinesia. Therefore anticholinergic drugs should be useful as pharmacologic probes in diagnosing cases of tardive dyskinesia. In addition, they can be used as predictors of treatment responses to cholinergic drugs (Casey & Denney, 1977).

Conclusion

From this review we can conclude that antiparkinsonian drugs have not been shown to increase the incidence of tardive dyskinesia, as previously suggested (Klawans 1973). However, they have been found to aggravate and/or uncover preexisting tardive dyskinesia. Thus, at present, it is recommended that they be discontinued, if clinically possible, for those patients in whom tardive dyskinesia is observed.

References

Altamura, A. C., Cavallaro, R., & Regazzetti, M. G. (1990). Prevalence and risk factors for tardive dyskinesia: a study in an Italian population of chronic schizophrenics. *Eur. Arch. Psychiatry Clin. Neurosci.* 240:9–12.

Asnis, G., Leopold, M., & Duvoisin, R. (1977). A survey of tardive dyskinesia in psychiatric outpatients. *Am. J. Psychiatry* 134:1367–70.

Barnes, T. R., Kidger, T., & Gore, S. M. (1983). Tardive dyskinesia: a 3-year follow-up study. *Psychol. Med.* 13:71–81.

Bédard, P. J., Mancilla, B. G., Blanchette, P., Gagnon, C., & DiPaolo, T. (1992). Levodopa-induced dyskinesia: facts and fancy. What does the MPTP monkey model tell us? *Can. J. Neurol. Sci.* 19:134–7.

Bell, R. C., & Smith, R. C. (1978). Tardive dyskinesia: characterization and prevalence in a statewide system. *Dis. Nerv. Syst.* 39:39–50.

Berger, P. A., & Dunner, M. J. (1985). Tardive dyskinesia: the major problem with antipsychotic maintenance therapy. In *Antipsychotics,* ed. D. G. Burrows, T. R. Norman, & B. Davis, pp. 185–212. New York: Elsevier.

Birket-Smith, E. (1974). Abnormal involuntary movements induced by anticholinergic drugs. *Acta Neurol. Scand.* 50:801–11.

Branchey, M., & Branchey, L. (1984). Patterns of psychotropic drug use and tardive dyskinesia. *J. Clin. Psychopharmacol.* 4:41–5.

Burke, R. E., Fahn, S., & Jankovic, J. (1982). Tardive dystonia: late-onset and persistent dystonia caused by antipsychotic drugs. *Neurology* 32:1335–46.

Burnett, G. B., Prange, A. J., & Wilson, I. C. (1980). Adverse effects of anticholinergic antiparkinsonian drugs in tardive dyskinesia. *Neuropsychobiology* 6:109–20.

Casey, D. E., & Denney, D. (1977). Pharmacological characterization of tardive dyskinesia. *Psychopharmacology* 54:1–8.

Chacko, R. C., Root, L., & Marmion, J. (1985). The prevalence of tardive dyskinesia in gerontopsychiatric outpatients. *J. Clin. Psychiatry* 46:55–7.

Chien, C.-P., Ross-Townsend, A., & Donnelly, M. (1980). Past history of drug and somatic treatment in tardive dyskinesia. In *Tardive Dyskinesia: Research and Treatment*, ed. W. E. Fann, R. C. Smith, J. M. Davis, & E. F. Domino, pp. 297–308. New York: SP Medical & Scientific Books.

Chouinard, G., Annable, L., Mercier, P., & Ross-Chouinard, A. (1986). A five-year follow-up study of tardive dyskinesia. *Psychoparmacol. Bull.* 22:259–63.

Chouinard, G., DeMontigny, C., & Annable, L. (1979). Tardive dyskinesia and antiparkinsonian medication. *Am. J. Psychiatry* 136:228–9.

Crane, G. E. (1980). Neuroleptic drugs and other factors predisposing to tardive dyskinesia. In *Tardive Dyskinesia: Research and Treatment*, ed. W. E. Fann, R. C. Smith, J. M. Davis, & E. F. Domino, pp. 281–90. New York: SP Medical & Scientific Books.

Davis, W. A. (1975). Dyskinesia associated with chronic antihistamine use. *N. Engl. J. Med.* 294:113.

Doongaji, D. R., Jeste, D. V., & Jape, N. M. (1982). Tardive dyskinesia in India: a prevalence study. *J. Clin. Psychopharmacol.* 2:341–4.

Ezrin-Waters, C., Seeman, M. V., & Seeman, P. (1981). Tardive dyskinesia in schizophrenic outpatients: prevalence and significant variables. *J. Clin. Psychiatry* 42:16–22.

Fleischhauer, J., Kocher, R., & Hobi, V. (1985). Prevalence of tardive dyskinesia in a clinic population. *Psychopharmacology* (*Suppl. 2*), pp. 162–72.

Gardos, G., Cole, J. O., & Labrie, R. A. (1977). Drug variables in the etiology of tardive dyskinesia: application of discriminant function analysis. *Prog. Neuropsychopharmacol.* 1:147–55.

Gardos, G., Samm, I., & Kollos, M. (1980). Absence of severe tardive dyskinesia in Hungarian schizophrenic outpatients. *Psychopharmacology* 71:29–34.

Good, M. I. (1981). Reversibility of long-term tardive dyskinesia associated with antiparkinsonian medication: a case report. *Am. J. Psychiatry* 138:1112–13.

Greil, W., Haag, H., & Rossangl, G. (1984). Effect of anticholinergics on tardive dyskinesia: a controlled discontinuation study. *Br. J. Psychiatry* 145:304–10.

Holden, T. J. (1987). Tardive dyskinesia in long-term hospitalized Zulu psychiatric patients. *S. Afr. Med. J.* 71:88–90.

Holden, T. J., Sandler, R., & Myslobodsky, M. (1984). Tardive dyskinesia: prevalence and subtypes at Valkenberg Hospital, Cape Town. *S. Afr. Med. J.* 66:132–4.

Imada, T., Ohnishi, K., Kamisada, M., Matsuda, G., & Tajima, O. (1991). A prospective study of tardive dyskinesia in Japan. *Eur. Arch. Psychiatry Clin. Neurosci.* 240:250–4.

Itil, T. M., Reisberg, B., & Hughe, M. (1981). Clinical profiles of tardive dyskinesia. *Compr. Psychiatry* 22:282–90.

Itoh, M., Fugui, Y., & Kanusada, M. (1984). Recent trend on the prevalence of tardive dyskinesia in Japan. *Prog. Neuropsychopharmacol. Biol. Psychiatry* 8:39–49.

Jeste, D. V., & Wyatt, R. J. (1982). *Understanding and Treating Tardive Dyskinesia.* New York: Guilford Press.

Jus, A., Pineau, P., & Lachance, R. (1976). Epidemiology of tardive dyskinesia. *Dis. Nerv. Syst.* 37:210–14.

Kane, J. M., & Smith, J. M. (1982). Tardive dyskinesia: prevalence and risk factors. *Arch. Gen. Psychiatry* 39:473–81.

Kane, J. M., Woerner, M., Weinhold, P., Wegner, J., & Kinon, B. (1984). Incidence of tardive dyskinesia: five-year data from a prospective study. *Psychopharmacol. Bull.* 20:387–9.

Kennedy, P. F., Herson, M. I., & McGuire, R. J. (1971). Extrapyramidal disorders after prolonged phenothiazine therapy. *Br. J. Psychiatry* 118:509–18.

Kiloh, L. G., Smith, J. S., & Williams, S. E. (1973). Antiparkinson drugs as causal agents in tardive dyskinesia. *Med. J. Aust.* 2:591–3.

Klawans, H. L. (1973). The pharmacology of tardive dyskinesia. *Am. J. Psychiatry* 130:82–6.

Klawans, H. L., Goetz, C., & Perlik, S. (1980). Tardive dyskinesia: review and update. *Am. J. Psychiatry* 137:900–8.

Kok, L. P., & Christopher, Y. S. (1985). Tardive dyskinesia in schizophrenic outpatients. *Ann. Acad. Med. Singapore* 14:87–90.

Kolakowska, T., Williams, A. O., & Arden, M. (1985). Tardive dyskinesia and current dose of neuroleptic drugs. *Arch. Gen. Psychiatry* 42:925.

Kulhanek, F., Schwitzer, J., Hebenstreit, G., Hinterhuber, H., & Schuber, H. (1984). Tardive dyskinesia and correlating factors in a mental hospital in Austria. *Neuropsychiatr. Clin.* 3:281–7.

McCreadie, R. G., Barron, E. T., & Winslow, G. S. (1982). The Nithsdale schizophrenia survey. II. Abnormal movements. *Br. J. Psychiatry* 140:587–90.

Mallya, A., Jose, C., & Brig, M. (1977). Antiparkinsonian neuroleptics and tardive dyskinesia. *Biol. Psychiatry* 14:645–9.

Morgenstern, H., Galzer, W. M., Gibowski, L. D., & Holmberg, S. (1987). Predictors of tardive dyskinesia: results of a cross-sectional study in an outpatient population. *J. Chronic Dis.* 40:319–27.

Nomoto, M., Thompson, P. D., & Sheehy, M. P. (1987). Anticholinergic induced chorea in the treatment of focal dystonia. *Mov. Disord.* 2:53–6.

Perényi, A., & Arato, M. (1980). Tardive dyskinesia on Hungarian psychiatric wards. *Psychosomatics* 21:904–9.

Perris, C., Dimitrijevic, P., & Jacobsson, J. (1979). Tardive dyskinesia in psychiatric patients treated with neuroleptics. *Br. J. Psychiatry* 135:509–14.

Ramsay, F. M., & Millard, P. M. (1985). Tardive dyskinesia in the elderly. *Age and Ageing* 15:145–50.

Rao, J. M., Cowie, V. A., & Mathew, B. (1987). Tardive dyskinesia in neuroleptic-medicated mentally handicapped subjects. *Acta Psychiatr. Scand.* 76:507–13.

Reunanen, M., Kaartinen, P., & Varsanen, E. (1982). The influence of anticholinergic treatment on tardive dyskinesia caused by neuroleptic drugs. *Acta Neurol. Scand.* (*Suppl. 90*) 65:278–9.

Rey, J. M., Hient, G. E., & Johnson, G. F. S. (1981). Assessment of tardive dyskinesia in psychiatric outpatients, using a standardized rating scale. *Aust. N.Z. J. Psychiatry* 15:33–7.

Saltz, B., Woerner, M. G., Kane, J. M., Lieberman, J. A., & Alvir, J. (1991). Prospective study of tardive dyskinesia incidence in the elderly. *JAMA* 266:2402–6.

Simpson, G. M., Varga, E., Lee, J. H., & Gardos, G. (1978). Tardive dyskinesia and psychotropic drug history. *Psychopharmacology* 58:117–24.

Smith, R. E., & Domino, E. F. (1980). Dystonic and dyskinetic reactions induced by H_1 antihistamine medication. In *Tardive Dyskinesia: Research and Treatment*, ed. W. E. Fann, R. C. Smith, J. M. Davis, & E. F. Domino, pp. 325–32. New York: SP Medical and Scientific Books.

Sramek, J., Roy, S., Ahrens, T., Pinanong, P., Cutler, N., & Pi, E. (1991). Prevalence of tardive dyskinesia among three ethnic groups of chronic psychiatric patients. *Hosp. Community Psychiatry* 42:590–2.

Thacht, B. T., Chase, T. N., & Basma, J. F. (1975). Oral-facial dyskinesia associated with prolonged use of antihistaminic decongestants. *N. Engl. J. Med.* 293:486–7.

Waddington, J. L., & Youssef, H. (1986). Involuntary movements and cognitive dysfunction in late onset schizophrenic outpatients. *Irish Med. J.* 79:347–50.

Warne, R. W., & Gubbay, S. S. (1979). Choreiform movements induced by anticholinergic therapy. *Med. J. Aust.* 1:465.

West, R. R., & Newgreen, D. B. (1979). Choreiform movements induced by anticholinergic therapy. *Med. J. Aust.* 2:87–8.

Williams, R., Naya, A., & Dalby, J. T. (1986). Tardive dyskinesia in outpatient schizophrenics treated with depot phenothiazines. *J. Clin. Psychopharmacol.* 6:318–19.

Wojeik, J. D., Gelenberg, A. J., & Labrie, R. A. (1980). Prevalence of tardive dyskinesia in an outpatient population. *Compr. Psychiatry* 21:370–80.

Yassa, R. (1985). Antiparkinsonian medication withdrawal in the treatment of tardive dyskinesia: a report of three cases. *Can. J. Psychiatry* 30:440–2.

Yassa, R. (1988). Tardive dyskinesia and anticholinergic drugs: a critical review of the literature. *Encephale* 14:233–9.

Yassa, R., Ananth, J., Cordozo, S., & Ally, J. (1983). Tardive dyskinesia in an outpatient population: prevalence and predisposing factors. *Can. J. Psychiatry* 28:391–4.

Yassa, R., Camille, Y., & Belzile, L. (1987). Tardive dyskinesia in the course of antidepressant therapy: a prevalence study and review of the literature. *J. Clin. Psychopharmacol.* 7:243–6.

Yassa. R., Ghadirian, A. M., & Schwartz, G. (1985). Tardive dyskinesia: developmental factors. *Can. J. Psychiatry* 30:344–7.

Yassa, R., & Nair, V. (1988). The association of tardive dyskinesia and pseudoparkinsonism. *Prog. Neuropsychopharmacol. Biol. Psychiatry* 12:909–14.

Yassa, R., Nair, V., & Iskandar, H. (1990). Factors in the development of severe forms of tardive dyskinesia. *Am. J. Psychiatry* 147:1156–63.

Yassa, R., Nair, V., & Schwartz, G. (1986). Early versus late onset psychosis and tardive dyskinesia. *Biol. Psychiatry* 21:1291–7.

Yassa, R., Nastase, C., Dupont, D., & Thibeau, M. (1992). Tardive dyskinesia in a psychogeriatric population: a 5-year study. *Am. J. Psychiatry* 149:1206–11.

Part III
Mechanisms Underlying Tardive Dyskinesia

Part III

11

Neurochemistry of the Basal Ganglia

N.P.V. NAIR, M.D.,
and T.E.G. WEST, Ph.D.

Until recently, it was believed that the basal ganglia had a small role in behavior limited to the control of motor behavior. Research during the past decade, however, suggests that the basal ganglia are involved in a wide range of behaviors, including not only skeletomotor and oculomotor activities but also limbic, affective, and cognitive functions. These changes in our understanding of the organization and function of the basal ganglia have followed important advances deriving from anatomic, pharmacologic, and physiologic studies.

Structures of the Basal Ganglia

The basal ganglia include the caudate, putamen, and ventral striatum, as well as the globus pallidus, subthalamic nucleus, and substantia nigra. Together, the caudate, putamen, and ventral striatum form the neostriatum; they also constitute the input stage of the basal ganglia. The globus pallidus, which is divided into internal (GPi) and external (GPe) segments, lies medial to the putamen. The substantia nigra has two components: the pars compacta (SNc) and the pars reticulata (SNr). The SNr and the GPi are cytologically similar and often are considered as a single structure. Both the SNr and GPi are recognized as major sources of the basal-ganglia output (Nauta, 1979).

Input to the Basal Ganglia

The neostriatum is the largest and most important receptive region of the basal ganglia. Inputs to the neostriatum originate mainly in the cortex, thalamus, and SNc, with less prominent inputs arising in the globus pallidus, subthalamic nucleus (STN), dorsal raphe, and pedunculopontine tegmental nucleus. The most prominent input to the neostriatum is from the cortex (corticostriatal pathway).

The corticostriatal pathway has cell bodies distributed throughout most of the cerebral cortex, including the association, limbic, motor, premotor, and sensory areas. Topographically organized areas of the cortex project to the neostriatum (Kemp & Powell, 1970). For example, whereas the motor and somatosensory cortices send topographic projections to the putamen (Kemp & Powell, 1970; Jones et al., 1977; Künzle, 1975, 1977), the frontal and supplementary eye fields send projections to the caudate nucleus (Künzle & Akert, 1977; Künzle, 1978; Selemon & Goldman-Rakic, 1985, 1988). Projections from the frontal association cortex descend to the caudate, and particular regions of the cingulate, frontal, and temporal cortex send projections to the ventral striatum (Selemon & Goldman-Rakic, 1985, 1988).

The neostriatum also receives topographic projections from several areas of the thalamus, including the centromedian, parafascicular, ventralis anterior pars magnocellularis, and ventralis lateralis pars orals nuclei (Nakano, et al., 1991; Sadikot, Parent, & François, 1992).

In addition to the projections from the cortex and thalamus, the neostriatum receives input from the substantia nigra. This pathway originates in the SNc and projects through the medial forebrain bundle, terminating diffusely throughout the neostriatum (Bjorklund & Lindvall, 1984).

Output of the Basal Ganglia

The neostriatum projects massively to both components of the globus pallidus and to the SNr. The SNr and GPi project directly to target nuclei in the thalamus, and the GPe projects to the STN. The STN, in turn, is connected with the substantia nigra and both segments of the pallidum (Szabo, 1962; Carpenter et al., 1981; Smith & Parent, 1986; Groenewegen & Berendse, 1990; Selemon & Goldman-Rakic, 1990). The STN also receives projections from the cortical region (Von Monakow, Akert, & Künzle, 1978; Romansky et al., 1979; Kitai & Deniau, 1981). The projection from the SNr and GPi to the thalamus is considered to represent the major output pathway of the basal ganglia.

Circuitry of the Basal Ganglia

The current view of the organization of the basal ganglia seems to be that the basal ganglia, along with their cortical and thalamic connections, are organized into separate parallel circuits (Alexander, DeLong, & Strick, 1986; Alexander, Crutcher, & DeLong, 1990; cf. Parthasarathy, Schall, & Graybiel, 1992). Although the anatomic evidence is incomplete, it appears that each circuit leads from the cerebral cortex through the basal ganglia, by way of the thalamus, to the frontal lobe. Each circuit engages specific areas of the cerebral cortex, neostriatum, pallidum, and thalamus. Alexander and Crutcher (1990) have suggested that there may be as many as five separate circuits: the motor, oculomotor, and limbic circuits and two prefrontal circuits.

Because reviews of this topic have been presented in detail elsewhere (Alexander et al. 1986, 1990; Alexander & Crutcher, 1990), we shall give only a brief description of each circuit.

Motor Circuit

The motor, premotor, and somatosensory areas project to the putamen (Künzle, 1975, 1977, 1978; Selemon & Goldman-Rakic, 1985). The putamen, in turn, sends projections to specific portions of the GPi and GPe, as well as to the SNr (Szabo, 1967; Johnson & Rosvold, 1971; Parent, Bouchard, & Smith, 1984). The "motor" portions of the GPi and SNr project to specific nuclei of the thalamus (Nauta & Mehler, 1966; Parent & DeBellefeuille, 1982). A connection between the thalamic nuclei and the premotor and motor cortex closes the circuit (Strick, 1976; Kievit & Kuypers, 1977; Schell & Strick, 1984; Matelli et al., 1989). The motor circuit is believed to be involved in both the preparation and execution of movement.

Oculomotor Circuit

The frontal and supplementary eye fields project to the caudate nucleus (Künzle & Akert, 1977; Künzle, 1978; Selemon & Goldman-Rakic, 1985, 1988). The caudate nucleus then projects to selected areas of the thalamus by way of the SNr and GPi (Carpenter, Nakano, & Kim, 1976; Parent et al., 1984). The oculomotor circuit is closed with connections between the thalamus and the frontal and supplementary eye fields (Kievit & Kuypers, 1977). This circuit seems to be involved in the control of eye movements.

Prefrontal Circuits

The prefrontal circuits include the dorsolateral prefrontal circuit and the lateral orbitofrontal circuit. The dorsolateral prefrontal circuit links the association and dorsolateral prefrontal cortices with parts of the caudate (Goldman & Nauta, 1977; Selemon & Goldman-Rakic, 1985, 1988). The caudate projects to specific thalamic nuclei by way of the SNr and GPi (Johnson & Rosvold,

1971; Kuo & Carpenter, 1973; Parent et al., 1984). The circuit is closed by connections between each thalamic nucleus and the dorsolateral prefrontal cortex. It is believed that this circuit is concerned with specific aspects of spatial memory.

The lateral orbitofrontal circuit includes a projection from the orbitofrontal cortex to part of the caudate nucleus (Selemon & Goldman-Rakic, 1985). The caudate projects to the SNr and the GPi (Szabo, 1962; Johnson & Rosvold, 1971), which in turn make connections with several thalamic nuclei (Carpenter et al., 1976). The thalamic nuclei project to the lateral orbitofrontal area of the cortex (Goldman-Rakic & Porrino, 1985). There is some suggestion that obsessive/compulsive behavior may be related to this circuit.

Limbic Circuit

The anterior cingulate area (ACA), the medial orbitofrontal cortex (MOFC), and the temporal cortex project to the ventral striatum (Selemon & Goldman-Rakic, 1985, 1988; Berendse, Galis-de Graaf, & Groenewegen, 1992). The ventral striatum projects to parts of the thalamus by way of the ventral pallidum (Kuo & Carpenter, 1973; Nauta & Cole, 1978). This circuit is closed by the projection from the thalamus back to the ACA and MOFC (Groenewegen, 1988). There is speculation that the limbic circuit may play a role in emotional or motivational processes (Butters et al., 1973).

Identified Neurotransmitters of Basal-Ganglia–Thalamocortical Circuitry

The proposed basal-ganglia–thalamocortical circuits are believed to share several common features (Figure 11.1). The input stage of each circuit arises from fast-conducting, excitatory glutaminergic cortical neurons (Spencer, 1976; Divac, Fonnum, & Storm-Mathisen, 1977; Perschak & Cuenod, 1990). The glutaminergic neurons project to different areas of the neostriatum, including the caudate, putamen, and ventral striatum (Nauta, 1979; Graybiel, 1990). The additional components of each circuit include two parallel pathways: a *direct* pathway and an *indirect* pathway. Both pathways originate in the neostriatum and are believed to produce differential effects on the output of the basal ganglia.

The direct pathway consists of a striatal projection to the GPi and to the SNr. This projection is inhibitory and appears to contain γ-aminobutyric acid (GABA) and substance P (Graybiel & Ragsdale, 1983; Albin, Young, & Penney, 1989b).

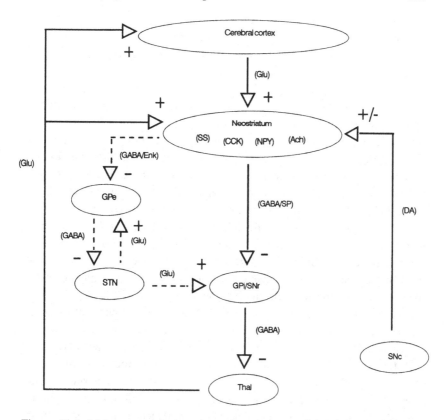

Figure 11.1. Major connections and neurotransmitters of basal-ganglia–thalamo-cortical circuitry, including the direct (solid line) and indirect (dotted lines) pathways from the neostriatum to the GPi and SNr. Inhibitory neurons are indicated by minus signs, and excitatory neurons by plus signs. Abbreviations: Ach, acetylcholine; CCK, cholecystokinin; DA, dopamine; Enk, enkephalin; GABA, γ-aminobutyric acid; Glu, glutamate; NPY, neuropeptide Y; NT, neurotensin; SS, somatostatin; Thal, thalamus.

The indirect pathway consists of a projection from the striatum to the GPe. The striatal projection is inhibitory and contains both the inhibitory transmitter GABA and the inhibitory peptide enkephalin (Graybiel & Ragsdale, 1983). The sole projection from the GPe is to the STN and is mediated by GABA (Parent, 1990). The STN, in turn, projects back to the GPe and GPi by excitatory, glutaminergic-containing neurons (Carpenter et al., 1981; Kita & Kitai, 1987; Nakanishi, Kita, & Kitai, 1987; Albin et al., 1989a).

The major output for both the direct and indirect pathways arises from the GPi and SNr and is inhibitory and GABAergic (Nauta, 1979; Penney & Young, 1981; Chevalier et al., 1985). The GPi and SNr project principally to the ventrolateral thalamus and also to the brain stem (Parent, 1990). The GPi appears to have greater influence on the thalamus, whereas the SNr has more influence on the brain stem. The areas of the thalamus that receive input from the GPi and SNr send glutaminergic projections to different regions of the cortex.

The direct and indirect pathways are considered to have opposite effects on the GPi/SNr and thus on their targets in the thalamus (Alexander & Crutcher, 1990). Activation of the direct pathway by glutaminergic cortical neurons excites GABAsubstance-P striatal neurons, which in turn cause disinhibition of the GABAergic neurons of the GPi/SNr. Disinhibition of GPi/SNr GABA-ergic neurons results in the activation of thalamic neurons. The activation of thalamic neurons causes increased excitation of cortical neurons. This pathway is believed to facilitate and maintain ongoing motor behavior.

In comparison, activation of the indirect pathway by glutaminergic cortical neurons stimulates the striatal inhibitory GABA/enkephalin projection, resulting in suppression of GABAergic neuronal activity. The suppression of GABAergic neurons causes disinhibition of STN excitatory glutaminergic neurons, thereby triggering the GPi/SNr inhibitory GABAergic output projections to inhibit their target nuclei in the thalamus. The inhibition of thalamic neurons results in decreased excitation of cortical neurons (Alexander & Crutcher, 1990). This pathway is believed to suppress motor activity.

Disturbances in the activity of either pathway are believed to be responsible for many disorders of movement. Overactivity of the indirect pathway and underactivity of the direct pathway are believed to result in hypokinesia. In contrast, overactivity of the direct pathway and underactivity of the indirect pathway seem to cause hyperkinesia.

An important element of the basal-ganglia circuitry is the nigrostriatal dopaminergic pathway. The nigrostriatal pathway, which originates in the SNc and projects to the neostriatum through the medial forebrain bundle, appears to modulate the activities of the direct and indirect pathways differentially by activation of different dopamine receptors. Dopaminergic neurons, which synapse on striatal GABA/substance-P neurons, appear to excite the direct pathway by activation of the D_1 receptor. In comparison, dopaminergic neurons synapsing on striatal GABA/enkephalin neurons appear to inhibit the indirect pathway by activation of the D_2 receptor (Albin et al., 1989b; Gerfen et al., 1990).

Other neurotransmitters, including acetylcholine, somatostatin, neuropeptide Y (NPY), cholecystokinin (CCK), and neurotensin, appear to influence the activity of the basal ganglia. The majority of these neurotransmitters project to, or are located within, the neostriatum.

Acetylcholine (cholinergic) neurons reside within the neostriatum (Bolam,

Ingham, & Smith, 1984; Satoh & Fibiger, 1985) and are largely interneurons (Phelps, Houser, & Vaughn, 1985). There appears to be an important association between acetylcholine and dopamine in the neostriatum. Both dopaminergic and cholinergic neurons synapse on the same output neuron of the neostriatum (possibly efferent GABAergic projections), but not on each other (Izzo & Bolam, 1988).

Somatostatinergic neurons, like cholinergic neurons, are believed to be primarily interneurons in the neostriatum (Chesselet & Graybiel, 1986; Desjardins & Parent, 1992). It has been speculated that the somatostatinergic interneurons play an integrative role between the motor and limbic compartments of the striatum (Gerfen, 1984; Gerfen, Baimbridge, & Thibeault, 1987).

In the neostriatum, NPY neurons appear to be co-localized with somatostatin and the enzyme nicotinamide adenine dinucleotide phosphate diaphorase (NADPH-D) (Chronwall, Chase, & O'Donohue, 1984; Smith & Parent, 1986), although some NPY neurons may coexist with GABA (Hendry et al., 1984; Smith & Parent, 1986). NPY neurons generally receive few inputs, but make contact with many neurons in their vicinity, including GABA. Kerkerian-Le Goff et al. (1991) have postulated that NPY neurons have an important role in regulating striatal GABAergic function.

CCK is located in the neostriatum (Takagi et al., 1984) and may be co-localized within the afferents of midbrain dopaminergic neurons (Hökfelt et al., 1980). Although most neurons containing CCK appear to originate from outside the neostriatum, there is evidence to suggest that some neurons intrinsic to the neostriatum may contain CCK (Takagi et al., 1984).

Neurotensin appears to play an important role in modulating the activities of dopamine (Blaha et al., 1990; Drumheller et al., 1990; Chapman, 1992) and acetylcholine (Torocsik et al., 1993) in the neostriatum.

Patch-and-Matrix Organization in the Neostriatum

The neostriatum consists of two distinct compartments, called patches (or striosomes) and the matrix. These two compartments have been identified on the basis of the distribution of markers for various neurotransmitters, enzyme systems, and receptors (Gerfen, 1984, 1985; Graybiel, 1990). For example, patches are rich in μ-opiate receptors, enkephalin, and substance P, whereas the matrix is rich in cholinesterase, calbindin, dopamine D_2 receptors, and somatostatin fibers. The patches compose the smaller of the two compartments and are located within the matrix.

There appears to be an association between the compartmental organization of corticostriatal inputs and the cortical area of origin. The prelimbic cortex projects to the patch compartment, whereas many of the cortical regions, including the visual and motor cortices, project to the matrix.

The patch compartment sends projections to the dopaminergic neurons in the SNc and possibly to neighboring regions (Graybiel, 1990). The matrix projects mainly to the pallidum and to the SNr, but not to the SNc.

These findings suggest that the patch compartment and its association with the limbic system may play a role in modulating the dopaminergic system, possibly in relation to motivational information from the limbic system (Graybiel, 1990). The matrix appears to play a role in motor and cognitive behaviors.

References

Albin, R. L., Aldridge, J. W., Young, A. B., & Gilman, S. (1989a). Feline subthalamic nucleus neurons contain glutamate-like but not GABA-like or glycine-like immunoreactivity. *Brain Res*. 491:185–8.

Albin, R. L., Young, A. B., & Penney, J. B. (1989b). The functional anatomy of basal ganglia disorders. *Trends Neurosci*. 12:366–75.

Alexander, G. E., & Crutcher, M. D. (1990). Functional architecture of basal ganglia circuits: neural substrates of parallel processing. *Trends Neurosci*. 13:266–71.

Alexander, G. E., Crutcher, M. D., & DeLong, M. R. (1990). Basal ganglia–thalamocortical circuits: parallel substrates for motor, oculomotor, "prefrontal" and "limbic" functions, *Prog. Brain Res*. 85:119–46.

Alexander, G. E., DeLong, M. R., & Strick, P. L. (1986). Parallel organization of functionally segregated circuits linking basal ganglia and cortex. *Ann. Rev. Neurosci*. 9:357–81.

Berendse, H. W., Galis-de Graff, & Groenewegen, H. J. (1992). Topographical organization and relationship with ventral striatal compartments of prefrontal corticostriatal projections in the rat. *J. Comp. Neurol*. 316:314–47.

Bjorklund, A., & Lindvall, O. (1984). Dopamine-containing systems in the CNS. In *Handbook of Chemical Neuroanatomy. Vol. 2: Classical Transmitters in the CNS*, part 1, ed. A. Bjorklund & T. Hökfelt, pp. 55–122. Amsterdam: Elsevier.

Blaha, C. D., Coury, A., Fibiger, H. C., & Phillips. A. G. (1990). Effects of neurotensin on dopamine release and metabolism in the rat striatum and nucleus accumbens: cross-validation using in vivo voltammetry and microdialysis. *Neuroscience* 34:699–705.

Bolam, J. P., Ingham, C. A., & Smith, A. D. (1984). The section-Golgi-impregnation procedure. 3. Combination of Golgi impregnation with enzyme histochemistry and electron microscopy to characterize acetylcholinesterase-containing neurons in the rat neostriatum. *Neuroscience* 12:687–709.

Bolam, J. P., Powell, J. F., Wu, J.-Y., & Smith, A. D. (1985). Glutamate decarboxylase-immunoreactive structures in the rat neostriatum: a correlated light and electron microscopic study including a combination of Golgi impregnation and immunohistochemistry. *J. Comp. Neurol*. 237:1–20.

Butters, N., Butter, C., Rosen, J., & Stein, D. (1973). Behavioral effects of sequential and one-stage ablations of orbital prefrontal cortex in the monkey. *Exp. Neurol.* 39:204–14.

Carpenter, M. B., Carleton, S. C., Keller, J. T., & Conté, P. (1981). Connections of the subthalamic nucleus in the monkey. *Brain Res.* 224:1–29.

Carpenter, M. B., Nakano, K., & Kim, R. (1976). Nigrothalamic projections in the monkey demonstrated by autoradiographic technics. *J. Comp. Neurol.* 165:401–16.

Chapman, M. A. (1992). Neurotensin increases extracellular striatal dopamine levels in vivo. *Neuropeptides* 22:175–83.

Chesselet, M. F., & Graybiel, A. M. (1986). Striatal neurons expressing somatostatin-like immunoreactivity: evidence for a peptidergic interneuronal system in the cat. *Neuroscience* 17:547–71.

Chevalier, G., Vacher, S., Deniau, J. M., & Desban, M. (1985). Disinhibition as a basic process in the expression of striatal functions. I. The striato-nigral influence on tecto-spinal/tecto-diencephalic neurons. *Brain Res.* 334:215–26.

Chronwall, B. M., Chase, T. N., & O'Donohue, T. L. (1984). Coexistence of neuropeptide Y and somatostatin in rat and human cortical and rat hypothalamic neurons. *Neurosci. Lett.* 52:213–17.

Desjardins, C., & Parent, A. (1992). Distribution of somatostatin immunoreactivity in the forebrain of the squirrel monkey: basal ganglia and amygdala. *Neuroscience* 47:115–33.

Divac, I., Fonnum, F., & Storm-Mathisen, J. (1977). High affinity uptake of glutamate in terminals of corticostriatal axons. *Nature* 266:377–8.

Drumheller, A. D., Gagne, M. A., St.-Pierre, S., & Jolicoeur, F. B. (1990). Effects of neurotensin on regional concentrations of dopamine, serotonin and their main metabolites. *Neuropeptides* 15:169–78.

Gerfen, C. R. (1984). The neostriatal mosaic: compartmentalization of corticostriatal input and striatonigral output systems. *Nature* 311:461–4.

Gerfen, C. R.(1985). The neostriatal mosaic. I. Compartmental organization of projections from the striatum to the substantia nigra in the rat. *J. Comp. Neurol.* 236:454–76.

Gerfen, C. R., Baimbridge, K. G., & Thibeault, J. (1987). The neostriatal mosaic. II. Biochemical and developmental dissociation of patch-matrix mesostriatal systems. *J. Neurosci.* 7:3935–44.

Gerfen, C. R., Engber, T. N., Mahan, L. C., Susel, Z., Chase, T. N., Monsma, F. J., & Sibley, D. R. (1990). D_1 and D_2 dopamine receptor-regulated gene expression of striatonigral and striatopallidal neurons. *Science* 250:1429–32.

Goldman, P. S., and Nauta, W. J. H. (1977). An intricately patterned prefrontocaudate projection in the rhesus monkey. *J. Comp. Neurol.* 171:369–86.

Goldman-Rakic, P. S., & Porrino, L. J. (1985). The primate mediodorsal (MD) nucleus and its projection to the frontal lobe. *J. Comp. Neurol.* 242:535–60.

Graybiel, A. M. (1990). Neurotransmitters and neuromodulators in the basal ganglia. *Trends Neurosci.* 13:244–54.

Graybiel, A. M., & Ragsdale, C. W. (1983). Biochemical anatomy of the striatum. In *Chemical Neuroanatomy*, d. P. C. Emson, pp. 427–504. New York: Raven Press.

Groenewegen, H. J. (1988). Organization of the afferent connections of the mediodorsal thalamic nucleus in the rat, related to mediodorsal-prefrontal topography. *Neuroscience* 24:379–431.

Groenewegen, H. J., & Berendse, H. W. (1990). Connections of the subthalamic nucleus with ventral striatopallidal parts of the basal ganglia in the rat. *J. Comp. Neurol.* 294:607–22.

Hendry, S. H. C., Jones, E. G., De Felipe, J., Schmechel, D., Brandon, C., & Emson, P. C. (1984). Neuropeptide-containing neurons of the cerebral cortex are also GABAergic. *Proc. Nat. Acad. Sci. USA* 81:6526–30.

Hökfelt, T., Skirboll, L., Rehfeld, M. F., Goldstein, M., Markey, K., & Dann, O. (1980). A subpopulation of mesencephalic dopamine neurons projecting to limbic areas contains a cholecystokinin-like peptide. Evidence from immunhistochemistry combined with retrograde tracing. *Neuroscience* 5:2093–124.

Izzo, P. N., & Bolam, J. P. (1988). Cholinergic synaptic input to different parts of spiny striatonigral neurons in the rat. *J. Comp. Neurol.* 269:219–34.

Johnson, T. N., & Rosvold, H. E. (1971). Topographic projections of the globus pallidus and the substantia nigra selectively placed lesions in the precommisural caudate nucleus and putamen in the monkey. *Exp. Neurol.* 33:584–96.

Jones, E. G., Coulter, J. D., Burton, H., & Porter, R. (1977). Cells of origin and terminal distribution of corticostriatal fibers arising in the sensory-motor cortex of monkeys. *J. Comp. Neurol.* 173:53–80.

Kemp, J. M., & Powell, T. P. S. (1970). The cortico-striate projection in the monkey. *Brain* 93:525–46.

Kerkerian-Le Goff, L., Salin, P., Vuillet, J., & Nieoullon, A. (1991). Neuropeptide Y neurons in the striatal network. Functional adaptive responses to impairment of striatal inputs. In *The Basal Ganglia, III*, ed. G. Bernardi et al., pp. 49–61. New York: Plenum Press.

Kievit, J., & Kuypers, H. G. J. M. (1977). Organization of the thalamo-cortical connexions to the frontal lobe in the rhesus monkey. *Exp. Brain Res.* 29:299–322.

Kita, H., & Kitai, S. J. (1987). Efferent projections of the subthalamic nucleus in the rat: light and electron microscopic analysis with the PHA-L method. *J. Comp. Neurol.* 260:435–52.

Kitai, S. T., & Deniau, J. M. (1981). Cortical inputs to the subthalamus: intracellular analysis. *Brain Res.* 214:411–15.

Künzle, H. (1975). Bilateral projections from precentral motor cortex to the putamen and other parts of the basal ganglia. An autoradiographic study in *Macaca fascicularis. Brain Res.* 105:253–67.

Künzle, H. (1977). Projections from the primary somatosensory cortex to basal ganglia and thalamus in the monkey. *Exp. Brain Res.* 30:481–92.

Künzle, H. (1978). An autoradiographic analysis of the efferent connections from premotor and adjacent prefrontal regions (areas 6 and 9) in *Macaca fascicularis. Brain Behav. Evol.* 15:185–234.

Künzle, H., & Akert. K. (1977). Efferent connections of cortical area 8 (frontal eye field) in *Macaca fascicularis.* A reinvestigation using the autoradiographic technique. *J. Comp. Neurol.* 173:147–163.

Kuo, J. S., & Carpenter, M. B. (1973). Organization of pallido-thalamic projections in rhesus monkey. *J. Comp. Neurol.* 151:201–36.

Matelli, M., Luppino, G., Fogassi, L., & Rizzolatti, G. (1989). Thalamic input to inferior area 6 and area 4 in the macaque monkey. *J. Comp. Neurol.* 280:468–88.

Nakanishi, H., Kita, H., & Kitai, S. T. (1987). Intracellular study of rat substantia nigra pars reticulata neurons in an in vitro slice preparation: electrical membrane properties and response to characteristics to subthalamic stimulation. *Brain Res.* 437:45–55.

Nakano, K., Hasegawa, Y., Kayahara, T., & Kuga, Y. (1991). Topographical organization of the thalamostriatal projection in the Japanese monkey, *Macaca fuscata*, with special reference to the centromedian-parafascicular and motor thalamic nuclei. In *The Basal Ganglia, III*, ed. G. Bernardi et al., pp. 63–72. New York: Plenum Press.

Nauta, W. J. H. (1979). A proposed conceptual organization of the basal ganglia and telencephalon. *Neuroscience* 4:1875–81.

Nauta, W. J. H., & Cole, M. (1978). Efferent projections of the subthalamic nucleus: an autoradiographic study in monkey and cat. *J. Comp. Neurol.* 180:1–16.

Nauta, W. J. H., & Mehler, W. R. (1966). Projections of the lentiform nucleus in the monkey, *Brain Res.* 1:3–42.

Parent, A. (1990). Extrinsic connections of the basal ganglia. *Trends Neurosci.* 13:254–8.

Parent, A., Bouchard, C., & Smith, Y. (1984). The striatopallidal and striatonigral projections: two distinct fiber systems in primate. *Brain Res.* 303:385–90.

Parent, A., & DeBellefeuille, L. (1982). Organization of efferent projections from the internal segment of globus pallidus in primate as revealed by fluorescence retrograde labelling method. *Brain Res.* 245:201–14.

Parthasarathy, H. B., Schall, J. D., & Graybiel, A. M. (1992). Distributed but convergent ordering of corticostriatal projections: analysis of the frontal eye field and the supplementary eye field in the macaque monkey. *J. Neurosci.* 12:4468–88.

Penney, J. B., & Young, A. B. (1981). GABA as the pallidothalamic neurotransmitter: implications for basal ganglia function. *Brain Res.* 207:195–9.

Perschak, H., & Cuenod, M. (1990). In vivo release of endogenous glutamate and aspartate in the rat striatum during stimulation of the cortex. *Neuroscience* 35:283–7.

Phelps, P. E., Houser, C. R., & Vaughn, J. E. (1985). Immunocytochemical localization of choline acetyltransferase within the rat neostriatum: a correlated light and electron microscopic study of cholinergic neurons and synapses. *J. Comp. Neurol.* 238:286–307.

Romansky, K. V., Usunoff, K. G., Ivanov, D. P., & Galabov, G. P. (1979). Corticosubthalamic projection in the cat: an electron microscopic study. *Brain Res.* 163:319–22.

Sadikot, A. F., Parent, A., & François, C. (1992). Efferent connections of the centromedian and parafascicular thalamic nuclei in the squirrel monkey: a PHA-L study of subcortical projections. *J. Comp. Neurol.* 315:137–59.

Satoh, K., & Fibiger, H. C. (1985). Distribution of central cholinergic neurons in the baboon (*Papio*). I. General morphology. *J. Comp. Neurol.* 236:197–214.

Schell, G. R., & Strick, P. L. (1984). The origin of thalamic inputs to the arcuate premotor and supplementary motor areas. *J. Neurosci.* 4:539–60.

Selemon, L. D., & Goldman-Rakic, P. S. (1985). Longitudinal topography and interdigitation of cortico-striatal projections. *J. Neurosci.* 5:776–94.

Selemon, L. D., & Goldman-Rakic, P. S. (1988). Common cortical and subcortical targets of the dorsolateral prefrontal and posterior parietal cortices in the rhesus monkey: evidence for a distributed neural network subserving spatially guided behavior. *J. Neurosci.* 8:4049–68.

Selemon, L. D., & Goldman-Rakic, P. S. (1990). Topographic intermingling of striatonigral and striatopallidal neurons in the rhesus monkey. *J. Comp. Neurol.* 297:359–76.

Smith, Y., & Parent, A. (1986). Neuropeptide Y immunoreactive neurons in the striatum of cat and monkey: morphological characteristics, intrinsic organization and co-localization with somatostatin. *Brain Res.* 372:241–53.

Spencer, H. J. (1976). Antagonism of corticol excitation of striatal neurons by glutamic acid diethylester: evidence for glutamic acid as an excitatory transmitter in the rat striatum. *Brain Res.* 102:91–101.

Strick, P. L. (1976). Anatomical analysis of ventrolateral thalamic input to primate motor cortex. *J. Neurophysiol.* 39:1020–31.

Szabo, J. (1962). Topical distribution of striatal efferents in the monkey. *Exp. Neurol.* 5:21–36.

Szabo, J. (1967). The efferent projections of the putamen in the monkey. *Exp. Neurol.* 19:463–76.

Takagi, H., Mizuata, H., Matsuda, T., Inagaki, S., Tateishi, K., & Hamaoka, T. (1984). The occurrence of cholecystokinin-like immunoreactive neurons in rat neostratum: light and electron microscopic analysis. *Brain Res.* 309:346–9.

Torocsik, A., Rakovska, A., Gorcs, T., & Vizi, E. S. (1993). Effect of neurotensin and immunneutralization with anti-neurotensin-serum on dopaminergic–cholinergic interaction in the striatum. *Brain Res.* 612:306–12.

Von Monakow, H., Akert, K., & Künzle, H. (1978). Projections of the precentral motor cortex and other cortical areas of the frontal lobe to the subthalamic nucleus in the monkey. *Exp. Brain Res.* 33:395–403.

12

A Reanalysis of the Dopamine Theory of Tardive Dyskinesia: The Hypothesis of Dopamine D_1/D_2 Imbalance

LINDA PEACOCK, M. D., and JES GERLACH, M.D.

Today, more than 30 years after the first descriptions of neuroleptic-induced involuntary movements (Schonecker, 1957; Uhrbrand & Faurbye, 1960), a definitive understanding of the pathophysiology of the syndrome is lacking. In fact, the very number of theories offered to explain the basis of tardive dyskinesia is testimony to the absence of a fundamental, unifying explanation for the propensity of neuroleptics to induce tardive dyskinesia. Indeed, it remains uncertain that there ever will be one unifying explanation.

The classic explanation of the pathogenesis of tardive dyskinesia is the dopamine-hypersensitivity theory (Klawans & Rubovits, 1972; Tarsy & Baldessarini, 1973). According to this theory, chronic blockade of the postsynaptic dopamine receptors by neuroleptics results in adaptive dopamine-receptor hypersensitivity and cholinergic hypofunction, changes that result in chronic dyskinesia. Acute dyskinesia, on the other hand (i.e., dyskinesia occurring at the onset of dopamine blockade), has been believed to be a direct result of the dopamine blockade itself (i.e., acute dopamine hypofunction and cholinergic hyperfunction) (Gerlach, 1979). Because further development of the dopamine-hypersensitivity theory has focused mainly on the examination and manipulation of dopamine D_2 receptors in rodents, it could more properly be termed the dopamine D_2-hypersensitivity theory of tardive dyskinesia. In recent years, this theory has been criticized for lack of confirmation of its postulates in humans (Fibiger & Lloyd, 1984; Gerlach, 1985; Casey, 1991).

We intend to reanalyze the role of the dopaminergic system in the pathogenesis of tardive dyskinesia. Because our experimental model is a nonhuman-primate model for oral tardive dyskinesia, corresponding to the buccolinguomasticatory (BLM) syndrome in humans, this chapter will concentrate on that syndrome. More specifically, we shall present arguments for the role of a dopamine D_1/D_2 imbalance in favor of dopamine D_1 in the pathophysiology of the BLM syndrome, whether acute or chronic. Throughout this chapter, we use the terminology D_1 and D_2 as all-inclusive for the dopamine D_1- and D_2-receptor families. The implications of the recently discovered subtypes of dopamine D_1 and D_2 receptors are discussed in the final section on areas for future research.

Clinical Dyskinesia Paradigms

Our analysis revolves around four basic syndromes of clinical dyskinesia:

Acute or Initial Dyskinesia. This form of dyskinesia, which can occur after short-term neuroleptic treatment (days to weeks), often includes involuntary movements of the extremities, as well as oral movements. It may be accompanied by subjective discomfort in the form of psychomotor unrest (akathisia), may involve dystonic features (indeed, it may be a mild variant of dystonia), may be relieved by reduction of the neuroleptic dosage and/or by addition of an anticholinergic, and may indicate that the individual is predisposed to develop tardive dyskinesia (Gerlach, 1979).

Chronic Dyskinesia. This kind of dyskinesia, which appears after longer-term treatment with neuroleptics (months to years), is often restricted to the oral region. In many cases it is not accompanied by subjective discomfort unless others have made the patient aware of the disfigurement; it may be worsened by or may first appear after a decrease in dosage or discontinuation of the neuroleptic. It may also be worsened by the addition of an anticholinergic (to relieve parkinsonism). It is induced primarily (perhaps only) in predisposed individuals and is especially prone to occur with increasing age (Crane, Naranjo, & Chase, 1971; Gerlach, 1979; Casey, 1991).

Acute-in-Chronic Dyskinesia. This is a term used to describe patients who are known to have chronic dyskinesia as well as an overlying element of acute dyskinesia. For such patients, reduction of the neuroleptic dosage and/or addition of an anticholinergic will relieve the akathisia and reduce the degree of dyskinesia, although the underlying chronic dyskinesia will persist (Gerlach, 1979, 1985).

Spontaneous Dyskinesia. This form of dyskinesia can occur, independent of neuroleptic treatment, in the elderly or in patients with certain disease states such as schizophrenia.

Animal Models

Rodents

Animal models for tardive dyskinesia, usually involving rats, often are considered to be unsatisfactory in that they do not sufficiently emulate human tardive dyskinesia (Waddington, 1990; Casey, 1991). Two major points of contention have emerged: (1) A majority of rats will develop perioral movements, in some cases after very short periods of neuroleptic treatment. (2) Often the perioral movements appear only after a dopamine-agonist challenge (generally with mixed D_1/D_2 agonists such as apomorphine), and they are reversible. In contrast, in nonhuman primates (discussed later) and humans, the development of tardive dyskinesia requires neuroleptic treatment for months or years, occurs only in predisposed individuals, appears without dopamine-agonist challenge, and often is irreversible.

One proposed model for tardive dyskinesia in rats has been the spontaneous, vacuous-chewing model (Waddington et al., 1983). This syndrome has been described as developing after months of neuroleptic treatment, persisting for long periods of time, and occurring more markedly in senescent animals, which also have higher tardive dyskinesia scores at baseline. However, other investigators have reported similar oral movements after very short periods of treatment and have interpreted the phenomenon as related more to dystonia (Rupniak, Jenner, & Marsden, 1985; Waddington & Molloy, 1987; Waddington, 1990). We are in a quandary whether or not models based on rats can sufficiently replicate clinical experience. This dilemma can be resolved, however, if two postulates can be accepted. The first is that rats are, to a greater extent than nonhuman primates and humans, "preprimed" to react to various stimuli with increased oral activity (thus the term "rodent," derived from the Latin *rodere*, meaning to gnaw). In other words, rats are, per se, "predisposed individuals." The second postulate is that acute dyskinesia and tardive dyskinesia are not separate phenomena, as hitherto assumed, but represent aspects of a continuum (Gerlach & Hansen, 1992).

There have been several studies implicating a D_1/D_2 imbalance, in favor of D_1, in the pathophysiology of oral dyskinesia in rats. The first proposal of such a mechanism came from Rosengarten, Schweitzer, and Friedhoff (1983). In that study, administration of either a D_2 antagonist or a D_1 agonist resulted in oral dyskinesia. Combining a D_2 antagonist with the D_1 agonist further enhanced the oral dyskinesia, whereas combining a D_2 agonist with the D_1 agonist abolished the oral dyskinesia. In a subsequent study in rats it was found that a D_1 agonist induced oral activity, whereas a D_2 agonist suppressed it (Johansson et al., 1987). Later, Glenthøj, Arnt, and Hyttel (1990a) reported that rats previously exposed to D_2-antagonist treatment showed increased responses to a D_1 agonist (induction of tongue protrusions), as compared with controls. In fact, some investigators have distinguished between two main syndromes of D_1 agonism: (1) vacuous chewing movements (dyskinesia model), occurring primarily in animals with D_2 hypofunction (e.g., due to senescence or simultaneous D_2 antagonism), and (2) grooming activity, occurring in rats without such D_2 hypofunction (Waddington, 1986; Waddington & O'Boyle, 1987; Daly & Waddington, 1992).

In summary, there is no question that D_1 agonism induces increased oral activity in rats. It is also tempting to conclude that when the D_2 system is relatively intact, a grooming syndrome is induced, and that when the D_2 system is relatively hypoactive (e.g., due to age or to ongoing or previous neuroleptic treatment, as discussed later), a syndrome more closely resembling dyskinesia is induced. Two questions, however, remain: whether or not the two oral syndromes are indeed different, and how they relate to tardive dyskinesia in humans (Glenthøj et al., 1990b; Waddington, 1990).

Nonhuman Primates

Animal models involving nonhuman primates introduce the element of individual susceptibility to the development of dyskinesia, thereby mimicking clinical experience more clearly than in the rodent models (Casey, 1991). Thus, in monkeys, as in humans, some individuals are remarkably resistant, and others sensitive, to development of dyskinesia. In other words, whereas rodent models offer sensitivity, monkey models offer specificity in determining dyskinetic potential. Let us look at some laboratory results involving two groups of eight *Cebus apella* monkeys: one drug-naive, and one neuroleptic-primed.

Drug-Naive Monkeys. Eight male *Cebus apella* monkeys were treated in a crossover study for a 14-week period with increasing doses of a D_1 antagonist, NNC 756 (NNC group), or a D_2 antagonist, raclopride (RAC group) (Gerlach & Hansen, 1993). After a 12-week washout period, each group was given the other antagonist for 14 weeks. Before and after the antagonist treatments, the monkeys underwent acute testing with the D_1 agonist SKF 81297 and the D_2 agonist quinpirole. Whereas the group that had received gradually increasing dosages of NNC 756 first (NNC group) showed no dystonia (although parkinsonism was seen), the group that received raclopride first (RAC group) showed dystonia. When the NNC group was switched to raclopride, high single-test doses of raclopride did not produce dystonia; during continued treatment, however, the animals became sensitized, requiring smaller doses to avoid dystonia. When the RAC group was given NNC 756, dystonia developed, although tolerance to that effect did develop eventually. During treatment with each dopamine antagonist, acute oral dyskinesia was seen; it tended to increase during raclopride treatment and decrease during treatment with NNC 756. After withdrawal of the dopamine antagonists, oral dyskinesia (tardive dyskinesia) was more pronounced following raclopride treatment, whereas grooming was more pronounced after treatment with NNC 756. After treatment, testing with the dopamine antagonists showed that subsequent to treatments with both raclopride and NNC 756, supersensitivity to the D_2 agonist had developed, presenting as increased arousal, anxiousness, and body stereotypies. After treatments with both NNC 756 and raclopride, although supersensitivity also developed toward the D_1 agonist, the character of the supersensitivity was different: Whereas after NNC 756, SKF 81297 induced a special grooming behavior, after raclopride it induced oral dyskinesia, with less grooming.

Primed Monkeys. Another group of *Cebus apella* monkeys, 5 females and 3 males, were treated with haloperidol for 2 years in order to develop a tardive dyskinesia model. In 5 of the monkeys, a mild BLM syndrome was induced. Using that model, we carried out a study of the acute effects of D_1 and D_2 agonists and antagonists (Peacock, Lublin, & Gerlach, 1990).

That study showed that subdystonic doses of raclopride (D_2 antagonist) aggravated oral dyskinesia in the animals with tardive dyskinesia. However, although small doses of SCH 23390 (D_1 antagonist) increased oral dyskinesia in the entire group of monkeys, inhibition of preexisting tardive dyskinesia was seen at subdystonic doses. The study also showed that when given alone, SKF 81297 (D_1 agonist) produced oral dyskinesia in all the monkeys, the reaction being extreme (>100 mouth movements in 90 seconds) in animals with tardive dyskinesia. No significant increase in grooming, however, was seen. As for quinpirole (D_2 agonist) given alone, it had no significant effects on oral dyskinesia, although a tendency toward suppression was seen. Interestingly, both the D_1 antagonist and the D_2 agonist, given in combination with SKF 81297, caused suppression of the oral dyskinesia induced by the D_1 agonist.

Neither a combination of raclopride with SKF 81297 nor a twofold increase in the dose of SKF 81297 produced further exacerbation of the oral dyskinesia, probably because the animals were already maximally stimulated.

The findings in those two studies and in other monkey studies indicate the following:

- Treatment with a D_2 antagonist results in long-term, irreversible increased sensitivity to D_2- and D_1-antagonist treatment in the form of dystonia and dyskinesia (Lublin, Gerlach, & Peacock, 1993).
- During long-term treatment with a D_1 antagonist, tolerance develops toward the dystonic potential; thus high dosages can be given without producing dystonia (Christensen, 1990; Coffin, Barnett, & McHugh, 1991; Lublin et al., 1993). Given in acute high doses to drug-naive *Cebus* monkeys, a D_1 antagonist (SCH 23390) will produce dystonia (Casey, 1992).
- In drug-naive monkeys and in primed monkeys, treatment with both D_2 and D_1 antagonists can induce oral dyskinesia in the acute treatment phase (acute dyskinesia), as discussed later. Whereas a slight tolerance appears to develop to this effect during ongoing treatment with a D_1 antagonist, increasing dyskinesia develops during D_2-antagonist treatment (Lublin, Gerlach, & Mørkenberg, 1994).
- After withdrawal of long-term D_2-antagonist treatment, typical chronic oral dyskinesia (tardive dyskinesia) may be seen. Long-term D_1-antagonist treatment, at high dosages, may also induce tardive dyskinesia, if the "grooming syndrome" that appears after such treatment is a tardive dyskinesia correlate. When given at lower dosages, so-called clinical doses, a D_1 antagonist does not induce a grooming syndrome (Lublin et al., 1994). Therefore, the risk for tardive dyskinesia after D_1-antagonist treatment, if any, appears to be lower than that with a D_2 antagonist.
- Both D_2-antagonist treatment and (high-dosage) D_1-antagonist treatment will confer increased sensitivity to D_1-agonist effects. In the case of D_2-antagonist treatment, again this is expressed chiefly as oral dyskinesia, whereas in the case of (high-dosage) D_1-antagonist treatment, grooming-like behavior emerges. However, treatment with "clinical" dosages of a D_1 antagonist elicits no increased sensitivity to a D_1 agonist (Lublin et al., 1994).
- In primed monkeys, treatment with a D_1 agonist promotes oral dyskinesia, even in animals otherwise not presenting that behavior spontaneously. However, in animals with preexisting tardive dyskinesia, the oral dyskinesia becomes particularly extreme. Addition of a D_1 antagonist or a D_2 agonist to the D_1-agonist treatment counteracts the oral dyskinesia. These findings support the hypothesis that an imbalance of D_1/D_2 activity in favor of D_1 results in oral dyskinesia; they also indicate that the monkeys with tardive dyskinesia have relative D_1 hypersensitivity.
- The aggravated oral hyperkinesia in those monkeys with preexisting tardive dyskinesia (acute-in-chronic dyskinesia) that receive acute treatment with a D_2 antagonist at subdystonic doses can be explained by presynaptic D_2

blockade, resulting in increased release of dopamine. As the postsynaptic dopamine D_2 receptors are blocked, the dopamine stimulates the D_1 receptors, resulting in aggravation of tardive dyskinesia. Another implicated mechanism is the action of the direct postsynaptic blockade of a subset of D_2 receptors, which in itself causes acute dyskinesia and, in the long term, tardive dyskinesia, as discussed later.

• The fact that acute treatment with a D_1 antagonist at subdystonic doses diminishes preexisting tardive dyskinesia again points to a role for D_1 activity in tardive dyskinesia: When sufficient numbers of D_1 receptors are blocked, tardive dyskinesia is alleviated. But how do small doses of a D_1 antagonist increase oral dyskinesia in animals without preexisting tardive dyskinesia? It has been shown that a D_1 antagonist can increase both dopamine release (Imperato, Mulas, & Di Chiara, 1987) and the firing rate of dopaminergic neurons (Mereu et al., 1985). It has also been shown that a D_1 antagonist can reduce agonist binding to the D_2 receptor (Seeman et al., 1989). It is therefore conceivable that in a situation in which small numbers of D_1 receptors are blocked and in which the D_2 receptors are less efficient in binding dopamine, the increased stimulation of the dopaminergic system would result in preferential expression of the D_1 receptors, resulting in oral dyskinesia. As mentioned earlier, another mechanism implicated might be the direct blockade of a subset of D_1 receptors, which in itself can induce dyskinesia, as discussed later.

Clinical Studies

Most clinical studies have tried to manipulate the dopaminergic system on the basis of the D_2-hypersensitivity theory of tardive dyskinesia. However, the variable and generally disappointing results of such trials, as well as the lack of biochemical evidence, have led to rejection of that hypothesis (Fibiger & Lloyd, 1984; Gerlach, 1985). Later studies shifted their focus, determining that although alleviation of tardive dyskinesia usually can be achieved by D_2-receptor blockade and/or dopamine depletion (Gerlach, 1979; Fog, 1985), such methods seldom lead to total suppression (Nordic Dyskinesia Study Group, 1986; Lublin et al., 1991). In fact, in some cases, acute aggravation of tardive dyskinesia occurs during D_2 blockade. According to this line of reasoning, discontinuation of a D_2 antagonist does not always lead to aggravation of tardive dyskinesia; in many cases tardive dyskinesia decreases or remains unchanged. Furthermore, if D_2 hypersensitivity were responsible for tardive dyskinesia, it would be expected that D_2 antagonism would show more consistent and more effective suppressive effects, just as discontinuation should more consistently lead to aggravation. In effect, when D_2 antagonism has been found to alleviate tardive dyskinesia, the alleviation has, in most cases, been found to correspond to a concordant induction of parkinsonism. That D_2 antagonism may further aggravate tardive dyskinesia, and its withdrawal alleviate tardive dyskinesia, indicates that relative D_1 hypersensitivity rather than D_2 hypersensitivity may play a role in tardive dyskinesia.

So far, specific manipulations of the D_1 system have been too limited to confirm or refute the D_1/D_2-imbalance hypothesis. Nonetheless, the findings in two areas of clinical research may indirectly support the D_1/D_2-imbalance hypothesis.

In the first area, different dosage regimens for Madopar (levodopa with benserazide, a peripheral decarboxylase inhibitor) have shown that higher dosages of this drug tend to increase tardive dyskinesia during treatment, whether or not the patients are also taking neuroleptics (Alpert, Diamond, & Friedhoff, 1982; Casey, Gerlach, & Bjørndal, 1982). During a 5-week follow-up period, the tardive dyskinesia scores for patients also taking neuroleptics remained fixed, whereas neuroleptic-free patients showed modest-to-good improvements in their tardive dyskinesia scores. The best effect, total resolution, occurred in the youngest patient, a 45-year-old who had had tardive dyskinesia for 1 year. In terms of the D_1/D_2-imbalance hypothesis, those findings can be explained as follows: First the fact that acute high doses of levodopa tended to aggravate tardive dyskinesia is reconcilable with a D_1/D_2 imbalance in favor of D_1, for in such situations the effect of the increased dopamine, if any, will be to stimulate the D_1 receptors relatively more than the D_2 receptors. Second, the finding that tardive dyskinesia decreased after levodopa treatment in neuroleptic-free patients is attributable to the free exposure of both the D_1 and D_2 receptors, thereby allowing the increased dopamine to normalize their sensitivities and restore the D_1/D_2 balance. In elderly patients, however, in whom the D_1/D_2 balance is further disturbed by a relative loss of D_2 receptors, the balance is only partially restored. Moreover, the balance is not restored at all in neuroleptic-treated patients, because the ongoing D_2 blockade continues the process, via the D_2 system, that has promoted tardive dyskinesia.

In the second area, clinical experience with clozapine offers support for the D_1/D_2-imbalance hypothesis of tardive dyskinesia. Clozapine is a unique antipsychotic in that it does not cause dystonia, and its use apparently entails minimal, if any, risk of promoting tardive dyskinesia (Gerlach & Hansen, 1992; Peacock et al., 1996); for a review of clozapine's pharmacology, see Coward (1992). Treatment with clozapine may even allow resolution of tardive dyskinesia (Lieberman et al., 1991; Peacock et al., in press). In contrast to traditional neuroleptics, clozapine causes modest and balanced blockades of both D_1 and D_2 receptors (Farde et al., 1992). In rats, receptor-binding studies, as well as biochemical and behavioral studies, all indicate that clozapine is more like a D_1 antagonist than a D_2 antagonist (Jenner, Rupniak, & Marsden, 1985; La Hoste et al., 1991). That offers further support for the hypothesis that eliciting D_1 antagonism entails less risk of promoting tardive dyskinesia than does D_2 antagonism.

Receptor Studies

In animals and in humans, studies of the dopamine receptors in relation to spontaneous dyskinesia and dopamine-antagonist-induced dyskinesia have yielded conflicting results. Many of the studies were carried out prior to recognition of the D_1 and D_2 systems, without the availability of specific agonists and antagonists. They often focused either on receptor number and binding or on function alone, rather than on both these aspects. The functional biochemical studies that have been conducted have concentrated on the D_1 receptor's stimulation and the D_2 receptor's inhibition of adenylate cyclase; function in relation to other effector systems has not been examined. Although the findings are inconclusive and controversial, we shall outline the studies that have elucidated D_1/D_2-receptor changes of possible relevance to the pathogenesis of tardive dyskinesia.

Rosengarten et al. (1983) were the first researchers to postulate a role for D_1/D_2 imbalance in the pathogenesis of tardive dyskinesia. In 1986, that same group found an increased incidence of spontaneous oral movements in rats with higher D_1/D_2-receptor ratios, due to genetic predisposition, senescence, or in utero biochemical manipulation.

Memo et al. (1987) concluded that long-term haloperidol (D_2 antagonist) treatment in rats resulted in increased efficiency for both D_1 and D_2 recognition sites (function was studied, not receptor number or binding), with increased effects of the D_1 agonist in stimulating adenylate cyclase, and the D_2 agonist in inhibiting adenylate cyclase. The two systems remained balanced; the results of stimulation with dopamine did not differ from those for saline with regard to effects on adenylate cyclase.

The majority of studies have reported up-regulation of D_2-receptor number and increased ability of D_1 agonists to stimulate adenylate cyclase (i.e., increased D_1 function, through without increased D_1-receptor number or affinity) in response to long-term D_2 antagonism (Waddington & O'Boyle,

1987). Long-term treatment of rats with SCH 23390 (D_1 antagonist) has been found to result not only in up-regulation of D_1 receptors but also in increased behavioral responses to quinpirole (D_2 agonist) (Hess et al., 1986).

In general, the findings in receptor studies among humans have been contradictory and inconclusive, largely because of the methodological problems mentioned at the beginning of this section. Postmortem studies of humans, in particular, have suffered from insufficient registration of the subjects' tardive dyskinesia during life.

With positron-emission tomography (PET) one can obtain synchronized tardive dyskinesia ratings and evaluations of relative receptor densities. At the time of this writing, however, only three studies (all studies of D_2 receptors only) involving small numbers of subjects in different diagnostic categories have been published; no definitive conclusions can be drawn concerning differences in D_1- and D_2-receptor densities between patients with tardive dyskinesia and those without. For example, Losonczy et al. (1989) found significantly lower D_2-receptor numbers in patients with tardive dyskinesia than in controls (all schizophrenic patients). Blin et al. (1989), on the other hand, found a positive correlation between densities of D_2 receptors and orofacial AIMS scores (mostly patients with diagnoses of depression). And Andersson et al. (1990) found no significant differences in D_2-receptor binding rates between tardive dyskinesia patients (mainly with organic psychoses) and controls (healthy volunteers, plus patients with organic psychoses and pituitary adenomas). It must be emphasized that one limitation of PET is indeed critical, because behavioral and biochemical variations can occur without changes in receptor numbers or affinities; PET can provide indications of only receptor binding characteristics, not receptor function.

As for age, several postmortem studies have found decreases in D_2-receptor numbers and activity with aging, although the findings regarding D_1 receptors have been conflicting. The majority of studies point to increasing D_1/D_2-receptor ratios with increasing age (Waddington & O'Boyle, 1987). Because age has long been recognized as a predisposing factor for both spontaneous dyskinesia and neuroleptic-related oral dyskinesia, the possibility of a relative decrease in D_2-receptor activity in relation to D_1-receptor activity with increasing age would support the hypothesis of tardive dyskinesia being related to a D_1/D_2 imbalance in favor of D_1.

Proposed Models for D_2- and D_1-Antagonist-Induced Dyskinesia

We propose the following four models for D_2- and D_1-antagonist-induced dyskinesia, as well as a model combining aspects of models 2, 3, and 4.

Model 1

According to the original dopamine-hypersensitivity theory of tardive dyskinesia, conceived at a time when there was no knowledge of dopamine-receptor subtypes, acute neuroleptic blockade of dopamine receptors and a simultaneous increase in acetylcholine turnover should result in parkinsonism, whereas chronic dopamine blockade should result in compensatory dopamine hypersensitivity and cholinergic hyposensitivity, leading to decreasing manifestations of parkinsonism and thus to tardive dyskinesia (Klawans & Rubovits, 1972; Tarsy & Baldessarini, 1973; Gerlach, 1979) (Figure 12.1a). One implication of that model would be that parkinsonism and tardive dyskinesia are at opposite poles, and possibly are mutually exclusive.

Model 2

In view of the evidence from both monkey studies and clinical observations that acute dopamine blockade by neuroleptics can evoke dyskinesia (especially in individuals previously exposed to neuroleptics) and that parkinsonism and tardive dyskinesia often occur simultaneously, a second model hypothesizes that blockade of one subset of D_2 receptors will result in dyskinesia, whereas blockade of another subset will result in parkinsonism (Gerlach, 1985; Scheel-Krüger & Arnt, 1985; Gerlach & Casey, 1988) (Figure 12.1b). According to this model, acute D_2-receptor blockade will result in an admixture of hypokinesia (parkinsonism) and hyperkinesia (acute dyskinesia, or, in severe cases, dystonia). The degree of expression of the individual effects will depend on the degrees of antagonism of the receptor subsets. Long-term D_2-antagonist treatment can result in reversible or irreversible dysfunction of the receptor subsets, leading to tardive dyskinesia, tardive dystonia, and tardive parkinsonism. This model is still viable.

Model 3

With the development of a range of D_1- and D_2-selective agonists and antagonists, it was found that the D_1 and D_2 systems play opposing roles in relation to oral dyskinesia: D_1 activity promoting, and D_2 activity opposing, such behavior. All this leads to a model in which an imbalance in the D_1/D_2-receptor ratio in favor of D_1 results in dyskinesia (Rosengarten et al., 1983; Peacock et al., 1990; Gerlach, 1991). This model adequately explains the acute effects of neuroleptics, with D_2 blockade resulting in parkinsonism and, at the same time, in relatively increased stimulation of the D_1 receptors, which in turn results in dyskinesia (Figure 12.1c). The model is also in accord

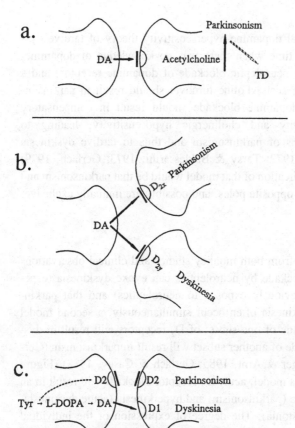

Figure 12.1. Schematic representations of dopamine synapses, illustrating previous hypotheses regarding tardive dyskinesia (TD). (a) Acute dopamine blockade increases acetylcholine turnover, resulting in parkinsonism. Chronic dopamine blockade results in dopamine hypersensitivity and cholinergic hyposensitivity, resulting in decreased parkinsonism and tardive dyskinesia. (b) Acute blockade of one subset of D_2 receptors results in dyskinesia, and blockade of another subset results in parkinsonism. Parkinsonism and dyskinesia are intermixed to varying degrees, depending on the relative degrees of antagonism of the D_2-receptor subsets. According to this model, tardive dyskinesia may be the result of induction of long-term dysfunction (mimicking blockade) of a D_2 receptor subset. (c) D_1 activity promotes, and D_2 activity opposes, dyskinesia. Blockade of presynaptic D_2 receptors increases dopamine release. As the postsynaptic D_2 receptors are also blocked, the dopamine stimulates the D_1 receptors, resulting in dyskinesia. The postsynaptic D_2 blockade can also lead to parkinsonism.

with the increasing prevalence of spontaneous dyskinesia with increasing age (where there is a relative decrease in D_2 receptors relative to D_1 receptors) and the greater susceptibility of the elderly to dyskinesia.

Model 4

A model for a change in the relative D_1/D_2-receptor ratios is inadequate, for it does not conform with what is known about changes in the numbers of D_1 and D_2 receptors after long-term D_1- or D_2-antagonist treatment and the propensities of these antagonists to induce tardive dyskinesia. Thus, long-term D_1-antagonist treatment, which increases the number of D_1 receptors, entails an apparently lesser risk of promoting tardive dyskinesia, in contrast to D_2-antagonist treatment, which increases the number of D_2 receptors and carries an apparently greater risk of promoting tardive dyskinesia (Glenthøj, Bolwig, & Hemmingsen, 1991, 1993; Lublin et al., 1994). In light of the foregoing, the effects of D_1 and D_2 antagonists on the efficacies of the D_1 and D_2 receptors must be considered. The phrase "efficacy of the receptor" is used in a broad sense, encompassing the effects of the binding of dopamine on the receptor's immediate effector and the effector's participation in the subsequent cascade of reactions, which also involves interactions with other neurotransmitter systems.

A model that could explain the propensity of D_2 antagonists to promote tardive dyskinesia would have to show that such treatment would increase the efficacy of the D_1 receptors in promoting oral dyskinesia and at the same time would promote ongoing D_2 blockade that would disallow the expression of any increased D_2 sensitivity that would otherwise oppose dyskinesia (Figure 12.2b). If the D_2 blockade were discontinued, increased expression of D_2 activity and normalization of D_1 activity would allow gradual resolution of the tardive dyskinesia, though in some individuals the imbalance would persist and the tardive dyskinesia would be irreversible. Such individuals with persistent tardive dyskinesia may have an endogenous imbalance in D_1/D_2-receptor numbers or efficacies.

Acute D_1-antagonist treatment can result in transitory acute dyskinesia. This effect is most often seen when small doses are given (Peacock et al., 1990). The mechanism of this paradoxical effect is unknown. One possible explanation is that there may be subsets of D_1 receptors whose direct blockade will cause dyskinesia or parkinsonism (analogous to the D_2-receptor subsets mentioned for model 2). Another possible explanation is that even a relatively small level of D_1 blockade might cause relatively greater indirect D_2 antagonism and, at the same time, increased dopamine activity, the net result of

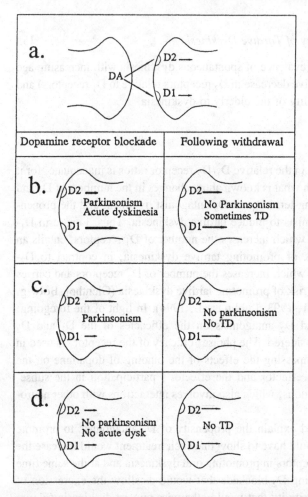

Figure 12.2. Schematic representation of new tardive dyskinesia hypotheses encompassing changes in the efficacies of the blocked postsynaptic receptors and the associated dopamine neuron systems. (a) D_1 activity promotes, and D_2 activity inhibits, dyskinesia. Normally, the activities of the D_1 and D_2 receptors are in balance, and there is no dyskinesia. (b) Long-term D_2-antagonist treatment increases the efficacy of D_1 receptors in promoting dyskinesia. The ongoing D_1 blockade disallows the expression of any increased D_2 sensitivity, and acute dyskinesia may result. After withdrawal of the D_2 antagonist, increased expression of D_2 activity and normalization of D_1 activity allow gradual resolution of tardive dyskinesia. In some individuals the imbalance persits, and the tardive dyskinesia is irreversible. (c) Acute D_1-antagonist treatment can cause transitory acute dyskinesia. Although the mechanism of this paradoxical dyskinesia is unclear, there are several possible explanations. Long-term D_1-antagonist treatment mildly increases the efficacy of the D_2 receptors in opposing dyskinesia. The ongoing D_1 blockade disallows the expression of any increased D_1 sensitivity. When the D_1 blockade is discontinued, D_1 hypersensitivity is held in check by the concomitant D_2 hypersensitivity, and there is no tardive dyskinesia. (d) Clozapine produces balanced and relatively weak blockade of both D_1 and D_2 receptors. The sensitivities of the D_1 and D_2 receptors remain balanced both during and after treatment, so that neither acute nor tardive dyskinesia is induced.

154

which would be increased expression of the unblocked D_1 receptors (as discussed in the section on nonhuman-primate studies). Long-term D_1-antagonist treatment results in mildly increased efficacy of the D_2 receptors to oppose dyskinesia; at the same time, the ongoing blockade of the D_1 receptors disallows the expression of any increased D_1 sensitivity (Figure 12.2c). When the D_1 blockade is discontinued, D_1 hypersensitivity is either (1) completely checked by the concomitant D_2 hypersensitivity (after treatment with "clinical" dosages of a D_1 antagonist), with no resultant dyskinesia, or (2) only partially checked (after treatment with "supraclinical" dosages), resulting in a "grooming" syndrome that resolves with the normalization of D_1 sensitivity.

Clozapine treatment, which results in balanced and relatively weak blockade of both D_1 and D_2 receptors, permits a continual balance between D_1 and D_2 activities, thereby entailing lesser risk of promoting both acute dyskinesia and chronic dyskinesia (Figure 12.2d).

Combination Model

A combination of models 2, 3, and 4 may be operative as well. Model 3 can explain the acute effects of D_1 and D_2 antagonists and an individual predisposition to develop spontaneous and tardive dyskinesia. D_2-antagonist treatment can induce tardive dyskinesia both by causing long-term dysfunction of a subset of D_2 receptors (model 2) and by increasing the efficacy of D_1 receptors (model 3). Although blockade of a subset of D_1 receptors may result in acute dyskinesia, no long-term dysfunction of these receptors is seen, and tolerance develops rapidly. Furthermore, any induction of hypersensitivity of D_1 receptors that would promote dyskinesia (which appears to be minimal after clinical dosages of a D_1 antagonist) is checked by concomitantly increased efficacy of D_2 receptors opposing dyskinesia.

Conclusions and Areas for Future Research

In this chapter we have presented the evidence that supports a role for an imbalance in D_1/D_2 activities in the pathophysiology of tardive dyskinesia. Specifically, we have proposed that whereas traditional neuroleptic treatment (i.e., D_2-antagonist treatment) induces an increase in the number of D_2 receptors, it also increases the efficacy of D_1 receptors. In individuals predisposed to tardive dyskinesia, D_1 activity predominates. In such individuals, preexisting relative D_2 hyposensitivity or D_1 hypersensitivity will be unmasked by acute D_2-antagonist treatment, thereby promoting acute dyskinesia. A subsequent further imbalance in D_1- and D_2-receptor activities due to long-term treatment will promote the induction of chronic oral dyskinesia (tardive dyskinesia). During ongoing D_2-antagonist treatment, the tardive dyskinesia can either be masked by the ensuing parkinsonism or be aggravated because the D_2 blockade allows greater expression of D_1 activity (acute in chronic tardive dyskinesia). A further mechanism whereby D_2 antagonism may cause acute dyskinesia entails a direct effect of the blockade of a subset of D_2 receptors. Long-term D_2 antagonism may induce reversible or irreversible dysfunction of this D_2-receptor subset, resulting in tardive dyskinesia.

The development of clinically efficacious D_1 antagonists may be one answer to the problem of preventing tardive dyskinesia. We propose that D_1 antagonism, by promoting increased D_2 efficacy, allows a counteraction for any D_1-receptor up-regulation induced by this treatment, thereby avoiding domination of D_1 activity. Clinical trials with D_1 antagonists must be undertaken so that the clinical implications of this "counterbalanced" D_1 hypersensitivity can be elucidated. Such trials are under way, but as yet neither the short- nor long-term findings are known. As with D_2 antagonists, however, understanding the long-term effects may require many years of use.

During recent years there has been a tremendous increase in the number of studies to elucidate the nature of the dopaminergic system in the CNS. Thus, whereas this chapter speaks in terms of dopamine D_1 and D_2 receptors, it is now known that at least five dopamine-receptor subtypes exist: the D_2 subtypes l and s (long and short); the D_3 and D_4, belonging to the D_2 family; and the D_1 and D_5, belonging to the D_1 family (Sibley & Monsma, 1992). Increasing insight into these receptor subtypes may well explain individual susceptibility/resistance to tardive dyskinesia, clarify the pathogenesis of this syndrome, and lead to preventive measures through the development of more selective dopamine antagonists. It can already be hypothesized that genetic polymorphisms, altered regulation at the level of DNA or mRNA, postribosomal modifications of protein synthesis, and regional differences in the expression of dopamine-receptor subtypes may be able to account for individual susceptibility/resistance to tardive dyskinesia, as well as the capacity of neuroleptics to produce long-term side effects.

It must be emphasized, however, that although the dopaminergic system does play a role in the pathophysiology of tardive dyskinesia, it may not play the title role. The CNS is composed of a multitude of neurotransmitter systems, all acting on one another and counteracting each other in a fine balance, with different and often opposing interactions occurring at different anatomic sites. Changes in the balance within one system will invariably effect changes in the balance within another. Therefore, the primary sensitivity to tardive dyskinesia, or the imbalance resulting in tardive dyskinesia, may well be found in another transmitter system, whether GABAergic, cholinergic, peptidergic, or some other system. Also, imbalances in different neurotransmitter systems may account for the heterogeneous pathophysiology of tardive dyskinesia.

References

Alpert, M., Diamond, F., & Friedhoff, A. J. (1982). Receptor sensitivity modification in the treatment of tardive dyskinesia. *Psychopharmacol. Bull.* 18:90–92.

Andersson, U., Eckernas, S.-Å., Hatvig, P., Ulin, J., Långstrom, B., & Haggstrom, J.-E. (1990). Striatal binding of ^{11}C-NMSP studied with positron emission tomography in patients with persistent tardive dyskinesia: no evidence for altered dopamine D_2 receptor binding. *J. Neural Transm. Gen. Sec.* 79:215–26.

Blin, J., Baron, J. C., Cambon, H., Bonnet, A. M., Dubois, B., Loc'h, C., Maziere, B., & Agid, Y. (1989). Striatal dopamine D_2 receptors in tardive dyskinesia: PET study. *J. Neurol. Neurosurg. Psychiatry* 52:1248–52.

Casey, D. E. (1991). Neuroleptic drug-induced extrapyramidal syndromes and tardive dyskinesia. *Schizophr. Res.* 4:109–20.

Casey, D. E. (1992). Dopamine D_1 (SCH 23390) and D_2 (haloperidol) antagonists in drug-naive monkeys. *Psychopharmacology* 107:18–22.

Casey, D. E., Gerlach, J., & Bjørndal, N. (1982). Levodopa and receptor sensitivity modification in tardive dyskinesia. *Psychopharmacology* 78:89–92.

Christensen, A. V. (1990). Long-term effects of dopamine D_1 and D_2 antagonists in vervet monkeys. *Behav. Neurol.* 3:49–60.

Coffin, V. L., Barnett, A., & McHugh, D. T. (1991). Reversal of extrapyramidal side effects with SCH 23390, a dopamine D_1 receptor antagonist. In *Abstracts of Panels and Posters*, 30th annual meeting of the American College of Neuropharmacology, San Juan, Puerto Rico, December 9–13.

Coward, D. M. (1992). General pharmacology of clozapine. *Br. J. Psychiatry* (*Suppl. 17*) 160:5–11.

Crane, G. E., Naranjo, E. R., & Chase, C. (1971). Motor disorders induced by neuroleptics: a proposed new classification. *Arch. Gen. Psychiatry* 24:179–84.

Daly, S. A., & Waddington, J. L. (1992). D-1 dopamine receptors and the topography of unconditioned motor behaviour: studies with the selective, "full efficacy" benzazepine D-1 agonist SKF 83189. *J. Psychopharmacol.* 6:50–60.

Farde, L., Nordstrom, A.-L., Wiesel, F.-A., Pauli, S., Halldin, C., & Sedvall, G. (1992). Positron emission tomographic analysis of central D_1 and D_2 dopamine receptor occupancy in patients treated with classical neuroleptics and clozapine. *Arch. Gen. Psychiatry* 49:538–44.

Fibiger, H. C., & Lloyd, K. G. (1984). Neurobiological substrates of tardive dyskinesia: the GABA hypothesis. *Trends Neurosci.* 7:462–4.

Fog, R. (1985). The effect of dopamine antagonists in spontaneous and tardive dyskinesia. In *Dyskinesia: Research and Treatment*, ed. D. E. Casey, T. N. Chase, A. V. Christensen, & J. Gerlach, pp. 118–21. Berlin: Springer-Verlag.

Gerlach, J. (1979). Tardive dyskinesia. *Dan. Med. Bull.* 46:209–45.

Gerlach, J. (1985). Pathophysiological mechanisms underlying tardive dyskinesia. In *Dyskinesia: Research and Treatment*, ed. D. E. Casey, T. N. Chase, A. V. Christensen, & J. Gerlach, pp. 98–103. Berlin: Springer-Verlag.

Gerlach, J. (1991). Current views on tardive dyskinesia. *Pharmacopsychiatry* 24:47–8.

Gerlach, J., & Casey, D. E. (1988). Tardive dyskinesia. *Acta Psychiatr. Scand.* 77:369–78.

Gerlach, J., & Hansen, L. (1992). Clozapine and D_1/D_2 antagonism in extrapyramidal functions. *Br. J. Psychiatry (Suppl. 17)* 160:34–7.

Gerlach, J., & Hansen, L. (1993). Effect of chronic treatment with NNC 756, a new D-1 receptor antagonist, or raclopride, a D-2 receptor antagonist, in drug-naive *Cebus* monkeys: dystonia, dyskinesia and D_1/D_2 supersensitivity. *J. Psychopharmacol.* 7:355–64.

Glenthøj, B., Arnt, J., & Hyttel, J. (1990a). Effect of a dopamine D-1 agonist in rates treated chronically with zuclopenthixol. *Life Sci.* 47:1339–46.

Glenthøj, B., Bolwig, T. G., & Hemmingsen, R. (1991). Continuous versus discontinuous neuroleptic treatment in an animal model of tardive dyskinesia. In *Biological Psychiatry*, vol. 1, ed. G. Racagni, N. Brunello, & T. Fukada, pp. 602–4. Amsterdam: Elsevier.

Glenthøj, B., Bolwig, T. G., & Hemmingsen, R. (1993). Effects of chronic discontinuous and continuous treatment of rats with a dopamine D_1 receptor antagonist (NNC-756). *Eur. J. Pharmacol.* 242:283–91.

Glenthøj, B., Hemmingsen, R., Allerup, P., & Bolwig, T. G. (1990b). Intermittent versus chronic neuroleptic treatment in a rat model. *Eur. J. Pharmacol.* 190:275–86.

Hess, E. J., Albers, L. J., Hoang, L., & Creese, I. (1986). Effects of chronic SCH 23390 treatment on the biochemical and behavioral properties of D_1 and D_2 dopamine receptors: potentiated behavioral responses to a D_2 dopamine agonist after selection D_1 dopamine receptor upregulation. *J. Pharmacol. Exp. Ther.* 238:846–54.

Imperato, A., Mulas, A., & Di Chiara, G. (1987). The D_1 antagonist SCH 23390 stimulates while the D_1 agonist SKF 38393 fails to affect dopamine release in the dorsal caudate of freely-moving rats. *Eur. J. Pharmacol.* 142:177–81.

Jenner, P., Rupniak, N. M. J., & Marsden, C. D. (1985). Differential alteration of striatal D-1 and D-2 receptors induced by the long-term administration of haloperidol, sulpiride or clozapine in rats. In *Dyskinesia: Research and Treatment*, ed. D. E. Casey, T. N. Chase, A. V. Christensen, & J. Gerlach, pp. 174–81. Berlin: Springer-Verlag.

Johansson, P., Levin, E., Gunne, L., & Ellison, G. (1987). Opposite effects of a D_1 and a D_2 agonist on oral movements in rats. *Eur. J. Pharmacol.* 134:83–8.

Kistrup, K., & Gerlach, J. (1987). Selective D-1 and D-2 receptor manipulation in *Cebus* monkeys: relevance for dystonia and dyskinesia in humans. *Pharmacol. Toxicol.* 61:157–61.

Klawans, H. L., & Rubovits, R. (1972). An experimental model of tardive dyskinesia. *J. Neural Transm.* 33:235–46.

La Hoste, G. J., O,Dell, S. J., Widmark, C. B., Shapiro, R. M., Potkin, S. G., & Marshall, J. F. (1991). Differential changes in dopamine and serotonin receptors induced by clozapine and haloperidol. In *Advances in Neuropsychiatry and Psychopharmacology. Vol. 1: Schizophrenia Research*, ed. C. A. Tamminga & S. C. Schultz, pp. 351–61. New York: Raven Press.

Lieberman, J. A., Saltz, B., Johns, C. A., Pollack, S., Borenstein, M., & Kane, J. (1991). The effects of clozapine on tardive dyskinesia. *Br. J. Psychiatry* 158:503–10.

Losonczy, M. F., Davidson, M., Lobel, D., Fowler, J., Crispman, D., Wolf, A. P., & Davis, K. L. (1989). Methodological issues in PET scan evaluation of dopamine supersensitivity in tardive dyskinesia. *Schizophr. Res.* 2:112.

Lublin, H., Gerlach, J., Hagert, U., Meidahl, B., Mølbjerg, C., Pedersen, V.,

Rendtorff, C., & Tolvanen, E. (1991). Zuclopenthixol, a combined dopamine D_1/D_2 antagonist, versus haloperidol, a dopamine D_2 antagonist, in tardive dyskinesia. *Eur. Neuropsychopharmacol.* 1:541–8.

Lublin, H., Gerlach, J., & Mørkeberg, F. (1994). Long-term treatment with clinical doses of the D_1 antagonist NNC 756 and the D_2 antagonist raclopride in monkeys previously exposed to dopamine antagonists. *Psychopharmacology* 114:495–504.

Lublin, H., Gerlach, J., & Peacock, L. (1993). Chronic treatment with the D-1 receptor antagonist, SCH 23390, and the D-2 receptor antagonist, raclopride, in Cebus monkeys withdrawn from previous haloperidol treatment: extrapyramidal syndromes and dopaminergic supersensitivity. *Psychopharmacology* 112:389–97.

Memo, M., Pizzi, M., Missale, C., Carruba, C. O., & Spano, P. F. (1987). Modification of the function of D_1 and D_2 dopamine receptors in striatum and nucleous accumbens of rats chronically treated with haloperidol. *Neuropharmacology* 26:477–80.

Mereu, G., Collu, M., Ongini, E., Biggio, G., & Gessa, G. L. (1985). SCH 23390, a selective dopamine D_1 antagonist, activates dopamine neurons but fails to prevent their inhibition by apomorphine. *Eur. J. Pharmacol.* 111:393–6.

Nordic Dyskinesia Study Group (1986). Effect of different neuroleptics in tardive dyskinesia and parkinsonism: a video-controlled multicenter study with chlorprothixene, perphenazine, haloperidol and haloperidol + biperiden. *Psychopharmacology* 90:423–9.

Peacock, L., Lublin, H., & Gerlach, J. (1990). The effects of dopamine D_1 and D_2 receptor agonists and antagonists in monkeys withdrawn from long-term neuroleptic treatment. *Eur. J. Pharmacol.* 186:49–59.

Peacock, L., Solgaard, T., Lublin, H., & Gerlach, J. (1996). Clozapine versus typical antipsychotics: a retro- and prospective study of extrapyramidal side effects. *Psychopharmacology* 124:188–196.

Rosengarten, H., Schweitzer, J. W., & Friedhoff, A. J. (1983). Induction of oral dyskinesias in naive rats by D-1 stimulation. *Life Sci.* 33:2479–82.

Rosengarten, H., Schweitzer, J. W., & Friedhoff, A. J. (1986). Selective dopamine D_2 receptor reduction enhances a D_1 mediated oral dyskinesia in rats. *Life Sci.* 39:29–35.

Rupniak, N. M. J., Jenner, P., & Marsden, C. D. (1985). Pharmacological characterization of spontaneous or drug-associated purposeless chewing movements in rats. *Psychopharmacology* 85:71–9.

Scheel-Krüger, J., & Arnt, J. (1985). New aspects on the role of dopamine, acetylcholine and GABA in the development of tardive dyskinesia. In *Dyskinesia: Research and Treatment*, ed. D. E. Casey, T. N. Chase, A. V. Christensen, & J. Gerlach, pp. 98–103. Berlin: Springer-Verlag.

Schonecker, M. (1957). Ein eigentumliches Syndrom in oralen Bereich bei Megaphen-applikation. *Nervenartz* 28:35–6.

Seeman, P., Niznik, H. B., Guan, H. C., Booth, G., & Ulpian, C. (1989). Link between D_1 and D_2 receptors is reduced in schizophrenia and Huntington diseased brain. *Proc. Natl. Acad. Sci. USA* 86:10156–60.

Sibley, D. R., & Monsma, F. R., Jr. (1992). Molecular biology of dopamine receptors. *Trends Pharmacol. Sci.* 13:61–9.

Tarsy, D., & Baldessarini, R. J. (1973). Pharmacologically-induced behavioral supersensitivity to apomorphine. *Nature* 245:262–3.

Uhrbrand, L., & Faurbye, A. (1960). Reversible and irreversible dyskinesia after treatment with perphenazine, chlorpromazine, reserpine and electroconvulsive therapy. *Psychopharmacologia* 1:408–18.

Waddington, J. L. (1986). Behavioural correlates of the action of selective D-1 dopamine receptor antagonists; impact of SCH 23390 and SKF 83566, and functionally interactive D-1 : D-2 receptor systems. *Biochem. Pharmacol.* 35:3661–7.

Waddington, J. L. (1990). Spontaneous orofacial movements induced in rodents by very long-term neuroleptic drug administration: phenomenology, pathophysiology and putative relationship to tardive dyskinesia. *Psychopharmacology* 101:431–47.

Waddington, J. L., Cross, A. J., Gamble, S. J., & Bourne, R. C. (1983). Spontaneous orofacial dyskinesia and dopaminergic function in rats after 6 months neuroleptic treatment. *Science* 220:530–2.

Waddington, J. L., & Molloy, A. G. (1987). The status of late-onset vacuous chewing/perioral movements during long-term neuroleptic treatment in rodents: tardive dyskinesia or dystonia? *Psychopharmacology* 91:136–7.

Waddington, J. L., & O'Boyle, K. M. (1987). The D-1 dopamine receptor and the search for its functional role: from neurochemistry to behavior. *Rev. Neurosci.* 1:157–84.

13

Tardive Dyskinesia and Phenylalanine Metabolism: Risk-Factor Studies

MARY ANN RICHARDSON, Ph.D., CHERYL FLYNN, Ph.D., LAURA READ, Ph.D., MARGARET REILLY, Ph.D., and RAYMOND SUCKOW, Ph.D.

Continuing research on tardive dyskinesia has considerably broadened the classic hypothesis of dopamine-receptor supersensitivity, proposed more than 20 years ago (Klawans, 1973). Roles for other neurotransmitter systems (GABA and norepinephrine) have been postulated (Tamminga, Crayton, & Chase, 1979; Wagner et al., 1982; Fibiger & Lloyd, 1984; Gunne, Häggström, & Sjöquist, 1984; Jeste, Doongaji, & Linnoila, 1984; Stahl et al., 1985; Kaufman et al., 1986; Thaker et al., 1987; Andersson et al., 1989; Thaker, Nguyen, & Tamminga, 1989), and there is a newer hypothesis suggesting that cellular damage mediated by free radicals underlies tardive dyskinesia (Lohr et al., 1988, 1990; Cadet & Lohr, 1989). Demographic and psychiatric variables, such as gender, age, and concomitant affective disorder, have also been identified as risk factors (Smith & Baldessarini, 1980; Jeste & Wyatt, 1982; Kane & Smith, 1982; Richardson et al., 1985; Kane et al., 1986; Weiner & Lang, 1989). Increasingly, these disparate variables support the concept that tardive dyskinesia, like most brain dysfunctions, may involve multiple abnormalities and that vulnerability to it may be multifactorial. In this chapter we summarize our findings concerning risk factors for tardive dyskinesia that suggest that amino acid metabolism – particularly that of the large neutral amino acid phenylalanine (Phe) – may play a role in vulnerability to tardive dyskinesia.

Four Studies

The first of our studies associating tardive dyskinesia with the metabolism of Phe was a large-scale (N = 211) cross-sectional, point-prevalence study of mentally retarded adult residents in a state developmental center (Richardson et al., 1986, 1989). We found that phenylketonuria (PKU) was a significant risk factor for tardive dyskinesia, given that 86% of those with PKU in the sample had tardive dyskinesia, as compared with 28% of the non-PKU population. Variables related to the duration and dosage of neuroleptic treatment were not significant discriminators for tardive dyskinesia status. PKU is a severe hyperphenylalaninemia (HPA) that along with milder HPA variants is caused by structural mutations in the genes coding for phenylalanine-4-hydroxylase or, more rarely, dihydropteridine reductase, located on chromosome 12 (Lidsky et al., 1984; Ledley, Levy, & Woo, 1986) and chromosome 4, respectively (Brown & Dahl, 1987). Phenylalanine-4-hydroxylase converts Phe to tyrosine, and dihydropteridine reductase regenerates the tetra-hydrobiopterin cofactor (Danks et al., 1978). Affected individuals have elevated plasma and tissue concentrations of Phe and its metabolites: phenylethylamine (PEA), phenyllactic acid (PLA), and phenylacetic acid (PAA). These metabolites, found in trace amounts in normal individuals, are derived from the transformation of the alanine side chain of Phe by alternative pathways (Knox & Hsia, 1957; Pardridge & Choi, 1986). Defects found in patients with PKU include depressed protein and lipid syntheses and deficient myelination (Proud, Hsia, & Wolf, 1989). The neurological symptoms of the disorder include mental retardation, seizures, spasticity, and electroen-cephalographic (EEG) irregularities. Associated psychiatric and behavioral symptoms include anxiety, restlessness, hyperactivity, and irritability (Knox, 1972).

A second investigation, a case–control (N = 32) study of male schizophrenics, focused on the associations between affective symptoms and tardive dyskinesia (Richardson et al., 1985, 1989). In that study, multivariate analysis found that "activation" and "hostility-suspiciousness," factors in the Brief Psychiatric Rating Scale (BPRS) (Overall & Gorham, 1962), could discriminate positive tardive dyskinesia status independently. That risk-factor finding and several significant univariate tardive dyskinesia associations from the study – the "inappropriate affect" item from the Affective Flattening Scale (Andreasen, 1979), a history of manic symptoms (according to the criteria of the *Diagnostic and Statistical Manual of Mental Disorders*, third edition [DSM-III]), a history of grandiose delusions, and the "suicide" item from the Hamilton Psychiatric Rating Scale for Depression (Hamilton, 1960) – generated a vulnerability profile that defined male schizophrenics with secondary mania-like affective symptoms as significantly at risk for tardive dyskinesia. Those findings are in agreement with the findings in several other studies reporting associations between affective disorder and tardive dyskinesia (Davis, Berger, & Hollister, 1976; Rosenbaum et al., 1979; Cutler & Post, 1982; Rush, Diamond, & Alpert, 1982; Yassa et al., 1992).

Of particular interest in regard to these findings were the previous reports of abnormally high urinary concentrations of PEA in manic patients (Fischer & Heller, 1972). PEA had been proposed as a neuromodulator (Boulton & Juorio, 1982; Boulton, Juorio, & Paterson, 1990), influencing arousal, mood, and libido. Elevated concentrations have been associated with mania, and low concentrations have been associated with depressive disorder (Sabelli & Mosnaim, 1974; Sabelli et al., 1983a,b, 1986). In one study, 5 women with bipolar affective disorder periodically excreted very high urinary concentrations of PEA (Karoum et al., 1982). The PEA excretion rate did not correlate with mood ratings, but seemed to be a trait condition. Those patients also manifested inappropriate affect. In another study, 3 women with rapidly cycling bipolar disorder and depression-dependent dyskinesia also had abnormally high concentrations of PEA (Linnoila et al., 1983). In another study, schizoaffective/manic patients (DSM-III-R) had significantly higher 24-hour PAA excretion rates than did schizophrenics (Sabelli et al., 1989). In fact, the psychiatric-symptom profiles for the patients from those studies who excreted abnormally high concentrations of PEA and PAA (although the patients were generally not from the same diagnostic group) closely resembled the profile for tardive dyskinesia vulnerability defined in our study of male schizophrenics. Because that suggested a relationship between PKU-like defects in Phe metabolism and a manic affective profile, we hypothesized that schizophrenics and PKU patients may share Phe-related risk factors for tardive dyskinesia.[6]

To examine that hypothesis, schizophrenic males ($n = 53$) and females ($n = 17$) were administered a high-protein breakfast, containing a mean Phe load per subject of 50 mg/kg. Plasma concentrations of PEA, Phe, and other large neutral amino acids (LNAA) were measured before and after the meal. Logistic regression analysis indicated that higher post-loading plasma Phe concentrations and Phe/LNAA ratios were risk factors for tardive dyskinesia, independent of age, in male schizophrenics ($n = 53$). The "activation" factor of the BPRS was also a significant factor in predicting tardive dyskinesia, in agreement with our prior finding. Although tardive dyskinesia was as prevalent in our pilot sample of females ($n = 17$, 71%) as it was for males (64%), no associations between tardive dyskinesia and Phe variables for the females, similar to those found for males, appeared.

In a subsequent study, we tested more rigorously the Phe risk-factor finding by administering a challenge of pure Phe (100 mg/kg) measured exactly for each patient. In males ($n = 209$), the Phe challenge yielded significantly greater differentiation between patients with tardive dyskinesia and those without, as compared with the protein load, again eliciting significantly higher post-loading plasma Phe concentrations and Phe/LNAA ratios in those with tardive dyskinesia. Besides finding that post-challenge Phe variables are predictors of tardive dyskinesia, the overall logistic regression models (for males) predicted that older age and a higher Hamilton Psychiatric Rating Scale for Depression (HAM-D) score were risk factors for tardive dyskinesia. Significant gender differences were again found in the relationship between Phe variables and tardive dyskinesia status for females ($n = 103$); no significant relationships between their tardive dyskinesia status and plasma Phe variables were found, except for a trend toward higher fasting Phe concentrations in those with tardive dyskinesia.

We thus found the Phe risk factor for tardive dyskinesia in males to be reproducible, as were the gender differences and the affective disorder components. Recently, Gardos et al. (1992) found an association between the severity of tardive dyskinesia symptoms and 2-hour-post-loading plasma concentrations of Phe in unipolar depressed patients given an oral Phe challenge (100 mg/kg). Neither of these novel findings indicate the mechanism linking Phe metabolism with tardive dyskinesia, but by using PKU as a model, we speculate that a defect, perhaps genetic, in Phe metabolism may influence the supply of amino acids to the brain.

Amino Acid Transport in Brain and PKU

The brain, separated from the peripheral circulation by the blood–brain barrier, relies on facilitated diffusion from plasma for its supply of amino acids for protein and neurotransmitter synthesis. Tryptophan and tyrosine, precursors for the monoamine neurotransmitters dopamine, norepinephrine, epinephrine, and serotonin, enter the brain via a neutral amino acid transporter, designated the L-system (for leucine). This transport system competitively mediates the bidirectional flux of all the neutral amino acids (Phe, tryptophan, tyrosine, leucine, isoleucine, valine, threonine, methionine, and histidine) between the blood and brain. This high-affinity, low-capacity system is normally unsaturated; thus entry of a given amino acid into the brain is determined by a combination of its concentration in plasma, its relative affinity for the carrier, and the concentrations of the competing amino acids (Fernstrom & Faller, 1978). The ratio of the concentration of a single amino acid to the concentrations of the other LNAA is a simplified, commonly used index for the entry of that amino acid into the brain, one that corrects for the competition of the other LNAA at the blood–brain barrier. Using Phe as an example, it is calculated as follows (Pardridge & Choi, 1986):

$$\text{Phe/LNAA} = \frac{[\text{Phe}]}{[\text{isoleucine} + \text{leucine} + \text{valine} + \text{tyrosine} + \text{tryptophan} + \text{methionine} + \text{histidine}]}$$

A further refinement of this equation will correct for the affinities of the various amino acids for the carrier, which vary by more than 500% (Pardridge, 1988). Because Phe has the highest affinity of all the neutral amino acids, its transport is somewhat more efficient than that predicted by this equation. Phe is therefore the most potent of the LNAA in decreasing the availability of other amino acids, such as tyrosine and tryptophan, to the brain (Daniel, Moorhouse, & Pratt, 1976).

The concentration of Phe in plasma is determined not only by diet but also by the efficiency of the liver phenylalanine-4-hydroxylase complex that converts Phe to tyrosine. Normally, about half of ingested Phe is converted to tyrosine. As a rule, the brain is protected from large changes in circulating concentrations of amino acids caused by diet, because normal foodstuffs contain relatively stable proportions of amino acids. Concomitant intake of fats and carbohydrates, as usually occurs, also influences the amino acid concentrations in plasma, mostly because of the effects of insulin, which increases the uptake of branched-chain amino acids (valine, isoleucine, and leucine) into muscle from plasma. However, in the presence of conditions such as diabetes, hepatic encephalopathy, and certain inborn errors of metabolism such as PKU, or in situations where there is selective ingestion of one or more amino acids, resultant disproportionate plasma concentrations of amino acids are reflected in brain and cerebrospinal fluid (CSF) concentrations of amino acids; such disproportionate concentrations can alter neurotransmitter synthesis, causing neurological and psychiatric symptoms.

As a directly relevant example, studies of CNS neurotransmitter function in patients with PKU have shown that elevated plasma concentrations of Phe will profoundly decrease the plasma, urine, and CSF concentrations of 5-hyrdroxyindoleacetic acid, homovanillic acid, 3-methoxy-4-hydroxyphenylglycol, vanillylmandelic acid, dopamine, norepinephrine, epinephrine, and serotonin (Weil-Malherbe, 1955; Pare, Sandler, & Stacey, 1957; Nadler & Hsia, 1961; Cession-Fossion et al., 1966; Butler et al., 1981; Curtius et al., 1981). Moreover, postmortem analyses have shown that there are 30–40% decreases of tyrosine and tryptophan in PKU brain tissue (McKean, 1972). Brain serotonin concentrations seem particularly vulnerable to PKU, for serotonin synthesis is at least threefold more sensitive to inhibition by elevated Phe concentrations than is dopamine synthesis (Curtius et al., 1981; Hommes, 1989). Similarly, deficiencies of dihydrobiopterine synthetase can reduce dopamine excretion by 50% and that of serotonin by 90% (Curtius et al., 1981).

Although the neurological consequences of severe HPA are conspicuous, there are data from both psychiatric patients and treated PKU subjects suggesting that smaller changes in Phe concentrations have measurable effects on cognitive function, EEG activity, and neurotransmitter concentrations (Branchey et al., 1984; Bjerkenstedt et al., 1985; Krause et al., 1985, 1986, 1988; Epstein et al., 1989). Such changes can be reversed by restricting Phe intake and usually are found in patients under good metabolic control with normal development and without baseline neurological signs or EEG abnormalities. Those studies suggest that the CNS is sensitive to Phe concentrations throughout life, not just during development. An investigation of schizophrenics (Bjerkenstedt et al., 1985) showed that increased CSF concentrations of Phe were significantly associated with decreased CSF concentrations of tyrosine, tryptophan, homovanillic acid, and 5-hydroxyindoleacetic acid. The data in that study suggested a defect in L-system transport in patients with schizophrenia. In depressed alcoholic patients (Branchey et al., 1984), increased plasma concentrations of Phe and tyrosine were associated with significantly lower tryptophan concentrations and tryptophan/LNAA ratios than in nondepressed alcoholics or control subjects.

Phe Metabolites and Neurological Function

Although an elevated plasma concentration of Phe appears to be the primary etiological factor in neurotransmitter abnormalities in patients with PKU (Greengard & Wolfe, 1987), the metabolites PEA, PLA, and PAA also inhibit the activities of tyrosine hydroxylase, tryptophan hydroxylase, and dopa decarboxylase (Fellman, 1956; Knox & Hsia, 1957; Oates et al., 1963; Curtius et al., 1981; Pardridge & Choi, 1986), as well as syntheses of melanin, acetyl-CoA, and GABA (Scriver & Rosenberg, 1973). In particular, PEA, a lipophilic trace amine that readily traverses the blood–brain barrier (Oldendorf, 1971), may be a more proximal mediator of Phe-mediated abnormalities, even when conventionally defined HPA is absent. PEA induces a motor syndrome in animals and augments dopamine release in several areas of the rat brain (Perlow et al., 1980; Philips, 1985). Long-term PEA administration sensitizes animals to PEA-induced behavioral effects (Dourish, 1981), and long-term treatment with haloperidol enhances behavioral sensitivity to PEA administration (Stoff et al., 1984). Those findings, if pertinent to humans, would provide a consistent rationale for PEA involvement with movement disorders in those patients sensitized by long-term typical neuroleptic treatment. It is interesting that clozapine, an atypical neuroleptic associated with a low incidence of extrapyramidal symptoms, blocks the effects of PEA in animals, but haloperidol does not (Dourish, 1981).

PEA is also a congener of amphetamine, abuse of which produces a psychosis resembling paranoid schizophrenia (Young & Scoville, 1938; Snyder, 1973). The psychotogenic potential of PEA, coupled with observations of a high prevalence of schizophrenia in families of PKU patients, prompted a number of studies to examine the roles of Phe, PEA, and other Phe metabolites in schizophrenia. Although some negative findings were reported (Perry & Tischler, 1966; Blumenthal, 1967; Larson & Nyman, 1968), several early studies suggested that PKU heterozygotes and other relatives were at risk for schizophrenia-like illness and affective disorder (Folling, 1934; Penrose & Camb, 1935; Thompson, 1957; Kuznetsova, 1974). Of particular interest was the conclusion by Vogel (1985) that late-onset schizophrenia with affective features is more common in PKU heterozygotes than in the general population. An early study (Poisner, 1960) reported higher fasting serum concentrations of Phe in schizophrenics than in control subjects, and another reported no differences between normal subjects and schizophrenics in the plasma concentrations of Phe or PEA (Szymanski, Naylor, & Karoum, 1987). A later study concluded that CSF concentrations of Phe were significantly higher in schizophrenic patients than in control subjects (Reveley et al., 1987). Potkin et al. (1983), however, could not detect differences in plasma concentrations of Phe between schizophrenics and normal subjects after an oral Phe challenge. Other investigators have shown that there are differences between schizophrenic subgroups: In addition to the schizoaffective/manic patients (DSM-III-R) with higher PAA excretion rates mentioned earlier (Sabelli et al., 1989), urinary PAA concentrations (total and conjugated) were found to be significantly lower in nonparanoid schizophrenics than in control subjects (Karoum et al., 1984), and CSF concentrations of PAA were found to be higher in paranoid schizophrenics than in nonparanoid schizophrenics (Faull et al., 1989). More recently, schizophrenics (DSM-III-R, $n = 41$) were found to have significantly higher plasma concentrations of PEA than normal subjects ($n = 34$), although there were no differences between the patient groups as classified by either psychopathologic variables or paranoid and nonparanoid designations (O'Reilly et al., 1991). Those data hint that defects in Phe metabolism may exist in a subgroup of psychiatric patients who are selectively vulnerable to neuroleptic-induced movement disorders.

Tardive Dyskinesia and Gender

Thus far, we have found the Phe risk factor for males only. These findings are consistent with data demonstrating gender differences in amino acid metabolism for both normal subjects and psychiatric patients (Bremer et al., 1981). As examples, female plasma and urine amino acid profiles have been shown to fluctuate with the estrus cycle (Bremer et al., 1981), and Hagenfeldt et al. (1984) found significantly lower plasma concentrations of valine, isoleucine, leucine, Phe, and tryptophan in normal females than in males. Bjerkenstedt et al. (1985) reported significant gender differences for plasma concentrations of amino acids in schizophrenics, and they found differences in CSF concentrations of isoleucine and leucine only for schizophrenic females versus normal subjects. Rao et al. (1990), when analyzing several biochemical variables for differences between normal subjects and schizophrenics, found gender differences in serum concentrations of cysteine, methionine, lysine, serine, glutamine, proline, valine, isoleucine, leucine, lysine, norepinephrine, epinephrine, prolactin, and growth hormone in both normal subjects and schizophrenics. The similar gender differences we have found in our studies may indicate underlying gender-based differences in the pathophysiology of tardive dyskinesia. Alternatively, the indices of the disorder measurable in males may be masked in females by unrelated gender-based differences in metabolism.

Conclusion

We have found relationships among plasma Phe variables, affective disorder, and tardive dyskinesia in male psychiatric patients. Although the goal of research into tardive dyskinesia historically has been to identify a single primary etiological factor, the accumulating data suggest that multiple factors operate simultaneously. Although it may furnish only a partial picture of the vulnerability to tardive dyskinesia, we are hopeful that an examination of the relationship between Phe metabolism and tardive dyskinesia will lead to progress in teasing apart the elements of this complex disorder.

Acknowledgment

These studies were partially funded by National Institute of Mental Health grants RO1MH44153-03 and RO3MH40629.

References

Andersson, U., Häggström, J.-E., Levin, E. D., Bondesson, U., Valverius, M., & Gunne, L. M. (1989). Reduced glutamate decarboxylase activity in the subthalamic nucleus in patients with tardive dyskinesia. *Mov. Disord.* 4:37–46.

Andreasen, N. C. (1979). Affective flattening and the criteria for schizophrenia. *Am. J. Psychiatry* 136:944–7.

Bjerkenstedt, L., Edman, G., Hagenfeldt, L., Sedvall, G., & Wiesel, F.-A. (1985). Plasma amino acids in relation to cerebrospinal fluid monamine metabolites in schizophrenic patients and health controls. *Br. J. Psychiatry* 147:276–82.

Blumenthal, M. D. (1967). Mental illness in parents of phenylketonuric children. *J. Psychiatr. Res.* 5:59–74.

Boulton, A. A., & Juorio, A. V. (1982). Brain trace amines. In *Handbook of Neurochemistry*, vol. 1, ed. A. Lajtha, pp. 189–222. New York: Plenum.

Boulton, A. A., Juorio, A. V., & Paterson, I. A. (1990). Phenylethylamine in the CNS: effects of monoamine oxidase inhibiting drugs, deuterium substitution and lesions and its role in the neuromodulation of catecholaminergic neurotransmission. *J. Neural Transm. (suppl.)* 29:119–29.

Branchey, L., Branchey, M., Shaw, S., & Lieber, C. S. (1984). Relationship between changes in plasma amino acids and depression in alcoholic patients. *Am. J. Psychiatry* 141:1212–15.

Bremer, H. J., Duran, M., Kamerling, J. P., Przyrembel, H., & Wadman, S. K. (1981). *Disturbances of Amino Acid Metabolism: Clinical Chemistry and Diagnosis.* Baltimore: Urban & Schwarzenberg.

Brown, R. M., & Dahl, H. H. (1987). Localization of the human dihydropteridine reductase gene to band p15.3 of chromosome 4 by in situ hybridization. *Genomics* 1:67–70.

Butler, I. J., O'Flynn, M. E., Seifert, W. E., & Howell, R. R. (1981). Neurotransmitter defects and treatment of disorders of hyperphenylalaninemia. *J. Pediatrics* 98:729–33.

Cadet, J. L., & Lohr, J. B. (1989). Possible involvement of free radicals in neuroleptic-induced movement disorders. Evidence from treatment of tardive dyskinesia with vitamin E. *Ann. N. Y. Acad. Sci.* 570:176–85.

Cession-Fossion, A., Vandermeulen, R., Dodinval, P., & Chantraine, J. M. (1966). Elimination urinaire de l'adreniline, de la noradrenaline, et de l'acide vanillyl-mandelique chez enfants oligophrenes phenylpyruviques. *Pathol. Biol. (Paris)* 14:1157–9.

Curtius, H.-C., Niederwieser, A., Visconti, M., Leimbacher, W., Wegmann, H., Blehova, B., Ray, F., Schaub, J., & Schmidt, H. (1981). Serotonin and dopamine synthesis in phenylketonuria. *Adv. Exp. Med. Biol.* 133:277–91.

Cutler, N. R., & Post, R. M. (1982). State-related cyclical dyskinesias in manic depressives. *J. Clin. Psychopharmacol.* 2:350–4.

Daniel, P. M., Moorhouse, S. R., & Pratt, O. E. (1976). Amino acid precursors of monoamine neurotransmitters and some factors influencing their supply to the brain. *Psychol. Med.* 6:277–86.

Danks, D. M., Bartholome, K., Clayton, B. E., Curtius, H.-C., Grabe, H., Kaufman, S., Leeming, R. J., Pfleiderer, W., Rembold, H., & Ray, F. (1978). Malignant hyperphenylalaninaemia. Current status. *J. Inherit. Metab. Dis.* 1:49–53.

Davis, K. L., Berger, P. A., & Hollister, L. E. (1976). Tardive dyskinesia and depressive illness. *Psychopharmacol. Commun.* 2:125–30.

Dourish, C. T. (1981). Behavioural effects of acute and chronic β-phenylethylamine administration in the rat: evidence for the involvement of 5-hydroxytryptamine. *Neuropharmacology* 20:1067–72.

Epstein, C. M., Trotter, J. F., Averbook, A., Freeman, S., Kutner, M. H., & Elsas, L. J. (1989). EEG mean frequencies are sensitive indices of phenylalanine effects on normal brain. *Electroencephalogr. Clin. Neurophysiol.* 72:133–9.

Faull, K. F., King, R. J., Barchas, J. D., & Csernansky, J. G. (1989). CSF phenylacetic acid and hostility in paranoid schizophrenia. *Psychiatry Res.* 30:111–18.

Fellman, J. H. (1956). Inhibition of dopa decarboxylase by aromatic acids associated with phenylpyruvic oligophrenia. *Proc. Soc. Exp. Biol. Med.* 93:413–14.

Fernstrom, J. D., & Faller, D. V. (1978). Neutral amino acids in the brain: changes in response to food ingestion. *J. Neurochem.* 30:1531–8.

Fibiger, H. C., & Lloyd, K. G. (1984). Neurobiological substrates of tardive dyskinesia: the GABA hypothesis. *Trends Neurosci.* 7:462–4.

Fischer, E., & Heller, B. (1972). Phenylethylamine as a neurohumoral agent in brain. *Behav. Neuropsychiatry* 4:8–11.

Folling, A. (1934). Ueber Ausscheidung von phenylbrenztrauben Saure in den Harn als Stoffwechselanomalie in Verbindurg mit Imbeziliat. *Physiol. Chem.* 127:167–76.

Gardos, G., Cole, J. O., Matthews, J. D., Nierenberg, A. A., & Dugan, S. J. (1992). The acute effects of a loading dose of phenylalanine in unipolar depressed patients with and without tardive dyskinesia. *Neuropsychopharmacology* 6:241–7.

Greengard, O., & Wolfe, J. (1987). Cerebral serotonin regulation by phenylalanine analogues and during hyperphenylalaninemia. *Biochem. Pharmacol.* 36:965–70.

Gunne, L. M., Häggström, J. E., & Sjöquist, B. (1984). Association with persistent neuroleptic-induced dyskinesia of regional changes in brain GABA synthesis. *Nature* 309:347–9.

Hagenfeldt, L., Bjerkenstedt, L., Edman, G., Sedvall, G., & Wiesel, F.-A. (1984). Amino acids in plasma and CSF and monoamine metabolites in CSF: interrelationship in health subjects. *J. Neurochem.* 42:833–7.

Hamilton, M. (1960). A rating scale for depression. *J. Neurol. Neurosurg. Psychiatry* 23:56–62.

Hommes, F. A. (1989). The role of the blood–brain barrier in the aetiology of permanent brain dysfunction in hyperphenylalaninaemia. *J. Inherit. Ment. Dis.* 12:41–6.

Jeste, D. V., Doongaji, D. R., & Linnoila, M. (1984). Elevated cerebrospinal fluid noradrenaline in tardive dyskinesia. *Br. J. Psychiatry* 144:177–80.

Jeste, D. V., & Wyatt, R. J. (1982). *Understanding and Treating Tardive Dyskinesia*. New York: Guilford Press.

Kane, J. M., & Smith, J. M. (1982). Tardive dyskinesia: prevalence and risk factors 1959 to 1979. *Arch. Gen. Psychiatry* 39:473–81.

Kane, J. M., Woerner, M., Borenstein, M., Wegner, J., & Lieberman, J. (1986). Integrating incidence and prevalence of tardive dyskinesia. *Psychopharmacol. Bull.* 22:254–8.

Karoum, F., Linnoila, M., Potter, W. Z., Chuang, L.-W., Goodwin, F. K., &

Wyatt, R. J. (1982). Fluctuating high urinary phenylethylamine excretion rate in some bipolar affective disorder patients. *Psychiatry Res.* 6:215–22.

Karoum, F., Potkin, S., Chuang, L. W., Murphy, D. L., Liebowitz, M. R., & Wyatt, R. J. (1984). Phenylacetic acid excretion in schizophrenia and depression: the origins of PAA in man. *Biol. Psychiatry* 19:165–78.

Kaufman, C. A., Jeste, D. V., Shelton, R. C., Linnoila, M., Kafka, M. S., & Wyatt, R. J. (1986). Noradrenergic and neuroradiological abnormalities in tardive dyskinesia. *Biol. Psychiatry* 21:799–812.

Klawans, H. L. (1973). The pharmacology of tardive dyskinesia. *Am. J. Psychiatry* 130:82–6.

Knox, W. E. (1972). Phenylketonuria. In *The Metabolic Basis of Inherited Disease*, 2nd ed., ed. J. B. Stanbury, J. B. Wyngaarden, & D. S. Frederickson, pp. 263–94. New York: McGraw-Hill.

Knox, W. E., & Hsia, D. Y. (1957). Pathogenetic problems in phenylketonuria. *Am. J. Med.* 22:687.

Krause, W., Epstein, C., Averbook, A., Dembure, P., & Elsas, L. (1986). Phenylalanine alters the mean power frequency of electroencephalograms and plasma L-dopa in treated patients with pheylketonuria. *Pediatr. Res.* 20:1112–61.

Krause, W., Halminski, M., McDonald, L., Dembure, P., Salvo, R., Freides, D., & Elsas, L. (1985). Biochemical and neuropsychological effects of elevated plasma phenylalanine in patients with treated phenylketonuria. *J. Clin. Invest.* 75:40–8.

Krause, W. L., Halminski, M., Naglak, M., McDonald, L., Salvo, R., Freides, D., Epstein, C., Dembure, P., Averbook, A., & Elsas, L. J. (1988). Effects of high plasma phenylalanine concentration in older early-treated PKU patients: performance, neurotransmitter synthesis, and EEG mean power frequency. In *Dietary Phenylalanine and Brain Function*, ed. R. J. Wurtman & E. Ritter-Walker, pp. 179–86. Boston: Birkhauser.

Kuznetsova, L. I. (1974). Frequency and phenotypic manifestations of schizophrenia in the patients with phenylketonuria. *Sov. Genetics* 8:554–5.

Larson, C. A., & Nyman, G. E. (1968). Pheylketonuria: mental illness in heterozygotes. *Psychiatria Clinica* 1:367–74.

Ledley, F. D., Levy, H. L., & Woo, S. L. C. (1986). Molecular analysis of the inheritance of phenylketonuria and mild hyperphenylalaninemia in families with both disorders. *N. Engl. J. Med.* 314:1276–80.

Lidsky, A. S., Robson, K. J. H., Thirumalachary, C., Barker, P. E., Ruddle, F. H., & Woo, S. L. C. (1984). The PKU locus in man is on chromosome 12. *Am. J. Hum. Genet.* 36:527–33.

Linnoila, M., Karoum, F., Cutler, N. P., & Potter, W. Z. (1983). Temporal association between depression-dependent dyskinesias and high urinary phenylethylamine output. *Biol. Psychiatry* 18:513–17.

Lohr, J. B., Cadet, J. L., Lohr, M. A., Larson, L., Wasli, E., Wade, L., Hylton, R., Vidoni, C., Jeste, D. V., & Wyatt, R. J. (1988). Vitamin E in the treatment of tardive dyskinesia: the possible involvement of free radical mechanisms. *Schizophr. Bull.* 14:291–6.

Lohr, J. B., Kuczenski, R., Bracha, H. S., Moir, M., & Jeste, D. V. (1990). Increased indices of free radical activity in the cerebrospinal fluid of patients with tardive dyskinesia. *Biol. Psychiatry* 28:535–9.

McKean, C. M. (1972). The effects of high phenylalanine concentrations on serotonin and catecholamine metabolism in the human brain. *Brain Res.* 47:469–76.

Nadler, H. L., & Hsia, D. Y. (1961). Epinephrine metabolism in phenylketonuria. *Proc. Soc. Exp. Biol. Med.* 107:721–3.

Oates, J. A., Nirenberg, P. Z., Jepson, J. B., Sjöerdsma, A., & Udenfriend, S. (1963). Conversion of phenylalanine to phenylethylamine in patients with PKU. *Proc. Soc. Exp. Biol. Med.* 112:1078–81.

Oldendorf, W. H. (1971). Brain uptake of radio labelled amino acids, amines and hexoses after arterial infusion. *Am. J. Physiol.* 221:1629–39.

O'Reilly, R., Davis, B. A., Durden, D. A., Thorpe, L., Machnee, H., & Boulton, A. A. (1991). Plasma phenylethylamine in schizophrenic patients. *Biol. Psychiatry* 30:145–50.

Overall, J. E., & Gorham, D. R. (1962). The brief psychiatric rating scale. *Psychol. Rep.* 10:799–812.

Pardridge, W. M. (1988). Phenylalanine transport at the human blood–brain barrier. In *Dietary Phenylalanine and Brain Function*, ed. R. J. Wurtman & E. Ritter-Walker, pp. 55–62. Boston: Birkhauser.

Pardridge, W. M., & Choi, T. B. (1986). Neutral amino acid transport at the human blood–brain barrier. *Fed. Proc.* 45:2073–8.

Pare, C. M. B., Sandler, M., & Stacey, R. S. (1957). 5-Hydroxytryptamine deficiency in phenylketonuria. *Lancet* 1:551–3.

Penrose, L. S., & Camb, M. D. (1935). Inheritance of phenylpyruvic amentia (phenylketonuria). *Lancet* 2:192–4.

Perlow, M. J., Chiueh, C. C., Lake, C. R., & Wyatt, R. J. (1980). Increased dopamine and norepinephrine concentrations in primate CSF following amphetamine and phenylethylamine administration. *Brain Res.* 186:469–73.

Perry, T. L., & Tischler, B. (1966). Pheylketonuria in a woman of normal intelligence and her child. *N. Engl. J. Med.* 274:1018–19.

Philips, S. R. (1985). In vivo release of endogenous dopamine from rat caudate nucleus by phenylethylamine. In *Neuropsychopharmacology of the Trace Amines*, ed. A. A. Boulton, P. R. Bieck, L. Maitre, & P. Riederer, pp. 229–34. Clifton: Humana Press.

Poisner, A. M. (1960). Serum phenylalanine in schizophrenia: biochemical genetic aspects. *J. Nerv. Ment. Dis.* 131:74–6.

Potkin, S. G., Cannon-Spoor, H. E., Delisi, L. E., Neckers, L. M., & Wyatt, R. J. (1983). Plasma phenylalanine, tyrosine, and tryptophan in schizophrenia. *Arch. Gen. Psychiatry* 40:749–52.

Proud, V. K., Hsia, Y. E., & Wolf, B. (1989). Disorders of amino acid metabolism. In *Basic Neurochemistry: Molecular, Cellular, and Medical Aspects*, 4th ed., ed. G. J. Siegel, B. Agranoff, R. W. Albers, & P. Molinoff, pp. 733–63. New York: Raven Press.

Rao, M. L., Gross, G., Strebel, B., Braunig, P., Huber, G., & Klosterkotter, J. (1990). Serum amino acids, central monoamines, and hormones in drug-naive, drug-free, and neuroleptic-treated schizophrenic patients and health subjects. *Psychiatry Res.* 34:243–57.

Reveley, M. A., DeBelleroche, J., Recordati, A., & Hirsch, S. R. (1987). Increased CSF amino acids and ventricular enlargement in schizophrenia: a preliminary study. *Biol. Psychiatry* 22:413–20.

Richardson, M. A., Haugland, G., Pass, R., & Craig, T. J. (1986). The prevalence of tardive dyskinesia in a mentally retarded population. *Psychopharmacol. Bull.* 22:243–9.

Richardson, M. A., Pass, R., Bregman, Z., & Craig, T. J. (1985). Tardive dyskinesia and depressive symptoms in schizophrenics. *Psychopharmacol. Bull.* 21:130–5.

Richardson, M. A., Suckow, R., Whittaker, R., Boggiano, W., Sziraki, I., Kushner, H., & Perumal, A. (1989). The plasma phenylalanine/large neutral amino acid ratio: a risk factor for tardive dyskinesia. *Psychopharmacol. Bull.* 25:47–51.

Rosenbaum, A. H., Maruta, T., Jiang, N., Auger, R. G., de la Fuente, J. R., & Duane, D. D. (1979). Endocrine testing in tardive dyskinesia: preliminary report. *Am. J. Psychiatry* 136:102–3.

Rush, M. Diamond, F., & Alpert, M. (1982). Depression as a risk factor in tardive dyskinesia. *Biol. Psychiatry* 17:387–92.

Sabelli, H. C., Durai, U. N., Fawcett, J., & Javaid, J. I. (1989). High phenylacetic acid differentiates schizoaffective from schizophrenic patients. *J. Neuropsychiatry Clin. Neurosci.* 1:37–9.

Sabelli, H. C., Fawcett, J., Gusovsky, F., Edwards, J., Jeffriess, H., & Javaid, J. (1983a). Phenylacetic acid as an indicator in bipolar affective disorders. *J. Clin. Psychopharmacol.* 3:268–70.

Sabelli, H. C., Fawcett, J., Gusovsky, F., Javaid, J., Edwards, J., & Jeffriess, H. (1983b). Urinary phenylacetate: a diagnostic test for depression? *Science* 220:1187–8.

Sabelli, H. C., Fawcett, J., Gusovsky, F., Javaid, J. I., Wynn, P., Edwards, J., Jeffriess, H., & Kravitz, H. (1986). Clinical studies on the phenylethylamine hypothesis of affective disorder: urine and blood phenylacetic acid and phenylalanine dietary supplements. *J. Clin. Psychiatry* 47:66–70.

Sabelli, H. C., & Mosnaim, A. D. (1974). Phenylethylamine hypothesis of affective behavior. *Am. J. Psychiatry* 131:695–9.

Scriver, C. R., & Rosenberg, L. E. (1973). *Amino Acid Metabolism and Its Disorders*. Philadelphia: Saunders.

Smith, J. M., & Baldessarini, R. J. (1980). Changes in prevalence, severity, and recovery in tardive dyskinesia with age. *Arch. Gen. Psychiatry* 37:1368–73.

Snyder, S. H. (1973). Amphetamine psychosis: a "model" schizophrenia mediated by catecholamines. *Am. J. Psychiatry* 130:61–7.

Stahl, S. M., Thornton, J. E., Simpson, M. L., Gerger, P. A., & Napoliello, M. J. (1985). Gamma-vinyl-GABA treatment of tardive dyskinesia and other movement disorders. *Biol. Psychiatry* 20:888–92.

Stoff, D. M., Jeste, D. V., Gillin, J. C., Moja, E. A., Cohen, L., Stauderman, K. A., & Wyatt, R. J. (1984). Behavioral supersensitivity to β-phenylethylamine after chronic administration of haloperidol. *Biol. Psychiatry* 19:101–6.

Szymanski, H. V., Naylor, E. W., & Karoum, F. (1987). Plasma phenylethylamine and phenylalanine in chronic schizophrenic patients. *Biol. Psychiatry* 22:194–8.

Tamminga, C. A., Crayton, J. W., & Chase, T. N. (1979). Improvement in tardive dyskinesia after muscimol therapy. *Arch. Gen. Psychiatry* 36:595–8.

Thaker, G. K., Nguyen, J. A., & Tamminga, C. A. (1989). Increased saccadic distractibility in tardive dyskinesia: functional evidence for subcortical GABA dysfunction. *Bio. Psychiatry* 25:49–59.

Thaker, G. K., Tamminga, C. A., Alphs, L. A., Lafferman, J., Ferraro, T. N., & Hare, T. A. (1987). Brain γ-aminobutyric acid abnormality in tardive dyskinesia. *Arch. Gen. Psychiatry* 44:522–9.

Thompson, J. H. (1957). Relatives of phenylketonuric patients. *J. Ment. Defic. Res.* 1:67–78.

Vogel, F. (1985). Phenotypic deviations in heterozygotes of phenylketonuria (PKU). *Prog. Clin. Biol. Res.* 177:337–49.

Wagner, R. L., Jeste, D. V., Phelps, B. H., & Wyatt, R. J. (1982). Enzyme studies in tardive dyskinesia. 1. One-year biochemical follow-up. *J. Clin. Psychopharmacol.* 2:312–14.

Weil-Malherbe, H. (1955). The concentration of adrenaline in human plasma and its relation to mental activity. *J. Ment. Sci.* 101:733–55.

Weiner, W. J., & Lang, A. E. (1989). *Movement Disorders: A Comprehensive Survey*, pp. 645–84. Mount Kisco: Futura.

Yassa, R., Nastase, C., Dupont, D., & Thibeau, M. (1992). Tardive dyskinesia in elderly psychiatric patients: a 5 year study. *Am. J. Psychiatry* 149:1206–11.

Young, D., & Scoville, W. B. (1938). Paranoid psychosis in narcolepsy and the possible danger of benzadrine treatment. *Med. Clin. North Am.* 22:637–46.

14

Neuroendocrinological Studies of Tardive Dyskinesia

MARGOT ALBUS, M.D., Ph.D.

Recent research supports the idea that tardive dyskinesia is an etiologically heterogeneous disorder, with multiple neurochemical abnormalities contributing to its pathophysiology. A neurotransmitter imbalance has been the most frequently suggested pathophysiological mechanism, referring mainly to dopaminergic hyperactivity, GABAergic deficiency, or serotonergic imbalance (Ebadi & Hama, 1988).

The dopamine-supersensitivity hypothesis has been shown to be inadequate as a unitary explanation (Fibiger & Lloyd, 1984; Stoessl, Dourish, & Iversen, 1989). Some current proposals suggest that dopamine-receptor supersensitization resulting from chronic blockade by neuroleptics may be the first step in the pathogenesis of tardive dyskinesia, followed by necessary processes (not yet identified) in other neurochemical systems (Cassady et al., 1992).

Involvement of the GABA system in the development of persistent dyskinesia accounts for some of the evidence unexplained by the hypothesis of dopamine-receptor supersensitivity (Scheel-Krüger, 1986; Thaker et al., 1989b). Recent studies have supported the idea of GABA neuronal hypofunction in the substantia nigra pars reticulata (Monteleone et al., 1988; Thaker et al., 1989b).

There is also evidence for a serotonergic abnormality in patients with tardive dyskinesia. Much of our information suggests an inhibitory role for serotonin (5-HT) on nigrostriatal dopaminergic functioning (Sandyk, 1989). It seems that, in contrast to classic neuroleptics, clozapine does not induce tardive dyskinesia, the reason being that it is a potent 5-HT_2 antagonist, the role of which is to release tonic inhibition of dopaminergic transmission and prevent depolarization inactivation at the presynaptic dopaminergic neuron, as well as to prevent denervation supersensitivity at the postsynaptic dopaminergic neuron (Coward, 1992).

Other studies have suggested that tardive dyskinesia may involve abnormal neurotransmitter function in the noradrenergic system. However, it seems unlikely that noradrenergic dysfunction plays a central role in the pathophysiology of tardive dyskinesia.

In addition to examining these neurotransmitter systems, investigators have focused on a possible role for the opiate system, as well as involvements of melatonin, glucose metabolism, free radicals, and estrogens, in the pathophysiology of movement disorders.

Another possible approach to evaluation of underlying pathophysiological mechanisms would be to determine, on the basis of peripheral neuroendocrine alterations, just where the regulation process suffers central dysfunction. In this chapter, studies based on that strategy, as well as strategies that focus on neuroendocrine findings, will be reviewed with regard to their impact on the pathophysiology of tardive dyskinesia.

The Dopaminergic Systems

Homovanillic Acid and Dopamine-β-hydroxylase

Three dopaminergic pathways can be assessed: the nigrostriatal, the mesolimbic, and the tuberoinfundibular. Changes in the major dopamine metabolite, homovanillic acid (HVA), in cerebrospinal fluid (CSF) and plasma can be used as indicators of activity in the nigrostriatal and mesolimbic pathways. Because the nigrostriatal pathway is believed to be involved in the development of tardive dyskinesia, the hypothesis of dopamine-receptor supersensitivity suggests that concentrations of HVA should be lower in patients with tardive dyskinesia than in patients without tardive dyskinesia. However, several investigators have found no increased CSF concentrations of HVA in patients with tardive dyskinesia, who showed no differences when compared with control subjects (Pind & Faurbye, 1970; Bowers, Moore, & Tarsy, 1979; Nagao et al., 1979). Also, it has been suggested that plasma concentrations of HVA may, under certain circumstances, reflect central dopaminergic activity, thereby providing another approach to assessment of dopaminergic systems in patients with tardive dyskinesia (Muscettola et al., 1990). In one study (Kirch et al., 1983), plasma concentrations of HVA were reported to correlate with the severity of involuntary movements in medicated patients with tardive dyskinesia; however, that finding could not be replicated by Moore et al. (1983). Those authors reported a robust correlation between age and plasma concentrations of HVA in tardive dyskinesia patients, but no significant correlations between plasma concentrations of HVA and tardive dyskinesia, as measured by the Abnormal Involuntary Movement Scale (AIMS) (Guy, 1976).

Investigating the changes in CSF or plasma concentrations of HVA after discontinuation of neuroleptics is another approach to the study of potential differences in dopaminergic tone between patients with and without tardive dyskinesia. Perényi et al. (1985), investigating schizophrenic patients after discontinuation of neuroleptics, found that patients who did not develop withdrawal dyskinesia tended to have had nonsignificantly higher CSF concentrations of HVA before neuroleptic withdrawal than had patients who developed withdrawal dyskinesia. Whereas the reported decreases in CSF concentrations of HVA during the first 14 days after neuroleptic withdrawal were significantly smaller than those in patients who did not develop withdrawal dyskinesia, the elevations in CSF concentrations of HVA following neuroleptic discontinuation remained for longer periods in patients who developed withdrawal dyskinesia. Pérenyi et al. (1985) suggested that the prolonged elevations in CSF concentrations of HVA indicated permanent increases in dopamine turnover that were necessary for the development of both withdrawal dyskinesia and tardive dyskinesia in parallel with denervation hypersensitivity. In contrast, Glazer et al. (1989) found that patients who developed withdrawal-exacerbated tardive dyskinesia did not differ from patients without withdrawal-exacerbated tardive dyskinesia in terms of mean plasma HVA concentrations or changes in plasma HVA concentrations after discontinuation of neuroleptics. If circulating plasma concentrations of HVA are indicators of central dopaminergic function, those authors were unable to show that dopaminergic function in patients who developed withdrawal-exacerbated tardive dyskinesia differed from dopaminergic function in those without it.

Two studies have indicated a relationship between high plasma activities of dopamine-β-hydroxylase (DBH) and development of tardive dyskinesia (Arato et al., 1980; Jeste et al., 1981a). According to Jeste and Wyatt (1982), the high plasma DBH activity seen in patients suffering from tardive dyskinesia may be a risk factor for development of tardive dyskinesia. Accepting that supposition, higher plasma DBH activities would be expected in patients who develop withdrawal dyskinesia than in patients who do not. However, Perényi et al. (1985) failed to find such a correlation.

Muscettola et al. (1990) undertook a naturalistic study of 16 schizophrenic patients with moderately severe tardive dyskinesia, comparing them with a group of 14 patients without tardive dyskinesia who had not taken neuroleptics for a mean of 32.9 months. Whereas in patients with orofacial tardive dyskinesia, plasma HVA concentrations were significantly lower than in controls without tardive dyskinesia, in other dyskinetic patients the plasma HVA concentrations were not significantly different. Those data support the contention that orofacial dyskinesia is a relatively unitary syndrome distinct from other dyskinesias. Those authors therefore proposed that the low plasma concentrations of HVA may have reflected reduced presynaptic dopaminergic activity, perhaps in response to neuroleptic-induced supersensitivity of dopamine receptors, but only in orofacial tardive dyskinesia. Because the authors of the other studies cited did not differentiate between the different subgroups of tardive dyskinesia patients, the data of Muscettola et al. (1990) may provide an explanation for the discrepant findings reported thus far. Their data suggest that the inconsistency in the findings can be partially attributed to the fact that tardive dyskinesia is a heterogeneous disorder and that only the orofacial form of tardive dyskinesia is caused predominantly by dopaminergic supersensitivity in the nigrostriatal dopaminergic pathway.

Prolactin

The activity of the third dopaminergic pathway, the tuberoinfundibular, can be assessed indirectly by measuring the blood concentrations of prolactin (Csernansky et al., 1986a). Dopamine tonically inhibits prolactin secretion from lactotropic cells in the anterior pituitary via the tuberoinfundibular dopaminergic pathway. Thus, blood prolactin concentrations may inversely reflect the activity of tuberoinfundibular dopaminergic neurons or the sensitivity of the pituitary dopamine receptors.

According to Brown (1983), if neuroleptic-induced dopaminergic supersensitivity develops concurrently in the various brain dopaminergic pathways, lower prolactin concentrations may be associated with symptoms of tardive dyskinesia. However, several studies to examine the potential relationship between prolactin responses and tardive dyskinesia have yielded only negative findings. Tripodianakis, Markianos, and Garelis (1983) found no correlation between prolactin concentrations and tardive dyskinesia in patients undergoing long-term neuroleptic treatment. Also, Asnis et al. (1979) found no relationship between tardive dyskinesia and prolactin concentrations during neuroleptic treatment or after its withdrawal, nor any relationship between increased severity of tardive dyskinesia and changes in prolactin concentrations after an acute challenge with haloperidol. Additionally, Naber et al. (1980), Jeste et al. (1981b), Arato et al. (1984), Müller-Spahn et al. (1984), and Albus et al. (1985) reported no association between the severity of tardive dyskinesia and serum prolactin concentrations. In addition to the negative findings from studies that searched for a possible relationship between prolactin concentrations and tardive dyskinesia, Smith et al. (1978) found no evidence for a greater reduction of prolactin after an apomorphine challenge in patients with tardive dyskinesia. Moreover, the findings in several other studies – Ettigi et al. (1976), Tamminga et al. (1977), Cohen, Cooper, and Altshul (1979), Brown and Laughren (1980), Arato et al. (1980), and Wolf et al. (1982) – that focused primarily on the prolactin responses to various pharmacologic interventions in patients with tardive dyskinesia were inconclusive. Csernansky et al. (1986b) used prolactin-index (PI) values, calculated as the ratio of plasma prolactin concentration to neuroleptic concentration, as individual measures of patients' tuberoinfundibular dopamine sensitivities, corrected for a given amount of circulating neuroleptic concentration. The PI values correlated with tardive dyskinesia and paranoid symptoms in younger patients, but not in older neuroleptic-treated schizophrenics. Those authors concluded that tardive dyskinesia may have a different pathologic mechanism in older patients, in whom it is less often reversible. The correlations among PI values, tardive dyskinesia and psychotic symptoms led those authors to suggest that changes in PI values might parallel the development of dopaminergic supersensitivity in the mesolimbic and nigrostriatal pathways.

There is evidence that regulation of the dopamine-receptor response is different in the pituitary as compared with the striatum. Perhaps the supersensitivity that develops after long-term neuroleptic treatment occurs on a regional basis within the CNS (Lieberman et al., 1989), thus rendering prolactin an invalid measure for nigrostriatal activity. Moreover, prolactin secretion seems to be influenced by other factors besides supersensitivity of dopaminergic neurons, one of them being an alteration in GABAergic tone (Monteleone et al., 1988). This renders it questionable to use prolactin as an indicator for dopaminergic activity. Also, gender-related differences make it difficult to interpret any correlation between prolactin concentrations and tardive dyskinesia.

A gender-related association between prolactin concentrations and the severity of tardive dyskinesia has been shown by Glazer et al. (1981) and Lenox, Weaver, and Saran (1985), with both groups reporting that female patients with tardive dyskinesia tended to have higher mean prolactin concentrations than male patients with tardive dyskinesia. The principal finding in those studies was that postmenopausal women with severe tardive dyskinesia had higher serum prolactin concentrations than postmenopausal women with mild tardive dyskinesia. Those findings focused attention on a potential association between estrogens and tardive dyskinesia.

The Role of Estrogens

Hormones such as estrogens have been shown to modulate dopamine receptors (Hruska & Silbergeld, 1980). DiPaolo and Falardeau (1985) demonstrated that small doses of estradiol could facilitate dopaminergic transmission in the striatum. In a monkey model of dyskinesia, Bédard and Boucher (1986) found that simultaneous initial exposure to haloperidol and estradiol seemed to prevent rebound sensitivity to apomorphine. Thus, estrogen may affect tardive dyskinesia in at least two ways. Furthermore, when given with a neuroleptic, it can reduce the behavioral manifestations of the dyskinesia, probably at the same time increasing the number of striatal D_2 receptors (Hruska & Silbergeld, 1980).

Among humans, tardive dyskinesia occurs in both sexes, but is more frequent in postmenopausal women (Smith et al., 1978). Villeneuve, Cazejust, and Coté (1980), Bédard et al. (1984), and Glazer et al. (1985) have reported some improvement during estrogen administration for both men and women with tardive dyskinesia, as well as substantial increases in their serum estradiol concentrations during treatment. However, no obvious pattern of improvement was shown in tardive dyskinesia scores as a function of serum estrogen or prolactin concentration. From those findings, one must conclude that the relationships among estrogen, prolactin, striatal dopamine-receptor supersensitivity, and tardive dyskinesia are still unclear.

In the studies of Glazer and associates, a significant relationship between plasma concentrations of HVA and the severity of tardive dyskinesia could be found only in postmenopausal women (Glazer et al., 1983). Earlier, Glazer et al. (1981) had reported an association between elevated serum prolactin concentrations and the severity of tardive dyskinesia in postmenopausal women on neuroleptic medication. In the former study, Glazer et al. (1983) examined tardive dyskinesia patients for evidence of relationships among baseline plasma concentrations of estradiol, prolactin, and HVA. They found that compared with male patients with tardive dyskinesia, female patients with tardive dyskinesia had significantly lower mean serum estradiol concentrations and significantly higher mean plasma HVA concentrations, as well as a tendency toward higher serum prolactin concentrations. Although that study indicated that more than half of the hyperprolactinemic women had estradiol deficiencies, no association could be found between randomly sampled morning circulating estradiol or prolactin concentrations and the severity of tardive dyskinesia in that group. Thus, although a hypogonadal state may be a factor influencing the severity of tardive dyskinesia, the findings in that study suggest that the degree of hypogonadism is not important. Also, the higher HVA concentrations in women would suggest a relationship between tardive dyskinesia and dopaminergic function in postmenopausal women, but not in men. In summary, although they do not show a correlation between serum estradiol concentrations and the severity of tardive dyskinesia, those studies suggest that a hypoestrogenic state may in part explain the gender-specific association between dopaminergic function and tardive dyskinesia.

The GABAergic System

Several studies of γ-aminobutyric acid (GABA) transmission have indicated that a dysfunction in GABA-mediated neuronal transmission occurs in the basal ganglia as a consequence of long-term neuroleptic treatment (Scheel-Krüger, 1986; Monteleone et al., 1988). During long-term administration of neuroleptics, the turnover rate of the nigrostriatal GABAergic pathway decreases, and GABA receptors become supersensitive. Consequently, GABA concentrations decrease in the substantia nigra pars reticulata (Coward, 1982).

GABA

Consistent with the hypothesis of GABAergic supersensitivity is the observation that when GABA concentrations in CSF from the lumbar spine were measured in neuroleptic-free schizophrenics, some with and some without tardive dyskinesia, significant reductions were seen in patients with tardive dyskinesia (Thaker et al., 1987). Those authors reported that a GABA-mimetic drug, γ-vinyl-γ-aminobutyric acid (GVG), produced consistent antidyskinetic effects. During treatment with GVG, lumbar CSF concentrations of GABA showed a twofold increase. The finding of reductions in CSF GABA concentrations in schizophrenic patients with tardive dyskinesia, as compared with schizophrenics without tardive dyskinesia (Thaker et al., 1987), suggests that supersensitivity of GABA receptors may be operative in the pathophysiology of tardive dyskinesia. Assuming that subcortical GABA dysfunction exists, one can predict that schizophrenics with tardive dyskinesia may have an abnormality in this system that results in decreased tonic inhibition and increased saccadic distractibility. Consequently, Thaker, Nguyen, and Tamminga (1989a) investigated saccadic distractibility in patients with and without tardive dyskinesia. They found that tardive dyskinesia patients had significantly more inappropriate saccades than did patients without tardive dyskinesia or normal controls. Those authors proposed that the increased distractibility seen in patients with tardive dyskinesia resulted from reduced GABA activity in the nigrotectal tract. That clinical hypothesis, which is remarkably consistent with findings in animal models, would localize the supposed GABA deficit in tardive dyskinesia patients in the nigrotectal pathway.

There is also indirect evidence for a correlation between the activity of the GABAergic system and tardive dyskinesia. Case studies of patients with rapid-cycle affective disorder have detailed more marked dyskinetic symptoms during periods of depression than during mania. Those changes in dyskinetic symptoms are paralleled by state-dependent fluctuations in the CSF GABA concentrations, with low GABA concentrations during depressive phases (Post et al., 1980).

Prolactin

Besides dopamine, which tonically inhibits prolactin secretion, GABA has been shown to modulate prolactin secretion from the anterior pituitary gland (Racagni et al., 1982). Therefore, indirect assessments of endogenous GABAergic activity can be made by investigating plasma prolactin responses to GABAergic pharmacologic challenges. Monteleone et al. (1988) examined the effects of the GABA-mimetic drug sodium valproate on plasma prolactin concentrations in schizophrenic patients with and without tardive dyskinesia, as well as in healthy control subjects. They reported that whereas in the healthy controls and in the schizophrenic patients with tardive dyskinesia the sodium valproate induced significant decreases in plasma prolactin concentrations, no significant changes were observed in patients without tardive dyskinesia.

The normal neuroendocrine responsiveness and the positive correlations between plasma prolactin responses and AIMS scores reported in dyskinetic patients, indicating supersensitivity at postsynaptic sites in the tuberoinfundibular GABAergic system, are intriguing findings. However, because of the various factors that influence prolactin secretion, any explanation must remain speculative at this time. Further investigations are needed to clarify the role of GABAergic supersensitivity in tardive dyskinesia patients.

The Noradrenergic System

Several earlier studies have suggested that the noradrenergic system may play a role in the pathophysiology of tardive dyskinesia. The major metabolite of norepinephrine, methoxyhydroxyphenylglycol (MHPG), which has been shown to reflect central noradrenergic function, has been found at nonsignificantly elevated concentrations in the plasma of patients with tardive dyskinesia, as compared with patients without tardive dyskinesia (Glazer, Charney, & Heninger, 1987). Other investigators (Albus et al., 1985) have reported nonsignificantly elevated baseline serum concentrations of norepinephrine in patients with severe tardive dyskinesia, as compared with patients without tardive dyskinesia, when both groups were on long-term maintenance treatment with neuroleptics. In addition to those studies that have investigated a possible relationship between baseline concentrations of norepinephrine or MHPG and tardive dyskinesia, one study has focused on the relationship between tardive dyskinesia and changes in CSF norepinephrine after discontinuation of neuroleptics.

Perényi et al. (1985) reported that the decreases in CSF norepinephrine concentrations after neuroleptic discontinuation were significantly smaller in patients who had developed withdrawal dyskinesia than in those who had not. More recently, Glazer et al. (1989), in studying the effects of neuroleptic discontinuation on tardive dyskinesia and MHPG concentrations, reported that patients who exhibited withdrawal-exacerbated tardive dyskinesia after neuroleptic discontinuation had had significantly lower plasma MHPG concentrations at baseline. Although the noradrenergic system appears to play a less significant role in tardive dyskinesia than do other systems, these findings suggest that in a presumed subtype of tardive dyskinesia, namely, in withdrawal-exacerbated tardive dyskinesia, this system may be implicated.

There has been one treatment study of clozapine whose findings support a possible involvement of the noradrenergic system in tardive dyskinesia (Lieberman et al., 1989). Those authors reported that the clozapine-induced elevations in CSF norepinephrine concentrations were more pronounced in tardive dyskinesia patients than in patients without tardive dyskinesia. Together with the findings of Jeste, Doongaji, and Linnoila (1984) and Jeste et al. (1986), who reported elevated CSF norepinephrine concentrations in patients with tardive dyskinesia, as compared with patients without tardive dyskinesia, these data tentatively suggest that there is increased responsiveness of the α-adrenergic receptor system to the α-adrenolytic effects of neuroleptics in tardive dyskinesia patients.

Thus far, the evidence for involvement of the noradrenergic system in tardive dyskinesia remains speculative. Not only do the α-adrenolytic effects of the neuroleptics influence norepinephrine secretion, as well as MHPG secretion, but also the neuroleptics differ in their α-adrenolytic potencies. Therefore, the findings suggesting a correlation between norepinephrine or MHPG and tardive dyskinesia are undermined by the different α-adrenolytic effects of the neuroleptics, and thus interpretation of the data is difficult.

Studies of Glucose Metabolism

Insulin may act as a neuromodulator, affecting the release of catecholamines from the hypothalamus (Young, Kuhar, & Roth, 1980). Thus, a decrease in central hypothalamic insulin release could increase the risk for tardive dyskinesia for lowering the neurons' threshold of resistance to lasting damage by neuroleptics (Mukherjee, Bilder, & Sakeim, 1986). That assumption is supported by the findings in a study by Lozovski, Kopin, and Saller (1985), who showed that the usual haloperidol-induced increases in the numbers of dopamine receptors were not seen in rats treated with insulin at dosages sufficient to elicit pronounced hypoglycemia.

Mukherjee et al. (1986) found 75% of an elderly diabetic psychiatric population to have tardive dyskinesia – a prevalence much higher than would be expected on the basis of the literature reports – and also found delayed recovery curves following administration of a standard glucose load to the patients with tardive dyskinesia; that was not observed in age-matched controls without tardive dyskinesia. Furthermore, a study by Ganzini et al. (1991) demonstrated a significantly higher prevalence and greater severity of tardive dyskinesia among a neuroleptic-treated diabetic population than among a similar neuroleptic-treated nondiabetic population.

In another study, Mukherjee et al. (1989) examined the relationships among tardive dyskinesia, glucose tolerance, and family medical history for 22 non-insulin-dependent diabetics. During neuroleptic treatment, fasting blood glucose concentrations were significantly higher in tardive dyskinesia patients than in patients without tardive dyskinesia. However, that finding did not hold when patients were drug-free. Also, there were no significant differences in post-loading glucose concentrations between patients in the group given neuroleptic treatment and those in the drug-free group. Nevertheless, for patients with a family history of non-insulin-dependent diabetes mellitus, there was a positive correlation with the development of tardive dyskinesia. All those studies suggest that disorders of glucose metabolism may be associated with the onset of tardive dyskinesia, although the mechanisms of interaction between these two physiological processes are unknown.

Mouret et al. (1991) reported that treatment with low dosages of insulin produced clear and long-lasting attenuation of tardive dyskinesia induced by long-term neuroleptic treatment in schizophrenics. Because insulin stimulates dopamine release both in vitro and in vivo (Sauter et al., 1983), dopamine-receptor sensitivity may have been reversed through that mechanism. Those data favor a role for decreased glucose availability in reversing receptor hypersensitivity, in concordance with the data from animal models (Lozovski et al., 1985).

The reported association between decreased glucose availability and reversal of dopamine-receptor hypersensitivity may support the hypothesis that tardive dyskinesia is a consequence of dopamine-receptor hypersensitivity resulting from neuroleptic-induced dopamine denervation in striatal regions. In animals, there is evidence that hyperglycemia results in diminished dopaminergic transmission and increased sensitivity of postsynaptic dopamine receptors (Saller & Chiodo, 1980). Thus, in neuroleptic-treated patients, the addition of diabetes to the neuroleptic treatment may be more likely to impair striatal dopaminergic transmission and produce dopamine receptor hypersensitivity, with an increased incidence of tardive dyskinesia as a possible consequence.

Studies of the Hypothalamic-Pituitary Axis

Secretion of pituitary hormones, such as adrenocorticotropic hormone (ACTH) and growth hormone (GH), is controlled by hypothalamic releasing factors and by a negative-feedback loop entailing adrenal cortisol secretion. A failure of dexamethasone to suppress plasma cortisol concentrations is believed to indicate hyperactivity of the hypothalamic-pituitary-adrenal (HPA) axis. The assumption that hyperactivity of the HPA axis may be partially due to dopamine-receptor supersensitivity in neuroleptic-treated schizophrenic patients (Dewan, Pandurangi, & Levy, 1985) led several investigators to examine the relationship between the activity of the HPA axis and tardive dyskinesia. However, the evidence for the assumption of a correlation between the activity of the HPA axis and tardive dyskinesia is weak, for no difference in plasma concentrations of GH (Jeste et al., 1981b) or in GH responses to apomorphine (Müller-Spahn et al., 1984) have been found in patients with tardive dyskinesia, as compared with patients without tardive dyskinesia. Lenox et al. (1985) reported that baseline GH concentrations were within the normal range in patients with tardive dyskinesia, again demonstrating no evidence for dopaminergic supersensitivity in the hypothalamic-pituitary axis in patients with chronic tardive dyskinesia. Aleem, Kulkarni, and Yeragani (1988) used the dexamethasone suppression test (DST) in 10 patients with and 10 without symptoms of tardive dyskinesia. Although there was no significant difference in frequency of DST suppression of cortisol between patients with and those without tardive dyskinesia, there was a significant positive correlation between post-DST plasma cortisol concentrations and the movement-disorder scales. Those authors concluded that the stronger correlation between tardive dyskinesia and post-DST concentrations of cortisol suggested a relationship between tardive dyskinesia and dexamethasone nonsuppression. However, because the HPA axis is influenced by the noradrenergic, cholinergic, and dopaminergic systems, the finding of differences in HPA activity between patients with tardive dyskinesia and those without does not further elucidate the pathophysiological mechanisms relevant to the development of tardive dyskinesia.

Studies of Melatonin and Serotonin

Attention has also focused on the role of melatonin in patients with tardive dyskinesia. Several studies have reported spontaneous mood-dependent alterations in the severity of tardive dyskinesia, depression being associated with spontaneous exacerbation of tardive dyskinesia, and mania with its attenuation (DePotter, Linowski, & Mendlewicz, 1983). Because mania is associated with increased melatonin secretion, and depression with decreased melatonin secretion (Miles & Philbrick, 1988), those findings support the hypothesis that diminished melatonin secretion facilitates the emergence of tardive dyskinesia (Sandyk & Fisher, 1989a; Sandyk, 1990a). Consequently, some authors have suggested that the increased prevalence of tardive dyskinesia among depressed and elderly schizophrenic patients may be associated with diminished melatonin-mediated disinhibition of the HPA axis (Kane, Woerner, & Lieberman, 1988; Sandyk & Fisher, 1989a).

The studies published thus far, however, provide only indirect evidence for a hypothesis of melatonin deficiency contributing to tardive dyskinesia. Sandyk (1990b) reported an association between pineal calcification (PC) and axial dyskinesias. Because the findings of Trentini et al. (1987) indicated an inverse correlation between PC and melatonin secretion in humans, it was thought that PC might be associated with markedly reduced melatonin secretion. Sandyk's findings would then tentatively suggest that the emergence of axial dyskinesias might be associated with reduced melatonin secretion.

Another approach has focused on the possibility of abnormal hypothalamic-pituitary regulation of melanocyte-stimulating hormone (MSH) being implicated in the pathophysiology of tardive dyskinesia. Sorokin et al. (1988) suggested that the emergence of tardive dyskinesia may be associated with abnormalities in the activities of MSH peptides. To investigate the role of MSH in tardive dyskinesia, Sandyk (1989) examined the relationship between the severity of tardive dyskinesia and seborrheic dermatitis in 3 patients. Whereas low tardive dyskinesia scores were associated with the presence of mild seborrheic lesions, the increasing severity of tardive dyskinesia following neuroleptic discontinuation was associated with marked exacerbation of the seborrheic skin lesions. Sandyk (1989) concluded that increased pituitary MSH release, which exacerbates seborrheic dermatitis, parallels the severity of tardive dyskinesia. However, that conclusion was questioned by Charlton (1990). He argued that in order to establish a link between tardive dyskinesia and MSH, the concentrations of the hormone itself would have to be measured and correlated with the severity of tardive dyskinesia. Because that step has not yet been taken, the evidence for an association between MSH or melatonin secretion and tardive dyskinesia remains weak.

Sandyk and Fisher (1989b) sought to examine any linkage among melatonin secretion, opioid peptides, and tardive dyskinesia. They tested the effects of naloxone, alone or in combination with melatonin, on the severity of tardive dyskinesia in a rat model. Because naloxone was ineffective for reducing dyskinetic movements in pinealectomized rats, their findings indicate that the antidyskinetic effects of naloxone are mediated, at least in part, through the action of melatonin. Because naloxone requires the presence of melatonin to affect tardive dyskinesia, and melatonin has been shown to regulate brain serotonin metabolism, Sandyk and Fisher (1989b) speculated that serotonergic neurons may also be involved in mediating naloxone's effects in tardive dyskinesia patients.

Several animal studies have demonstrated that serotonin (5-HT) synthesis in the midbrain and hypothalamus is closely regulated by melatonin (Aldegunde, Miquez, & Veira, 1985). Reduced melatonin secretion is believed to be associated with diminished cerebral serotonin activity, a decrease that may ultimately contribute to the emergence of tardive dyskinesia. Korsgaard, Gerlach, and Christensson (1985) reported alterations in the severity of nonoral stereotypies produced by pharmacologic manipulations of the serotonin system. Those observations suggest that the activity of the serotonin system may be important in the expression of dystonic movements. Because serotonin functions are reduced in some depressed patients (van Praag, 1986), and nighttime serum melatonin concentrations are lower in depressed patients (Frazer et al., 1986), it is conceivable that the state of depression may be linked to abnormalities in melatonin regulation of serotonin in tardive dyskinesia patients. In addition, psychiatric patients who have developed dyskinetic symptoms while receiving neuroleptics have had significantly lower CSF concentrations of serotonin metabolites than patients not manifesting dyskinesia, despite similar drug exposure (Chase, Schnur, & Gordon, 1970).

The findings in the previously cited studies partially support the hypothesis of a role for abnormal melatonin and serotonin regulation in dyskinetic symptoms. Nevertheless, the data available again provide only indirect evidence for an involvement of abnormal melatonin and serotonin activities in the pathogenesis of tardive dyskinesia.

Studies of Free Radicals

It has been theorized that persistent tardive dyskinesia is caused by free-radical toxicity in the basal ganglia (Cadet, Lohr, & Jeste, 1986). Also, neuroleptics have been shown to increase, at least initially, the turnover of catecholamines in the brain (Mackay et al., 1982), and increased metabolism of catecholamines probably is associated with increased free-radical formation (Lohr, 1991). The findings in several studies support an involvement of free radicals in the pathogenesis of tardive dyskinesia. Horrobin et al. (1989) reported consistently greater reductions in essential fatty acids in the plasma phospholipids of schizophrenic patients with tardive dyskinesia. Horrobin et al. (1989) also speculated that free radicals might be involved in the damage to fatty acids seen in patients with tardive dyskinesia. Recently, Lohr et al. (1990) reported increased CSF indices of lipid peroxidation in patients with tardive dyskinesia, as compared with control patients without tardive dyskinesia.

On the basis of those findings, one might expect that vitamin E, which possesses antioxidant properties, would neutralize the damaging effects of those free radicals (Lohr, 1991). Lohr et al. (1988), in a double-blind, placebo-controlled study in which 15 patients with tardive dyskinesia or tardive dystonia were treated with vitamin E, found significant reductions in AIMS scores after treatment with vitamin E, but not after treatment with the placebo. Elkashef et al. (1990) reported that vitamin E had a modest suppressive effect on tardive dyskinesia and that patients with either buccolingual tardive dyskinesia or dystonia improved the most. However, two recent studies have failed to show a therapeutic effect of vitamin E on tardive dyskinesia (Egan et al., 1991; Shriqui et al., 1991). Thus far, the evidence for involvement of free radicals in tardive dyskinesia is inconclusive. Further studies will be necessary to evaluate the potential involvement of free radicals in the different subtypes of tardive dyskinesia.

Miscellaneous Findings

Another metabolic approach to an understanding of tardive dyskinesia derives from studies carried out to evaluate phenylalanine metabolism. Disturbances in phenylalanine metabolism have been described as risk factors for the development of tardive dyskinesia (Richardson et al., 1988). Those authors speculated that chronically higher concentrations of phenylalanine may lead to lower concentrations of dopamine, norepinephrine, and serotonin, which, in combination with the effects of neuroleptics, would lead to a greater risk for developing tardive dyskinesia. In a comparison of patients with tardive dyskinesia versus patients without tardive dyskinesia, Richardson et al. (1989) reported a significant positive correlation between plasma phenylalanine concentrations and tardive dyskinesia after a high-protein diet. Lieberman et al. (1989) also found that phenylethylamine levels were consistently, albeit nonsignificantly, higher in patients with tardive dyskinesia than in those without.

A report by Canoso, Romero, and Yunis (1986) suggested that it is possible to identify individuals susceptible to tardive dyskinesia by classifying patients according to their human leucocyte antigen (HLA) types. Those authors found that subjects who were positive for HLA-B44 and autoantibodies had moderate-to-severe dyskinesia. Brown and White (1991) were unable to replicate that finding; however, as Wright (1991) pointed out, their sample had not been large enough to confirm or refute an association between HLA-B44 and tardive dyskinesia. Although Metzer, Newton, and Steele (1990) also failed to confirm a significant association between tardive dyskinesia and HLA-B44, they reported that possession of the DR4 antigen increased the relative risk for tardive dyskinesia and that all their patients with the extended haplotype B44-DR4 had neuroleptic-induced movement disorders. Those data indicate that the extended B44-DR4 haplotype predisposes to both schizophrenia and tardive dyskinesia. Future research will be necessary to elucidate the importance of those findings.

Conclusion

The previously cited studies, focusing as they did on neuroendocrinological alterations in the different pathways that are assumed to be involved in the development of tardive dyskinesia, were far from conclusive. Even though several peripheral indices of central dopaminergic and GABAergic activity tentatively suggest a more pronounced supersensitivity of dopaminergic and/or GABAergic neurons in patients with tardive dyskinesia, the findings do not elucidate the pathophysiological mechanisms underlying tardive dyskinesia. What eludes explanation is the highly complex pathophysiology of tardive dyskinesia that balances the multiple neurotransmitter systems. The majority of studies have evaluated the metabolites of different neurotransmitter systems, without taking into consideration the interrelationships among these monoamine neurotransmitters. That has been a shortcoming in many investigations, for Lu et al. (1989) have demonstrated that the ratios between different monoamine metabolites show significant imbalances in patients with tardive dyskinesia.

As the complexities of the potentially involved neuronal pathways become increasingly evident, the less likely it appears that we will be able to find specific alterations in the peripheral neuroendocrine parameters with which to illuminate the pathophysiology of tardive dyskinesia. Indeed, assessments of the peripheral neuroendocrine parameters are beset by many confounding factors, such as gender, age, type of neuroleptic administered, and duration of neuroleptic treatment. Considering the small numbers of patients investigated in most of the studies, we are unlikely to be able to determine even clear-cut differences in the parameters investigated. Moreover, there is increasing evidence that tardive dyskinesia is a heterogeneous disorder. Assuming that the different subtypes of tardive dyskinesia are caused by abnormal activities in different central pathways, we should not be surprised that investigations not differentiating between those subtypes fail to detect differences.

The majority of neuroendocrinological studies concerning tardive dyskinesia were carried out in the early and middle 1980s. Since then, new techniques have been developed that can allow direct evaluation of central neurotransmitter systems. Such a centralized approach would appear to be more promising than would evaluations of peripheral neuroendocrine parameters for revealing the pathophysiological mechanisms underlying tardive dyskinesia.

References

Albus, M., Naber, D., Müller-Spahn, F., Douillet, P., Reinertshofer, T., & Ackenheil, M. (1985). Tardive dyskinesia: relation to computer-tomographic, endocrine, and psychopathological variables. *Biol. Psychiatry* 20:1082–9.

Aldegunde, M., Miquez, I., & Veira, J. (1985). Effects of pinealectomy on regional brain serotonin metabolism. *Int. J. Neurosci.* 26:9–13.

Aleem, A., Kulkarni, A., & Yeragani, V. K. (1988). Dexamethasone suppression test, schizophrenia and movement disorder. *Acta Psychiatr. Scand.* 78:689–94.

Arato, M., Bagdy, G., Perényi, A., & Béla, A. (1984). Comparative neurochemical investigations of tardive dyskinesia and neuroleptic-induced parkinsonism. *Psychiatry Res.* 11:347–51.

Arato, M., Perényi, A., Fekete, M. I. K., Bagdy, G., & Erdós, A. (1980). Neuroendocrine investigations in tardive dyskinesia. *Neuroendocrinol. Lett.* 2:315–20.

Asnis, G. M., Sachar, E. J., Langer, G., Halpern, F. S., & Fink, M. (1979). Normal prolactin responses in tardive dyskinesia. *Psychopharmacology* 66:247–50.

Bédard, P. J., & Boucher, R. (1986). Estradiol can suppress haloperidol-induced supersensitivity in dyskinetic monkeys. *Neurosci. Lett.* 64:206–10.

Bédard, P. J., Bouchar, R., Daigle, M., & DiPaolo, T. (1984). Similar effect of estradiol and haloperidol on experimental dyskinesia in monkeys. *Psycho-neuroendocrinology* 9:375–9.

Bowers, M. B., Moore, D. C., & Tarsy, D. (1979). Tardive dyskinesia: a clinical test of the supersensitivity hypothesis. *Psychopharmacology* 61:137–41.

Brown, W. A. (1983). Prolactin levels and effects of neuroleptics. *Psychosomatics* 24:569–81.

Brown, W. A., & Laughren, T. (1980). Growth hormone release and the tardive dyskinesia of neuroleptic withdrawal. *Lancet* 1:259.

Brown, K. W., & White, T. (1991). Human leucocyte antigens and tardive dyskinesia. *Br. J. Psychiatry* 158:270–2.

Cadet, J. L., Lohr, J. B., & Jeste, D. V. (1986). Free radicals and tardive dyskinesia. *Trends Neurosci.* 9:107–8.

Canoso, R. T., Romero, J. A., & Yunis, E. J. (1986). Immunogenetic markers of chlorpromazine induced tardive dyskinesia. *J. Neuroimmunol.* 12:247–52.

Cassady, S., Thaker, G., Moran, M., Layne, J., & Tamminga, C. (1992). GABA-ergic involvement in persistent tardive dyskinesia – a late and persistent process? *Biol. Psychiatry* 31:159A.

Charlton, B. C. (1990). Melanocyte-stimulating hormone in tardive dyskinesia. *Biol. Psychiatry* 27:676–8.

Chase, T. N., Schnur, J. A., & Gordon, E. K. (1970). Cerebral spinal fluid monoamine catabolites in drug-induced extrapyramidal diseases. *Neuropharmacology* 9:265–8.

Cohen, K. L., Cooper, R. A., & Altshul, S. (1979). Prolactin levels in tardive dyskinesia. *N. Engl. J. Med.* 301:300–4.

Coward, D. M. (1982). Classical and non-classical neuroleptics induce supersensitivity of nigral GABAergic mechanisms in the rat. *Psychopharmacology* 78:180–4.

Coward, D. M. (1992). General pharmacology of clozapine. *Br. J. Psychiatry* 160:5–11.

Csernansky, J. G., Prosser, E., Kaplan, J., Mahler, E., Berger, P. A., & Hollister, L. E. (1986a). Possible associations among plasma prolactin levels, tardive dyskinesia, and paranoia in treated schizophrenics. *Biol. Psychiatry* 21:632–42.

Csernansky, J. G., Vinogradov, S., Prosser, E., Kaplan, J., Berger, P. A., & Hollister, L. E. (1986b). Associations among plasma prolactin levels, tardive dyskinesia, and paranoia in treated schizophrenics: relevance to supersensitivity psychosis. *Biol. Psychiatry* 22:897–9.

DePotter, R. W., Linowski, P., & Mendlewicz, J. (1983). State-dependent tardive dyskinesia in manic–depressive illness. *J. Neurol. Neurosurg. Psychiatry* 46:666–8.

Dewan, M. J., Pandurangi, A. K., & Levy, B. F. (1985). Are schizophrenics with abnormal dexamethasone test results a distinct subgroup? *Acta Psychiatr. Scand.* 72:274–7.

DiPaolo, T., & Falardeau, P. (1985). Modulation of brain and pituitary dopamine receptors by estrogens and prolactin. *Prog. Neuro-Psychopharmacol. Biol. Psychiatry* 8:473–80.

Ebadi, M., & Hama, Y. (1988). Dopamine, GABA, cholecystokinin and opioids in neuroleptic-induced tardive dyskinesia. *Neurosci. Behav. Rev.* 12:179–87.

Egan, M. F., Hyde, T., Albers, G., Elkashef, A., Alexander, R. C., & Wyatt, R. J. (1991). Treatment of tardive dyskinesia with vitamin E (abstract). In

Program and Abstracts of the American Psychiatric Association Meeting, NR37. Washington, DC: American Psychiatric Association.

Elkashef, A. M., Ruskin, P. E., Bacher, N., & Barrett, D. (1990). Vitamin E in the treatment of tardive dyskinesia. *Am. J. Psychiatry* 147:505–6.

Ettigi, P., Nair, N. P. V., Lall, S., Cervantes, P., & Guyda, H. (1976). Effect of apomorphine on growth hormone and prolactin secretion in schizophrenic patients with or without oral dyskinesia, withdrawn from chronic neuroleptic therapy. *J. Neurol. Neurosurg. Psychiatry* 39:870–6.

Fibiger, H. C., & Lloyd, K. G. (1984). Neurobiological substrates of tardive dyskinesia: the GABA hypothesis. *Trends Neurosci.* 7:462–4.

Frazer, A., Brown, R., Kocsis, J., & Caroff, S. (1986). Patterns of melatonin rhythms in depression. *J. Neural Transm.* 21:269–90.

Ganzini, L., Heintz, R. T., Hoffman, W. F., & Casey, D. E. (1991). The prevalence of tardive dyskinesia in neuroleptic-treated diabetics. *Arch. Gen. Psychiatry* 48:259–64.

Glazer, W. M., Bowers, M. B., Charney, D. S., & Heninger, G. R. (1989). The effect of neuroleptic discontinuation on psychopathology, involuntary movements, and biochemical measures in patients with persistent tardive dyskinesia. *Biol. Psychiatry* 26:224–33.

Glazer, W. M., Charney, D. S., & Heninger, G. R. (1987). Noradrenergic function in schizophrenia. *Arch. Gen. Psychiatry* 44:898–904.

Glazer, W. M., Moore, D. C., Bowers, M. B., & Brown, W. A. (1981). Serum prolactin and tardive dyskinesia. *Am. J. Psychiatry* 138:1493–6.

Glazer, W. M., Naftolin, F., Moore, D., Bowers, M. B., & MacLusky, N. J. (1983). The relationship of circulating estradiol to tardive dyskinesia in men and post-menopausal women. *Psychoneuroendocrinology* 8:429–34.

Glazer, W. M., Naftolin, F., Morgenstern, H., Barnea, E. R., MacLusky, N. J., & Brenner, L. M. (1985). Estrogen replacement and tardive dyskinesia. *Psychoneuroendocrinology* 10:345–50.

Guy, W. (ed.) (1976). *ECDEU Assessment Manual for Psychopharmacology*, rev. ed., pp. 534–7. Publication ADM 76-338. Washington, DC: U.S. Department of Health, Education, and Welfare.

Horrobin, D. F., Manku, M. S., Morse-Fisher, N., Vaddadi, K. S., Courtney, P., Glen, A. I. M., Glen, E., Spellman, M., & Bates, C. (1989). Essential fatty acids in plasma phospholipids in schizophrenics. *Biol. Psychiatry* 25:562–8.

Hruska, R. E., & Silbergeld, E. K. (1980). Estrogen treatment enhances dopamine receptor sensitivity in the rat striatum. *Eur. J. Pharmacol.* 61:397–400.

Jeste, D. V., DeLisi, L. E., Zaloman, S., Wise, C. D., Phelps, B. H., Rosenblatt, J. E., Potkin, S. G., Bridge, T. P., & Wyatt, R. J. (1981a). A biochemical study of tardive dyskinesia in young male patients. *Psychiatry Res.* 4:327–31.

Jeste, D. V., Doongaji, D. R., & Linnoila, M. (1984). Elevated cerebrospinal fluid noradrenaline in tardive dyskinesia. *Br. J. Psychiatry* 144:177–80.

Jeste, D. V., Lohr, J. B., Kaufmann, C. A., & Wyatt, R. J. (1986). Pathophysiology of tardive dyskinesia; evaluation of supersensitivity theory and alternative hypotheses. In *Tardive Dyskinesia and Neuroleptics: From Dogma to Reason*, ed. D. E. Casey & G. Gardos, pp. 15–32. Washington, DC: American Psychiatric Press.

Jeste, D. V., Neckers, L. M., Wagner, R. L., Wise, C. D., Staub, R. A., Rogol, A., Potkin, S. G., Bridge, T. P., & Wyatt, R. J. (1981b). Lymphocyte monoamine oxidase and plasma prolactin and growth hormone in tardive dyskinesia. *J. Clin. Psychiatry* 42:75–7.

Jeste, D. V., & Wyatt, R. J. (1982). Biochemical theories. In *Understanding and Treating Tardive Dyskinesia,* ed. D. V. Jeste & R. J. Wyatt, pp. 107–50. New York: Guilford Press.

Kane, J. M., Woerner, M., & Lieberman, J. (1988). Tardive dyskinesia: prevalence, incidence, and risk factors. *J. Clin. Psychopharmacol.* 8:52S–6S.

Kirch, D., Hattox, S., Bell, J., Murphy, R., & Freedman, R. (1983). Plasma homovanillic acid and tardive dyskinesia during neuroleptic maintenance and withdrawal. *Psychiatry Res.* 9:217–23.

Korsgaard, S., Gerlach, J., & Christensson, E. (1985). Behavioral aspects of serotonin–dopamine interaction in the monkey. *Eur. J. Pharmacol.* 118:245–52.

Lenox, R. H., Weaver, L. A., & Saran, B. M. (1985). Tardive dyskinesia: clinical and neuroendocrine response to low dose bromocriptine. *J. Clin. Psychopharmacol.* 5:291–2.

Lieberman, J., Johns, C., Cooper, T., Pollack, S., & Kane, J. (1989). Clozapine pharmacology and tardive dyskinesia. *Psychopharmacology* 99:54–9.

Lohr, J. B. (1991). Oxygen radicals and neuropsychiatric illness. *Arch. Gen. Psychiatry* 48:1097–106.

Lohr, J. B., Cadet, J. L., Lohr, M. A., Larson, L., Wasli, E., Wade, L., Hylton, R., Vidoni, C., Jeste, D. V., & Wyatt, R. J. (1988). Vitamine E in treatment of tardive dyskinesia: the possible involvement of free radical mechanisms. *Schizophr. Bull.* 14:291–6.

Lohr, J. B., Kuczenski, R., Bracha, H. S., Moir, M., & Jeste, D. V. (1990). Increased indices of free radical activity in the cerebrospinal fluid of patients with tardive dyskinesia. *Biol. Psychiatry* 28:535–9.

Lozovski, D. B., Kopin, I. J., & Saller, C. F. (1985). Modulation of dopamine receptor supersensitivity by chronic insulin: implication in schizophrenia. *Brain Res.* 343:190–3.

Lu, R. B., Ko, H. C., Lin, W. L., Lin, Y. T., & Ho., S. L. (1989). CSF neurochemical study in tardive dyskinesia. *Biol. Psychiatry* 25:717–24.

Mackay, A. V. P., Iversen, L. L., Rossor, M., Spokes, E., Bird, E., Arregui, A., Creese, I., & Snyder, S. (1982). Increased brain dopamine and dopamine receptors in schizophrenia. *Arch. Gen. Psychiatry* 39:991–7.

Metzer, W. S., Newton, J. E., & Steele, R. W. (1990). HLA antigens in tardive dyskinesia. *J. Neuroimmunol.* 26:179–81.

Miles, A., & Philbrick, D. R. S. (1988). Melatonin and psychiatry. *Biol. Psychiatry* 23:405–15.

Monteleone, P., Maj, M., Ariano, M. G., Iovino, M., Fiorenza, L., & Steardo, L. (1988). Prolactin response to sodium valproate in schizophrenics with and without tardive dyskinesia. *Psychopharmacology* 96:223–6.

Moore, D. C., Glazer, W. M., Bowers, M., & Heninger, G. R. (1983). Tardive dyskinesia and plasma homovanillic acid. *Biol. Psychiatry* 18:1399–402.

Mouret, J., Khomais, M., Lemoine, P., & Sebert, P. (1991). Low doses of insulin as a treatment of tardive dyskinesia: conjuncture or conjecture? *Eur. Neurol.* 31:199–203.

Mukherjee, S., Bilder, R. M., & Sakeim, H. A. (1986). Tardive dyskinesia and glucose metabolism (letter). *Arch. Gen. Psychiatry* 43:193.

Mukherjee, S., Roth, S. D., Sandyk, R., & Schnaer, D. B. (1989). Persistent tardive dyskinesia and neuroleptic effects on glucose tolerance. *J. Psychiatr. Res.* 29:17–27.

Müller-Spahn, F., Ackenheil, M., Albus, M., May, G., Naber, D., Welter, D., &

Zander, K. (1984). Neuroendocrine effects of apomorphine in chronic schizophrenic patients under long term neuroleptic therapy and after drug withdrawal. Relations to psychopathology and tardive dyskinesia. *Psychopharmacology* 84:436–40.

Muscettola, G., Barbato, G., de Bartolomes, A., Monteleone, P., & Pickar, D. (1990). Plasma HVA, tardive dyskinesia and psychotic symptoms in long-term drug-free inpatients with schizophrenia. *Psychiatry Res.* 33:259–67.

Naber, D., Finkbeiner, C., Fischer, B., Zander, K. J., & Ackenheil, M. (1980). Effect of long-term neuroleptic treatment on prolactin and norepinephrine levels in serum of chronic schizophrenics: relations to psychopathology and extrapyramidal symptoms. *Neuropsychobiology* 6:181–9.

Nagao, T., Oshimo, T., Mitsunobu, K., Sato, M., & Otsuki, S. (1979). Cerebrospinal fluid monoamine metabolites and cyclic nucleotides in chronic schizophrenic patients with tardive dyskinesia or drug-induced tremor. *Biol. Psychiatry* 14:509–23.

Perényi, A., Frecska, E., Bagdy, G., & Réval, K. (1985). Changes in mental condition, hyperkinesis and biochemical parameters after withdrawal of chronic neuroleptic treatment. *Acta Psychiatr. Scand.* 72:430–5.

Pind, K., & Faurbye, K. (1970). Concentration of HVA and 5HIAA in the CSF after treatment with probenecid in patients with drug-induced tardive dyskinesia. *Acta Psychiatr. Scand.* 46:323–6.

Post, R. M., Ballenger, J. C., Hare, T. A., Goodwin, F. K., Laker, C. R., Jimerson, D. C., & Bunney, W. E. (1980). CSF GABA in normals and patients with affective disorder. *Brain Res. Bull.* 5:755–9.

Racagni, G., Apud, J. A., Cocchi, D., Locatelli, V., & Müller, E. E. (1982). GABAergic control of anterior pituitary hormone secretion. *Life Sci.* 31:823–38.

Richardson, M. A., Suckow, R., Whittacker, R., Boggiano, W., Sziraki, I., Kushner, H., & Perumal, A. (1989). The plasma phenylalanine large neutral amino acid ratio: a risk factor for tardive dyskinesia. *Psychopharmacol. Bull.* 25:47–51.

Richardson, M. A., Suckow, R., Whittacker, R., Perumal, A., Boggiano, W., Szirak, I., & Kushner, H. (1988). Phenylalanine, phenylethylamine and tardive dyskinesia in psychiatric patients. In *Trace Amines: Comparative and Clinical Neurobiology*, ed. A. A. Boulton, A. V., Juorio, & R. Downer, pp. 409–22. Totowa: Humana Press.

Saller, C. F., & Chiodo, L. A. (1980). Glucose suppresses basal firing and haloperidol-induced increases in the firing rate of cerebral dopaminergic neurons. *Science* 210:1269–71.

Sandyk, R. (1989). Melanocyte-stimulating hormone in tardive dyskinesia. *Biol. Psychiatry* 26:213–41.

Sandyk, R. (1990a). Melanocyte-stimulating hormone and persistent tardive dyskinesia: a hypothesis. *Int. J. Neurosci.* 51:45–52.

Sandyk, R. (1990b). The association of pineal calcification with drug-induced dystonic movements. *Int. J. Neurosci.* 53:217–22.

Sandyk, R., & Fisher, H. (1989a). The relationship of serotonin metabolism and melatonin secretion to the pathophysiology of tardive dyskinesia. *Int. J. Neurosci.* 48:133–6.

Sandyk, R., & Fisher, H. (1989b). Melatonin mediates the antidyskinetic effects of naloxone in tardive dyskinesia. *J. Clin. Psychopharmacol.* 9:147–8.

Sauter, A., Goldstein, M., Engel, J., & Ueta, K. (1983). Effect of insulin on central catecholamines. *Brain Res.* 260:330–3.

Scheel-Krüger, J. (1986). Dopamine–GABA interactions: evidence that GABA transmits, modulates, and mediates dopaminergic functions in the basal ganglia and the limbic system. *Acta Neurol. Scand.* 107:1–5.

Shriqui, C. L., Bradwein, J., Jones, B. D., & Annable, L. (1991). Vitamin E in the treatment of tardive dyskinesia (abstract). In: *Program and Abstracts of the American Psychiatric Association Meeting*, NR80. Washington, DC: American Psychiatric Association.

Smith, J. M., Oswald, W. T., Kucharski, T., & Waterman, L. J. (1978). Tardive dyskinesia, age and sex differences in hospitalized schizophrenics. *Psychopharmacology* 58:207–11.

Sorokin, J. E., Giordani, B., Mohs, R. C., Losonczu, M. F., Davidson, M., Slever, L. J., Ryan, T. A., & Davis, K. L. (1988). Memory impairment in schizophrenic patients with tardive dyskinesia. *Biol. Psychiatry* 23:129–35.

Stoessl, A. J., Dourish, C. T., & Iversen, S. D. (1989). Chronic neuroleptic-induced mouth movements in the rat: suppression by CCK and selective dopamine D_1 and D_2 receptor antagonists. *Psychopharmacology* 98:372–9.

Tamminga, C. A., Smith, R. C., Pandey, G., Frohman, L. A., & Davis, J. M. (1977). A neuroendocrine study of supersensitivity in tardive dyskinesia. *Arch. Gen. Psychiatry* 34:1199–203.

Thaker, G. K., Nguyen, J. A., & Tamminga, C. A. (1989a). Saccadic distractibility in schizophrenic patients with tardive dyskinesia. *Arch. Gen. Psychiatry* 46:755–6.

Thaker, G. K., Tamminga, C. A., Alphs, L. D., Lafferman, J., Ferraro, T. N., & Hare, T. A. (1987). Brain gamma-aminobutyric acid abnormality in tardive dyskinesia. *Arch. Gen. Psychiatry* 44:522–9.

Thaker, G. K., Wagman, A. M., Kirkpatrick, B., & Tamminga, C. A. (1989b). Alterations in sleep polygraphy after neuroleptic withdrawal: a putative supersensitive dopaminergic mechanism. *Biol. Psychiatry* 25:75–86.

Trentini, G. P., De Gaetani, C. F., Criscuolo, M., Migaldi, M., & Ferrari, G. (1987). Pineal calcification in different physiopathological conditions in humans. In *Fundamentals and Clinics in Pineal Research*, ed. G. P. Trentini, C. De Gaetani and P. Pevet, pp. 291–304. New York: Raven Press.

Tripodianakis, J., Markianos, M., and Garelis, E. (1983). Neurochemical studies on tardive dyskinesia. Urinary homovanillic acid and plasma prolactin. *Biol. Psychiatry* 18:337–45.

Villeneuve, A., Cazejust, T., & Cote, M. (1980). Estrogens in tardive dyskinesia in male psychiatric patients. *Neuropsychobiology* 6:145–51.

Wolf, M. E., Bowie, L., Keener, S., & Mosnaim, A. D. (1982). Prolactin response in tardive dyskinesia. *Biol. Psychiatry* 17:485–90.

Wright, P. (1991). Tardive dyskinesia and HLA. *Br. J. Psychiatry* 159:863–4.

Young, W., Kuhar, M. J., & Roth, J. (1980). Radiohistochemical localization of insulin receptors in the adult and developing rat brain. *Neuropeptides* 1:15–22.

15

Cognitive Deficits and Tardive Dyskinesia

MARION E. WOLF, M.D., ALAN S. DEWOLFE, Ph.D.,
and ARON D. MOSNAIM, Ph.D.

An understanding of the multifaceted neurological disorder known as tardive dyskinesia, including its association with cognitive deficits, requires a global conceptualization. In this context, we must view tardive dyskinesia as an illness, the etiology of which follows the well-established biological scheme of a host (having various degrees of predisposing factors), a noxious agent (the neuroleptic drug), and an environment in which the first two components interact. Although studies abound concerning the roles of vulnerability factors, as well as antipsychotic agents, in the development of tardive dyskinesia (Kane & Smith, 1982; Singh & Simpson, 1988), research on environmental factors is scarce. Thus, before turning to our main review, we shall first briefly examine two sociological studies: one conducted in an inpatient setting, the other in an outpatient setting.

Two Sociological Studies

In the inpatient setting, it was the nursing staff who initially resisted our attempts to implement the recommendations of the American Psychiatric Association (1979) task-force report on the late neurological effects of antipsychotic drugs. The nurses were opposed to instituting the APA's suggested drug-free periods for patients on long-term neuroleptic treatment. We conducted many extra meetings and workshops to convince staff personnel on all shifts that such intervention was medically sound, safe, and feasible. But the nurses feared, even expected, that patients would experience clinical decompensation, and in the beginning they tended to consider any change in a patient's behavior during drug discontinuation to be indicative of deterioration. After repeated drug-free periods, however, the staff realized that patients rarely became assaultive or posed significant management problems. Furthermore, some patients actually showed improvement when excessive doses of neuroleptics were discontinued. Gradually, with experience, and after direct involvement in drug-free periods and educational activities, the nurses changed their point of view.

As for the outpatient setting, which involved a community-care placement program in which discharged chronic psychiatric patients lived in the private homes of nonprofessional community sponsors, we found that the sponsors were quite concerned at the prospect of discontinuing or decreasing the dosages of antipsychotics or antiparkinsonian drugs. There was a 50% increase in unscheduled visits and a 30% increase in after-hours visits by the sponsors, in addition to repeated telephone calls to request additional psychotropic medications for the patients. Also, when staff members made home visits to the patients and their sponsors, the sponsors expressed fears that reductions or withdrawals of medications would undermine the stability not only of the patients whose medications were to be reduced or withdrawn but also of other patients under their care. The sponsors were reassured that the community-placement clinic would follow the patients closely, that negative outcomes were not expected, and that a sponsor's role in the patients' care was considered essential. Educational activities for the sponsors were subsequently organized at our medical center; there, the effects and problems of psychotropic drugs were discussed in plain language. In the end, the educational activities facilitated smooth operation of the program. It may be, then, that a more comprehensive approach to the social issues will reduce the pressure on physicians to revert to often excessive neuroleptic prescriptions when difficulties arise because of changes in treatment.

Tardive Dyskinesia in Context

Our studies clearly indicate that biased opinions on the part of both the public and mental-health professionals can interfere with the prevention and management of tardive dyskinesia (Wolf & Brown, 1987). Moreover, studies in developing countries where labor is cheap and goods expensive, as reflected in the psychiatric-hospital settings by a relative abundance of personnel (i.e., nursing staff) and a restricted allocation of antipsychotic drugs (monthly quotas on oral and intramuscular neuroleptic agents), have shown that the prevalence of tardive dyskinesia is very low, as compared with that found in industrialized countries (Wolf & Puente, 1989). Perhaps tardive dyskinesia is, to a large extent, an illness of the underprivileged in affluent Western societies, where the economics of supply and demand for labor and goods are reversed from the pattern seen in developing countries.

Studies have also shown that tardive dyskinesia often coexists with drug-induced parkinsonism (Wolf et al., 1983a; Kolakowska et al., 1986) and that acute extrapyramidal side effects in the early phases of neuroleptic treatment may constitute a predisposing factor for the development of tardive dyskinesia (Kane et al., 1986). There is currently a dilemma, however, in defining the extent to which early and late extrapyramidal side effects represent different entities or are diverse manifestations of an "extrapyramidal diathesis" that reveals itself in polymorphous ways, that is, according to intervening factors such as age and the nature and duration of psychotropic drug treatment (Wolf, DeWolfe, & Mosnaim, 1991). Indeed, researchers have addressed the difficulties of controlling for spontaneous development of abnormal movements in the absence of neuroleptic treatment, attempting to determine the extent to which the movements are expressions of the basic schizophrenic process itself. Another confounding factor is that nonneuroleptic drugs can induce extrapyramidal signs; of particular importance in this category is lithium. Moreover, several investigators have established that patients with affective disorder (AD) are more vulnerable than schizophrenic patients to the development of tardive dyskinesia (Rosenbaum, Niven, & Hanson, 1977; Yassa, Ghadirian, & Schwartz, 1983; Gardos & Casey, 1984; Wolf et al., 1985). Clearly, this AD population is also exposed to the many varied effects of lithium. Also, it has been observed that the neuroleptic malignant syndrome, the clinical symptoms of which can include tardive dyskinesia, can be precipitated by lithium alone (Susman & Addonizio, 1987). Pharmocologic data also support the notion that neuroleptics potentiate the actions of lithium, and vice versa (Pandey, Goel, & Davis, 1979; Ostrow, Southam, & Davis, 1980; Wolf & Mosnaim, 1986; Wolf et al., 1992). Although it is difficult to draw clear conclusions from such complex clinical findings, in this chapter we attempt to isolate the variables involved in tardive dyskinesia and cognitive functions and review the nature of such associations.

Tardive Dyskinesia and Cognitive Functions: Four Studies

Methods

In this section we discuss the methods and statistical treatments used in four studies selected from our series of studies dealing with tardive dyskinesia (Wolf, Ryan, & Mosnaim, 1983b; Wolf, Koller, & Mosnaim, 1984; Wolf et al., 1985; DeWolfe, Ryan, & Wolf, 1988). Underlying our choices of these methods and statistical approaches was the need for maximum clarity of interpretation, as well as direct clinical relevance of the findings. To that end we took great care in selecting appropriate subjects for both the tardive dyskinesia group and the control group and in choosing statistical analyses that would simplify eventual applications of our findings to clinical practice.

Case Selection. In all four studies we selected patients for the tardive dyskinesia groups only after a minimum of 3 weeks of continuous evaluation. Initially, the subjects were chosen on the basis of the criteria of Jeste, Neckers, and Wagner (1981). They were then assessed for 3 weeks using the Simpson Rating Scale (Simpson, Lee, & Zoubok, 1979). Whereas we assigned to the tardive dyskinesia groups only those patients who showed tardive dyskinesia symptoms at every assessment, we assigned to the control groups only patients who showed no tardive dyskinesia symptoms at any of the assessments. Patients were maintained on the minimal neuroleptic dosages consistent with their clinical conditions, with AD patients being maintained on lithium. The memory functions of AD patients were tested during phases when they were free from depression, as indicated by clinical evaluation and by the Overall and Gorham (1962) Brief Psychiatric Rating Scale.

Subclassification of Tardive Dyskinesia Patients. Because of the clinically relevant differences among tardive dyskinesia patients based on their diagnoses (i.e., schizophrenia vs. AD), we subdivided the patients in all four studies into schizophrenic and AD groups, based on the Research Diagnostic Criteria (RDC) (Spitzer, Endicott, & Robbins, 1978). In the study by De-Wolfe et al. (1988), patients with tardive dyskinesia symptoms were classified on the basis of the locations of their motor symptoms. Their motor symptoms were rated for severity in the facial area, extremities (limbs), and trunk independently, via the Simpson Rating Scale.

Matching. When control groups without tardive dyskinesia were used (Wolf et al., 1983b, 1984), we compared the tardive dyskinesia groups and the control groups within diagnosis only. Thus, any differences in tardive dyskinesia status would not be confounded by differences in diagnoses. In the study by DeWolfe et al. (1988), the AD and schizophrenic groups did not differ significantly in regard to age, education, full-scale IQ, memory quotient, or severity ratings for tardive dyskinesia symptoms (total, facial, extremity, or trunkal). Thus, the differences found among the diagnostic groups and among the motor-symptom groups (facial, extremity, and trunkal) vis-à-vis the relationship between the severity of tardive dyskinesia symptoms and the degrees of cognitive deficits were not due to preexisting differences in age, education, degree of severity of tardive dyskinesia, or cognitive deficits in the subgroups.

Measures. As with our selection of the methods and statistical procedures to be used, we chose evaluative measures for both their clinical relevance and scientific merit. The Wechsler Adult Intelligence Scale (WAIS) (Wechsler, 1955), the Wechsler Memory Scale (WMS) (Wechsler, 1945), the Rey Auditory Verbal Learning Test (Lezak, 1976), the Mini-Mental State (MMS) examination (Folstein & Folstein, 1975), and the Simpson Rating Scale (Simpson et al., 1979) are all commonly used clinical measures, as are age, institutionalization history, and presence or absence of alcoholism and drug-induced parkinsonism. By using such highly reliable tests as the WAIS and WMS and subclassifying tardive dyskinesia patients by diagnosis and location of tardive dyskinesia symptoms, we combined high clinical relevance with a strong capacity to enhance statistical power.

Statistics. The statistics used in these studies permitted direct, straightforward analysis of clinically relevant data (e.g., IQ, memory quotient, diagnosis, severity of localized tardive dyskinesia symptoms, presence or absence of alcoholism and drug-induced parkinsonism) with as much statistical power as the level of data (e.g., nominal vs. interval data) and data distributions (e.g., normal vs. nonnormal) would permit. The statistics used (e.g., F, t, χ^2, and r) allowed us to keep the data in their most clinically useful form; for example, scores were not transformed, and β weighting was not needed.

Results

Diagnosis. In all three studies that focused on cognitive functions, the diagnoses were significantly related to the tardive dyskinesia symptoms. Diagnoses were significantly related to vulnerability (Wolf et al., 1985; Wolf, DeWolfe, & Mosnaim, 1987) inasmuch as age and institutionalization were related to vulnerability for schizophrenic patients but not for AD patients, and the MMS scores, the presence of alcoholism, and the presence of drug-induced parkinsonism were related to vulnerability for AD patients but not for schizophrenics.

Wolf, Ryan, and Mosnaim (1982) and Wolf et al. (1983b) found that whereas AD patients with tardive dyskinesia had poorer scores for memory and verbal learning than did AD patients without tardive dyskinesia, no such difference was found for schizophrenic patients with and without tardive dyskinesia. Subsequently, DeWolfe et al. (1988) found marked differences between the schizophrenic and AD groups with tardive dyskinesia in terms of the relationship between the severity of motor symptoms of tardive dyskinesia and the degree of cognitive deficits. For schizophrenic patients, these same researchers found frequent (10 of 22 *r* values) and strong correlations between the severity of motor symptoms of tardive dyskinesia and the degree of cognitive deficits for both intelligence and memory measures. However, for AD patients, they found only one significant correlation between the severity of motor symptoms of tardive dyskinesia and the degree of cognitive deficits.

Only in an electrophysiological study (Wolf et al., 1984) was it found that diagnoses were unrelated to the differences in how motor symptoms of tardive dyskinesia were related to experimental data. Those EEG findings indicated that schizophrenic patients with tardive dyskinesia did not differ from schizophrenic patients without tardive dyskinesia and that AD patients with tardive dyskinesia did not differ from AD patients without tardive dyskinesia. The only significant result in this study was that patients receiving both lithium and neuroleptics were significantly more likely to show EEG abnormalities than were patients receiving lithium or neuroleptics alone.

Location of Tardive Dyskinesia Symptoms. DeWolfe et al. (1988) found that the locations of motor symptoms of tardive dyskinesia were directly related to cognitive deficits and that locations also interacted with diagnoses in terms of how the relationship between motor-symptom severity and cognitive deficits was affected. In addition, whereas the severity of facial symptoms of tardive dyskinesia was strongly related to the degree of cognitive deficits (19 of 22 *r* values were significant), the severities of motor symptoms in the extremities and trunk were rarely related to the degrees of cognitive deficits (2 of 22 *r* values, and 1 of 22 *r* values, respectively, were significant). Table 15.1 summarizes the findings in the studies cited.

Discussion

The findings in our initial studies that suggested an association between cognitive deficits and tardive dyskinesia in AD patients have been confirmed by several investigators (Wegner et al., 1985; Wade et al., 1987; Waddington & Youssef, 1988). Although we did not find an association between cognitive dysfunction and tardive dyskinesia in schizophrenic patients in our preliminary studies, such an association was identified in subsequent studies. It appears that given the severe intellectual impairments among the initial schizophrenic population studied, the differences in the cognitive parameters examined for patients with and without tardive dyskinesia could not be detected with the psychometric instruments employed. Factors of this nature, or failure to control for age, duration of illness, and other confounding variables, may account for the negative findings reported by other investi-

Table 15.1. *Summary of findings in four studies cited*

Issue and study	Findings
Cognitive functions (Wolf et al., 1983b)	AD patients with tardive dyskinesia symptoms score significantly poorer on memory and verbal learning than do AD patients without tardive dyskinesia; schizophrenic patients, with and without tardive dyskinesia, show no significant differences.
Cognitive functions and symptom locations (DeWolfe et al., 1988)	The severity of motor symptoms is highly related to the severity of cognitive deficits for schizophrenic patients only. The severity of motor symptoms in the facial area is far more closely related to cognitive impairment than is the severity of motor symptoms in the extremities or trunk.
Electrophysiological data (Wolf et al., 1984)	EEG findings in AD and schizophrenic patients with tardive dyskinesia do not differ from those in matched controls without tardive dyskinesia. Patients taking both lithium and neuroleptics show more EEG abnormalities than do those taking either drug alone.
Vulnerability to tardive dyskinesia (Wolf et al., 1985)	A low MMS score, the presence of alcoholism, and the presence of drug-induced parkinsonism are indicators of vulnerability for AD patients only. Increasing age and a long history of institutionalization are indicators of vulnerability for schizophrenic patients only.

gators (Richardson et al., 1985; Kolakowska et al., 1986). The majority of researchers, however, have reported associations between tardive dyskinesia and cognitive deficits in schizophrenic patients (Struve & Wilner, 1983; Thomas & McGuire, 1986; Waddington & Youssef, 1986; Wade et al., 1987; Sorokin et al., 1988) that have been stronger for buccal-facial dyskinesias than for limb-trunk dyskinesias.

Our EEG data indicated that the tardive dyskinesia in schizophrenic patients and AD patients was not associated with specific EEG abnormalities. Furthermore, we noted that approximately 25% of patients on neuroleptics or lithium had abnormal EEG findings. Those findings are related to the controversial issue of lithium-neuroleptic neurotoxicity (Prakash, Kelwala, & Ban, 1982; Addy et al., 1986; Goldney & Spence, 1986; Wolf & Mosnaim, 1986; Miller & Menninger, 1987), an issue that has received increasing attention in recent years, given the increased risk for development of the neuroleptic malignant syndrome in patients receiving combinations of neuroleptics and lithium (Addonizio, 1985; Lazarus, Mann, & Caroff, 1989; Wolf & Mosnaim, 1991). Our pharmacokinetic data suggest that lithium may potentiate the effects of neuroleptics (Wolf & Mosnaim, 1986, 1991) and thus contribute to increased vulnerability to neuroleptic side effects, such as tardive dyskinesia and the neuroleptic malignant syndrome. Perhaps further integration of cognitive, EEG, and pharmacokinetic data will help us to understand the lithium-neuroleptic neurotoxicity seen at the clinical level as a continuum, ranging from cases resembling lithium neurotoxicity to cases indistinguishable from the neuroleptic malignant syndrome. Further studies are needed to assess the association between tardive dyskinesia and the neuroleptic malignant syndrome.

The nature of the association between cognitive deficits and tardive dyskinesia remains an enigma. It is not clear from the research reported thus far whether preexisting cognitive deficits predispose to the development of tardive dyskinesia or whether tardive dyskinesia is related to the appearance of a dementing process. Wegner et al. (1985), in a prospective study, found that schizophrenic and AD patients with tardive dyskinesia had more preexisting cognitive deficits than did their respective controls without tardive dyskinesia. Those authors also noted their surprise in finding that AD patients had poorer baseline conceptual-analysis test scores than did schizophrenics, for the latter, as a group, traditionally perform worse than AD patients on psychometric testing. As previously indicated, those investigators suggested that AD patients with cognitive deficits are particularly vulnerable to the development of tardive dyskinesia. Moreover, the natural course of AD (as opposed to schizophrenia) does not include spontaneous development of abnormal involuntary movements. We therefore wonder if a diagnosis of AD, the development of acute extrapyramidal symptoms with neuroleptic treatment and possibly also lithium treatment, the presence of preexisting cognitive deficits, and the development of tardive dyskinesia may all be parts of a common diathesis.

In our studies (Wolf et al., 1985), we have found that a low MMS score constitutes a risk factor for the development of tardive dyskinesia in AD patients, but not in schizophrenic patients. Wegner et al. (1985), in a prospective study, found that schizophrenic and AD patients with tardive dyskinesia had more preexisting cognitive deficits than did their respective controls without tardive dyskinesia, the finding being particularly robust for the AD patients. It would thus appear that in AD patients, cognitive deficits precede the appearance of tardive dyskinesia and constitute a vulnerability factor for subsequent appearance of the movement disorder.

A different picture emerges for schizophrenic patients. Waddington (1989) found that the initial levels of cognitive functioning in schizophrenic patients without tardive dyskinesia were not associated with manifestations of involuntary movements 5 years later. However, whereas those patients in whom tardive dyskinesia emerged over that 5-year period showed significant deteriorations in their cognitive functioning, no such impairments were evident among those in whom the movement disorder did not appear. In schizophrenic patients, for whom the development of abnormal involuntary movements and cognitive impairments is part of the natural course of the illness, there seems to be an association between the concomitant appearances of abnormal involuntary movements and cognitive deficits. Thus, although the clinical picture of tardive dyskinesia in schizophrenic patients is similar to that in AD patients, the association between cognitive deficits and tardive dyskinesia appears to follow different patterns in these two diagnostic categories, reflecting different pathophysiological mechanisms.

Additional prospective neuropsychological, brain-imaging, and EEG studies are needed to elucidate this challenging enigma.

References

Addonizio, G. (1985). Rapid induction of extrapyramidal side effects with combined use of lithium and neuroleptics. *J. Clin. Psychopharmacol.* 5:296–8.

Addy, R. O., Foliart, R. H., Saran, A. S., & Schubert, D. S. (1986). EEG observations during combined haloperidol-lithium treatment. *Biol. Psychiatry* 21:170–6.

American Psychiatric Association (1979). *Report of Task Force on Late Neurological Effects of Antipsychotic Drugs.* Washington, DC: American Psychiatric Association.

DeWolfe, A. S., Ryan, J. J., & Wolf, M. E. (1988). Cognitive sequelae of tardive dyskinesia. *J. Nerv. Ment. Dis.* 176:270–4.

Folstein, M. D., & Folstein, S. (1975). Mini Mental State: a practice and method for grading cognitive states of patients for the clinician. *J. Psychiatr. Res.* 12:189–98.

Gardos, G., & Casey, D. E. (1984). *Tardive Dyskinesia and Affective Disorders.* Washington, DC: American Psychiatric Press.

Goldney, R. D., & Spence, N. D. (1986). Safety of the combination of lithium and neuroleptic drugs. *Am. J. Psychiatry* 143:882–4.

Jeste, D. V., Neckers, L. M., & Wagner, R. L. (1981). Lymphocyte monoamine oxidase and plasma prolactin and growth hormone in tardive dyskinesia. *J. Clin. Psychiatry* 42:75–7.

Kane, J. M., & Smith, J. M. (1982). Tardive dyskinesia prevalence risk factors. *Arch. Gen. Psychiatry* 39:473–81.

Kane, J. M., Woerner, M., Borenstein, M., Wegner, J., & Lieberman, J. (1986). Integrating incidence and prevalence of tardive dyskinesia. *Psychopharmacol. Bull.* 22:254–8.

Kolakowska, T., Williams, A. O., Arden, M., & Reveley, M. A. (1986). Tardive dyskinesia in schizophrenics under 60 years of age. *Biol. Psychiatry* 21:161–9.

Lazarus, A., Mann, S. C., & Caroff, S. N. (eds.) (1989). *The Neuroleptic Malignant Syndrome*. Washington, DC: American Psychiatric Press.

Lezak, M. D. (1976). *Neuropsychological Assessment*. Oxford University Press.

Miller, F., & Menninger, F. (1987). Correlation of neuroleptic dose and neurotoxicity in patients given lithium and a neuroleptic. *Hosp. Community Psychiatry* 38:1219–21.

Ostrow, D. G., Southam, A. S., & Davis, J. M. (1980). Lithium–drug interactions altering the intracellular lithium level: an in vitro study. *Biol. Psychiatry* 15:723–39.

Overall, J. E., & Gorham, D. R. (1962). The Brief Psychiatric Rating Scale. *Psychol. Rep.* 10:799–812.

Pandey, G. N., Goel, L., & Davis, J. M. (1979). The effect of neuroleptic drugs on lithium uptake by human erythrocyte. *Clin. Pharmacol. Ther.* 26:96–102.

Prakash, R., Kelwala, S., & Ban, T. A. (1982). Neurotoxicity with combined administration of lithium and a neuroleptic. *Compr. Psychiatry* 23:567–71.

Richardson, M. A., Pass, R., Bregman, Z., & Craig, T. J. (1985). Tardive dyskinesia and depressive symptoms in schizophrenics. *Psychopharmacol. Bull.* 21:130–5.

Rosenbaum, H. N., Niven, R. G., & Hanson, N. P. (1977). Tardive dyskinesia: relationships with primary affective disorder. *Dis. Nerv. Syst.* 38:423–7.

Simpson, G. M., Lee, J. H., & Zoubok, B. (1979). A rating scale for tardive dyskinesia. *Psychopharmacology* 64:171–9.

Singh, H., & Simpson, G. M. (1988). Tardive dyskinesia: clinical features. In *Tardive Dyskinesia: Biological Mechanisms and Clinical Aspects*, ed. M. E. Wolf & A. D. Mosnaim, pp. 67–86. Washington, DC: American Psychiatric Press.

Sorokin, J. E., Giordoni, B., Mohs, R. C., Losonczy, M. F., Davidson, M., Siever, L. J., Ryan, T. A., & Davis, K. L. (1988). Memory impairment in schizophrenic patients with tardive dyskinesia. *Biol. Psychiatry* 23:129–35.

Spitzer, R. L., Endicott, J., & Robbins, E. (1978). *Research Diagnostic Criteria (RDC) for a Selected Group of Functional Disorders*, 3rd ed. New York: Biometrics Research, New York State Psychiatric Institute.

Struve, F. A., & Wilner, A. E. (1983). Cognitive dysfunction and tardive dyskinesia. *Br. J. Psychiatry* 143:597–600.

Susman, V. L., & Addonizio, G. (1987). Reinduction of neuroleptic malignant syndrome by lithium. *Clin. Psychopharmacol.* 7:339–41.

Thomas, P., & McGuire, R. (1986). Orofacial dyskinesia, cognitive function and medication. *Br. J. Psychiatry* 149:16–22.

Waddington, J. L. (1989). Schizophrenia, affective psychosis, and other disorders treated with neuroleptic drugs: the enigma of tardive dyskinesia, its neurobiological determinants and the conflict of paradigms. *Int. Rev. Neurobiol.* 31:297–353.

Waddington, J. L., & Youssef, H. A. (1986). Late onset involuntary movements in chronic schizophrenia: relationship of tardive dyskinesia to intellectual impairment and negative symptoms. *Br. J. Psychiatry* 149:616–20.

Waddington, J. L., & Youssef, H. A. (1988). Tardive dyskinesia in bipolar affective disorder: aging, cognitive dysfunction, course of illness, and exposure to neuroleptics and lithium. *Am. J. Psychiatry* 145:613–16.

Wade, J. B., Taylor, M. A., Kasprisin, A., Rosenberg, S., & Fiducia, D. (1987). Tardive dyskinesia and cognitive impairment. *Biol. Psychiatry* 22:393–5.

Wechsler, D. (1945). A standardized memory scale for clinical use. *J. Psychology* 19:87–9.

Wechsler, D. (1955). *Manual for the Wechsler Adult Intelligence Scale.* New York: Psychological Corporation.

Wegner, J. T., Catalano, F., Gibralter, J., & Kane, J. M. (1985). Schizophrenics with tardive dyskinesia. Neuropsychological deficits and family psychopathology. *Arch. Gen. Psychiatry* 42:860–5.

Wolf, M. E., & Brown, P. (1987). Overcoming institutional and community resistance to a tardive dyskinesia management program. *Hosp. Community Psychiatry* 38:65–8.

Wolf, M. E., Chevesich, J., Lehrer, E., & Mosnaim, A. D. (1983a). The clinical association of tardive dyskinesia and drug induced parkinsonisms. *Biol. Psychiatry* 18:1181–8.

Wolf, M. E., DeWolfe, A. S., & Mosnaim, A. D. (1987). Risk factors for tardive dyskinesia according to primary psychiatric diagnosis. *Hillside Clin. Psychiatry* 9:3–11.

Wolf, M. E., DeWolfe, A. S., & Mosnaim, A. D. (1991). The association of tardive dyskinesia with cognitive deficits: a review. *Res. Commun. Psychol. Psychiatry Behav.* 16:15–27.

Wolf, M. E., DeWolfe, A. S., Ryan, J. J., Lips, O., & Mosnaim, A. D. (1985). Vulnerability to tardive dyskinesia. *Clin. Psychiatry* 46:367–8.

Wolf, M. E., Koller, W. C., & Mosnaim, A. D. (1984). Electroencephalogram in tardive dyskinesia. *Clin. Electroencephalogr.* 15:222–5.

Wolf, M. E., & Mosnaim, A. D. (1986). Lithium and molindone interactions: pharmacokinetic studies. *Res. Commun. Psychol. Psychiatry Behav.* 11:23–8.

Wolf, M. E., & Mosnaim, A. D. (1991). Lithium–neuroleptic interactions: implications for the neuroleptic malignant syndrome. Presented at the American Psychiatric Association meeting, New Orleans.

Wolf, M. E., & Mosnaim, A. D. (1994). Improvement of axial dystonia with the administration of clozapine. *Int. J. Clin. Pharmacol. Ther.* 32:282–3.

Wolf, M. E., Mosnaim, G., Farinha, P., & Mosnaim, A. D. (1992). Reinduction of neuroleptic malignant syndrome by lithium. *Res. Commun. Psychol. Psychiatry Behav.* 17:69–72.

Wolf, M. E., & Puente, J. (1989). Prevalence of tardive dyskinesia in a state psychiatric hospital in Chile. Presented at the Fourth Latinoamerican Congress of Cellular Biology, Viña del Mar, Chile.

Wolf, M. E., Ryan, J. J., & Mosnaim, A. D. (1982). Organicity and tardive dyskinesia. *Psychosomatics* 23:475–80.

Wolf, M. E., Ryan, J. J., & Mosnaim, A. D. (1983b). Cognitive functions in tardive dyskinesia. *Psychol. Med.* 13:671–4.

Yassa, R., Ghadirian, A. M., & Schwartz, G. (1983). Prevalence of tardive dyskinesia in affective disorder patients. *Clin. Psychiatry* 43:410–12.

16

Studies of Tardive Dyskinesia Using Computed Tomography and Magnetic-Resonance Imaging

CHRISTIAN L. SHRIQUI, M.D., M.Sc., F.R.C.P.C.

Tardive dyskinesia is an involuntary hyperkinetic movement disorder associated with long-term exposure to antipsychotic medication (Casey, 1987). Its prevalence, estimated at 15–20% overall, is considerably higher among elderly subjects (Kane & Smith, 1982; Kane et al., 1984; Woerner et al., 1991; Yassa et al., 1992), and because of its variable outcomes, the absence of any effective treatment, and the potential for legal implications, tardive dyskinesia is of considerable concern to clinicians who prescribe maintenance antipsychotic drugs (Jeste & Wyatt, 1982a; Jeste et al., 1988; Shriqui, 1988; Bergen et al., 1989; Shriqui, Bradwejn, & Jones, 1990; Casey, 1991; Kane et al., 1992; Yassa & Nair, 1992).

Despite considerable research efforts, the pathophysiology and neuroanatomic picture of tardive dyskinesia remain largely unknown (Jeste & Wyatt, 1982b; Kane et al., 1984; Casey, 1991). Although dopaminergic supersensitivity may be an essential component in the emergence of tardive dyskinesia, recent hypotheses involving other neurotransmitters (e.g., γ-aminobutyric acid, norepinephrine, serotonin, acetylcholine), iron metabolism, diminished melatonin secretion, and free-radical neurotoxicity have been advanced (Jeste et al., 1986; Cadet, Lohr, & Jeste, 1987; Sandyk & Fischer, 1988; Lohr et al., 1990; Sandyk, 1990a; Shriqui & Jones, 1990; Lohr, 1991).

Neuropathological studies of tardive dyskinesia patients have reported increased nigral degeneration and gliosis (Christensen, Moller, & Faurbye, 1970; Arai et al., 1987). Pineal-gland calcification has also been reported and suggested as a potential neuroradiologic marker of persistent tardive dyskinesia in schizophrenic and bipolar patients (Sandyk, Awerbuch, & Kay, 1990; Sandyk, 1990b).

More recently, increased iron deposits in the basal ganglia in tardive dyskinesia patients (Hunter et al., 1968; Campbell et al., 1985) have been associated with magnetic-resonance imaging (MRI) findings of shortened T_2 relaxation times in the basal ganglia in patients with tardive dyskinesia (Drayer et al., 1986; Drayer, 1987; Rutledge et al., 1987; Bartzokis et al., 1990, 1991; Lohr, 1991). According to that hypothesis, cytotoxic free radicals, whose production is enhanced by neuroleptic drugs, would be active in iron–neuroleptic-drug interactions in tardive dyskinesia patients (Bartzokis et al., 1990; Lohr, 1991).

Scans from x-ray computed tomography (CT) and, more recently, MRI have been used to investigate neuroanatomic abnormalities in patients with tardive dyskinesia. Because of its widespread availability and lower cost, CT is the brain-imaging technique most frequently used to investigate patients who may have tardive dyskinesia. Nevertheless, MRI offers greater sensitivity and superior image resolution for investigating patients with tardive dyskinesia.

Since 1976, 9 of 24 English-language CT studies and 6 of 9 English-language MRI studies have reported significant abnormal findings in patients with tardive dyskinesia. These findings are summarized in Table 16.1 and Table 16.2, respectively. In general, the CT studies have been inconsistent in reporting structural abnormalities in patients with tardive dyskinesia. The MRI studies have tended to show neuroanatomic abnormalities more consistently, particularly those involving the basal ganglia, in cases of tardive dyskinesia. The current evidence from the CT and MRI studies combined suggests that neuroanatomic abnormalities are frequently associated with tardive dyskinesia. However, because of several confounding factors, no characteristic neuroanatomic picture of tardive dyskinesia can be derived from the available studies.

CT Studies of Tardive Dyskinesia

The vast range of abnormal findings revealed by CT includes cortical atrophy (Albus et al., 1985; Gimenez-Roldan, Mateo, & Bartolomy, 1985; Cooper et al., 1991; McClelland et al., 1991), increased ventricular brain ratios (Owens et al., 1985; Waddington et al., 1985; Johnstone et al., 1989; McClelland et al., 1991), decreased ventricular brain ratios (Gold et al., 1991), increased ventricular indices (Famuyiwa et al., 1979), increased third-ventricle widths (Bartels & Themelis, 1983; Johnstone et al., 1989), and caudate atrophy (Bartels & Themelis, 1983).

Sandyk et al. (1990) conducted a CT study of 129 chronically institutionalized schizophrenic patients (56 males, 73 females) with a mean age of 47 years. Forty-eight patients met the Research Diagnostic Criteria (RDC)

Table 16.1. CT studies of tardive dyskinesia (TD), 1976–91

Study	TD patients (n)	Controls (n)	Method of TD diagnosis	Mean age (years)	Psychiatric diagnosis	Method of psychiatric diagnosis	Neuroleptic status	CT method	Association with TD	p	Post hoc statistical power	Finding	Notes
Gelenberg (1976)	8	None	AIMG $\geq$ 2	Age range 17–56	Schizophrenia	Not specified	Not specified	Inspection	No caudate atrophy; nonsignificant mild cortical atrophy in 1 patient	NS	—	Negative	
Famuyiwa et al. (1979)	15	30	Clinical	49	Schizophrenia	Feighner	On	Manual	Huckman's number VIR/cella media index	NS NS	No	Positive	a
									↑ % abnormal ventricular index	<0.05			
Jeste et al. (1980a)	12 (females only)	12 (females only)	AIMG $\geq$ 3	70	Mixed (mainly schizophrenia)	Not specified	Mixed	Manual	BF-BC/VIR/Huckman's number	NS	No	Negative	b
								Manual planimetry	VBR	NS			
Jeste et al. (1980b)	6 (males only)	6 (males only)	AIMG $\geq$ 3	<50	Schizophrenia	Not specified	Not specified	Manual	BF-BC/VIR/Huckman's number	NS	—	Negative	
								Manual planimetry	VBR	NS			
Jeste et al. (1982)	17 (females only)	17 (females only)	AIMG $\geq$ 3	72	Schizophrenia	RDC (chart)	On	Manual	BF-BC	NS	No	Negative	c
								Manual planimetry	VBR	NS			
Brainin et al. (1983)	15		AIMS	45	?Mixed	Not specified	On	Manual	VIR/VWR	NS	—	Negative	
Bartels & Themelis (1983)	29	29	AIMS	66	Schizophrenia	ICD9 (chart)	Not specified	Computer assisted	↑ Intracaudate distance	<0.05	Yes	Positive	d
								Computer assisted	↑ Third-ventricle width	<0.05			
								Computer assisted	↑ Caudate atrophy	<0.05			
								Computer assisted	Ventricular index	NS			
								Computer assisted	Cella media index	NS			

(continued)

209

Table 16.1. *Continued*

Study	TD patients (n)	Controls (n)	Method of TD diagnosis	Mean age (years)	Psychiatric diagnosis	Method of psychiatric diagnosis	Neuroleptic status	CT method	Association with TD	p	Post hoc statistical power	Finding	Notes
Albus et al. (1985)	17 (males only)	10 (males only)	SADS > 1	48	Schizophrenia	DSM-III (interview)	On	Computer assisted / Computer assisted / Computer assisted / Computer assisted	Third-ventricle width / VBR / Anterior-horn width / Huckman's criteria for cortical atrophy	NS / NS / NS / <0.01	Yes	Positive	e
Gimenez-Roldan et al. (1985)	7	None	AIMS ≥ 4	62	Not specified	Not specified	On	Inspection	Moderate-to-severe degrees of diffuse atrophy in 5 patients (71%)	—	—	Positive	f
Owens et al. (1985)	136 patients (not designated as TD or non-TD)		AIMS/RDS	56	Schizophrenia	Feighner (interview)	Not specified	Computer assisted	↑ VBR	Sig.	Yes	Positive	g
Waddington et al. (1985)	4	12	S&K AIMS ≥ 2	44	Schizophrenia	Feighner (chart)	On	Manual planimetry	↑ VBR	<0.05	No	Positive	
Kolakowska et al. (1986)	12	26	AIMS ≥ 2	34	Schizophrenia	RDC (interview)	On	Semiautomated	VBR > mean ± 1 SD of the matched control group, defined as "large"	NS	—	Negative	h
Kaufman et al. (1986)	32	57	AIMS ≥ 2	46	Schizophrenia	RDC (interview)	Mixed	Manual planimetry / Manual planimetry	VBR / BF-BC	NS / NS	No	Negative	i
Hoffman et al. (1986)	28 patients (not designated as TD or non-TD)		S&K	63	Schizophrenia	DSM-III (interview)	On	Computer assisted	VBR	NS	No	Negative	
Hoffman et al. (1987)	19 patients (not designated as TD or non-TD)		S&K	62	Schizophrenia	DSM-III (interview)	On	Computer assisted	Third-ventricle width	NS	No	Negative	
Sorokin et al. (1988)	11 (males only)	16 (males only)	AIMS	40	Schizophrenia	DSM-III (interview)	Mixed	Computer assisted	VBR	NS	No	Negative	j
Swayze et al. (1988)	18	27	S&K AIMS	35	Schizophrenia	DSM-III (interview)	On	Manual planimetry / Manual planimetry	VBR / Frontal-horn VBR	NS / NS	No	Negative	k

Study	n	TD scale	n	Diagnosis	Criteria	Medication	Method	Finding	Significance	Power	Result
Johnstone et al. (1989)	127 patients (not designated as TD or non-TD)	AIMS/RDS	56	Schizophrenia	Feighner (interview)	Not specified	Computer assisted	↑ VBR / Frontal-horn VBR / Third-ventricle area	0.05 / 0.05 / 0.05	Yes	Positive
Barr et al. (1989)	17	S&K	24	Schizophrenia	DSM-III (interview)	Mixed	Computer assisted	VBR	NS	—	Negative
Gold et al. (1991)	25	Retrospective using S&K	27	Schizophrenia	DSM-III (interview)	Mixed	Manual planimetry / Manual planimetry	↓ lateral ventricles / ↓ VBR	<0.03 / Sig.	—	"Negative" [l]
Hoffman et al. (1991b)	19 patients (not designated as TD or non-TD)	AIMS S&K	64	Schizophrenia	DSM-III (interview)	On	Computer assisted	No significant change in VBR or volume index at follow-up	NS	—	Negative [m]
Cooper et al. (1991)	42	AIMS	37	Schizophrenia	DSM-III	NA	NA	VBR / ↑ Cortical atrophy	NS / Sig.	—	Positive [n]
McClelland et al. (1991)	12 (females only)	Only facial dyskinesia assessed	11 (females only)	Mixed (15 with schizophrenia)	DSM-III (chart)	Mixed	Computer assisted	↑ VBR / ↑ Frontal atrophy	Sig. / Sig.	—	Positive [o]
Sandyk & Kay (1991)	22	S&K	6	Schizophrenia	DSM-III (interview)	On	Computer assisted	VBR	NS	—	Negative [p]

Notes: *n*, number of subjects having had CT scan; NA, not available; NS, nonsignificant; sig., significant; VBR, ventricular brain ratio; VIR, ventricular index ratio; VWR, ventricular waist ratio; BF-BC, bifrontal bicaudate ratio; AIMS, Abnormal Involuntary Movement Scale; AIMG, AIMS global; S&K, Schooler and Kane criteria for TD; SADS, Simpson and Angus dyskinesia scale (1970); RDS, Rockland dyskinesia scale (1979). Post hoc statistical power (with alpha set to 0.05) as calculated by Hoffman and Casy (1990): "Yes" indicates power ≥0.8; "No" indicates power <0.8. Feighner = Feighner Criteria; RDC = Research Diagnostic Criteria; ICD9 = ICD9 Criteria; DSM-III = DSM-III Criteria.

[a] 45 of 50 patients (17 TD, 33 controls) were scanned. TD correlated with markedly low paired-associated learning. Patients over 60 years old were excluded.

[b] TD group had long-standing history of severe TD.

[c] CT indices of TD patients were compared with reference values from normal populations.

[d] Patients had moderate to severe TD.

[e] 27 of 36 patients (21 TD, 15 controls) were scanned. Cortical atrophy using Huckman's criteria for sulci enlargement significantly correlated with TD severity.

[f] 7 of 13 severe TD patients had either CT scan (n = 4) or pneumoencephalogram (n = 3).

[g] VBR measurements were also conducted for 51 nonschizophrenic patients not reported here. Linear relationship between increased VBR and TD.

[h] 38 of 91 subjects (23 TD, 68 controls) were scanned.

[i] 89 of 111 subjects (41 TD, 70 controls) were scanned. TD patients with plasma dopamine-β-hydroxylase (DBH) activity below mean level had significantly larger ventricles than non-TD patients with low DBH activity.

[j] 27 of 40 subjects were scanned.

[k] 45 of 49 subjects were scanned. S&K criteria for probable TD met for 9 TD patients.

[l] Although differences in CT variables between TD and control patients were significant, the study finding is "negative" in the sense that TD patients had smaller lateral ventricles and VBR indices than controls.

[m] Patients reexamined with CT after 2–4 years of follow-up. Different CT scan instruments were used initially and at follow-up, but they had comparable image resolution. Patients over 55 included.

[n] TD and control patients did not differ in age, gender, length of illness, or duration of treatment. TD group had more negative symptoms, cognitive impairments, and poorer prognoses.

[o] Global facial dyskinesia was assessed on a five-point scale. For the under-65 group (n = 9), mean age was 57; for the over-65 group (n = 14), mean age was 77.

[p] TD and non-TD patients showed no differences in neuroradiological measures of prefrontal cortical atrophy or parieto-occipital atrophy.

Table 16.2. *MRI studies of tardive dyskinesia (TD), 1987–92*

Studies	TD patients (n)	Psychiatric controls (n)	Normal controls (n)	Method of TD diagnosis	Mean age (years)	Psychiatric diagnosis	Method of psychiatric diagnosis	Neuroleptic status	MRI method	Findings	p	Notes
Besson et al. (1987)	15	6	15	AIMS	36	Schizophrenia	DSM-III	On	Computer-assisted T_1 measurements	TD and non-TD patients had increased basal-ganglia T_1 measures compared with controls	Sig.	Non-TD patients had significantly higher RBG and LBG T_1 measures than TD patients; MRI scans performed using and 0.08-T magnet.
										Increased ventricular dilatation in TD patients	NS	
Heinz et al. (1988)	7	0	0	AIMS	51	Schizophrenia, except for 1 patient with degenerative dementia	Not specified	Not specified	Inspection	Abnormal findings in 5 of 7 patients, but no consistent abnormalities	—	Small sample size; all patients had moderately severe TD; age range 24–77; MRI scans conducted on a 1.5-T magnet
Bartzokis et al. (1990)	9 (males only)	5 (males only)	0	AIMS S&K	36	Schizophrenia	DSM-III (interview)	On, except for 1 patient	Computer-assisted T_2 measurements	TD patients had shortened T_2 in LCN, LGP, and RGP	Sig.	Patients with less than 3 months of neuroleptic exposure (n = 4) had significant LCN T_2 variability; MRI scans conducted on a 1.5-T magnet
										TD patients had shortened T_2 in RCN	Approached significance	
Williamson et al. (1991)	14	10	0	ESRS	37	Schizophrenia	SCID	On	Computer-assisted T_1 and T_2 measurements	TD patients showed no differences from non-TD patients in T_1 or T_2 values in either right or left lentiform nucleus	NS	MRI scans conducted on a 1.5-T magnet
Mion et al. (1991)	16	16	16	S&K AIMS	32	Schizophrenia	DSM-III	On	Computer-assisted volumetric measurements	TD patients had smaller caudate-nucleus volumes than non-TD patients and controls	Sig.	Young study sample with age range 19–48; MRI scans conducted on a 1.5-T magnet

212

Study						Diagnosis	Diagnostic criteria	Medication	Measurement	Findings	Sig.	Comments
Harvey et al. (1991)	8	34	35	AIMS ≥ 2	31	Schizophrenia	RDC (chart)	3 patients were off medication	Computer-assisted T_1 measurements	No group differences in basal-ganglia T_1 values	NS	Within-patients T_1 values not related to TD; MRI scans conducted on a 0.5-T magnet
Bartzokis et al. (1991)	20 (males only)	20 (males only)	0	S&K AIMS	NA	Schizophrenia	DSM-III	?On	Computer-assisted T_2 values	Caudate T_2 values in non-TD patients > probable TD patients > persistent TD patients	Sig.	Probable TD patients ($n = 8$); persistent TD patients ($n = 12$); caudate T_2 values: average of left and right; MRI scans conducted on a 1.5-T magnet
Elkashef et al. (1991)	8	16	0	AIMS	NA	Schizophrenia	NA	?On	Computer-assisted volumetric measurements	TD patients had smaller right-putamen volumes than non-TD patients	Sig.	Similar trends for reduced volumes in TD patients observed for left putamen, globus pallidus, body of caudate nucleus; significant age difference between TD and non-TD patients
Nasrallah et al. (1992)	12	88	0	AIMS ≥ 2	33	Schizophrenia	DSM-III-R SCID-R (interview)	On	Computer-assisted volumetric measurements	No group differences in MRI brain measures (cerebral volume, lateral ventricular and third-ventricle volumes)	NS	MRI scans conducted on a 1.5-T magnet

Notes: n, number of subjects having had MRI scan; NA, not available; NS, nonsignificant; Sig., significant; RBG, right basal ganglia; LBG, left basal ganglia; LCN left caudate nucleus; RCN, right caudate nucleus; LGP, left globus pallidus; RGP, right globus pallidus; AIMS, Abnormal Involuntary Movement Scale; S&K, Schooler and Kane criteria for TD; ESRS, Extrapyramidal Symptom Rating Scale; DSM-III, DSM-III criteria; SCID, Structured Clinical Interview for DSM-III; RDC, Research Diagnostic Criteria; DSM-III-R, DSM-III revised criteria; SCID-R, Structured Clinical Interview for DSM-III-R.

(Schooler & Kane, 1982) for persistent tardive dyskinesia. The groups with and without tardive dyskinesia were comparable for age, gender, duration of illness, current neuroleptic dosage, and cumulative length of neuroleptic exposure. Pineal-gland calcification was found in 51% of patients ($n = 66$) and was positively correlated with the presence of tardive dyskinesia.

In a comprehensive review of 18 CT studies of patients with tardive dyskinesia published between 1976 and 1989, Hoffman and Casey (1991) noted that the 4 studies with adequate post hoc statistical power (Bartels & Themelis, 1983; Albus et al., 1985; Owens et al., 1985; Johnstone et al., 1989) reported significant abnormal findings (Table 16.1).

MRI Studies of Tardive Dyskinesia

MRI is a sensitive and noninvasive brain-imaging technique that has the following advantages: It does not produce any ionizing radiation; imaging of the brain can be accomplished in multiple planes, thereby allowing for three-dimensional reconstruction of brain regions; it produces excellent grey–white resolution; and it is not affected by bone artifacts. Because of its superior spatial resolution and anatomic resolution, MRI allows better visualization and measurement of basal-ganglia structures than does CT (Coffman & Nasrallah, 1986).

The limitations of MRI, as compared with CT, are its higher cost and longer scanning time. Those factors, as well as the more widespread availability of CT, are largely responsible for the predominance of CT for examination of tardive dyskinesia patients (Andreasen et al., 1989). Other factors that limit the use of MRI include the need to control the patient's dyskinetic movements and the potential for claustrophobic reactions during the MRI procedure (Andreasen et al., 1989). Our own experience in using MRI to examine tardive dyskinesia patients has shown that those claustrophobic reactions can be avoided through careful patient preparation and regular use of a short-acting benzodiazepine, such as 2 mg of lorazepam given sublingually approximately 30 minutes prior to the examination.

Differences in MRI tissue relaxation times (T_1 and T_2) reflect changes in the immediate environment of the protons and can provide biochemical information (Crooks, 1981). As mentioned earlier, a shortened T_2 in the extrapyramidal system is believed to reflect increased deposits of paramagnetic ferric iron (Drayer et al., 1986; Bartzokis et al., 1990).

The MRI findings in tardive dyskinesia patients have included shortened basal-ganglia T_1 values (Bessen et al., 1987), shortened basal-ganglia T_2 values (Bartzokis et al., 1990, 1991), reduced caudate-nucleus volumes

(Mion et al., 1991), reduced right-putamen volumes (Elkashef et al., 1991), and increased T_2 signals in the pons and medial temporal lobe (Heinz et al., 1988). Other studies have not shown significant differences between patients with and without tardive dyskinesia (Harvey et al., 1991; Williamson et al., 1991; Nasrallah et al., 1992).

Besson et al. (1987) conducted a study comparing 21 patients with schizophrenia and 15 normal controls. Of the 21 patients, 15 had tardive dyskinesia. The tardive dyskinesia patients had significantly shortened right- and left-basal-ganglia T_1 values, as compared with patients without tardive dyskinesia and with the normal controls.

Heinz et al. (1988) conducted a clinical morphological study of 7 long-term inpatients with moderately severe tardive dyskinesia between the ages of 24 and 77 years. Qualitative analysis revealed heterogeneous abnormalities in 5 of the 7 patients. Those findings included: marked cerebral atrophy, moderate-to-severe ventricular dilation, increased focal T_2 signal from the pons, and increased T_2 signal from the medial temporal lobe.

Bartzokis et al. (1990) studied 18 male patients with schizophrenia, 14 of whom each had a cumulative exposure to neuroleptics of more than 1 year, and 4 of whom each had less than 3 months of exposure. Nine of the group of 14 patients had tardive dyskinesia, showing significant T_2 shortening in the left caudate nucleus and in the left and right globus pallidus, as well as T_2 shortening that approached significance in the right caudate nucleus. The group of 4 patients, however, demonstrated significant variability in T_2 values for the left caudate nucleus.

Williamson et al. (1991) compared 14 schizophrenic patients with tardive dyskinesia and 10 diagnostically matched controls. The tardive dyskinesia patients showed no differences from the controls with regard to T_1 or T_2 values in either the right or left lentiform nucleus.

Mion et al. (1991) conducted a study involving three groups of subjects: 16 schizophrenic patients with tardive dyskinesia, 16 schizophrenic patients without tardive dyskinesia, and 16 normal control subjects. The tardive dyskinesia patients had smaller caudate-nucleus volumes than did either the patients without tardive dyskinesia or the controls.

Harvey et al. (1991) conducted a study of 42 patients with schizophrenia and 35 normal control subjects. Scans from 8 patients with tardive dyskinesia and 34 patients without tardive dyskinesia showed no group differences in basal-ganglia T_1 values.

Bartzokis et al. (1991) examined a total of 40 male schizophrenic patients, 20 of whom had tardive dyskinesia. Averaged caudate T_2 values in patients with persistent tardive dyskinesia were significantly shorter than were values in patients with probable tardive dyskinesia and those without tardive dyskinesia.

Elkashef et al. (1991) studied 8 schizophrenic patients with tardive dyskinesia and 16 diagnostically matched patients without tardive dyskinesia. The tardive dyskinesia patients had significantly reduced right-putamen volumes, as compared with the patients without tardive dyskinesia. Similar trends for reduced volumes in tardive dyskinesia patients were observed for the left putamen, the globus pallidus, and the body of the caudate nucleus.

Nasrallah et al. (1992) studied 100 schizophrenic patients, 12 of whom had tardive dyskinesia. No group differences were observed in cerebral volumes, lateral ventricular volumes, or third-ventricle volumes.

Confounding Factors

The potential confounding factors in brain-imaging studies of patients with tardive dyskinesia are numerous and have been addressed elsewhere (Krishnan, Ellinwood, & Rayasam, 1988; Hoffman & Casey, 1991). These factors, which are outlined next, will require greater scrutiny in future studies.

Patient Population and Control Groups

Most CT and MRI studies of patients with tardive dyskinesia have used psychiatric control groups matched for age, gender, and psychiatric diagnosis. Three of the nine MRI studies reviewed in Table 16.2 (Besson et al., 1987; Harvey et al., 1991; Mion et al., 1991) each employed an age- and gender-matched normal control group. None of the CT studies reviewed in Table 16.1, however, used a normal control group.

Whereas the mean age for subjects in the CT studies varied considerably, the subjects in the MRI studies tended to be younger, and the mean-age groups more homogeneous. A number of variables have not been adequately addressed: duration of illness, number and duration of hospitalizations, and matching of groups with and without tardive dyskinesia according to other variables such as education level, duration of neuroleptic treatment, current mean neuroleptic dosage, and height and weight. Nevertheless, some improvements in study designs have been made, particularly in MRI studies.

Method of Diagnosis

It is well known that both the presence and severity of tardive dyskinesia can fluctuate during the course of a depot neuroleptic injection cycle. In general, the studies reviewed did not specify a particular assessment time for the patients on depot neuroleptics. Although patients frequently are examined just prior to the next depot neuroleptic injection, tardive dyskinesia ratings can also be assessed at midpoint in the neuroleptic injection cycle, that is, when neuroleptic concentrations in plasma reach maximum stability. A potential risk with the latter method, however, is that tardive dyskinesia will go unrecognized because of a neuroleptic-masking effect of the neuroleptics.

The increased use of standardized rating scales for involuntary movements has significantly improved the reliability of tardive dyskinesia diagnoses. Although the Schooler and Kane (1982) RDC for tardive dyskinesia are frequently used, studies have employed various diagnostic criteria for tardive dyskinesia and thresholds of tardive dyskinesia severity.

Statistical Power

Statistical power has been a neglected consideration in brain-imaging studies of tardive dyskinesia. In a thorough assessment of this issue, Hoffman and Casey (1991) calculated post hoc statistical powers for 18 CT studies published between 1976 and 1989. They found that the post hoc power for most of those studies was low, except for four studies (Bartels & Themelis, 1983; Albus et al., 1985; Owens et al., 1985; Johnstone et al., 1989) in which the statistical power was adequate (Table 16.1).

Duration and Persistence of Tardive Dyskinesia

The duration and stability of tardive dyskinesia over time can vary considerably. Distinguishing between patients with persistent forms of tardive dyskinesia and those with fluctuating or withdrawal-emergent tardive dyskinesia is important, inasmuch as their pathophysiology and neuroanatomic pictures can differ. In an MRI study (Bartzokis et al., 1991) that distinguished subjects according to the presence of probable tardive dyskinesia, persistent tardive dyskinesia, or no tardive dyskinesia, patients with persistent tardive dyskinesia were found to have shorter T_2 values than patients with probable tardive dyskinesia. That finding supports the possibility that subtle structural brain alterations in tardive dyskinesia patients will vary according to the persistence and duration of the condition.

Type and Severity of Tardive Dyskinesia

In the CT and MRI studies of tardive dyskinesia, the analyses have rarely considered the severity and specific subtype of tardive dyskinesia (e.g., whether it is part of the buccofaciolingual syndrome, a peripheral or limb tardive dyskinesia, tardive dystonia, tardive akathisia, or a mixed form of tardive dyskinesia).

Effects of Medication

Although several of the CT and MRI studies reviewed here did not specify neuroleptic-medication status, the majority of the patients in those studies were on neuroleptics. In some cases, the groups included both neuroleptic-treated patients and untreated patients.

Although it is well known that neuroleptics can suppress tardive dyskinesia and that their withdrawal can unmask preexisting tardive dyskinesia, neuroleptics may also contribute to progressive structural brain changes that precede the onset of tardive dyskinesia. That there are differences in MRI T_2 values in the basal ganglia in patients with probable tardive dyskinesia, persistent tardive dyskinesia, and no tardive dyskinesia is consistent with that possibility. The number of years of neuroleptic exposure and the current neuroleptic dosage are two important variables to consider when matching patients without tardive dyskinesia, as well as those with probable or persistent tardive dyskinesia. Hoffman et al. (1991a) addressed this issue and reported that neuroleptic treatment obscured the correlation between tardive dyskinesia and ventricular brain ratio.

Antiparkinsonian anticholinergic agents are often said to exacerbate tardive dyskinesia, although they can be of benefit in certain tardive dyskinesia subtypes, such as tardive dystonia (Jeste et al., 1988). Given that antiparkinsonian anticholinergic medication has not been controlled for in most CT and MRI studies of tardive dyskinesia, one might wonder if concurrent use of those agents with neuroleptics could be interfering with associations between tardive dyskinesia and structural abnormalities. Three CT studies have reported effects of drug-induced parkinsonism on brain structure, with a positive correlation observed between drug-induced parkinsonism and ventricular brain ratio in schizophrenic patients (Hoffman, Labs, & Casey, 1986, 1987; Hoffman et al., 1991b).

Effect of Psychiatric Diagnosis

The vast majority of patients in the CT and MRI studies of tardive dyskinesia have had schizophrenia. The use of structured clinical interviews has greatly increased the reliability of psychiatric diagnoses in those studies.

Because patients with bipolar disorder are believed to be at increased risk for tardive dyskinesia (Kane & Smith, 1982; Yassa, Ghadirian, & Schwartz,

1983; Casey, 1991), the use of controlled brain-imaging studies of tardive dyskinesia in such patients might increase our understanding of the specificity of the neuroanatomic substrate of tardive dyskinesia.

Measurement Methods to Assess Neuroanatomic Changes

Differences in the scanning and measurement methods used in CT and MRI studies constitute another important source of variance. In MRI studies, the strength of the magnets used has varied from 0.08 to 1.5 tesla. In CT and MRI studies, the types and numbers of slices have differed markedly, as have the various morphometric assessment methods, which have included planimetric and semiautomated computer-based techniques (Ashtari et al., 1990). In addition, there has been considerable heterogeneity in the methods used to derive volume estimates for specific brain regions.

What is the Specificity of Recent Brain-Imaging Findings in Tardive Dyskinesia?

The characteristic neuroanatomic picture of tardive dyskinesia has become blurred by the increasing evidence from MRI studies of basal-ganglia abnormalities associated with schizophrenia and affective disorder. These findings include significant enlargement of the putamen and lesser enlargement of the caudate nucleus in male schizophrenic patients (Swayze et al., 1992), increased volume of the lenticular nucleus in schizophrenic patients (Jernigan et al., 1991), caudate atrophy in depressed patients (Krishnan et al., 1992), and bilateral caudate reduction in schizophrenic patients with marked negative symptoms (Young et al., 1991). In addition, at least one CT study has reported a decreased ventricular brain ratio and smaller lateral ventricles in schizophrenic patients with tardive dyskinesia (Gold et al., 1991).

Conclusion

Although we have not yet reached a clear understanding of the neuroanatomic substrate of tardive dyskinesia, the current evidence from CT and MRI studies indicates that structural brain abnormalities occur in a significant proportion of patients with tardive dyskinesia. In particular, the MRI studies of tardive dyskinesia patients have more frequently revealed abnormalities, particularly involving the basal ganglia, than have CT studies. This observation is consistent with the superior image resolution of MRI.

In addition to the many confounding factors already reviewed, it is important to consider the possibility that tardive dyskinesia represents a group of heterogeneous conditions that differ in terms of clinical manifestations, treatment responses, pathophysiology, and neuroanatomy.

Future controlled MRI brain-imaging studies should prospectively examine the neuroanatomic picture for schizophrenic patients recently started on neuroleptics. Repeated scanning of these patients at specified intervals could reveal progressive alterations, such as changes in T_2 values in the basal ganglia. Perhaps these changes could serve as potential clinical predictors for the occurrence of tardive dyskinesia. The issue of the specificity of MRI findings in nonschizophrenic patients with tardive dyskinesia requires further study as well.

Acknowledgment

This work was supported by a Career Development Award and by research grant 920852 from the Fonds de la Recherche en Santé du Québec (FRSQ).

References

Albus, M., Naber, D., Muller-Spahn, F., Douillet, P., Reinertshofer, T., & Ackenheil, M. (1985). Tardive dyskinesia: relation to computer-tomographic, endocrine, and psychopathological variables. *Bio. Psychiatry* 20:1082.

Andreasen, N. C., Ehrhardt, J., Yuh, W., Swayze, V., Ziebell, S., & Cohen, G. (1989). Magnetic resonance imaging in schizophrenia: an update. In *Schizophrenia: Scientific Progress*, ed. S. C. Schulz & C. A. Tamminga, pp. 207–15. Oxford University Press.

Arai, N., Amano, N., Iseki, E., Yokoi, S., Saito, A., Takekawa, Y., & Misugi, K. (1987). Tardive dyskinesia with inflated neurons of the cerebellar dentate nucleus. *Acta Neuropathol.* 73:38–42.

Ashtari, M., Zito, J. L., Gold, B. I., Lieberman, J. A., Borenstein, M. T., & Herman, P. G. (1990). Computerized volume measurement of brain structure. *Invest. Radiol.* 25:798–805.

Barr, W. B., Mukherjee, S., Degreef, G., & Corracci, G. (1989). Anomalous dominance and persistent tardive dyskinesia. *Biol. Psychiatry* 25:826–34.

Bartels, M., & Themelis, J. (1983). Computerized tomography in tardive dyskinesia. Evidence of structural abnormalities in the basal ganglia system. *Arch. Psychiatry Neurol. Sci.* 233:371–9.

Bartzokis, G., Garber, H. J., Marder, S. R., & Oldendorf, W. H. (1990). MRI in tardive dyskinesia. Shortened left caudate T_2. *Biol. Psychiatry* 28:1027–36.

Bartzokis, G., Marder, S. R., Oldendorf, W. H., Chang, F., & Mintz, J. (1991). Tardive dyskinesia: MRI implicates brain iron in hypothesized damage from oxydative processes. Presented at the Third International Congress on Schizophrenia Research, Tucson, Arizona.

Bergen, J. A., Eyland, E. A., Campbell, J. A., Jenkings, P., Kellehear, K., Richards, A., & Beumont, P. J. V. (1989). The course of tardive dyskinesia in patients on long-term neuroleptics. *Br. J. Psychiatry* 154:523–8.

Besson, J. A. O., Corrigan, F. M., Cherryman, G. R., & Smith, F. W. (1987). Nuclear magnetic resonance brain imaging in chronic schizophrenia. *Br. J. Psychiatry* 150:161–3.

Brainin, M., Reisner, T., & Zeithofer, J. (1983). Tardive dyskinesia: clinical correlation with computed tomography in patients aged less than 60 years. *J. Neurol. Neurosurg. Psychiatry* 46:1037–40.

Cadet, J. L., Lohr, J. B., & Jeste, D. V. (1987). Tardive dyskinesia and schizophrenic burnout: the involvement of cytotoxic free radicals. In *Handbook of Schizophrenia. Vol. 2: Neurochemistry and Neuropharmacology of Schizophrenia*, ed. F. A. Henn & L. E. DeLisi, pp. 425–38. Amsterdam: Elsevier.

Campbell, W. G., Raskind, M. A., Gordon, T., & Shaw, C. M. (1985). Iron pigment in the brain of a man with tardive dyskinesia. *Psychiatry* 142:364–5.

Casey, D. E. (1987). Tardive dyskinesia. In *Psychopharmacology: The Third Generation of Progress*, ed. H. Y. Meltzer, pp. 1411–19. New York: Raven Press.

Casey, D. E. (1991). Neuroleptic drug-induced extrapyramidal syndromes and tardive dyskinesia. *Schizophrenia* 4:109–20.

Christensen, E., Moller, J. E., & Faurbye, A. (1970). Neuropathological investigation of 28 brains from patients with dyskinesia. *Acta Psychiatr. Scand.* 46:14–23.

Coffman, J. A., & Nasrallah, H. A. (1986). Magnetic resonance brain imaging in schizophrenia. In *Handbook of Schizophrenia, Vol. 1: The Neurology of Schizophrenia*, ed. H. A. Nasrallah & D. R. Weinberger, pp. 251–66. Amsterdam: Elsevier.

Cooper, S. J., Doherty, M. M., Foster, J., & Waddington, J. (1991). The relationship of involuntary movements to treatment variables, symptomatology and CT scan variables in chronic schizophrenia. *Biol. Psychiatry* 29:4085.

Crooks, L. E. (1981) Overview of NMR imaging techniques. In *Nuclear Magnetic Resonance in Medicine*, ed. L. Kaufman, L. E. Crooks, & A. R. Margulis, pp. 30–52. Tokyo: Igaku-Shoin.

Drayer, B. P. (1987). Magnetic resonance imaging and brain iron: implications in the diagnosis and pathochemistry of movement disorders and dementia. *Br. Neuroimaging Quarterly* 3:15–30.

Drayer, B. P., Burger, P., Darwin, R., Riederer, S., Herfkens, R., & Johnson, G. A. (1986). MRI of brain iron. *Roentgenology* 147:103–10.

Elkashef, A. M., Buchanan, R. W., Munson, R. C., & Breier, A. (1991). Basal ganglia pathology in schizophrenia and tardive dyskinesia: a quantitative magnetic resonance imaging study. Presented at the Third International Congress on Schizophrenia Research, Tucson, Arizona.

Famuyiwa, O. O., Eccleston, D., Donaldson, A. A., & Garside, R. F. (1979). Tardive dyskinesia and dementia. *Br. J. Psychiatry* 135:500–4.

Gelenberg, A. J. (1976). Computerized tomography in patients with tardive dyskinesia. *Am. J. Psychiatry* 133:578–9.

Gimenez-Roldan, S., Mateo, D., & Bartolomy, P. (1985). Tardive dystonia and severe tardive dyskinesia. A comparison of risk factors and prognosis. *Acta Psychiatr. Scand.* 71:488–94.

Gold, J. M., Egan, M. F., Kirch, D. G., Goldberg, T. E., Daniel, D. G., Bigelow, L. B., & Wyatt, R. J. (1991). Tardive dyskinesia: neuropsychological, computerized tomographic, and psychiatric symptom findings. *Biol. Psychiatry* 30:587–99.

Harvey, I., Ron, M. A., Murray, R., Lewis, S., Barker, G., & McManus, D.

(1991). MRI in schizophrenia: basal ganglia and white matter T_1 times. *Psychol. Med.* 21:587–98.

Heinz, R., Rayasam, K., Krishnan, K. R. R., Wingfield, M., Irigaray, P., & Ellinwood, E. H. (1988). MRI scans in patients with tardive dyskinesia. *Biol. Psychiatry* 24:852–7.

Hoffman, W. F., Ballard, L. C., Keepers, G. A., Hansen, T. E., & Casey, D. E. (1991a). Neuroleptics obscure the correlation of tardive dyskinesia and ventricular brain ratio. In *New Research Program and Abstracts, 144th APA Annual Meeting*, NR477, p. 162. Washington, DC: American Psychiatric Association.

Hoffman, W. F., Ballard, L., Turner, E. H., & Casey, D. E. (1991b). Three-year follow-up of older schizophrenics: extrapyramidal syndromes, psychiatric symptoms, and ventricular brain ratio. *Biol. Psychiatry* 30:913–26.

Hoffman, W. F., & Casey, D. E. (1991). Computed tomographic evaluation of patients with tardive dyskinesia. *Schizophr. Res.* 5:1–12.

Hoffman, W. F., Labs, S. M., & Casey, D. E. (1986). Drug-induced parkinsonism: relationship to brain atrophy in older schizophrenics. In *Proceedings of the Society of Biological Psychiatry*, 41st annual meeting, Washington DC, p. 184. New York: Elsevier.

Hoffman, W. F., Labs, S. M., & Casey, D. E. (1987). Neuroleptic-induced parkinsonism in older schizophrenics. *Biol. Psychiatry* 22:427–39.

Hunter, R., Blackwood, W., Smith, M. C., & Cummings, J. N. (1968). Neuropathological findings in three cases of persistent dyskinesia following phenothiazine medication. *J. Neurol. Sci.* 7:263–73.

Jernigan, T. L., Zisook, S., Heaton, R. K., Moranville, J. T., Hesselink, J. R., & Braff, D. L. (1991). Magnetic resonance imaging abnormalities in lenticular nuclei and cerebral cortex in schizophrenia. *Arch. Gen. Psychiatry* 48:881–90.

Jeste, D. V., Kleinman, J. E., Potkin, S. G., Luchins, D. J., & Weinberger, D. R. (1982). Ex uno multi: subtyping the schizophrenic syndrome. *Biol. Psychiatry* 17:199–222.

Jeste, D. V., Lohr, J. B., Clark, K., & Wyatt, R. J. (1988). Pharmacological treatments of tardive dyskinesia in the 1980s. *J. Clin. Psychopharmacol.* (*Suppl.*) 8:38–48.

Jeste, D. V., Lohr, J. B., Kaufmann, C. A., & Wyatt, R. J. (1986). Pathophysiology of tardive dyskinesia; evaluation of supersensitivity theory and alternative hypotheses. In *Tardive Dyskinesia and Neuroleptics: From Dogma to Reason*, ed. D. E. Casey & G. Gardos, pp. 15–32. Washington, DC: American Psychiatric Press.

Jeste, D. V., Wagner, R. L., Weinberger, D. R., Rieth, K. G., & Wyatt, R. J. (1980a). Evaluation of CT scans in tardive dyskinesia. *Am. J. Psychiatry* 137:247–8.

Jeste, D. V., Weinberger, D. R., Zalcman, S., & Wyatt, R. J. (1980b). Computed tomography in tardive dyskinesia. *Br. J. Psychiatry* 136:606–8.

Jeste, D. V., & Wyatt, R. J. (1982a). Therapeutic strategies against tardive dyskinesia: two decades of experience. *Arch. Gen. Psychiatry* 39:803–16.

Jeste, D. V., & Wyatt, R. J. (1982b). *Understanding and Treating Tardive Dyskinesia*. New York: Guilford Press.

Johnstone, E. C., Owens, D. G. C., Bydder, G. M., Colter, N., Crow, T. J., & Frith, C. D. (1989). The spectrum of structural brain changes in schizophrenia: age of onset as a predictor of cognitive and clinical impairments and their cerebral correlates. *Psychol. Med.* 19:91–103.

Kane, J. M., Jeste, D. V., Barnes, T. R. E., Casey, D. E., Cole, J. O., Davis, J. M., Gualtieri, C. T., Schooler, N. R., Sprague, R. L., & Wettstein, R. M. (1992). *Tardive Dyskinesia: A Task Force Report of the American Psychiatric Association.* Washington, DC: American Psychiatric Association.

Kane, J. M., & Smith, J. M. (1982). Tardive dyskinesia prevalence and risk factors. 1959 to 1979. *Arch. Gen. Psychiatry* 39:473–81.

Kane, J. M., Woerner, M., Lieberman, J., & Kinon, B. (1984). Tardive dyskinesia. In *Neuropsychiatric Movement Disorders,* ed. D. V. Jeste & R. J. Wyatt, pp. 97–118. Washington, DC: American Psychiatric Press.

Kaufmann, C. A., Jeste, D. V., Shelton, R. C., Linnoila, M., Kafka, M. S., & Wyatt, R. J. (1986). Noradrenergic and neuroradiological abnormalities in tardive dyskinesia. *Biol. Psychiatry* 21:799–812.

Kolakowska, T., Williams, A. O., Ardern, M., & Reveley, M. A. (1986). Tardive dyskinesia in schizophrenics under 60 years of age. *Biol. Psychiatry* 21:161–9.

Krishnan, K. R. R., Ellinwood, E. H., & Rayasam, K. (1988). Tardive dyskinesia: structural changes in the brain. In *Tardive Dyskinesia: Biological Mechanisms and Clinical Aspects,* ed. M. E. Wolf & A. D. Mosnaim, pp. 167–77. Washington, DC: American Psychiatric Press.

Krishnan, K. R. R., McDonald, W. M., Escalona, P. R., Doraiswamy, P. M., Na, C., Husain, M. M., Figiel, G. S., Boyko, O. B., Ellinwood, E. H., & Nemeroff, C. B. (1992). Magnetic resonance imaging of the caudate nuclei in depression. Preliminary observations. *Arch. Gen. Psychiatry* 49:553–7.

Lohr, J. B. (1991). Oxygen radicals and neuropsychiatric illness. *Arch. Gen. Psychiatry* 48:1097–106.

Lohr, J. B., Kuczenski, R., Bracha, H. S., Moir, M., & Jeste, D. V. (1990). Increased indices of free radical activity in the cerebrospinal fluid of patients with tardive dyskinesia. *Biol. Psychiatry* 28:535–9.

McClelland, H. A., Metcalfe, T. A., Kerr, T. A., Dutta, D., & Watson, P. (1991). Facial dyskinesia: a 16-year follow-up study. *Br. J. Psychiatry* 158:691–6.

Mion, C. C., Andreasen, N. C., Arndt, S., Swayze, V. W., II, & Cohen, G. A. (1991). MRI abnormalities in tardive dyskinesia. *Psychiatry Res.* 40:157–66.

Nasrallah, H. A., Bornstein, R. A., Olson, S. C., Schwarzkopf, S. B., & Jurjus, G. (1992). Neuropsychobiological correlates of tardive dyskinesia. In *New Research Program and Abstracts, 145th Annual Meeting of the American Psychiatric Association,* p. 163. Washington, DC: American Psychiatric Association.

Owens, D. C., Johnstone, E. C., Crow, T. J., Frith, C. D., Jagoe, J. R., & Kreel, L. (1985). Lateral ventricular size in schizophrenia: relationship to the disease process and its clinical manifestations. *Psychol. Med.* 15:27–41.

Rutledge, J. N., Hilal, S. K., Silver, A. J., Defendini, R., & Fahn, S. (1987). Study of movement disorders and brain iron by MR. *Am. J. Neuroradiol.* 8:397–411.

Sandyk, R. (1990a). Pineal calcification and subtypes of tardive dyskinesia. *Int. J. Neurosci.* 53:223–9.

Sandyk, R. (1990b). The relationship of pineal calcification to subtypes of tardive dyskinesia in bipolar patients. *Int. J. Neurosci.* 54:307–13.

Sandyk, R., Awerbuch, G. I., & Kay, S. R. (1990). Pineal gland calcification and tardive dyskinesia. *Lancet* 23:1528.

Sandyk, R., & Fischer, H. (1988). Serotonin in involuntary movement disorders. *Int. J. Neurosci.* 42:185–205.

Sandyk, R., & Kay, S. R. (1991). The relationship of tardive dyskinesia to positive schizophrenia. *Int. J. Neurosci.* 56:107–39.

Schooler, N. R., & Kane, J. M. (1982). Research diagnoses for tardive dyskinesia. *Arch. Gen. Psychiatry* 39:486–7.

Shriqui, C. L. (1988). Dyskinésie tardive: mise à jour. *Revue Canadienne de Psychiatrie* 33:637–44.

Shriqui, C. L., Bradwejn, J., & Jones, B. D. (1990). Tardive dyskinesia: legal and preventive aspects. *Can. J. Psychiatry* 35:576–80.

Shriqui, C. L., & Jones, B. D. (1990). Free radicals and tardive dyskinesia. *Can. J. Psychiatry* 35:282–3.

Simpson, G. M., & Angus, J. W. S. (1970). A rating scale for extrapyramidal side effects. *Acta Psychiatr. Scand. (Suppl.)* 212.

Sorokin, J. E., Giordani, B., Mohs, R. C., Losonczy, M. F., Davidson, M., Siever, L. J., Ryan, T. A., & Davis, K. L. (1988). Memory impairment in schizophrenic patients with tardive dyskinesia. *Biol. Psychiatry* 23:129–35.

Swayze, V. W., II, Andreasen, N. C., Alliger, R. J., Yuh, W. T. C., & Ehrhardt, J. C. (1992). Subcortical and temporal structures in affective disorder and schizophrenia: a magnetic resonance imaging study. *Biol. Psychiatry* 31:221–40.

Swayze, V. W., II, Yates, W. R., Andreasen, N. C., & Alliger, R. J. (1988). CT abnormalities in tardive dyskinesia. *Psychiatry Res.* 26:51–8.

Waddington, J. L., O'Boyle, K. M., Molloy, A. G., Youssef, H. A., King, D. J., & Cooper, S. J. (1985). Neurotransmitter receptors and ageing: dopamine/ neuroleptic receptors, involuntary movements and the disease process of schizophrenia. In *Therapeutics in the Elderly*, ed. K. O'Malley & J. L. Waddington. Amsterdam: Elsevier.

Williamson, P., Pelz, D., Merskey, H., Morrison, S., & Conlon, P. (1991). Correlation of negative symptoms in schizophrenia with frontal lobe parameters on magnetic resonance imaging. *Br. J. Psychiatry* 159:130–4.

Woerner, M. G., Kane, J. M., Lieberman, J. A., Alvir, J., Bergmann, K. L., Borenstein, M., Schooler, N. R., Mukherjee, S., Rotrosen, J., Rubinstein, M., & Basavaraju, N. (1991). The prevalence of tardive dyskinesia. *J. Clin. Psychopharmacol.* 11:34–42.

Yassa, R., Ghadirian, A. M., & Schwartz, G. (1983). Prevalence of tardive dyskinesia in affective disorder patients. *J. Clin. Psychiatry* 44:410–12.

Yassa, R., & Nair, N. P. V. (1992). A 10-year follow-up study of tardive dyskinesia. *Acta Psychiatr. Scand.* 86:262–6.

Yassa, R., Nastase, C., Dupont, D., & Thibeau, M. (1992). Tardive dyskinesia in the elderly psychiatric patients: a 5-year study. *Am. J. Psychiatry* 149:1206–11.

Young, A. H., Blackwood, D. H. R., Roxborough, H., McQueen, J. K., Martin, M. J., & Kean, D. (1991). A magnetic resonance imaging study of schizophrenia: brain structure and clinical symptoms. *Br. J. Psychiatry* 158:158–64.

17

Rodent and Other Animal Models of Tardive Dyskinesia During Long-Term Neuroleptic-Drug Administration: Controversies and Implications for the Clinical Syndrome

JOHN L. WADDINGTON, Ph.D.

The prominence of tardive dyskinesia in some patients, juxtaposed against the difficulty of developing a valid (i.e., behaviorally homologous and pharmacologically isomorphic) animal model for this clinical syndrome, provides one of today's greater contradictions in neuroleptic psychopharmacology. It should be emphasized that conceptually, seeking such models for tardive dyskinesia – in terms of late-onset, usually orofacial, movements that emerge during very long term treatment with neuroleptic drugs – differs greatly from seeking to clarify the consequences of that treatment at the level of dopaminergic neurotransmission. In the latter situation, any relationship to tardive dyskinesia is indirect. Indeed, the well-established changes in neuronal function, such as striatal dopamine-receptor sensitivity, have been widely reported to occur in the absence of spontaneous behaviors akin to those of the clinical disorder whose putative pathophysiology is supposedly reproduced (Waddington, 1989, 1990).

The rodent studies of the 1980s – the first decade during which the attempt to find behavioral homology, as opposed to purported pathophysiology, was examined – have been reviewed elsewhere (Waddington, 1990). Among 21 relevant studies of orofacial function in rats administered neuroleptic drugs for substantial proportions of their adult lives, many showed late-onset oral movements, although no such effects (or sometimes even a very early onset of such movements) were apparent in others. To some extent, the phenomenology, pharmacologic characteristics, and pathophysiology of these late-onset movements paralleled clinical tardive dyskinesia, although a careful consideration of the methodological factors did not resolve the apparent inconsistencies (Waddington, 1990). The purpose of this chapter is to consider the more recent studies in this field and to clarify the extent to which they complement or contradict the notion that tardive dyskinesia can be validly modeled in rodents. Although the findings in studies of nonhuman primates (e.g.,

225

McKinney et al., 1980; Gunne, Häggström, & Sjöquist, 1984; Domino, 1985; Crossman, 1987; Lifshitz et al., 1991) are not a primary focus of this chapter, they will, on occasion, be considered.

Phenomenology

To varying extents, the findings in recent studies conform with proposed criteria for homologous/isomorphic animal models of tardive dyskinesia (Jeste & Wyatt, 1982; Waddington, 1990). In one study, when rats were given haloperidol orally via their drinking water, the spontaneous chewing movements, tongue protrusions, and buccal twitching that were seen after approximately 40 days endured for a total of 51 days of treatment (Kolenik, Hoffman, & Bowers, 1989). In a second study, 10 weeks after fluphenazine decanoate injections were begun at 3–4 week intervals, vacuous chewing and jaw tremors were observed; at 21–24 weeks of treatment, an anticholinergic challenge reduced, but did not abolish, the continuing excessive mouth movements in the depot neuroleptic group (Stoessl, Dourish, & Iversen, 1989). Similarly, in a third study, after 2–3 months of monthly injections of haloperidol decanoate, an excess of vacuous chewing movements was induced, which continued over 18 months of treatment (Johansson, 1990).

In another set of studies, haloperidol, when given to rats via a combination of drinking water and/or osmotic minipump, failed to influence either the observed oral movements or computer-scored oral movements in a restraining-tube test during 1 month of treatment although oral movements were observed at 1 month in an open cage. As for withdrawal, an excess of oral movements was observed in the tube test only immediately after withdrawal from an 8-month regimen or haloperidol treatment; with clozapine, oral movements were generally depressed; with raclopride, on the other hand, late-onset movements were induced, but only of very small amplitude, and they declined following drug withdrawal. In terms of the energy spectra of computer-scored oral "movelets," haloperidol was reported to induce increases at low frequencies (1–2 Hz) after 7 months of treatment and after subsequent withdrawal, whereas clozapine and raclopride tended to reduce movements at all frequencies (See & Ellison, 1990a). Such haloperidol-induced oral movements were weakly attenuated by an acute anticholinergic challenge (See & Chapman, 1991).

In still another set of studies, after administration of haloperidol to rats via drinking water, vacuous chewing was observed to be maximally induced by 8–12 weeks. That chewing continued at that level to 24 weeks of treatment, during which time an anticholinergic challenge reduced but did not abolish the movements, although they gradually remitted during the subsequent 2 weeks of withdrawal. At 24 weeks, 41% of haloperidol-treated rats manifested vigorous oral movements, 22% displayed mild or modest movements, and 38% failed to show any such movements (Tamminga et al., 1990). Similarly, twice-daily injections of haloperidol induced an excess of chewing episodes by days 21–28 of treatment, movements that persisted for at least 3 days following cessation of such injections (Diana et al., 1992). However, in complete contradiction, daily injections of haloperidol were also reported to induce an excess of jaw movements at 50–60 minutes following the *first* injection, which did not increase over nine subsequent daily injections thereafter and were reduced by co-injection of an anticholinergic (Steinpreis, Baskin, & Salamone, 1993).

Clearly, the cited studies showed some degree of consistency, in that the majority indicated the induction of various forms of spontaneous, late-onset orofacial movement(s) during continuous, long-term treatment with typical neuroleptic drugs, movements that could not be abolished with anticholinergics and that showed at least some measure of persistence following drug withdrawal. Although such findings conform to varying extents with proposed criteria for homologous/isomorphic animal models of tardive dyskinesia (Jeste & Wyatt, 1982; Waddington, 1990), we continue to see reports of apparently similar orofacial movements emerging very early in the course of neuroleptic treatment, and in a manner sensitive to attenuation by anticholinergics. That such findings are substantially inconsistent with those same criteria, showing a profile of phenomena more akin to acute extrapyramidal reactions such as parkinsonism and dystonia (Waddington, 1992), constitutes a major, enduring conundrum in the field (Rupniak, Jenner, & Marsden, 1986; Waddington & Molloy, 1987, Waddington, 1990). The question, then, is what underlies these reactions at the methodological and/or pathophysiological level.

Methods

A careful review of the initial rodent studies in the field has failed to isolate any specific procedural variations(s) that might account for their fundamental differences (Waddington, 1990). However, over the past few years, certain methodological factors have been shown to influence the sometimes diverse outcomes.

Continuous Versus Intermittent Paradigms

In a series of studies (Glenthøj & Hemmingsen, 1989; Glenthøj et al., 1990; Glenthøj, Bolwig, & Hemmingsen, 1991), investigators reported that continuity of administration of neuroleptic drugs appears to influence the prominence and persistence of orofacial movements in rodents. Whereas vacuous chewing and tongue protrusions were observed both in open cages and in restraining tubes early during the course of treatment with haloperidol via drinking water, those movements became more prominent during subsequent long-term treatment as well as more persistent following drug withdrawal after 15 weeks for animals that had received the drug on a discontinuous basis (i.e., 2 days out of 7 each week), as compared with a continuous basis. Those findings were interpreted in terms of sensitization/kindling phenomena and tended to be less evident in animals that were treated similarly with zuclopenthixol.

Using a different, though related, approach, See and Ellison (1990b) analyzed both observed oral movements and computer-scored oral movelets in animals receiving haloperidol (for 28 days or 8 months) on either an intermittent basis (one weekly injection) or a continuous basis (via drinking water and/or osmotic minipump). The two treatment paradigms resulted in distinct, though complex, profiles of effect over time. Those authors interpreted the continuous treatment as resulting in late-onset oral movements that had peak energy at 1–3 Hz and increased on drug withdrawal; they associated intermittent treatment with the emergence of large-amplitude oral movelets that had peak energy at 4–7 Hz. The former pattern was likened to tardive dyskinesia on the basis of time course and energy spectrum; in several reports have indicated that the clinical syndrome shows maximum energy in the 1–3-Hz band (Ellison & See, 1989). Conversely, the latter pattern was likened to the phenomenon of "primed dystonia," evident in nonhuman primates challenged intermittently with neuroleptics (Waddington, 1992).

Those same authors (See & Ellison, 1990b) have identified a third pattern of late-onset, withdrawal-enhanced oral movelets of very small amplitude that can be induced by both continuous and discontinuous treatment regimens; they regard that third pattern as distinct from either of the other two oral syndromes. Because that third pattern matches those authors' previous putative rodent model for tardive dyskinesia (Ellison et al., 1987), their changing perspective attests to the difficulty of interpreting increasingly complex, computer-derived data concerning oral movements. However, those authors are surely correct to emphasize (Waddington, 1990; Ellison, 1991) the dangers of interpreting "oral movements" as a homogeneous syndrome, as well as the capacity of continuous and discontinuous neuroleptic regimens in rats to induce different sets of effects. This has been noted previously for nonhuman primates and has been speculated on clinically (Waddington, 1989, 1992).

Strain Differences

Although a review of the previous literature has not shown the choice of a particular strain of rat to be a major factor in causing the differences between studies (Waddington, 1990), a systematic comparison of rat strains is needed to clarify this important issue.

Tamminga et al. (1990) reported that during 19 weeks of continuous halo-peridol administration via drinking water, late-onset vacuous chewing movements emerged in Sprague-Dawley, Long-Evans, and Wistar rats, although both baseline and haloperidol-associated degrees of oral movements were considerably higher in Long-Evans rats than in the other two strains. Sprague-Dawley rats tended to show the least variability in such movements and the greatest neuroleptic/control ratio for such movements, together with a somewhat slower rate of decline after neuroleptic withdrawal. Furthermore, the overall effect of an anticholinergic challenge to partially attenuate those movements appeared to vary according to the particular rat strains used.

These data suggest that vulnerability to such effects of long-term administration of neuroleptic drugs can be subject to genetic regulation. However, it remains to be determined if such regulation may have its basis in pharmacodynamic or pharmacokinetic processes. The extent to which genetic factors may influence vulnerability to tardive dyskinesia in the clinic remains controversial (Waddington, 1989; Chapter 5, this volume).

Psychosocial Environment

The roles of environmental factors in the emergence of orofacial movements during neuroleptic treatment in animals have yet to be investigated. However, Glenthøj and Hemmingsen (1991) have reported that rats subjected to the stress of uncontrollable loud noise show more spontaneous vacuous chewing movements than do control animals. Because there is evidence that the baseline degree of oral movement can be a determinant of the extent to which long-term neuroleptic treatment will increase such movements (Waddington, 1990, 1991), the psychosocial environment in which such rodent studies are conducted may help shape the outcome.

Pathophysiology

The Hypothesis of Dopamine-Receptor Supersensitivity

The longevity of the general hypothesis of dopamine-receptor supersensitivity as the cause of tardive dyskinesia contrasts sharply with the paucity of its direct supporting evidence. Indeed, only the clinical pharmacologic profile of tardive dyskinesia (attenuation by typical dopamine antagonists, exacerbation by conventional doses of dopamine agonists) is consistent with the hypothesis, and such indirect evidence may merely mean that dopaminergic activity is an important regulator of motor function, rather than a major pathophysiological factor in this movement disorder. Conversely, more direct examination of dopamine-receptor (D_1 and D_2) status, whether in postmortem brains from patients with movement disorders or in living patients examined by positron-emission tomography, has failed to indicate any excess dopamine-receptor supersensitivity in those with dyskinesia. In addition, the periodic coexistence of tardive orofacial dyskinesia and peripheral parkinsonism (classically a dopaminergic hypofunction disorder) makes the hypothesis more dubious (Gerlach & Casey, 1988; Waddington, 1989, 1992). In the animal arena, it seems well established that dopamine-receptor supersensitivity, evident in terms of both radioligand binding and behavioral responsivity to dopamine agonists, is readily induced after 1–2 weeks of neuroleptic treatment in the absence of any excess of spontaneous oral movements. Furthermore, when such oral movements have emerged during considerably longer periods of neuroleptic treatment, they have not shown the characteristics of dopaminergic hyperfunction phenomena (Waddington, 1990).

Greater tolerance to an increase in the dopamine metabolite homovanillic acid after an acute haloperidol injection has been reported in rats with, as opposed to those without, oral movements following 51 days of haloperidol administration via drinking water (Kolenik et al., 1989). That finding would be consistent with greater postsynaptic striatal dopamine-receptor supersensitivity in those animals with oral movements, leading to greater feedback inhibition of presynaptic dopamine release and/or greater depolarization inactivation. But what might be the net change in overall dopaminergic function in the face of such a putative juxtaposition of increased postsynaptic dopamine-receptor supersensitivity and reduced presynaptic dopamine release? Recently, Fields et al. (1991) reported that up-regulation of dopamine ("D_2-like") receptors after several procedures was associated with decreasing capacity for dopamine biosynthesis in rat striatum. They argued that such a compensatory mechanism might account for an initial absence of spontaneous behavioral signs of dopamine-receptor supersensitivity, but that if overtaxed during very long term neuroleptic treatment, it might fail and give rise to such phenomena subsequently. These notions clearly require further investigation.

The Hypothesis of D_1-Like-Receptor Involvement

A recent variant of the general dopaminergic hypothesis of hyperfunction/receptor supersensitivity holds that heightened (absolute or relative) activity through D_1-like receptors underlies tardive dyskinesia. That proposition had its origins in the ability of acute D_1-agonist challenges, but not D_2-agonist challenges, to induce oral movements/dyskinesia, particularly when D_2 receptors are concurrently blocked, and to exacerbate such movements in animals previously treated on a long-term basis with typical neuroleptics and/or selective D_1 and D_2 antagonists. Such data have been reported for both rodents and nonhuman primates (Rosengarten et al., 1988; Waddington, 1990; Gerlach, Hansen, & Peacock, 1991).

In rats treated for 1 month with haloperidol, vacuous chewing was inhibited by the selective D_1 antagonist SCH 23390; it was also suppressed both by acute challenge with haloperidol and by the dopamine-synthesis inhibitor α-methyl-p-tyrosine (AMPT). In AMPT-treated animals, vacuous chewing was reinstated by administering the selective D_1 agonist SKF 38393 (Diana et al., 1992). Those data would be consistent with the proposition that such oral movements have their basis in dopamine acting preferentially on D_1 receptors; they are complemented by evidence from higher species that basal-ganglia D_1 receptors are involved in mediating orofacial dyskinesia (Spooren, Piosik, & Cools, 1991).

However, whereas some authors have reported SCH 23390 to similarly suppress vacuous chewing that emerged during several months of treatment with fluphenazine decanoate in rats (Stoessl et al., 1989), others have noted such movements to be suppressed by the selective D_2 antagonist raclopride. In the acute situation, D_2 antagonists can enhance the action of D_1 agonists to induce oral movements, an activity that may involve D_2 interactions with a subtype of D_1-like receptor (Waddington et al., 1989; Daly & Waddington, 1993). Furthermore, there is recent evident that 8 months of treatment with haloperidol decanoate can reduce the density of rat striatal D_1 receptors (Laruelle et al., 1992) and that depletion of dopamine in the ventrolateral striatum with 6-hydroxydopamine can induce vacuous chewing that can be increased by an acute challenge with haloperidol (Jicha & Salamone, 1991). It is still unclear, however, how either the general formulation or any particular variant of the hypothesis of dopaminergic hyperfunction/receptor supersensitivity causing tardive dyskinesia can accommodate such complexities.

Nondopaminergic Mechanisms

There is increasing agreement that the search for the pathophysiology of tardive dyskinesia should not be confined to dopaminergic systems. The most prominent alternative hypothesis focuses on putative hypofunction in γ-aminobutyric acid (GABA) neurons (Gerlach & Casey, 1988; Waddington, 1989). Evidence to support the GABA-dysfunction hypothesis from previous rodent studies has been inconclusive (Waddington, 1990), although Kaneda et al. (1992) recently reported that coadministration of the GABAergic agent progabide attenuated the development of oral movements over 12 months of treatment with haloperidol. In nonhuman primates, the GABA hypothesis has been elaborated to encompass excitatory interactions of amino acids, GABA, and neuropeptides in the emergence of the syndrome (Johansson, et al., 1990; Mitchell et al., 1992; Gunne & Andren, 1993).

Physiological studies indicate that oral movements may be regulated by an extrastriatal, central pattern generator, with the final topography of such movements being controlled by two relatively independent but associated co-systems (Van Willigen et al., 1986; Zhang & Sasamoto, 1990). It has been argued that tardive dyskinesia constitutes an inappropriate and over-elaborated manifestation of such innate, fundamental motor patterns. Indeed, long-term treatment with neuroleptic drugs might progressively disrupt the function of that generator and/or any associated co-system(s) via their effects on basic cellular functions (Waddington, 1989, 1990). There are preliminary rodent data suggesting that such central dysfunction might at least in part be expressed via peripheral cholecystokinin/vagal mechanisms (Stoessl & Polanski, 1993).

Cerebral Dysfunction and Aging

Evidence from previous rodent studies has indicated that cortical lesions increase the baseline degree of oral movements, thereby heightening the effects of long-term neuroleptic treatment, and the baseline degree of such movements also increases with aging (Waddington, 1990, 1991). The most recent studies have indicated a specific role for the frontal cortex, rather than global cortical/subcortical damage (Johansson, 1990), and they have reported such an age effect both in rodents (Kaneda et al., 1992) and in primates (Rupniak et al., 1990). On the basis of these and related data, it has been argued that long-term neuroleptic treatment is more likely to induce oral movements in animals in which (frontal) cortical function has already been compromised; such treatment may not so much induce orofacial movements as precipitate or hasten a syndrome that can occur spontaneously with cerebral dysfunction and/or aging or senescence (Waddington, 1990; Chapter 5, this volume).

Neuropathology

Evidence that neuroleptic drugs disrupt a variety of basic cellular functions continues to emerge. Although many of the acute effects of this type are evident only at relatively high dosages, lower dosages of these drugs may cause significant disruption of such processes in a progressive manner if continued for very long terms (Waddington, 1989, 1990).

Previous studies of putative effects at the morphologic/neuropathologic level have proved contentious (Waddington, 1989; Jeste, Lohr, & Manley, 1992). However, recent studies have reevaluated the ultrastructural changes seen with electron microscopy (Vincent et al., 1991; Kerns et al., 1992; Meshul et al., 1992; See, Chapman, & Meshul, 1992) and the neuropathologic changes seen with light microscopy (Jeste et al., 1992) in striatal and extrastriatal regions, including frontal cortex, following various long-term neuroleptic treatments. The remaining issues include the extent to which such changes may be morphologic correlates of dopamine-receptor supersensitivity, or else may indicate "neurotoxic" effects, and the varying treatment periods and their continuities in relation to whether haloperidol and clozapine do or do not produce comparable profiles of effects in striatal and frontal cortical regions.

Conclusion

Since my previous reviews of these issues (Waddington, 1989, 1990), the majority of new studies have shown one or more late-onset orofacial movement syndrome(s) that emerge either during or after withdrawal from long-term neuroleptic treatment. However, paradoxical instances of apparently indistinguishable oral movements emerging very early in the course of such treatment continue to be reported periodically and require explanation. The pharmacologic profiles of these late-onset phenomena indicate partial sensitivity to attenuation by anticholinergics, and they should not be overlooked when adjudicating the extent of parallelism with the presumed profile of clinical tardive dyskinesia. Conversely, apparent differences between typical neuroleptics and new, atypical antipsychotics, and between continuous and discontinuous treatment paradigms, cannot yet be fully interpreted. More substantial clinical data are needed.

In relation to pathophysiology, variants of the hypothesis of dopaminergic hyperfunction continue to hold center stage. Direct evidence to support them, however, remains insubstantial. A new generation of morphologic/neuropathologic studies holds out the prospect of important information to help clarify these issues. It is essential to continue and to refine rodent studies in this area, alongside those in nonhuman primates, but to do so in a manner that will take fully into account the most recent information on, and changing perspectives of, the clinical syndrome for which an animal model is rightly sought, but which has yet to be validated.

Acknowledgment

The author's studies are supported by the Royal College of Surgeons in Ireland.

References

Crossman, A. R. (1987). Primate models of dyskinesia: the experimental approach to the study of basal ganglia-related involuntary movement disorders. *Neuroscience* 21:1–40.

Daly, S. A., & Waddington, J. L. (1993). Behavioural evidence for "D-1-like" dopamine receptor subtypes in rat brain using the new isochroman agonist A 68930 and isoquinoline antagonist BW 737C. *Psychopharmacology* 113:45–50.

Diana, M., Collu, M., Mura, A., & Gessa, G. L. (1992). Haloperidol-induced vacuous chewing in rats: suppression by α-methyl-tyrosine. *Eur. J. Pharmacol.* 211:415–19.

Domino, E. F. (1985). Induction of tardive dyskinesia in *Cebus apella* and *Macaca speciosa* monkeys: a review. In *Dyskinesia: Research and Treatment*, ed. D. E. Casey, T. N. Chase, A. V. Christensen, & J. Gerlach, pp. 217–23. Berlin: Springer-Verlag.

Ellison, G. (1991). Spontaneous orofacial movements in rodents induced by long-term neuroleptic administration: a second opinion. *Psychopharmacology* 104:404–8.

Ellison, G., & See, R. E. (1989). Rats administered chronic neuroleptics develop oral movements which are similar in form to those in humans with tardive dyskinesia. *Psychopharmacology* 98:564–6.

Ellison, G., See, R., Levin, E., & Kinney, J. (1987). Tremorous mouth movements in rats administered chronic neuroleptics. *Psychopharmacology* 92:122–6.

Fields, J. Z., Drucker, G. E., Wichlinski, L., & Gordon, J. H. (1991). Neurochemical basis for the absence of overt "stereotyped" behaviors in rats with up-regulated striatal D_2 dopamine receptors. *Clin. Neuropharmacol.* 14:199–208.

Gerlach, J., & Casey, D. E. (1988). Tardive dyskinesia. *Acta Psychiatr. Scand.* 77:369–78.

Gerlach, J., Hansen, L., & Peacock, L. (1991). D_1 dopamine hypothesis in tardive dyskinesia. In *Biological Psychiatry*, vol. 1, ed. G. Racagni, N. Brunello, & T. Fukuda, pp. 609–11. Amsterdam: Elsevier.

Glenthøj, B., Bolwig, T. G., & Hemmingsen, R. (1991). Continuous vs discontinuous neuroleptic treatment in an animal model of tardive dyskinesia. In *Biological Psychiatry*, vol. 1, ed. G. Racagni, N. Brunello, & T. Fukuda, pp. 602–4. Amsterdam: Elsevier.

Glenthøj, B., & Hemmingsen, R. (1989). Intermittent neuroleptic treatment induces long-lasting abnormal mouthing in the rat. *Eur. J. Pharmacol.* 164:393–6.

Glenthøj, B., & Hemmingsen, R. (1991). Development of vacuous chewing movements in rats: role of housing environment. *Life Sci.* 48:2137–40.

Glenthøj, B., Hemmingsen, R., Allerup, P., & Bolwig, T. G. (1990). Intermittent versus continuous neuroleptic treatment in a rat model. *Eur. J. Pharmacol.* 190:275–86.

Gunne, L. M., & Andren, P. E. (1993). An animal model for coexisting tardive dyskinesia and tardive parkinsonism: a glutamate hypothesis for tardive dyskinesia. *Clin. Neuropharmacol.* 16:90–5.

Gunn, L. M., Häggström, J. E., & Sjöquist, B. (1984). Association with persistent neuroleptic-induced dyskinesia of regional changes in brain GABA synthesis. *Nature* 309:347–9.

Jeste, D. V., Lohr, J. B., & Manley, M. (1992). Study of neuropathologic changes in the striatum following 4, 8 and 12 months of treatment with fluphenazine in rats. *Psychopharmacology* 106:154–60.

Jeste, D. V., & Wyatt, R. J. (1982). *Understanding and Treating Tardive Dyskinesia*. New York: Guilford Press.

Jicha, G. A., & Salamone, J. D. (1991). Vacuous jaw movements and feeding deficits in rats with ventrolateral striatal dopamine depletion: possible relation to parkinsonian symptoms. *J. Neurosci.* 11:3822–9.

Johansson, P. (1990). Methylazoxymethanol (MAM)-induced brain lesion and oral dyskinesia in rats. *Psychopharmacology* 100:72–6.

Johansson, P. E., Terenus, L., Häggström, J. E., & Gunne, L. (1990). Neuropeptide changes in a primate model (*Cebus apella*) for tardive dyskinesia. *Neuroscience* 37:563–7.

Kaneda, H., Shirakawa, O., Dale, J., Goodman, L., Bachus, S. E., & Tamminga, C. A. (1992). Co-administration of progabide inhibits haloperidol-induced oral dyskinesias in rats. *Eur. J. Pharmacol.* 212:43–9.

Kerns, J. M., Sierens, D. K., Kao, L. C., Klawans, H. L., & Carvey, P. M. (1992). Synaptic plasticity in the rat striatum following chronic haloperidol treatment. *Clin. Neuropharmacol.* 15:488–500.

Kolenik, S. A., Hoffman, F. J., & Bowers, M. B. (1989). Regional homovanillic acid levels and oral movements in rats following chronic haloperidol treatment. *Psychopharmacology* 98:430–1.

Laruelle, M., Jaskiw, G. E., Lipska, B. K., Kolachana, B., Casanova, M. F., Kleinman, J. E., & Weinberger, D. R. (1992). D_1 and D_2 receptor modulation in rat striatum and nucleus accumbens after subchronic and chronic haloperidol treatment. *Brain Res.* 575:47–56.

Lifshitz, K., O'Keeffe, R. T., Lee, K. K., Linn, G. S., Mase, D., Avery, J., Lo,

E. S., & Cooper, T. B. (1991). Effect of extended depot fluphenazine treatment and withdrawal on social and other behaviors of Cebus apella monkeys. Psychopharmacology 105:492–500.

McKinney, W. T., Moran, E. C., Kraemer, G. W., & Prange, A. J. (1980). Long-term chlorpromazine in rhesus monkeys: production of dyskinesias and changes in social behavior. Psychopharmacology 72:35–9.

Meshul, C. K., Janowsky, A., Casey, D. E., Stallbaumer, R. K., & Taylor, B. (1992). Effect of haloperidol and clozapine on the density of "perforated" synapses in caudate, nucleus accumbens, and medial prefrontal cortex. Psychopharmacology 106:45–52.

Mitchell, I. J., Crossman, A. R., Liminga, U., Andren, P., & Gunne, L. M. (1992). Regional changes in 2-deoxyglucose uptake associated with neuroleptic-induced tardive dyskinesia in the Cebus monkey. Mov. Disord. 7:32–7.

Rosengarten, H., Schweitzer, J. W., Egawa, M., & Friedhoff, A. J. (1988). Diminished D-2 dopamine receptor function and the emergence of repetitive jaw movements. In Central D-1 Dopamine Receptors, ed. M. Goldstein, K. Fuxe, & I. Tabachnick, pp. 159–67. New York: Plenum.

Rupniak, N. M. J., Jenner, P., & Marsden, C. D. (1986). Acute dystonia induced by neuroleptic drugs. Psychopharmacology 88:403–19.

Rupniak, N. M., Tye, S. J., Steventon, M. J., Boyce, S., & Iversen, S. D. (1990). Spontaneous orofacial dyskinesias in a captive cynomolgus monkey: implications for tardive dyskinesia. Mov. Disord. 5:314–18.

See, R. E., & Chapman, M. A. (1991). Cholinergic modulation of oral activity in drug-naive and chronic haloperidol-treated rats. Pharmacol. Biochem. Behav. 39:49–54.

See, R. E., Chapman, M. A., & Meshul, C. K. (1992). Comparison of chronic intermittent haloperidol and raclopride effects on striatal dopamine release and synaptic ultrastructure in rats. Synapse 12:147–54.

See, R. E., & Ellison, G. (1990a). Comparison of chronic administration of haloperidol and the atypical neuroleptics, clozapine and raclopride, in an animal model of tardive dyskinesia. Eur. J. Pharmacol. 181:175–86.

See, R. E., & Ellison, G. (1990b). Intermittent and continuous haloperidol regimens produce different types of oral dyskinesias in rats. Psychopharmacology 100:404–12.

Spooren, W. P. J. M., Piosik, P. A., & Cools, A. R. (1991). Dopamine D₁ receptors in the subcommissural part of the globus pallidus and their role in orofacial dyskinesia in cats. Eur. J. Pharmacol. 204:217–22.

Steinpreis, R. E., Baskin, P., & Salamone, J. D. (1993). Vacuous jaw movements induced by sub-chronic administration of haloperidol: interactions with scopolamine. Psychopharmacology 111:99–105.

Stoessl, A. J., Dourish, C. T., & Iversen, S. D. (1989). Chronic neuroleptic-induced mouth movements in the rat: suppression by CCK and selective dopamine D₁ and D₂ receptor antagonists. Psychopharmacology 98:372–9.

Stoessl, A. J., & Polanski, E. (1993). Neuroleptic-induced chewing movements in the rat are suppressed by peripherally but not centrally administered CCK and abolished by bilateral subdiaphragmatic vagotomy. Neuropharmacology 32:555–60.

Tamminga, C. A., Dale, J. M., Goodman, L., Kaneda, H., & Kaneda, N. (1990). Neuroleptic-induced vacuous chewing movements as an animal model of tardive dyskinesia: a study in three rat strains. Psychopharmacology 102:474–8.

Van Willigen, J. D., Jüch, P. J. W., Ballintijn, C. M., & Broekhuijsen, M. L. (1986). A hierarchy of neural control of mastication in the rat. *Neuroscience* 19:447–55.

Vincent, S. L., McSparren, J., Wang, R. Y., & Benes, F. M. (1991). Evidence for ultrastructural changes in cortical axodendritic synapses following long-term treatment with haloperidol or clozapine. *Neuropsychopharmacology* 5:147–55.

Waddington, J. L. (1989). Schizophrenia, affective psychoses and other disorders treated with neuroleptic drugs: the enigma of tardive dyskinesia, its neurobiological determinants, and the "conflict of paradigms." *Int. Rev. Neurobiol.* 31:297–353.

Waddington, J. L. (1990). Spontaneous orofacial movements induced in rodents by very long-term neuroleptic drug administration: phenomenology, pathophysiology and putative relationship to tardive dyskinesia. *Psychopharmacology* 101:431–47.

Waddington, J. L. (1991). Ageing and other determinants of baseline levels of spontaneous orofacial movements in rodents during long-term neuroleptic treatment. In *Biological Psychiatry*, vol. 1, ed. G. Racagni, N. Brunello, & T. Fukuda, pp. 612–14. Amsterdam: Elsevier.

Waddington, J. L. (1992). Mechanisms of neuroleptic-induced extrapyramidal side effects. In *Adverse Effects of Psychotropic Drugs*, ed. J. M. Kane & J. A. Lieberman, pp. 246–65. New York: Guilford Press.

Waddington, J. L., & Molloy, A. G. (1987). The status of late-onset vacuous chewing/perioral movements during long-term neuroleptic treatment in rodents: tardive dyskinesia or dystonia? *Psychopharmacology* 91:136–7.

Waddington, J. L., Murray, A. M., O'Callaghan, E., & Larkin, C. (1989). Orofacial dyskinesia: D-1/D-2 dopamine receptors in rodents, and familial/obstetric correlates of tardive dyskinesia in schizophrenia. In *Neural Mechanisms in Disorders of Movement*, ed. A. R. Crossman & M. A. Sambrook, pp. 359–66. London: Libbey.

Zhang, G., & Sasamoto, K. (1990). Projections of two separate cortical areas for rhythmical jaw movements in the rat. *Brain Res. Bull.* 24:221–30.

Part IV

Measurement of Tardive Dyskinesia

18

Instrument Measurements
of Tardive Dyskinesia

MICHAEL P. CALIGIURI, Ph.D.

The importance of a careful assessment of a patient with tardive dyskinesia cannot be overrated. Assessment of both the intensity and frequency of the disordered movements is necessary for a diagnosis of tardive dyskinesia. Measuring the severity of movements is important for documenting the course of the movement disorder and for evaluating the response to treatment, and sometimes even for prognosis. In fact, many clinical and medicolegal decisions are based solely on the findings in a thorough assessment. Unfortunately, reliable assessment of the severity of tardive dyskinesia presents a challenge. Gardos, Cole, and LaBrie (1977) noted that the absence of reliable, precise methods for assessment may be contributing to our inability to delineate the syndrome, to determine its prevalence, and to evaluate the efficacy of treatments; but the ability to monitor the severity and course of tardive dyskinesia is critical to our understanding and management of this disorder. A better understanding of the pathophysiology and pharmacology of tardive dyskinesia inevitably will depend on precise assessment of the distribution and variations of dyskinetic movements.

The earliest objective measurement for tremor was described in the literature more than 100 years ago (Peterson, 1889). Subsequent decades of research have produced several objective instrumentation approaches for assessment of parkinsonism (Evarts et al., 1979; Teravainen & Calne, 1980; Marsden & Schachter, 1981). Temporal and kinematic measurement of movements, measurements of frequency-domain spectral characteristics, and measurements of torque are now widely accepted approaches for assessment of bradykinesia, tremor, and rigidity, respectively. Similar attempts to achieve objective assessments of dyskinesia are relatively recent, having originated in the 1970s (Jus, Jus, & Villeneuve, 1973), when tardive dyskinesia was first beginning to be recognized as a significant clinical problem (Crane, 1973).

Since that time, the use of quantitative procedures for measuring tardive dyskinesia has received increasing attention (Lohr & Caligiuri, 1992).

Instruments for assessment have been designed to enhance our understanding of tardive dyskinesia and to facilitate our ability to prevent and treat it. Thus far, use of the instruments for quantification of dyskinesia (in fact, the instruments for quantification of all movement disorders) has been confined to the laboratory. Recently, however, the idea of objective clinical assessment of tardive dyskinesia has been gaining wider support, largely because of the problems associated with multi-item rating scales. The ready availability and ease of application of these subjective rating scales have increased their use as standard tools for assessing the severity of tardive dyskinesia. Nevertheless, their insensitivity, vulnerability to examiner bias, and inability to address the pathophysiological issues of tardive dyskinesia have tended to obscure their advantages.

This chapter seeks to outline the attributes of an instrumentation approach to assessment, to describe the technology and clinical applications of selected electromechanical procedures, and to offer a critical review of the literature dealing with electromechanical instruments for assessment. The literature review emphasizes pharmacologic studies because of their particular relevance to the management of tardive dyskinesia. The chapter concludes with recommendations for establishing a laboratory with instruments that can provide quantitative assessments of patients with tardive dyskinesia.

Attributes of Instrument Assessment Systems
Several attributes distinguish the use of an instrumentation approach from the use of traditional rating scales. These include the capability to provide linear measurements of the movements being studied, with sensitivity to subclinical abnormalities and selectivity to dyskinetic phenomena. In addition, many instrumentation approaches have high degrees of correlation with clinical assessment scales. These attributes are next discussed individually.

Linearity
Instrumentation systems are usually designed to measure movement abnormalities in terms of a continuous variable on an interval scale. In contrast, multi-item ordinal scales such as the Abnormal Involuntary Movement Scale (AIMS) (Guy, 1976) or the Rockland Tardive Dyskinesia Rating Scale (Simpson et al., 1979) categorize such movements on the basis of degrees of severity. Instrumentation systems are designed to yield linear measurements

of severity, that is, measurements in which the outcome variable is directly proportional to the input. For example, whereas an AIMS rating of 2 does not represent dyskinesia that is twice as severe as that represented by an AIMS score of 1, a score of 4 with an instrument quantification will be equivalent to twice 2, that is, once it is determined that the system gives linear measurements. Also, observer ratings produce ordinal or categorical data, whereas most instrumentation procedures yield continuous data.

Sensitivity

Instrument assessments can reveal subtle motor abnormalities below the threshold of detection that is possible during a clinical evaluation. This aspect of instrument quantification allows for potential determination of *subclinical* motor phenomena (May, Lee, & Bacon, 1983). In fact, several studies conducted in our laboratory involving neuroleptic-treated patients have demonstrated that electromechanical transduction of movements is sensitive to mild, subclinical motor abnormalities resembling dyskinesia. In a study of 28 neuroleptic-treated patients, 15 of whom did not have AIMS-based dyskinesia, we used fast Fourier analyses of lingual instability to reveal, in 4 patients, elevated spectral amplitudes within the tardive dyskinesia range (Caligiuri, Jeste, & Harris, 1989). Using the same analysis procedures for hand-force control, we found that whereas the mean spectral amplitude for 24 patients without tardive dyskinesia was significantly lower than the mean amplitude for 17 tardive dyskinesia patients, 21% of the patients without tardive dyskinesia had amplitudes greater than two standard deviations above the mean for normal control subjects (Caligiuri & Lohr, 1990). In still another study, we found that older patients without tardive dyskinesia exhibited greater hand-force instability than did younger patients without tardive dyskinesia or older neuroleptic-free controls (Caligiuri, Lohr, & Jeste, 1991b). Those findings suggest that advanced age and neuroleptic exposure together contribute to greater motor instability than would be expected from either advanced age or neuroleptic exposure alone.

The suggestion that instrument measurements of motor phenomena such as force instability can be sensitive to subclinical tardive dyskinesia will remain tenuous without prospective longitudinal studies. Such a study is currently under way and preliminary findings have been reported (Harris et al., 1992). Harris and associates, using instrument measurements to examine baseline motor function, followed 68 recently medicated patients (total lifetime exposure less than 1 month) for at least 6 months to study the incidence of tardive dyskinesia. They identified abnormal hand-force instability as a risk factor for predicting the presence of tardive dyskinesia within 6 months of neuroleptic exposure, having found that patients who developed tardive dyskinesia had a greater mean hand-force instability at baseline than did patients who did not develop tardive dyskinesia. That ongoing study suggests that electromechanical measurements of motor instability can provide useful information concerning the status of the motor system and its vulnerability to tardive dyskinesia, especially in older patients.

Selectivity

The appearance of other tardive syndromes in neuroleptic-treated patients raises an interesting question regarding assessment. As with tardive dyskinesia, akathisia and parkinsonism can have delayed onsets in some patients. These phenomena share a number of features associated with involuntary movements. In patients with tardive dyskinesia, the involuntary movements are random and seemingly purposeless. In akathisia, in contrast, the movements appear to be voluntary responses to subjective distress (Munetz & Cornes, 1983; Adler et al., 1989). Several investigators have noted the coexistence of signs and symptoms of akathisia and tardive dyskinesia (Chouinard, Annable, & Ross-Chouinard, 1982; Barnes & Braude, 1985) and parkinsonism and tardive dyskinesia (Jankovic & Casabona, 1987; Caligiuri et al., 1991a). As Barnes and Braude observed, in cases of coexisting akathisia and tardive dyskinesia, the problems of assessing the two are confounded by the absence of precise phenomenological descriptions for distinguishing one from the other. Clearly, comprehensive assessments of tardive dyskinesia and related disorders using multiple and parallel measurement procedures will be necessary for the development of precise phenomenology.

A careful differential diagnosis of dyskinesia in the presence of other drug-induced extrapyramidal side effects, such as tremor and akathisia, requires sensitive assessment procedures as well. Clinically, determining the simultaneous presence of different types of motor disorders in the same body region can often prove difficult. Nonetheless, although it is difficult to determine the simultaneous presence of tremor and tardive dyskinesia in the same body region, some instrument techniques are able to differentiate the two (Wirshing et al., 1989; Caligiuri et al., 1991a). Alpert, Diamond, and Friedhoff (1976), for instance, used spectral analyses to distinguish involuntary movements associated with tardive dyskinesia from those associated with parkinsonism. They located the concentration of spectral energy for hand movements in patients with tardive dyskinesia within the 0–3-Hz frequency range, whereas patients with parkinsonian tremors showed relatively little energy within that range. A number of instrument studies have confirmed the finding that dyskinesia is confined to frequencies less than 3 Hz (Bartzokis et al., 1989; Caligiuri et al., 1989; Wirshing et al., 1989; Caligiuri & Lohr, 1990). Electromyography (EMG) is another means used to differentiate between tardive dyskinesia and tremor. Normally, when an agonist muscle is active during voluntary movement, the antagonist is quiet. This reciprocal pattern of muscle activity, which is preserved in patients with parkinsonian tremor, is not seen with the involuntary movements of tardive dyskinesia patients (Hallett, 1983; Bathien, Koutlidis, & Rondot, 1984). This finding not only provides a means of differentiating between dyskinesia and parkinsonian tremor but also allows determination of the relative contributions of dyskinesia and tremor should both be present.

Concurrent Validity

Chien et al. (1977), in studying 9 tardive dyskinesia patients, compared the findings from five clinical rating scales with those from accelerometer measurements of buccolingual dyskinesia. They placed an accelerometer in a rubber bulb, which was then inserted into the patient's mouth. Involuntary movements produced pressure changes within the mouth that in turn affected the accelerometer. They reported that the accelerometer measurements were significantly correlated with AIMS scores ($r = .87$). They also reported that the accelerometer data were more closely related to actual movement counts ($r = .99$) than to subjective impressions of dyskinesia. Tryon and Pologe (1987), who used accelerometry to study 10 patients with tardive dyskinesia and 8 schizophrenic control patients without tardive dyskinesia, noted increased dyskinetic movements and more graph "spikes" (peak acceleration beyond 4 standard deviations from the mean) for the tardive dyskinesia patients than for the controls. Using discriminant analyses, all patients were correctly classified as either having or not having tardive dyskinesia, based on the number of accelerometric peaks.

Overall, investigators from three laboratories have reported high rates of concurrence between clinical ratings of dyskinesia and measurements of force instability (Caligiuri & Lohr, 1989, 1990; Vrtunski, Alphs, & Meltzer, 1991; Wirshing et al., 1991). Similar results were obtained using other instrument measurements of dyskinesia, including steady-state control of tongue position (Caligiuri et al., 1989), ultrasound-based counts of orofacial movements (Bartzokis et al., 1989), and counts of hand movements exceeding a specific displacement threshold (Trzepacz & Webb, 1987).

Limitations

Currently, there is no "gold standard" for assessing patients with tardive dyskinesia. Multi-item rating scales can provide useful information about the severity or amplitude of movements and their frequency of occurrence. Indeed, most rating scales combine the observed amplitude and frequency of occurrence into one score. Instrument measurements, on the other hand, have provided little information about the frequency of occurrence of dyskinesia, because of the relatively short periods during which the analyses have been made. Instrumentation procedures appear to be better suited for measuring the magnitudes of movements and their spectral properties.

Although instrumentation procedures can provide information that is difficult to obtain during clinical examination, they have a number of limitations. For example, they require the use of data-processing equipment and technical support, neither of which may be readily accessible. Also, although some instrument techniques are relatively inexpensive (e.g., force gauges, accelerometers), other techniques, such as ultrasound, can be very expensive. Instrument assessments, moreover, provide no information concerning the functional significance of the movement disorder, a characteristic that may be an important outcome variable in treatment studies. In addition, procedures such as EMG can be invasive and cumbersome to administer and can yield variable findings during repeated measurements. Finally, some patients, for reasons of paranoia or dementia, may be unable to participate in studies involving electronic apparatus.

Description of Apparatus and Analysis

Force measurements and accelerometry – two instrumentation procedures used to assess the severity of tardive dyskinesia – are discussed in this section. For various reasons, other procedures such as ultrasound, EMG, and electromechanical transduction of position, although sometimes used in the past to quantify the severity of tardive dyskinesia, have not gained wide acceptance in the clinical setting (Lohr & Caligiuri, 1992).

Force Procedures

Force gauges, or load cells, can be used to evaluate dyskinesia. The basic assumption underlying isometric force procedures is that dyskinetic movements are direct consequences of random muscle contractions and that these muscle contractions produce changes in force measurable over time (df/dt). In practice, dyskinetic movements can be transduced by using force procedures

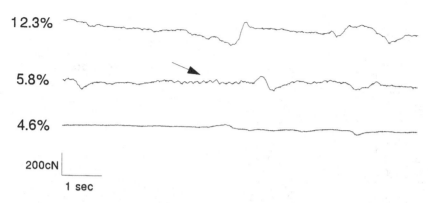

12.3%

5.8%

4.6%

200cN

1 sec

Figure 18.1. Examples of measurements of sustained force recorded from the hands of patients with moderate dyskinesia (top), mild dyskinesia (middle), and no dyskinesia (bottom). Dyskinesia severity was assessed using the AIMS. Values to the left of each waveform are coefficients of variability (SD/mean, percentages). Note the presence of parkinsonian tremor in the force waveform from the patient with mild tardive dyskinesia (arrow).

and engaging the patient in a steadiness task (Potvin et al., 1980; Vrtunski, Simpson, & Meltzer, 1989; Wirshing et al., 1989; Caligiuri & Lohr, 1989, 1990; Caligiuri et al., 1991a; Vrtunski et al., 1991). The procedures implemented in our laboratory require the patient to exert a small force on a rigid beam or platform instrumented with strain gauges and to maintain a constant force under isometric conditions for a set period of time. The force exerted by the patient is displayed on a computer monitor, as feedback, to assist in maintaining a constant pressure. Figure 18.1 shows typical force waveforms for various degrees of severity of tardive dyskinesia. The waveforms for sustained hand force came from individuals rated as having no tardive dyskinesia, mild tardive dyskinesia, and moderate–severe tardive dyskinesia. Their degrees of instability, scored as the coefficient of variability, were 4.6%, 5.8%, and 12.3%, respectively. Note the presence of tremor in the waveform for the patient with mild tardive dyskinesia (as indicated by the arrow).

Dyskinesia can also be relatively quantified from a force signal using time- or frequency-domain analysis. In our analyses, we have used both methods. For time-domain analysis, we obtain the mean and standard deviation for the medial 80% of the force array from each trial; the coefficient of variability (SD/mean) serves as the index of dyskinesia. For frequency-domain analysis, we use fast Fourier transform (FFT) procedures to examine the spectral characteristics. The FFT converts the time-domain waveform to a frequency-domain spectral plot, from which the relative power amplitudes associated

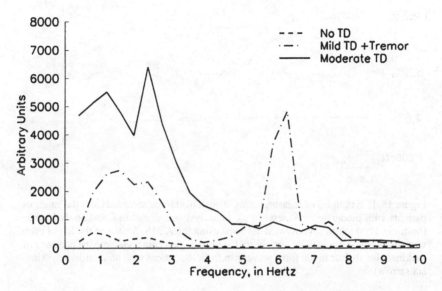

Figure 18.2. Results from FFT analyses of the data shown in Figure 18.1. The FFT waveforms emphasize the energy concentration within the 0–3-Hz range associated with tardive dyskinesia. The peak at 6 Hz exhibited by the patient with mild tardive dyskinesia is typical of parkinsonian tremor.

with specified frequency bins are extracted (e.g., 1–3 Hz in the case of dyskinesia). Previous studies have repeatedly demonstrated that dyskinesia is characterized by elevated spectral amplitudes within the 1–3-Hz range (Alpert et al., 1976; Caligiuri et al., 1989; Wirshing et al., 1989; Caligiuri & Lohr, 1990; Bravi, Moyle, & Chase, 1992). Figure 18.2 shows the associated FFT spectra for the three samples shown in Figure 18.1. Note the increase in spectral energy within the 0–3-Hz frequency range for the two tardive dyskinesia patients and the increase in spectral energy at 6 Hz for the patient with a parkinsonian tremor.

Accelerometry

Accelerometers are widely used to quantify hyperkinesias such as tremor and dyskinesia. An accelerometer is a miniature piezoelectric device or strain gauge that is responsive to acceleration in a single plane. The device can be attached to the finger, hand, foot, or leg without obstructing normal movements. A typical experimental accelerometer-based configuration for quantifying dyskinesia involves attaching a miniature accelerometer to the patient's chin, just below the lower lip, and recording orobuccal masticatory movements while the patient is engaged in manual activity, such as complet-

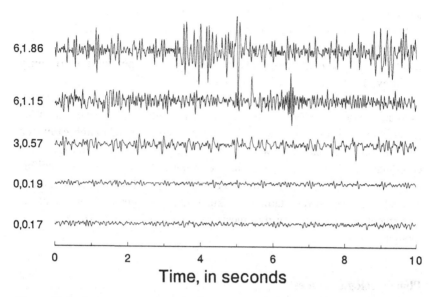

Figure 18.3. Examples of accelerometry waveforms from 5 patients (recorded from the chin), two with no dyskinesia (bottom two), one with mild dyskinesia (middle), and one with moderate-to-severe dyskinesia (top two). Values to the left of the waveforms consist of the AIMS score (sum of lip + jaw) and the peak-to-peak accelerometry amplitude (m/s²).

ing a pegboard test. It is common practice in our laboratory to record accelerometer readings from the chin while simultaneously recording hand-force instability. Such distraction maneuvers are intended to minimize the likelihood that the patient will deliberately suppress orofacial dyskinesia. Figure 18.3 shows typical accelerometer waveforms recorded from 5 patients (2 without and 3 with tardive dyskinesia) treated with neuroleptics.

Assessment of accelerometer data may involve both time-domain and frequency-domain analyses. Consider, for example, the data shown in Figure 18.3, for which the peak-to-peak amplitudes in meters per second per second (m/s²) were computed for each of the waveforms. As shown in Figure 18.3, accelerometer amplitudes for the 2 patients without tardive dyskinesia were less than 0.2 m/s², whereas the amplitudes for 2 of the 3 tardive dyskinesia patients exceeded 1.0 m/s².

Accelerometry has consistently demonstrated high sensitivity and close concurrence with observer ratings (Chien et al., 1977; Tryon & Pologe, 1987). Unpublished data from our laboratory concerning 38 patients with and without orobuccal masticatory tardive dyskinesia indicate that the peak-to-peak accelerometer amplitudes are highly correlated ($r = .77, p < .001$) with AIMS ratings. Published accelerometer studies have used spectral analyses to quantify dyskinesia and to differentiate between dyskinesia and tremor (Alpert et al., 1976; Nishikawa et al., 1986; Tryon & Pologe, 1987). Accelerometer data can also be converted to frequency counts, using automatic counters that count the number of peaks reaching threshold per unit time (Denney & Casey, 1975; Chien et al., 1977; Fann et al., 1977).

We recently completed a study that employed biaxial accelerometry to evaluate the degree of "randomness" associated with hand tardive dyskinesia (Lohr, Ing, & Caligiuri, 1990). Continuous recordings of thumb extension and opposition acceleration were made, and data were plotted on Cartesian coordinates. Patients with milder tardive dyskinesia exhibited greater uniformity in their spatial patterns of movement, as compared with the patterns seen for patients with severe tardive dyskinesia, suggesting that the abnormal movements of mild tardive dyskinesia may be less random than previously thought.

Pharmacologic Studies

Cholinergic Agonists and Antagonists

There is controversy concerning the beneficial effects of anticholinergic medication for reducing the severity of acute extrapyramidal symptoms, especially dystonia. Many patients who begin neuroleptic treatment are given anticholinergic agents prophylactically. No one knows, however, what proportion of such patients actually require anticholinergics. Nor are the effects of prolonged anticholinergic exposure on dyskinesia well understood. It is generally believed, however, that tardive dyskinesia patients who are taking anticholinergic medications will experience some relief from their tardive dyskinesia following withdrawal of the anticholinergic (Burnett et al., 1980; Greil et al., 1984).

Instrumentation techniques may be able to provide helpful information regarding the therapeutic and countertherapeutic effects of anticholinergic medication for patients with tardive dyskinesia. Klawans and Rubovits (1974), who compared the effects of physostigmine (an agent that increases the availability of acetylcholine) and scopolamine (an anticholinergic drug) on abnormal movements in patients with tardive dyskinesia, found that anticholinergic medication may exacerbate dyskinesia. In their study, a patient held a pocket flashlight whose filtered light beam was directed to a darkened wall. After time-exposure photography had recorded the light image, the area of the image was analyzed. Whereas physostigmine was found to decrease the amplitude (total area of the light image) of hand dyskinesia, scopolamine was found to increase the dyskinesia. Casey and Denney (1977), in a study of

2-(dimethylamino)ethanol (Deanol, a cholinergic agonist), attached an accelerometer to the diaphragm of a pressure transducer placed in a balloon inserted in the patient's mouth. They found that tardive dyskinesia patients who exhibited reduced severity of dyskinesia following Deanol administration also showed a reduction in the overall acceleration signal relative to the pretreatment condition. Somewhat later, using electromechanical measurements and spectral analyses, Wirshing et al. (1989) identified a subgroup of tardive dyskinesia patients who, unlike those of Casey and Denney, appeared to benefit from cholinergic antagonists: In 12 tardive dyskinesia patients, spectral analyses of machine-measured hand movements at rest were made prior to administration and 2 hours after administration of trihexyphenidyl hydrochloride. When comparisons were made with patients receiving placebo, treated patients showed marked reductions in the measured energy within the 0.5–3-Hz frequency range.

We recently studied 8 patients with various degrees of hand dyskinesia, using instrumentation procedures to evaluate whether or not anticholinergic withdrawal would have any effect on prevailing dyskinesia in patients who had been on long-term treatment (Lohr et al., 1990). Measurements of hand-force instability, recorded prior to abrupt withdrawal of anticholinergic (benztropine or trihexyphenidyl) and again at 1 month after withdrawal, constituted the baseline measurements. We found significant decreases in the scores for hand-force instability ($t = 6.3$, $p < .01$, using a paired-sample t test), findings that supported the contention that anticholinergic medications may exacerbate tardive dyskinesia. A follow-up study using spectral analysis with a larger patient sample indicated that the degree of improvement after withdrawal of anticholinergics (measured by the change in total spectral energy between 0 and 1.4 Hz associated with steady-state hand force) was proportional to the severity of the dyskinesia measured at baseline ($r = .79$, $p < .001$). Patients with more severe dyskinesia showed greter improvement after anticholinergic withdrawal.

The findings in these instrument studies exemplify the sensitivity of instrumentation procedures to changes in dyskinesia following pharmacologic manipulation. Three different approaches were undertaken, with each showing positive findings to different interventions. Neither instrument nor clinical studies of tardive dyskinesia have resolved the controversy over whether tardive dyskinesia patients benefit when anticholinergics are administered or withdrawn.

Masking of Tardive Dyskinesia by Neuroleptics

For a valid assessment of the persistence of tardive dyskinesia, consideration must be given to the suppressive effects of neuroleptics. Studies have shown that neuroleptic withdrawal can initially aggravate the intensity of dyskinesia

(Crane, Ruiz, & Kernahan, 1969; Turek et al., 1972; Jeste et al., 1979). This implies that in some patients, neuroleptics exert a suppressive effect on dyskinesia that is released by neuroleptic withdrawal. In one long-term study (44 weeks), Turek et al. (1972) compared the effects of neuroleptic withdrawal versus neuroleptic administration in terms of relief from tardive dyskinesia. They noted significant improvements in patients with dyskinesia during periods of neuroleptic administration but worsening of symptoms following neuroleptic withdrawal.

Using instrumentation procedures, we recently investigated the problem of neuroleptic masking, using 19 neuroleptic-treated patients. Eight of the patients underwent neuroleptic withdrawal, and the remaining 11 were maintained on stable neuroleptic dosages. Instrument measurements of hand dyskinesia (force instability) were made twice for all patients. The mean score (and SD) for force instability for the 11 stable patients was 3.9 (2.9) at the start of the study, and 3.7 (2.9) after 3 months. For patients undergoing neuroleptic withdrawal, the mean dyskinesia score, which was 4.5 (1.9) prior to neuroleptic withdrawal, increased significantly to 7.9 (4.9) following a 3-month withdrawal period ($t = 2.89, p < .05$). Clinical ratings over the same interval showed that the mean pre-withdrawal upper-extremity AIMS score of 0.82 (0.98) did not differ significantly from the post-withdrawal mean AIMS score of 0.36 (0.50). That preliminary study of the effects of neuroleptic withdrawal on upper-extremity dyskinesia suggests that instrument measurements are more sensitive to the masking effects of neuroleptics than are clinical ratings. Follow-up studies are under way to evaluate whether or not acute increases in force instability following neuroleptic withdrawal precede persistent, clinically observable tardive dyskinesia.

Summary and Conclusions

Several of the currently available instrument measurements appear to demonstrate high degrees of concurrence with clinical rating scales. Moreover, some procedures, especially measurements of sustained force, may be able to detect subclinical dyskinesia, whereas others, such as accelerometry, may help to differentiate tardive dyskinesia from other movement disorders. Also, instrument measurements can provide useful information about movement disorders that cannot be obtained from clinical ratings. With increasing selectivity, precision, and objectivity, the role of instrument assessments in the management of tardive dyskinesia doubtless will evolve from one of simple severity indexing to sophisticated procedures aimed at revealing underlying pathophysiology. But already the combination of subjective ratings and objective measurements of tardive dyskinesia frequently can provide more information about the disorder than can be obtained with a single procedure. The ideal assessment battery for patients with tardive dyskinesia probably should include both electromechanical procedures and clinical ratings.

The relative importance of the objective and subjective procedures will depend on the specific goal of the assessment. Early on in the course of neuroleptic treatment, greater emphasis should be placed on using sensitive, objective instrumentation procedures to document subclinical motor phenomena. However, if the goal of assessment is to document the emergence of tardive dyskinesia, the objective instrumentation findings should be supported by clinical ratings.

Careful planning and development will be essential if electromechanical assessment procedures are to be incorporated into a clinical setting serving patients with various psychiatric and cognitive abnormalities. A number of design factors should be considered prior to setting up a laboratory for instrument assessment of tardive dyskinesia. Such a laboratory must have (1) a transduction system that will be simple to construct, calibrate, and maintain, (2) a machine–patient interface that will be noninvasive, (3) procedural conditions that will not place excessive attentional or cognitive demands on the patient, and (4) procedures for data collection and analysis that will have high degrees of face, construct, and concurrent validity. With appropriate use, electromechanical quantifications of movements should advance our understanding of the pathophysiology of movement disorders. In the end, such procedures may even facilitate early detection and subsequent management of tardive dyskinesia.

Acknowledgments

This work was supported in part by USPHS grant R29-MH45959 and by the Department of Veterans Affairs Merit Review Program.

References

Adler, L. A., Angrist, B., Reiter, S., & Rotrosen, J. (1989). Neuroleptic-induced akathisia: a review. *Psychopharmacology* 97:1–11.

Alpert, M., Diamond, F., & Friedhoff, A. J. (1976). Tremographic studies in tardive dyskinesia. *Psychopharmacol. Bull.* 12:5–7.

Barnes, T. R. E., & Braude, W. M. (1985). Akathisia variants and tardive dyskinesia. *Arch. Gen. Psychiatry* 42:874–8.

Bartzokis, G., Wirshing, W. C., Hill, M. A., Cummings, J. L., Altshuler, L., & May, P. R. A. (1989). Comparison of electromechanical measures and observer ratings of tardive dyskinesia. *Psychiatry Res.* 27:193–8.

Bathien, N., Koutlidis, R. M., & Rondot, P. (1984). EMG patterns in abnormal involuntary movements induced by neuroleptics. *J. Neurol. Neurosurg. Psychiatry* 47:1002–8.

Bravi, D., Moyle, G. A., & Chase, T. N. (1992). Acute motor response to intravenous levodopa in parkinsonian patients. *Mov. Disord. (Suppl. 1)* 7:198.

Burnett, G. B., Prange, A. J., Wilson, I. C., Jolliff, L. A., Creese, I. C., & Synder, S. H. (1980). Adverse effects of anticholinergic antiparkinson drugs in tardive dyskinesia. An investigation of mechanism. *Neuropsychobiology* 6:109–20.

Caligiuri, M. P., Bracha, H. S., Lohr, J. B., & Jeste, D. V. (1991a). Clinical and instrumental assessment of neuroleptic-induced parkinsonism in patients with tardive dyskinesia. *Biol. Psychiatry* 29:139–48.

Caligiuri, M. P., Jeste, D. V., & Harris, M. J. (1989). Instrumental assessment of lingual motor instability in tardive dyskinesia. *Neuropsychopharmacology* 2:309–12.

Caligiuri, M. P., & Lohr, J. B.. (1989). A potential mechanism underlying the voluntary suppression of tardive dyskinesia. *J. Psychiatr. Res.* 23:257–66.

Caligiuri, M. P., & Lohr, J. B. (1990). Fine force instability: a quantitative measure of neuroleptic-induced dyskinesia in the hand. *J. Neuropsychiatry Clin. Neurosci.* 2:395–8.

Caligiuri, M. P., Lohr, J. B., & Jeste, D. V. (1991b). Instrumental evidence that age increases motor instability in neuroleptic-treated patients. *J. Gerontol. Biol. Sci.* 46:197–200.

Casey, D. E., & Denney, D. (1977). Deanol in the treatment of tardive dyskinesia. *Am. J. Psychiatry* 132:864–7.

Chien, C. P., Jung, K., Ross-Townsend, A., & Stearns, B. (1977). The measurement of persistent dyskinesia by piezoelectric recording and clinical rating scales. *Psychopharmacol. Bull.* 13:34–6.

Chouinard, G., Annable, L., & Ross-Chouinard, A. (1982). Fluphenazine enanthate and fluphenazine decanoate in the treatment of schizophrenic outpatients: extrapyramidal symptoms and therapeutic effect. *Am. J. Psychiatry* 139:213–18.

Crane, G. E. (1973). Persistent dyskinesia. *Br. J. Psychiatry* 122:395–405.

Crane, G. E., Ruiz, P., & Kernahan, W. J. (1969). Effects of drug withdrawal on tardive dyskinesia. *J. Neurol. Neurosurg. Psychiatry* 33:511–12.

Denney, D., & Casey, D. E. (1975). An objective method for measuring dyskinetic movements in tardive dyskinesia. *Electroencephalogr. Clin. Neurophysiol.* 38:645–6.

Evarts, E. V., Teravainen, H. T., Beuchert, D. E., & Calne, D. B. (1979). Pathophysiology of motor performance in Parkinson's disease. In *Dopaminergic Ergot Derivatives and Motor Performance*, ed. K. Fuxe & D. B. Calne, pp. 45–59. Elmsford, NY: Pergamon Press.

Fann, W. E., Stafford, J. R., Malone, R. L., Frost, J. D., & Richman, B. W. (1977). Clinical research techniques in tardive dyskinesia. *Am. J. Psychiatry* 134:759–62.

Gardos, G., Cole, J. O., & LaBrie, R. (1977). The assessment of tardive dyskinesia. *Arch. Gen. Psychiatry* 34:1206–12.

Greil, W., Haag, H., Rossnagl, G., & Ruther, E. (1984). Effect of anticholinergics on tardive dyskinesia: a controlled discontinuation study. *Br. J. Psychiatry* 145:304–10.

Guy, W. (ed.) (1976). *ECDEU Assessment Manual for Psychopharmacology*, rev.

ed. pp. 534–7. Publication ADM 76-338. Washington, DC: U.S. Department of Health, Education, and Welfare.

Hallett, M. (1983). Analysis of abnormal voluntary and involuntary movements with surface electromyography. In *Motor Control Mechanisms in Health and Disease,* ed. J. E. Desmedt, pp. 907–14. New York: Raven Press.

Harris, M. J., Panton, D., Caligiuri, M. P., Krull, A. J., Tran-Johnson, T., & Jeste, D. V. (1992). High incidence of tardive dyskinesia in older outpatients on low doses of neuroleptics. *Psychopharmacol. Bull.* 28:87–92.

Jankovic, J., & Casabona, J. (1987). Coexistent tardive dyskinesia and parkinsonism. *Clin. Neuropharmacol.* 10:511–27.

Jeste, D. V., Potkin, S. G., Sinha, S., Feder, S., & Wyatt, R. J. (1979). Tardive dyskinesia: reversible and persistent. *Arch. Gen. Psychiatry* 36:585–90.

Jus, K., Jus, A., & Villeneuve, A. (1973). Polygraphic profile of oral tardive dyskinesia and of rabbit syndrome: for quantitative and qualitative evaluation. *Dis. Nerv. Syst.* 34:27–32.

Klawans, H. L., & Rubovits, R. (1974). Effect of cholinergic and anticholinergic agents on tardive dyskinesia. *J. Neurol. Neurosurg. Psychiatry* 27:941–7.

Lohr, J. B., & Caligiuri, M. P. (1992). Quantitative instrumental assessment of tardive dyskinesia: a review. *Neuropsychopharmacology* 6:231–9.

Lohr, J. B., Ing, L., & Caligiuri, M. P. (1990). Are the movements in tardive dyskinesia truly random? *Soc. Neurosci. Abstracts* 16:1315.

Marsden, C. D., & Schachter, M. (1981). Assessment of extrapyramidal disorders. *Br. J. Clin. Pharmacol.* 11:129–51.

May, P. R. A., Lee, M. A., & Bacon, R. C. (1983). Quantitative assessment of neuroleptic-induced extrapyramidal symptoms: clinical and nonclinical approaches. *Clin. Neuropharmacol.* 6:S35–51.

Munetz, R. R., & Cornes, C. L. (1983). Distinguishing akathisia and tardive dyskinesia: a review of the literature. *J. Clin. Psychopharmacol.* 3:343–50.

Nishikawa, T., Tanaka, M., Tsuda, A., Kuwahara, H., Koga, I., & Uchida, Y. (1986). Effect of ceruletide on tardive dyskinesia: a pilot study of quantitative computer analyses on electromyogram and microvibration. *Psychopharmacology* 90:5–8.

Peterson, F. (1889). A contribution to the study of muscular tremor. *J. Nerv. Ment. Dis.* 16:9–12.

Potvin, A. R., Syndulko, K., Tourtellotte, W. W., Lemmon, J. A., & Potvin, J. H. (1980). Human neurologic function and the aging process. *J. Am. Geriatr. Soc.* 28:1–9.

Simpson, G. M., Lee, J. H., Zoubok, B., & Gardos, G. (1979). A rating scale for tardive dyskinesia. *Psychopharmacology* 64:171–9.

Teravainen, H., & Calne, D. N. (1980). Quantitative assessment of parkinsonian deficits. In *Parkinson's Disease – Current Progress, Problems and Management,* ed. U. K. Rinne, M., Klinger, & G. Stamm, pp. 145–64. Amsterdam: Elsevier.

Tryon, W. W., & Pologe, B. (1987). Accelerometric assessment of tardive dyskinesia. *Am. J. Psychiatry* 144:1584–7.

Trzepacz, P. T., & Webb, M. (1987). The choreometer: an objective test of chorea during voluntary movements. *Am. J. Psychiatry* 22: 771–6.

Turek, I. S., Kurland, A. A., Hanlon, T. E., & Bohm, M. (1972). Tardive dyskinesia: its relation to neuroleptic and antiparkinson drugs. *Br. J. Psychiatry* 121:605–12.

Vrtunski, P. B., Alphs, L. D., & Meltzer, H. Y. (1991). Isometric force control in schizophrenic patients with tardive dyskinesia. *Psychiatry. Res.* 37:57–72.

Vrtunski, P. B., Simpson, D. M., & Meltzer, H. Y. (1989). Voluntary movement dysfunction in schizophrenics. *Biol. Psychiatry* 25:529–39.

Wirshing, W. C., Cummings, J. L., Dencker, S. V., & May, P. R. A. (1991). Electromechanical characteristics of tardive dyskinesia. *J. Neuropsychiatry Clin. Neurosci.* 3:10–17.

Wirshing, W. C., Freidenberg, D. L., Cummings, J. L., & Bartzokis, G. (1989). Effects of anticholinergic agents on patients with tardive dyskinesia and concomitant drug-induced parkinsonism. *J. Clin. Psychopharmacol.* 9:407–11.

Part V

Tardive Dyskinesia in Different Populations

19

Cultural Aspects of Tardive Dyskinesia in Asia

SHIGETO YAMAWAKI, M.D., Ph.D., TERUO
HAYASHI, M.D., Ph.D., IKUO NAGAOKA, M.D.,
HIROSHI SAITOH, M.D., Ph.D., NORIO YOKOTA,
M.D., Ph.D., and YOSUKE UCHITOMI, M.D., PH.D.

Various neuroleptics have been widely used for treatment of schizophrenia in Asian countries, but long-term administration of these antipsychotic agents involves the risk of inducing complications, such as tardive dyskinesia. Sigwald, Bouttier, and Raymondeaud (1959) first described tardive dyskinesia in French hospitals, and Uhrbrand and Faurbye (1960) published a Danish epidemiologic study a year later.

In Asia, Japanese psychiatrists (Miyamoto et al., 1966) first described "mogue-mogue movement" as abnormal involuntary movements of the orofacial region in psychiatric patients; they concluded, however, that the abnormal movements were not related to administration of neuroleptics. That mogue-mogue movement was not dealt with again until the 1970s, when it was identified with tardive dyskinesia in a review by Kazamatsuri (1971) – a review that marked the beginning of public concern about tardive dyskinesia in Japan. In India, Pandurangi, Ananth, and Channabasavanna (1978) were the first to investigate the prevalence of tardive dyskinesia in mental hospitals. In China, an accurate epidemiologic study was carried out by a Chinese-American team (Ko et al., 1989). In Taiwan and Singapore, it was Lin and Chen (1980) and Kua, Ang, and Siew (1982), respectively, who first investigated tardive dyskinesia in chronic schizophrenia inpatients.

This chapter reviews the epidemiologic studies of tardive dyskinesia in Asia; it also discusses the clinical characteristics of tardive dyskinesia in Asian patients. The several epidemiologic studies of tardive dyskinesia carried out in Asian countries are important – both for clarifying the prevalence and risk factors for tardive dyskinesia, such as age and organic brain damage, and for understanding the cultural aspects of tardive dyskinesia in Asia.

Prevalence

Many reports have documented the prevalence of tardive dyskinesia among hospitalized and chronically ill adult psychiatric patients around the world.

Table 19.1. *Prevalences of tardive dyskinesia among neuroleptic-treated Asian patients*

Study	Total	Men	Women
Japan			
Miyamoto et al. (1966)	19.4% (69/356)	18.5% (41/222)	20.9% (28/124)
Kazamatsuri et al. (1973)	0.7% (7/1,073)	0.7% (4/611)	0.6% (3/462)
Ogita et al. (1975)	17.9% (22/123)	17.1% (12/70)	18.9% (10/53)
Itoh et al. (1980)	19.1% (435/2,274)	19.6% (190/969)	18.8% (245/1,305)
Takamiya (1985)	15.8% (78/495)	11.3% (32/282)	21.6% (46/213)
Koshino et al. (1992)	22.3% (144/647)	23.0% (83/361)	21.3% (61/286)
Hayashi et al. (1995)	43.8% (32/93)[a]	31.3% (10/32)[a]	46.3% (19/41)[a]
India			
Pandurangi et al. (1978)	5.0% (20/403)	3.6% (8/223)	6.6% (12/180)
Doongaji et al. (1982)	9.6% (173/1,801)	9.5% (108/1,141)	9.8% (65/660)
Singapore			
Kua et al. (1982)	2.5% (8/320)	2.0% (4/200)	3.3% (4/120)
Tan & Tay (1991)	27.6% (142/514)[a]	16.9% (35/207)[a]	34.9% (107/307)[a]
China			
Ko et al. (1989)	8.4% (73/866)	9.2% (59/641)	6.2% (14/225)
Taiwan			
Lin and Chen (1980)	4.5% (12/268)	5.1% (9/176)	3.3% (3/92)
Total	13.2% (1,215/9,213)	11.6% (595/5,135)	15.2% (617/4,078)

[a]Data from patients more than 60 years of age.

According to a review of 36 studies by Jeste and Wyatt (1981), its prevalence varies widely – from 2.9% to 46%.

Table 19.1 shows the reported prevalences of tardive dyskinesia among Asian neuroleptic-treated patients. Although the prevalence of tardive dyskinesia in Asian countries varies – ranging from 0.7% to 27.6% – it is relatively low compared with that in Western countries. But why is this so? Ko et al. (1989), who reported an 8.4% prevalence of tardive dyskinesia in a Chinese psychiatric hospital, concluded that the low prevalence may have been due to the use of relatively low dosages of neuroleptics in China. Similar findings have been reported in Indian studies (Pandurangi et al., 1978; Doongaji et al., 1982).

On the other hand, Tan and Tay (1991) investigated the prevalence of tardive dyskinesia among 514 elderly psychiatric patients of Chinese, Indian, Malay, and Eurasian backgrounds and found that the Eurasians had the highest prevalence (53.8%), followed by the Chinese (27.3%), Indians (25%), and Malayans (21.1%). Those authors suggested the possibility of underlying genetic differences in sensitivity to neuroleptics in Asian and European patients, inasmuch as similar practices had been used for both groups. Furthermore, two international comparative studies of the epidemiology of tardive dyskinesia have suggested that the severity of tardive dyskinesia in Japan is less than that in Western countries. First, Kazamatsuri, Matsushita, and Takemura (1973), in a comparison of the prevalence of tardive dyskinesia in Japanese and American psychiatric hospitals, found that severe cases were much more common in America than in Japan. Ogita, Yagi, and Itoh (1975), in a comparative study of tardive dyskinesia in Japan and France, found more severe cases in France, although the difference between tardive dyskinesia prevalences in Japan (17.9%) and France (18.3) was not significant. Binder and Levy (1981), however, reported that neuroleptic-induced extrapyramidal reactions were more frequent among Asians than among Americans, both white and black. It would be difficult at this time to draw any conclusions regarding relationships between genetic differences and the prevalence of tardive dyskinesia.

Age and Gender

Researchers agree that the risk for tardive dyskinesia increases with age. Patients more than 50 years of age are three times as likely to develop tardive dyskinesia as are those under age 50 (Jus et al., 1976). Jeste and Wyatt (1982) suggested that a patient's age at the time of beginning neuroleptic treatment is an important statistical determinant of relative risk. Similar results have been reported by several Asian researchers. Ogita (1981), for example, found that whereas the prevalence of tardive dyskinesia among young and middle-aged groups was 17.9%, among patients more than 60 years of age it was 78.3%. In our recent study, we reported that the incidence of tardive dyskinesia in newly treated Japanese elderly psychiatric patients is 44%, similar to that in the United States (Hayashi et al., 1995). Yagi et al. (1978) suggested that aging is related to the irreversibility of symptoms, rather than the prevalence of tardive dyskinesia. An Indian study reported that tardive dyskinesia was more common among the 41–50-year age group, after which it declined (Doongaji et al., 1982). That peak phenomenon was also reflected in Jeste and Wyatt's (1981) worldwide review.

In most Asian epidemiologic studies, the prevalence rate for females has been higher than that for males. Those results are approximately consistent with the data reported by other authors (Jeste & Wyatt, 1981). Takamiya (1985) speculated that the reason for the gender difference may have to do with differences in dopaminergic sensitivity, in that women are more sensitive than men in regard to both the prolactin response and neuroleptic-induced acute extrapyramidal symptoms. Koshino et al. (1992), however, reported that being female was not a risk factor, for they found no difference in male and female prevalences in their investigation.

Brain Organic Damage

Studies of the association between brain organic damage and tardive dyskinesia have yielded conflicting results. Yasuda et al. (1984) suggested that lobotomy is one of the relative risk factors, in that the prevalence and severity of tardive dyskinesia in lobotomized groups are higher than those in non-lobotomized groups. They speculated that neuroleptics may have provoked tardive dyskinesia after lobotomy had induced subclinical damage of the basal ganglia. Miyama, Itoi, and Tobo (1983), in a report of the autopsy of a patient who died of carbon monoxide poisoning and who showed parkinsonism and tardive dyskinesia induced by neuroleptics, suggested degeneration of the globus pallidus and substantia nigra as the background for the neuroleptic-induced tardive dyskinesia.

Several computed tomography (CT) studies have been carried out in tardive dyskinesia patients. Bartels and Themelis (1983), in CT studies of tardive dyskinesia patients, reported the presence of a wide third ventricle and narrowing of the caudate nucleus and lens nucleus. Jeste and Wyatt (1985) reported that their groups of patients with and without tardive dyskinesia did not differ in terms of ventricle-to-brain ratio (VBR) as revealed by CT; however, they reported that tardive dyskinesia patients with low plasma activities of dopamine-β-hydroxylase (DBH) had significantly larger VBRs than low-DBH patients without tardive dyskinesia. Takamiya et al. (1987), who also examined VBRs in schizophrenic patients on long-term neuroleptic treatment, observed no significant difference between the groups with and without tardive dyskinesia.

The association between neuroleptic-induced acute extrapyramidal symptoms and tardive dyskinesia has been discussed from several vantage points within the Asian literature. Yagi and Itoh (1973) described the association between neuroleptic-induced akathisia and tardive dyskinesia. Takamiya (1985) emphasized the association between neuroleptic-induced parkinsonism and tardive dyskinesia, noting that the appearance of parkinsonism that suggested vulnerability of striatal dopaminergic transmission might be a predictor of tardive dyskinesia in the future. Binder et al. (1987), in studying Japanese psychiatric inpatients, reported that smoking was associated with the prevalence of tardive dyskinesia and speculated that nicotine or some other active ingredient in cigarettes might be increasing dopaminergic activity either directly or indirectly.

Guy, Ban, and Wilson (1986), in an international survey of chronic schizophrenia that included Asian countries, found that patients with prominent negative symptoms had a high prevalence of tardive dyskinesia; they suggested that such patients might therefore tend to have had longer hospitalizations and neuroleptic treatments. McCreadie, Barron, and Winslow (1982), however, suggested that higher prevalences of tardive dyskinesia might be related to the type-2 syndrome of schizophrenia, where the organic brain damage could be an etiologic factor. In conclusion, tardive dyskinesia factors are associated not only with the length of hospitalization and the duration of neuroleptic therapy but also with the degree of brain organic damage.

Drug Factors

Although it is sometimes difficult to identify which drug induces tardive dyskinesia, there is no doubt that the main causative drugs are neuroleptics. It has been suggested that powerful dopamine-blocking neuroleptics may induce tardive dyskinesia (Kane & Smith, 1982) and that anticholinergic agents may induce tardive dyskinesia (Chouinard, Montigny, & Annable, 1979). Takamiya (1985) suggested a significant association between the prevalence of tardive dyskinesia and treatment with the combination of antiparkinsonian agents and neuroleptics. Indian psychiatrists (Chowdhury et al., 1991) described a patient with a complex movement disorder involving tardive dyskinesia, tardive dystonia, and tardive akathisia induced by a polymix of neuroleptics. Although the prevalence of tardive dyskinesia has been reported to be associated with the total amount of neuroleptics administered (Mukherjee et al., 1982) or the length of neuroleptic administration (Kane & Smith, 1982), Japanese researchers (Itoh et al., 1980) have reported that the prevalence of tardive dyskinesia is significantly correlated with the length of neuroleptic administration, but not with the total amount of neuroleptics administered.

Conclusion

Although additional studies unknown to us may have been reported in less prominent Asian journals, it appears that Asian countries, as compared with Western countries, have seen fewer systematic epidemiologic studies of tardive dyskinesia. Indeed, from this review, it would seem that the clinical features of tardive dyskinesia in Asian patients are quite similar to those seen in European or American patients.

Although methodologic differences such as diagnostic criteria and severity and type of tardive dyskinesia make it difficult to compare rates reported in various studies, the prevalence of tardive dyskinesia among Asian patients is, generally speaking, lower than that for European or American patients. In Asian countries, as compared with most Western countries, the smaller doses of neuroleptics traditionally prescribed seem to contribute to the low prevalence of tardive dyskinesia. Witness, for example, the relative average doses of neuroleptics: in China, 331.3 mg (chlorpromazine equivalent) (Ko et al., 1989); in Japan, 299 mg (Takamiya, 1985); in India, 240.5 mg (Doongaji et al., 1982). The genetic differences between Asian and European patients that might be underlying their sensitivities to neuroleptics should not be ignored, however (Tan & Tay, 1991). Clearly, further investigations in terms of genetic aspects are required.

References

Bartels, M., & Themelis, J. (1983). Computerized tomography in tardive dyskinesia. *Arch. Psychiatr. Nervenkrank.* 233:372–9.

Binder, R. L., Kazamatsuri, H., Nishimura, T., & McNiel, D. E. (1987). Smoking and tardive dyskinesia. *Biol. Psychiatry* 22:1280–2.

Binder, R. L., & Levy, R. (1981). Extrapyramidal reactions in Asians. *Am. J. Psychiatry* 138:1243–4.

Chouinard, G., Montigny, G., & Annable, L. (1979). Tardive dyskinesia and antiparkinsonian medication. *Am. J. Psychiatry* 136:228–9.

Chowdhury, K. L., Jalali, R. K., Abrol, A., Saproo, R. K., Shah, B. A., & Tramboo, R. (1991). Polypharmacy and tardive dyskinesia. *J. Assoc. Physicians India* 39:501–3.

Doongaji, D. R., Jeste, D. V., Jape, N. M., Sheth, A. S., Apte, J. S., Vahia, V. N., Desai, A. B., Vahora, S. A., Thatte, S., Vevaina, T., & Bharadwaj, J. (1982). Tardive dyskinesia in India: a prevalence study. *J. Clin. Psychopharmacol.* 2:341–4.

Guy, W., Ban, T. A., & Wilson, W. H. (1986). The prevalence of abnormal involuntary movements among chronic schizophrenics. *Int. Clin. Psychopharmacol.* 1:134–44.

Hayashi, T., Yamawaki, S., Nishikawa, T., & Jeste, D. V. (1995). Usage and side effects of neuroleptics in elderly Japanese patients. *Am. J. Geriatric Psychiatry* 3:308–16.

Itoh, H., Fujii, Y., Kaizawa, S., Kamisawa, M., Kamishima, K., Koga, Y., Masuda, Y., Miura, S., Nabeta, K., Nakano, Y., Ogita, K., Ohtsuka, N., Saitoh, F., Sakurai, S., Satoh, K., Suzuki, Y., Takamiya, M., Tanoue, S., Tateyama, M., Yamazumi, S., & Yoshida, H. (1980). Studies for prevention of neuroleptic-induced tardive dyskinesia. I: A new epidemiological approach. *Annual Report of Pharmacopsychiatry Research Foundation* 12:264–72 (in Japanese).

Jeste, D. V., & Wyatt, R. J. (1981). Changing epidemiology of tardive dyskinesia: an overview. *Am. J. Psychiatry* 138:297–309.

Jeste, D. V., & Wyatt, R. J. (1982). *Understanding and Treating Tardive Dyskinesia*. New York: Guilford Press.

Jeste, D. V., & Wyatt, R. J. (1985). Prevention and management of tardive dyskinesia. *J. Clin. Psychiatry* 46:14–18.

Jus, A., Peneau, R., Lachance, R., Pelchat, K., Jus, K., Pires, P., & Villeneuve, R. (1976). Epidemiology of tardive dyskinesia, part 1. *Dis. Nerv. Syst.* 37: 210–14.

Kane, J. M., & Smith, J. M. (1982). Tardive dyskinesia; prevalence and risk factors, 1959 to 1979. *Arch. Gen. Psychiatry* 39:473–81.

Kazamatsuri, H. (1971). Tardive dyskinesia: studies in foreign countries. *Seishin Igaku* 13:840–55 (in Japanese).

Kazamatsuri, H., Matsushita, M., & Takemura, M. (1973). Clinical studies on tardive dyskinesia (I). *Annual Report of Pharmacopsychiatry Research Foundation* 5:201–4 (in Japanese).

Ko, G. N., Zhang, L. D., Yan, W. W., Zhang, M. D., Buchner, D., Xia, Z. Y., Wyatt, R. J., & Jeste, D. V. (1989). The Shanghai 800: prevalence of tardive dyskinesia in Chinese psychiatric hospital. *Am. J. Psychiatry* 146:387–9.

Koshino, Y., Madokoro, S., Ito, T., Horie, T., Mukai, M., & Isaki, K. (1992). A survey of tardive dyskinesia in psychiatric inpatients in Japan. *Clin. Neuropharmacol.* 15:34–43.

Kua, E. H., Ang, P. C., & Siew, H. C. (1982). Tardive dyskinesia in chronic schizophrenic inpatients. *Singapore Med. J.* 23:19–21.

Lin, H. N., & Chen, C. (1980). Tardive dyskinesia inpatients treated with antipsychotics in chronic wards in Taipei. *J. Formosan Med. Assoc.* 79:332–7.

McCreadie, R. G., Barron, E. T., & Winslow, G. S. (1982). The Nithsdale schizophrenic survey. II: Abnormal movements. *Br. J. Psychiatry* 140:587–90.

Miyama, Y., Itoi, T., & Tobo, M. (1983). An autopsied case with progressive dementia, parkinsonism and oral dyskinesia following acute carbon monoxide poisoning. *Seishin Igaku* 25:748–51 (in Japanese).

Miyamoto, T., Yoshida, M., Iwata, T., Motoki, T., Oda, M., & Kawakami, H. (1966). Oral involuntary movement (mogue-mogue movement) in psychiatric inpatients. *Kyushu Seishin Igaku* 12:591–604 (in Japanese).

Mukherjee, S., Rosen, A. M., Cardenas, C., Varia, V., & Olarte, S. (1982). Tardive dyskinesia in psychiatric outpatients: a survey of prevalence and association with demographic, clinical and rug history variables. *Arch. Gen. Psychiatry* 39:466–9.

Ogita, K. (1981). Clinical factors predisposing to tardive dyskinesia. *Seishin Shinkei Yakuri* 3:727–39 (in Japanese).

Ogita, K., Yagi, G., & Itoh, H. (1975). Comparative analysis of persistent dyskinesia of long-term usage with neuroleptics in France and Japan. *Folia Psychiatrica Neurologica Japonica* 29:315–20.

Pandurangi, A. K., Ananth, J., & Channabasavanna, S. M. (1978). Dyskinesia in an Indian mental hospital. *Indian J. Psychiatry* 20:339–42.

Sigwald, J., Bouttier, D., & Raymondeaud, C. (1959). Quatre cas de dyskinésie facio-bucco-linguo-masticatoire à évolution prolongée secondaire à un traitement par les neuroleptiques. *Rev. Neurol.* 100:751–5.

Takamiya, M. (1985). Epidemiological study of tardive dyskinesia in psychiatric inpatients: risk factors for presence and severity. *Keio Igaku* 62:137–63 (in Japanese).

Takamiya, M., Tanoue, A., Sakura, K., Sakuma, K., Nakazato, H., & Itoh, H. (1987). CT study in tardive dyskinesia. *Seishin Igaku* 29:265–72 (in Japanese).

Tan, G. H., & Tay, L. K. (1991). Tardive dyskinesia in elderly psychiatric patients in Singapore. *Aus. N.Z. J. Psychiatry* 25:119–22.

Uhrbrand, I., & Faurbye, A. (1960). Reversible and irreversible dyskinesia after treatment with perphenazine, chlorpromazine, reserpine and electroconvulsive therapy. *Psychopharmacologia* 1:408–18.

Yagi, G., & Itoh, H. (1973). Neuroleptica-induced irreversibly extrapyramidal hyperkinesia: a case report with special reference to the onset, clinical course and pathogenesis of the syndrome. *Seishin Igaku* 15:727–34 (in Japanese).

Yagi, G., Itoh, H., Kamishima, K., Ogita, K., Otsuka, N., & Sakurai, S. (1978). Long-term prognosis of tardive dyskinesia: five year follow-up study on the severe and irreversible cases. *Rinsho Seichin Igaku* 7:707–14 (in Japanese).

Yasuda, M., Koyama, T., Kimura, N., Honma, H., & Ishizuka, N. (1984). Factors related to tardive dyskinesia: long-term effects of frontal leukotomy. *Seishin Igaku* 26:861–6 (in Japanese).

20

Tardive Dyskinesia in North Africa and the Middle East

DRISS MOUSSAOUI, M.D.

Psychiatry in North Africa and the Middle East, from Morocco to Iraq (excepting Israel), is a burgeoning specialty in an evolving medical field within developing countries. Currently it is beset by two main problems: insufficient numbers of physicians and trained staff and insufficient funding:

- Staff. A country like Morocco, with 27 million inhabitants, has no more than 200 psychiatrists, a few dozen clinical psychologists, and about 400 nurses specialized in psychiatry. However, in almost all of these countries, remarkable training efforts are under way and are steadily improving the situation.
- Funding. The number of beds available and the budget allocations for psychotropic medications are far behind the actual needs in these countries.

One of the consequences of this inadequate medical provision is that considerable proportions of the patients seen by psychiatrists in North Africa and the Middle East are psychotic, especially those seen in the public sector, for they represent most of the emergency cases. For example, in Casablanca, the second largest city in Africa, more than 80% of the hospitalized patients in psychiatric wards and about 60% of the patients seen in psychiatric outpatient clinics (representing more than 35,000 patients) are psychotic and are treated with neuroleptics. Nevertheless, in North Africa and the Middle East, there have been only a few studies of tardive dyskinesia, one of the most important iatrogenic effects of neuroleptics.

Although some studies have examined the extrapyramidal side effects of neuroleptics (Abd El Naby, Okasha, & Abo El Magd, 1963; Okasha et al., 1979), they have not addressed tardive dyskinesia. The main studies of tardive dyskinesia have been conducted in Morocco, Egypt, Tunisia, and Israel during the 1980s and 1990s. One of the reasons for the paucity of studies of tardive dyskinesia is that many psychiatrists believe that tardive dyskinesia is a rare condition among patients receiving neuroleptics. In fact, however, systematic studies conducted in some of these countries have shown tardive dyskinesia prevalence figures similar to those found in European and North American countries.

Another line of related research, under way in Casablanca, Morocco, is attempting to determine whether or not never-medicated schizophrenics show abnormal movements like those of tardive dyskinesia before contact with neuroleptics. Is schizophrenia a possible risk factor for tardive dyskinesia or for abnormal movements like those of tardive dyskinesia? In order to address that question and others, an international colloquium on tardive dyskinesia was held in Casablanca, Morocco, in 1987.

In this chapter we review the four kinds of tardive dyskinesia studies conducted in North Africa and the Middle East: epidemiologic studies, neuropsychological studies, therapeutic trials, and studies examining abnormal movements in never-medicated schizophrenics.

Epidemiologic Studies of Tardive Dyskinesia

General Prevalence

The first Egyptian study of dyskinesia (Abd El Naby et al., 1963) found a prevalence of acute dyskinesia of 1.3% in a sample of 317 patients treated with reserpine. However, there was no reference to tardive dyskinesia in this article. To our knowledge, the first paper on tardive dyskinesia in North Africa was published by Boucebci (1972). He described a 28-year-old female with acute delusional episodes and depressive features and a 46-year-old male with delusional paranoia, both of whom had abnormal involuntary movements of the lips and the face. The female patient also had abnormal movements of the neck, trunk, and limbs. Boucebci remarked that the prevalence of such movements is not well known and that antiparkinsonian medications were not helpful for those patients.

Since then, a study in Egypt and several others in Morocco and Tunisia have examined the epidemiology of tardive dyskinesia. The Egyptian study (Okasha et al., 1986), which involved 3,037 psychotic inpatients receiving long-term neuroleptic treatment, found only 52 dyskinetic cases (1.7%). Tardive dyskinesia was reported to have significant relationships to age (>40 years), female gender (>50 years), and long duration of hospitalization.

Moussaoui et al. (1988) reviewed the studies conducted in Morocco and Tunisia. The first study (Chorfi & Moussaoui, 1985), conducted with relatively small samples of three groups of 50 patients each (never-medicated schizophrenics, schizophrenics treated with neuroleptics, and nonpsychiatric patients), was designed to determine the prevalence of abnormal involuntary movements among never-medicated schizophrenics. Of 50 schizophrenic patients treated with neuroleptics, 10% had definite tardive dyskinesia. However, in a control group of 50 patients drawn from medical and surgical wards and matched for gender and age, none had tardive dyskinesia.

In a second study, conducted in 1985 in Casablanca, Morocco, A. Otarid examined 1,070 mainly schizophrenic and bipolar patients, treated with neuroleptics, and found 15.14% of them to have tardive dyskinesia (Moussaoui et al., 1988). A third study, conducted by B. Bentounsi in 1986, used a similar method with 400 treated outpatients and found a similar prevalence of 14.5%. The fact that the same types of patients showed similar results in studies with relatively large samples demonstrates good interrater reliability among members of the team working on tardive dyskinesia in Casablanca.

B. Bentounsi also examined 605 patients hospitalized in the oldest psychiatric hospital in Morocco (Berreshid) (Moussaoui et al., 1988). Many of those patients had been in that institution for at least 20–30 years. The prevalence of tardive dyskinesia among those patients was, surprisingly, among the highest reported in the literature (63.97%). That can be explained by a combination of factors: the patient population was elderly and had experienced long durations of treatment, which had been interrupted many times for various reasons; also, sometimes they had been given antiparkinsonian medication for years alone and had had antecedents of electroconvulsive treatment (ECT) and a high prevalence of organic brain syndrome. As a matter of fact, in Morocco, we see more and more patients with neurosyphilis.

However, the patients rated 3 or 4 on the Abnormal Involuntary Movement Scale (AIMS) represented only 1.5–3.92% of the total number of patients examined in Casablanca ($n = 1,470$) in these various studies. Those rated 4 (severe tardive dyskinesia) on the AIMS represented only 0–0.56%. Another study, in Tunis, conducted by S. Douki and L. Benamor using 200 patients receiving neuroleptics, found that the patients rated 3 and 4 represented 8%, whereas those rated 4 represented only 1.5% (Moussaoui et al., 1988).

Age and Tardive Dyskinesia

In the studies conducted in Casablanca and Berreshid, as well as in Tunis (Moussaoui et al., 1988), a significant relationship appeared between the occurrence of tardive dyskinesia and age: 8.75% of the tardive dyskinesia patients were under 30 years, and 40% were 50 years or older. However, B. Bentounsi found that the patients in Berreshid between the ages of 70 and 80 years showed a paradoxical slight decrease in the rate of tardive dyskinesia. In the study conducted by Otarid, there was a correlation between tardive dyskinesia rate and age and a correlation between tardive dyskinesia severity and age.

Gender and Tardive Dyskinesia

Douki and Benamor found that the occurrence of tardive dyskinesia was strongly correlated with female gender, the strongest risk factor for tardive dyskinesia. However, contrary to the findings reported in the literature, the studies of Otarid and Bentounsi showed no statistical difference between the two genders. Indeed, Otarid even found a significant excess of tardive dyskinesia among males, as compared with females. The explanation can be found in methodologic bias concerning the selection of patients.

Duration of Treatment and Tardive Dyskinesia

Douki and Benamor found neuroleptic treatment lasting more than 20 years to be the fourth most powerful predictor of the occurrence of tardive dyskinesia. Otarid and Bentounsi found a curvilinear relationship between length of neuroleptic treatment and occurrence of tardive dyskinesia.

Use of Antiparkinsonian Medication and Tardive Dyskinesia

The rate of tardive dyskinesia observed by Otarid and Bentounsi was significantly higher among patients receiving antiparkinsonian medication than among those not receiving such medication. It was not clear, however, whether antiparkinsonian medications represented a risk factor for tardive dyskinesia or aggravated a preexisting factor.

Other Possible Risk Factors for Tardive Dyskinesia

Douki and Benamor found other risk factors for tardive dyskinesia as well: presence of depressive disorders, discontinuation of neuroleptic treatment, and antecedents of ECT.

Neuropsychological Studies of Tardive Dyskinesia

In Egypt, El Sheshai and Rashed (1992) studied 280 inpatients undergoing neuroleptic treatment. Twelve patients were identified as having tardive dyskinesia (4.2%). They compared a control group of schizophrenic patients without tardive dyskinesia and patients with tardive dyskinesia and found that the latter performed significantly poorer on the comprehension, digit-span, and similarities subscales of the Wechsler Adult Intelligence Scale. Those investigators also found a significant correlation between lip movements and scores on the comprehension and digit-span subscales.

Therapeutic Tardive Dyskinesia Trials

Two therapeutic studies have been conducted in this field: one in Casablanca (a joint study between teams from Lyon, France, and Casablanca, Morocco) and one in Israel (a joint study between teams from California and Israel (Roberts et al., 1984). The latter was a double-blind, crossover, placebo-controlled study in which two schizophrenic women suffering from tardive dyskinesia were treated with naloxone intravenously every 4 hours, with the number of oral dyskinetic movements being measured after naloxone and placebo administration. Although a significant decrease in the number of dyskinetic movements was seen with low doses of naloxone (0.4 and 0.8 mg), especially at 20 minutes, a recrudescence of movements was seen 1 hour after injection of naloxone.

For the other clinical trial involving tardive dyskinesia patients in Morocco, Mouret et al. (1991) designed a double-blind, placebo-controlled study using low doses of insulin to treat tardive dyskinesia. The underlying hypothesis was that insulin would reduce postsynaptic dopaminergic hypersensitivity. Twenty schizophrenic patients were randomly assigned to either 10 units of standard insulin or placebo, with a daily injection until day 15, and then one injection every other week until day 90. At day 7, the insulin group showed a sharp decrease in the intensity of tardive dyskinesia symptoms, compared with the placebo group. That improvement persisted until day 90. The conclusion of those authors was that diminished glucose availability in the brain helps to decrease dopamine-receptor hypersensitivity.

Abnormal Involuntary Movements in Never-Treated Schizophrenics

In many developing countries, because of lack of medical services, it quite often happens that schizophrenic patients who have never seen a doctor and never received a neuroleptic are seen for the first time in a psychiatric ward or outpatient clinic, usually during an acute psychotic episode. Those kinds of patients can help us answer the question whether neuroleptics are the only risk factors for tardive dyskinesia or whether schizophrenia alone also represents a risk factor. That question is of interest because of descriptions of schizophrenic patients in the preneuroleptic era: "the spasmodic phenomena in the musculature of the face and of speech, which often appear, are extremely peculiar disorders. Some of them resemble movements of expression, wrinkling of the forehead, distortion of the corners of the mouth, irregular movements of the tongue and lips, twisting of the eyes, opening them wide, and shutting them tight . . . making faces or grimacing: they remind one of the corresponding disorders of choreic patients . . . smacking and clicking with the tongue, sudden sighing, sniffing, laughing, and clearing the throat" (Kraepelin, 1971).

Three studies have been conducted in Casablanca: Chorfi and Moussaoui (1985), A. Mamou (unpublished data), Kadri et al. (1994). In Chorfi and Moussaoui's study of 50 never-medicated schizophrenics, only 1 patient had doubtful abnormal movements of the lips and the periorbital region, as well as stereotypes in the upper limbs. The main criticism of that study was that the mean age of the patients was only 24.1 years. The second study (A. Mamou, unpublished data) assessed 20 never-medicated schizophrenics with a mean age of 28.3 years. In that sample, 1 patient had definite involuntary abnormal movements in the upper limbs.

The third study, a collaborative effort between teams from Casablanca, Morocco, and Portland, Oregon, looked at older patients, with longer durations of illness. The patients were assessed more than once and were systematically videotaped. To be sure that the patients were neuroleptic-free, those who had received any kind of medication that could not be clearly identified were excluded. The mean age was 28 ± 5.3 years, and the mean duration of illness 4.2 ± 2.6 years. Of 22 never-medicated schizophrenics, 3 (13.6%) met the diagnostic criteria for probable tardive dyskinesia. Mild movements were seen in an additional 5 patients, and the severity of movements increased with the duration of illness. The most frequently observed abnormal involuntary movements were in the extremities, contrary to the findings of Waddington and Youssef (1990), who reported that schizophrenics who had never received neuroleptics had abnormal movements mainly in the oral-facial region. However, the mean age for the patients in the Waddington and Youssef study was 88 years.

Kadri et al. (1994) suggested that although it appears that there is a relationship between the duration of illness and the severity of movements in the extremities, advanced age may play a greater role in the increased prevalence of oral-facial movements.

Conclusion

This quick review of studies conducted in North Africa and in the Middle East to examine tardive dyskinesia and related conditions delineates the beginning of interest in such topics in the 1970s, which increased in the 1980s and will certainly continue in the 1990s. Research in psychopharmacology in the region is, of necessity, developing steadily in parallel with psychiatry. Because these countries have the kinds of patients who are difficult to find in industrialized countries, particularly never-medicated schizophrenics, collaborative studies will be most welcome.

References

Abd El Naby, S., Okasha, A., & Abo El Magd, M. F. (1963). Side effects from reserpine therapy in Egyptian psychotics. *Egypt. J. Neurol. Psychiat. Neurosurg.* 4:57–69.

Boucebci, M. (1972). Syndrome extrapyramidal tardif aprés neuroleptiques. *Acta Psychiatr. Belg.* 72:233–40.

Chorfi, M., & Moussaoui, D. (1985). Les schizophrènes jamais traités n'ont pas de mouvements anormaux type dyskinésie tardive. *Encéphale* 11:263–5.

El Sheshai, A., & Rashed, S. (1992). Cognitive impairment secondary to tardive dyskinesia in chronic schizophrenia. Presented at the 5th Arab Congress of Psychiatry, Casablanca, Morocco.

Kadri, N., Fenn, D. S., Moussaoui, D., Hoffman, W. F., Bentounsi, B., Tilane, A., Khomeis, M., & Casey, D. E. (1994). Abnormal movements in never medicated schizophrenics. *Neuropsychopharmacology (Suppl. 2)* 10:134.

Kraepelin, E. (1971). *Dementia Praecox and Paraphrenia*. Huntington, NY: Robert Krieger.

Mouret, J., Khomais, M., Lemoine, P., & Sebert, P. (1991). Low doses of insulin as a treatment of tardive dyskinesia: conjuncture or conjecture? *Eur. Neurol.* 31:199–203.

Moussaoui, D., Douki, S., Bentounsi, B., Otarid, A., Chorfi, M., Mamou, A., & Benamor, L. (1988). Epidémiologie des dyskinésies tardives au Maghreb. *Encéphale* 14:203–8.

Okasha, A., El Okbi, H., Sadek, A., Lotaif, & Ashour, A. M. (1979). Drug-induced extrapyramidal side-effects in Egyptian schizophrenic patients. *Egypt. J. Psychiatry* 2:191–7.

Okasha, A., Khalil, A. H., Ashour, A., & Elfiky, M. R. (1986). Tardive dyskinesia in psychosis: a study of its prevalence, psychodemographic, and clinical aspects among neuroleptic-treated Egyptian patients. *Egypt. J. Psychiatry* 9:8–17.

Roberts, E., Munitz, H., Shalev, A., & Blum, I. (1984). The possible beneficial effect of naloxone in the treatment of tardive dyskinesia. Presented at the 14th C.I.N.P. Congress, February 19–23.

Waddington, J. L., & Youssef, H. A. (1990). The lifetime outcome and involuntary movements of schizophrenia never treated with neuroleptic drugs. *Br. J. Psychiatry* 156:106–8.

21

Tardive Dyskinesia in Europe

H. A. McCLELLAND, M.B., and T. A. KERR, M.D.

Persistent dyskinesia was first recognized in the late 1950s in Germany (Schonecker, 1957) and France (Sigwald et al., 1959). Amid the surge of publications from Germany, Denmark, and the United Kingdom that followed those early case studies, an influential Danish study (Faurbye et al., 1964) introduced the term "tardive dyskinesia."

This chapter reviews the studies from European countries that have examined the prevalence of tardive dyskinesia. Since the 1960s there has been a dearth of studies: Only three prevalence studies have come from Italy, and one each from Austria and Sweden; there have been none from Holland, Portugal, or Greece and, apart from Hungary, none from Eastern Europe. This review emphasizes the work from France, which had been excluded from recent major reviews (Jeste & Wyatt, 1982a; Kane & Smith, 1982; Morgenstern et al., 1987).

General Considerations

Genetic Factors

A genetic factor is likely to account for the predisposition to tardive dyskinesia. Family studies (Weinhold, Wegner, & Kane, 1981; Yassa & Ananth, 1981; Waddington & Youssef, 1988; Youssef, Lyster, & Youssef, 1989) have shown a concordance for tardive dyskinesia in first-degree relatives. This is not unexpected, for a familial genetic predisposition is found in drug-induced parkinsonism (Myrianthopoulos, Kurland, & Kurland, 1962).

A genetic ethnic component is also possible. Chinese populations reportedly have a lower prevalence of tardive dyskinesia than do those of Western countries (Chiu et al., 1992). A comparative study of Japanese and French

274

hospital patients (Ogita, Yagi, & Itoh, 1975) showed lower severities of tardive dyskinesia in the Japanese population, and a study in Bombay (Doongaji et al., 1982) revealed a low prevalence of tardive dyskinesia, the findings in both studies being attributed to the patterns followed in prescribing neuroleptics. A genetic component, however, may have been a contributory factor. Tan and Tay (1991) found that the prevalence of tardive dyskinesia in elderly psychiatric inpatients in Singapore was higher among Eurasians than among Chinese, Malays, or Indians. Moreover, primary dystonia is common in Jewish populations (Eldridge, 1970), which demonstrates a clear genetic factor. This possibility has rarely been investigated.

A genetic role may also be an unrecognized and confounding variable when tardive dyskinesia prevalences are compared for the various European ethnic groups.

A recent American study argues against this hypothesis. Sramek et al. (1991) found no difference in the prevalence rate (17%) for tardive dyskinesia among black, white, and Hispanic chronic psychiatric patients in an American state hospital.

Drug Use and Spontaneous Dyskinesia

Polypharmacy and the wide range in neuroleptic dosages used within local services and even hospitals constitute two factors that are common to all nations and continents. The uses of neuroleptics within countries will vary as well, depending on the diagnostic groups.

Often overlooked as a risk factor for tardive dyskinesia is a possible contribution from previous, unrecorded administration of neuroleptics. Such prior administrations can influence the prevalence of spontaneous dyskinesia, which Kane and Smith (1982) have suggested as being 5%. Consider, for example, the studies of elderly subjects that have distinguished between those "on" and "not on" neuroleptics, either during the period of examination or for a brief preceding period. Unless there is careful probing for a history of neuroleptic administration, a spuriously high rate of spontaneous dyskinesia can be reported.

The magnitude of the problem can be illustrated by the history of neuroleptic prescriptions in the Scandinavian countries. Grimsson et al. (1979) studied the use of psychotropic drugs in Finland, Iceland, Norway, and Sweden. In the first three countries, neuroleptic sales were similar, but sales were almost twice as high in Sweden, the result, possibly, of the 1970 Swedish recommendation that neuroleptics be employed as alternatives to hypnotics, sedatives, and tranquilizers. Grimsson et al. (1979) quoted a report from one Swedish health center where sleep disturbances and psychoneurosis accounted for about 50% of neuroleptic prescriptions, and such prescribing practices can influence tardive dyskinesia prevalence rates one to two decades later.

Because most prevalence studies have been carried out among patients with psychoses and organic brain syndromes, the extent to which tardive dyskinesia occurs in other psychiatric and medical patients is still uncertain. Two examples will suffice. First, several investigators (Katabia, Traube, & Marsden, 1978; Lavy, Melamed, & Penchas, 1978; Grimes, Hessan, & Preston, 1982) have shown that metoclopramide, a neuroleptic with a powerful antiemetic action but weak antipsychotic action, is a cause of tardive dyskinesia in medical patients. Also, a Swedish study (Wiholm et al., 1984) revealed that 11 cases of persistent dyskinesia (all women, over the age of 76 years) had been reported to the Adverse Drug Reaction Bureau – an incidence of 1/1,000 elderly patients on metoclopramide. Second, the first report of tardive dyskinesia in the United Kingdom (Evans, 1965) described 4 female patients who developed tardive dyskinesia after taking small doses of trifluoperazine for psychoneurosis. Such cases can influence the reported rates of spontaneous dyskinesia years later, because the dyskinesia may persist indefinitely after treatment has stopped.

Other studies have raised questions as well. The findings in a Belgian study by Delwaide and Desseilles (1977), as reworked by Kane and Smith (1982), were that 3% of elderly persons in a retirement home who had not been on neuroleptics and were without neurological signs had dyskinesia. However, the Belgian authors had checked for neuroleptic treatment only in regard to the preceding month. In a larger study (Woerner et al., 1991), 400 healthy volunteers were found to have a tardive dyskinesia prevalence rate of 1.3%. Again, insufficient details were given regarding past neuroleptic treatment. As for the French study of 270 elderly residents in a retirement home (Bourgeois, Boueilh, & Tignol, 1980a), in which the authors found tardive dyskinesia prevalence rates of 18% among non-neuroleptic-treated patients and 42% among those treated with neuroleptics, no details were given as to how far back the search for prior neuroleptic treatment had been pursued.

To date, given the difficulties of ascertaining whether or not there has been neuroleptic treatment, spontaneous dyskinesia cannot be said to have been clearly demonstrated in healthy elderly individuals. Indeed, Ticehurst (1990), in a small but thorough study of 105 elderly patients, found that 15 (14%) had no history of neuroleptic exposure and no dyskinesia, compared with a 45% tardive dyskinesia prevalence among those with a neuroleptic history.

To what extent dyskinesia spontaneously arises in schizophrenic patients never medicated with neuroleptics is a contentious issue. Confounding factors in comparing recent studies are age, length and severity of illness, and possibly ethnicity. Early writers, from Kraepelin and Bleuler, described abnormal movements, though not with the detail that would establish an unequivocal diagnosis of dyskinesia today. British investigators at Northwick Park were the first modern workers to claim a high spontaneous dyskinesia prevalence rate. They found (Owens, Johnstone, & Frith, 1982) a prevalence rate in a London mental hospital of 53% among 47 chronic schizophrenic patients (mean age 66 years) who had never received neuroleptics. The dyskinesia was mainly oro-facial. Other British investigators (McCreadie et al., 1996) examined 308 elderly Indian schizophrenic patients in the community with a minimum age of 50 years; 38% of those patients who had never received neuroleptics had typical dyskinesia. However, the control group of normal subjects, with a mean age of 63 years, had a dyskinesia prevalence rate of 15%. This is an unusually high rate that cannot readily be explained and must suggest some unknown cultural vulnerability. An American study of 100 neuroleptic-naive schizophrenic patients followed for more than 20 years (Fenton, Wyatt, & McGlashan, 1994) found an oro-facial dyskinesia prevalence rate of 15%. Yet McCreadie himself (McCreadie & Ohaeri, 1994), in a study on never-medicated Nigerian chronic schizophrenic patients (mean age 42 years), found no abnormal movements. The difference between the McCreadie studies in Nigeria and India is remarkable and is difficult to explain away simply on the basis of age. These studies contrast strongly with an American study (Chatterjee et al., 1995) that evaluated 89 neuroleptic-naive first-episode schizophrenic patients for extrapyramidal signs and spontaneous dyskinesia. Only 1 patient had spontaneous dyskinesia. All subjects were in their mid-20s.

A provisional conclusion is that spontaneous dyskinesia may occur in chronic schizophrenic patients in the higher age groups, particularly in those with negative symptoms; otherwise it is uncommon.

Neuroleptic Dosages in Patients with Psychoses

Among the benefits claimed for neuroleptic treatment of schizophrenics, using low or intermittent dosages, are reductions in the frequency and severity of tardive dyskinesia (Jolley et al., 1989). Follow-up studies in the United Kingdom have suggested that reductions in neuroleptic dosage can lead to lower prevalences of tardive dyskinesia (Gibson, 1978; Johnson et al., 1987). A French study (Fanget, Henry, & Aimard, 1986), using a very low neuroleptic dosage, reported an incidence rate of 3.8% over an average of 9 years of treatment among 52 patients whose average age was 42 years.

A greater awareness of the disadvantages of neurological side effects in general has not led to lower neuroleptic dosages. In a New York study (Reardon et al., 1989), the mean dosage at the time of patient discharge had increased between 1973 and 1982 because of a switch from low- to high-potency neuroleptics. When expressed in chlorpromazine equivalents (CPZE) (Appleton, 1982), the mean neuroleptic dosage at discharge was 880 mg/day in 1973, compared with 1,885 mg/day in 1982.

That emphasis on the use of high-potency neuroleptics can also be discerned in European studies. A study of a hospital serving a Paris arrondissement (Fombonne et al., 1989) found that for patients receiving neuroleptics, the average was 1.6 neuroleptic drugs being prescribed per patient. Thus polypharmacy was common: Whereas dosages of sedative neuroleptics such as chlorpromazine and thioridazine varied from 15 to 300 mg/day, with a mean of 168 mg/day, the dosages of "incisive" (high-potency) neuroleptics, such as trifluoperazine, varied from 20 to 600 mg/day (CZPE 400–12,000 mg/day), with a mean of 144 mg/day (CPZE 2,880 mg/day). Some patients were thus receiving high amounts of neuroleptics.

At a psychiatric teaching hospital in Berlin, Schmidt, Niemeyer, and Muller-Oerlinghausen (1983) reported that haloperidol was prescribed at a mean dosage of 16 mg/day (CPZE 800 mg/day), thioridazine at 180 mg/day, and perazine at 324 mg/day. In France, a study (Bourgeois, 1988) of tardive dyskinesia indicated an average dosage of 900 mg/day (CPZE). A 3-year follow-up study in England (Barnes, Kidger, & Gore, 1983) found that 30% of the patient population was receiving more than 1,000 mg/day (CPZE).

The few studies from other European countries indicate lower dosage regimens. In Hungary, Gardos et al. (1980) reported a mean dosage of 485 mg/day (CPZE). Another Hungarian prevalence study (Perényi & Arato, 1980) found a mean daily dosage of 365 mg (CPZE). A prevalence study of tardive dyskinesia in Italy (Altamura, Cavallaro, & Regazzetti, 1990) reported an average neuroleptic dosage of 382 mg/day (CPZE), and Topiar and Kanczucka (1975), examining neuroleptic dosage for newly admitted schizophrenic patients over a 6-week period in a Czech hospital, found a mean daily dose of chlorpromazine of 300 mg (range 150–600 mg).

French psychiatrists seem to prescribe the widest range of neuroleptic dosages, a tendency confirmed by a review of modern French textbooks. In Britain and Germany, neuroleptics appear to be prescribed at lower dosages than in the United States. In Hungary, Italy, and the Czech Republic, lower neuroleptic dosages are prescribed, as compared with the previously cited countries. As for Spain and Portugal, there is insufficient information in the relevant literature to characterize dosages.

Although high-potency neuroleptics have long been suspected of imposing increased risk for tardive dyskinesia, this has not been clearly demonstrated. Any association could be a consequence of disproportionately large (CPZE) dosages.

Prevalence Studies in European Countries

Early studies of the prevalence of tardive dyskinesia relied on the individual author's judgment of diagnosis and severity. By the 1970s, the standardization offered by the Abnormal Involuntary Movement Scale (AIMS) and Simpson's Rockland scales led to wide application of those measures; the French, however, used the scale developed by Villeneuve (Jus et al., 1978).

Jeste and Wyatt (1982a) reported data on the proportion of patients with moderate-to-severe dyskinesia, excluding those with mild and borderline symptoms. However, we have included minor grades in our review, for we believe that there is no *a priori* reason to suppose that mild cases of dyskinesia are not forms of tardive dyskinesia. Furthermore, follow-up studies (Barnes et al., 1983; Robinson & McCreadie, 1986; Yassa & Nair, 1989; McClelland et al., 1991) have shown that mild cases of dyskinesia can become persistent and worsen. Moreover, Yassa and Nair (1989) have concluded that mild tardive dyskinesia, even if involving only one body area, should be included in prevalence studies.

France and Belgium

France. Maurel, Ruel, and Kabare (1966) studied 208 female patients "of whom the majority had chronic psychoses." Of those on neuroleptics, 49.1% (83 of 169) suffered from persistent dyskinesia. In the majority of cases (90.3%), the dyskinesia was mild, the patients with severe dyskinesia being older (mean age 71 years). Buccolinguomasticatory movements were present in 68.6% of cases. Neuroleptic dosages were not given, the authors commenting that "usual doses were not exceeded." In three cases, the movements became worse once neuroleptics were withdrawn.

Twenty years later, a study from Lyon (Fanget et al., 1986) reported on 52 patients (30 men and 22 women) with chronic psychoses and an average age of 42 years. Neuroleptic treatment had been given for a mean period of 9 years, although nearly a third of the patients had had periods without neuroleptics for up to 9 months. Only 2 patients (3.8%) developed tardive dyskinesia, both women in their early sixties. That low incidence of dyskinesia was attributed to low-dosage neuroleptic treatment; average daily doses were 4 mg haloperidol (CPZE 200 mg), 57 mg chlorpromazine, and 38 mg levoprom-azine.

From the Aquitaine region, Bourgeois and colleagues have contributed major prevalence studies. However, they excluded minor dyskinesia as not being of clinical significance, reporting only "marked" movement disorders. The overall prevalence rate of 8.2% reported in their studies could therefore have been as much as three times higher if all grades had been included.

One of their studies (Bourgeois et al., 1977) involved 1,480 patients in three hospitals, and another (Bourgeois, Grau, & Arretche-Berthelot, 1976) involved 1,660 patients in two other hospitals; both studies are summarized by Bourgeois (1988). Between 15% and 20% of the patients were "estimated" as no longer receiving neuroleptics at the time of the examinations. Of the 3,140 patients, 49.2% suffered from chronic schizophrenia and paranoid psychoses, with 50.7% having other diagnoses, including affective and organic illness. An overall prevalence of 8.2% was found for "marked" dyskinesia, with female patients having a significantly higher rate (10.6%) than male patients (5.8%). Unfortunately, age was not considered, although it was clearly of importance, inasmuch as the mean age for women (64.9 years) was greater than that for men (54.0 years). The mean duration of neuroleptic treatment was 20 years. If one assumes that the 10 sample patients for whom the total neuroleptic dosage was cited were representative, the average neuroleptic dose per patient per day over the years would be 926 mg (CPZE). In 59% of cases, the dyskinesia was orofacial.

In that same study, Bourgeois (1988) quoted from a study by Delance, written as a memorandum in 1985 for the Université Paris Sud, from a psychiatric hospital, Henry Ey de Bonneval. In that study, 16% of 262 patients on neuroleptics had tardive dyskinesia.

In a comparison of tardive dyskinesia rates in French and Japanese hospitals, Ogita et al. (1975) found similar prevalences: 18.3% of 131 patients in France, and 17.9% of 123 patients in Japan. The Japanese cohort, compared with the French, had dyskinesia that was less severe and more intermittent, possibly attributable to the lesser amount of medication given to the Japanese patients. In the Japanese hospital, the average daily doses of chlorpromazine and haloperidol were 120 mg and 6.9 mg (CPZE 345 mg), respectively. No figures were quoted for the French hospital, with the exception of oral fluphenazine, which was given at daily doses of 200–300 mg (CPZE 14,000–21,000 mg); in Japan, the daily doses of oral fluphenazine were 1–6 mg (CPZE 70–420 mg).

When Bourgeois et al. (1980a,b) studied 270 elderly subjects in a retirement home, they found that 18% of those considered as not having received neuroleptics had dyskinesia, compared with 42% of those treated with neuroleptics.

Many French clinicians in the early decades of treating tardive dyskinesia (Flugel, 1956; Deniker, 1960) were tolerant regarding extrapyramidal side effects, considering them to be part of the antipsychotic effect. They therefore allowed large doses of neuroleptics to be prescribed.

The Fanget study (which claimed low neuroleptic dosages) and the Ogita study (which found that French dosages were higher than those in Japan) suggest that when differences in neuroleptic dosage regimens are present, the lower dosages will lead to lower prevalence rates of dyskinesia or less severe forms of dyskinesia.

Belgium. Delwaide and Desseilles (1977) studied two elderly populations: one cohort (55 patients) from a retirement home, and a second cohort, whose members had dementia (185 patients), from a psychogeriatric unit. Of the 240 patients, 64 were male and 176 were female. The selected patients were not on neuroleptics at the time, although the authors did not comment whether or not past treatment with neuroleptics had been excluded. Eighty-eight patients (36.7%) had dyskinesia, the rates in the retirement home and psychogeriatric unit being 29% and 38%, respectively. Dyskinesia was found to be three times more prevalent among the females. In 84% of those affected, the movements were confined to the orofacial region. Only 9% of the 88 patients with facial dyskinesia had no associated neurological signs. Thus, only 3.3% of the total sample were patients with dyskinesia who had otherwise healthy neurological systems.

Waddington (1989) has shown that dyskinesia rates among the elderly increase sharply in cohorts that have medical, neurological, and dementing disorders. Studies to examine specifically delineated normal, healthy elderly groups have consistently found very low dyskinesia rates, ranging from zero (Koller, 1982) to 4.0% (Kane et al. 1982). The healthy elderly patients in the Delwaide and Desseilles (1977) study therefore had a prevalence rate similar to those seen in other Western countries.

Scandinavian Countries

Denmark. Two important studies came from the St. Hans mental hospital in the early 1960s. The first (Uhrbrand & Faurbye, 1960) reported on 500 female patients, of whom 33 had prevalence dyskinesia, although the severity was not graded. In 29 patients, the syndrome was attributed to neuroleptics; in the other 4, electroconvulsive treatment (ECT) was judged the culprit, although those 4 patients had had neuroleptics in the past. Dyskinesia was more common in the elderly. In 11 of the 17 patients who had had their neuroleptics discontinued, the movements persisted during follow-up, and in two cases the dyskinesia continued after the neuroleptic dosage had been reduced.

In a more systematic prevalence survey from the same hospital (Faurbye et al., 1964), the authors studied 417 female patients with the buccolinguomasticatory (BLM) triad. Although it was a controlled trial, their definition of "spontaneous dyskinesia" referred only to patients who had not had drugs in the month prior to the onset of symptoms. The prevalence of the BLM triad in the 216 schizophrenic patients was established as 9.7%, the prevalence of "spontaneous dyskinesia" being 1.85%. Those authors, noting that dyskinesia increased with age (over 50 years), suggested ECT as a contributory factor.

Sweden. In a study carried out by Perris et al. (1979), patients were rated on the Simpson scale by three doctors trained in its use. The authors were satisfied as to interrater reliability. All 347 patients in the hospital were examined (213 male and 134 female). Tardive dyskinesia was found in 17.3%, with the higher prevalence being among females (29.8%, compared with 9.4% among males). The prevalence of tardive dyskinesia was seen to increase rapidly after 50 years of age. All patients had apparently been treated with neuroleptics. In their examination of 18 patients with tardive dyskinesia and 18 without, the authors sought to determine the neuroleptic and other drug treatments. They found that neither the duration of treatment nor the total amount of neuroleptics taken could distinguish between the groups, nor did either treatment variable correlate with the severity of tardive dyskinesia. The main psychiatric diagnoses were not stated.

Italy, Spain, Portugal, Holland, and Greece

With the exception of Italy, we have found no reports of relevant, original clinical research carried out in these countries. Even a review article on tardive dyskinesia from Spain (Gomez-Feria Prieto, 1989) contained no references indicating any work carried out in that country; the one original study on the prevalence of tardive dyskinesia in a Spanish journal came from Chile (Varela Guzman, Tapia Villanueva, & La Roche Olsen, 1984).

Using the criteria of the *Diagnostic and Statistical Manual of Mental Disorders,* third edition (DSM-III), Altamura et al. (1990) surveyed a schizophrenic population treated with neuroleptics, resident in a northern Italian psychiatric hospital. The patients had refused to leave, despite passage of a new law in 1978 that strongly encouraged community resettlement. Using the Rockland-Simpson rating scale, those investigators assessed 148 patients (80 male, 68 female) aged 28–87 years; 32% were found to be affected by tardive dyskinesia. Although the prevalence of tardive dyskinesia was seen to increase sharply after the age of 50 years, no gender difference was found. Neither was any correlation found between tardive dyskinesia and the duration of treatment, the total amount of neuroleptic, or the type of neuroleptic prescribed. The average duration of illness was 29.7 years. In general, such long-term institutionalized patients are expected to have a high prevalence of tardive dyskinesia. The members of the patient group were also elderly, more than one-third (36%) being older than 60 years. Those investigators arbitrarily reduced the prevalence rate from 37% to 32%, arguing that the rate of spontaneous dyskinesia was 5%. Thus, the true prevalence of dyskinesia was put at 37%. The average CPZE dosage was 380 mg/day, a dosage well within accepted prescribing limits.

A more recent Italian study by Muscettola et al. (1993) found a much lower prevalence rate (19%). Using the AIMS, they examined 1,745 patients (1,269 in hospital, 476 outpatients). More than 75% of the neuroleptic-treated patients received less than 400 mg (CPZE) per day; a further 21% received 401–800 mg/day; only 3% received more than 800 mg/day. Those investigators found, as have the majority of other studies, that female gender, advanced age, and high neuroleptic dosage were all significantly associated with increased risk for tardive dyskinesia. In both studies (Altamura et al., 1990; Muscettola et al., 1993), the evidence shows that Italian psychiatrists use comparatively low dosages of neuroleptics for the majority of their patients. The higher tardive dyskinesia prevalence in the Altamura study (37% or 32%), compared with the Muscettola study (19.1%), may in part be attributed to the older average age of the patients, the longer duration of illness, and the fact that all were inpatients, thereby suggesting a more disabled and more vulnerable group.

A follow-up study (Cavallaro et al., 1993) carried out over 3 years and involving 125 institutionalized schizophrenic patients confirmed that the prevalence of tardive dyskinesia increased over time (from 39.2% to 52.8%), but within those overall rates, 28.6% recovered and 30% improved. Such a finding confirms the fluctuating nature of the condition, as has been shown in other studies.

Eastern European Countries

There has been little research on tardive dyskinesia in the Eastern European countries, including the former Soviet Union. Apart from several reviews of Western research (Lerner, 1988) and a few case histories, we could not find any research on the prevalence of dyskinesia in the available Russian literature.

Hungary. The exception to that general statement concerns Hungary. In 1980, Perényi and Arato surveyed 200 inpatients diagnosed as schizophrenic according to the Feighner criteria (Feighner et al., 1972). All had been treated with neuroleptics for at least 2 years. Thirty-three patients not receiving neuroleptics at the time of the study were included. Using the AIMS rating, those authors found a tardive dyskinesia prevalence of 23.5% (31% among males, 16% among females), with the frequency and severity of tardive dyskinesia having increased with age. Indeed, they found that the older the patient was at the start of neuroleptic treatment, the more likely it was that tardive dyskinesia would develop.

If patients with mild tardive dyskinesia (score of 1 on AIMS) had been included, the prevalence would have risen from 23.5% to 49.5%. That study was unusual in that the prevalence of tardive dyskinesia was found to be significantly higher among men than among women. Also, the amount of neuroleptic prescribed was not associated with the presence of dyskinesia, the daily mean dose being 365 mg (CPZE).

Using the AIMS, Gardos et al. (1980) reported on the prevalence of tardive dyskinesia among 122 Hungarian schizophrenic outpatients. Although 16% of the patients had tardive dyskinesia, no case was severe. Of the 44% of patients with mild dyskinetic movements on the global-severity item, one-third were assessed as having tremor rather than tardive dyskinesia. The overall prevalence of tardive dyskinesia using that wider criterion (including mild cases, but excluding tremor) was 31%. Those authors attributed their 16% rate (better than the rates in North American studies) to greater use of ECT and avoidance of high-dosage neuroleptic treatment. The mean neuroleptic dosage for 106 of the patients was 574 mg/day (CPZE).

In 1988, Gardos et al. published a 7-year follow-up of the original patient cohort, two-thirds of whom were available for assessment. Although they noted that the prevalence of tardive dyskinesia had increased from 27% to 38.5% over the 7-year follow-up period, they found no severe cases of tardive dyskinesia. Nevertheless, the AIMS global rating had increased from a mean of 1.51 to 1.81 ($P < .01$). They also found that neither age nor neuroleptic dosage was associated with prognosis. The 10-year follow-up report (Gardos et al., 1994) showed a reduced prevalence rate (31%). However, of the 63 patients examined in that last survey, 11 had had remissions, and 12 who had developed tardive dyskinesia had been free of such movements at baseline. The fluctuating nature of the condition, with frequent remissions, is now well recognized and their study confirms that only a fraction of patients at risk, perhaps no more than 10%, have persistent or unremitting dyskinesia. Nevertheless, that long-stay population in Hungary had a prevalence rate for tardive dyskinesia as high as that found in western countries. That no severe tardive dyskinesia occurred in the outpatient study could be due to the lower neuroleptic dosages prescribed for even severely ill schizophrenic patients in Hungary.

Furthermore, without minimizing the potentially serious nature of tardive dyskinesia, this follow-up study confirms the fluctuating nature of the condition and, as the authors state, the feasibility of maintenance neuroleptic therapy for chronic psychotic patients.

Germany and Switzerland

Germany. Schonecker (1957) was the first to draw attention to an unusual and unexpected development in neuroleptic treatment: Among 4 cases of extrapyramidal reactions, in which 1 patient had an acute dyskinetic reaction, the other 3 patients (elderly women with senile dementia) had persistent movements that had started after neuroleptic administration and continued beyond withdrawal of medication.

As for prevalence, on the basis of a questionnaire sent to ward therapists, Hoff and Hoffmann (1967) reported a tardive dyskinesia prevalence rate of 0.5% among 10,000 patients. Eckmann (1968), however, reported a 4.1% prevalence rate of dyskinesia among non-neuroleptic-treated patients, but a 2.9% rate among those treated with neuroleptics. That lower dyskinesia rate among neuroleptic-treated patients than among non-neuroleptic-treated patients was a unique finding. Eckmann, who stated that the 1,392 patients had been examined over 24 hours, must have delegated the assessments to others.

Degkwitz and Wenzel (1967b), who surveyed two German hospitals, a nursing home, and a psychogeriatric ward, found, in one hospital, an overall dyskinesia rate of 17% for the 766 patients on neuroleptics (males 10.9%, females 21.0%); dyskinesia was mild in only 39 of the 91 affected patients. For those not on neuroleptics, the dyskinesia rate was 1.3%. In the other hospital, they found the dyskinesia rate for those on neuroleptics to be 23% (20.7% among males, 24.2% among females). In the nursing home for the nondemented aged, they found a prevalence rate of 1.2% among those not treated with neuroleptics. In the psychogeriatric ward, where the elderly demented patients had never received neuroleptics, they found a 1% dyskinesia rate. Those investigators therefore showed a tardive dyskinesia prevalence of 17–23% for patients treated with neuroleptics and a tardive dyskinesia prevalence of just over 1% for those not on neuroleptics. That study was among the first to show that a reduction in neuroleptic dosage (as distinct from complete cessation of neuroleptics) could uncover suppressed dyskinesia.

A detailed survey of 755 patients by Heinrich, Wegener, and Bender (1968) found a dyskinesia rate of 17% among those on neuroleptics and a 3% rate among those not on neuroleptics. Minor grades of dyskinesia were included. Those investigators found no correlation with age or dosage, although dosage reduction over a period of 15 months did result in an increase in prevalence. Oral dyskinesia was the predominant form. In their smaller study in a home for the elderly, the same authors found a 2% rate of spontaneous dyskinesia (i.e., among those who apparently had never been treated with neuroleptics).

Hippius and Lange (1970), in a survey of 668 inpatients at the Karl Bonhoeffer Clinic in Berlin, decided that the slightest movements – "some barely obvious rubbing of the fingers would be registered" – would be counted as dyskinesia. They found an overall dyskinesia rate among 530 neuroleptic-treated patients of 34.3%, with no gender difference in the rates. But if one analyzes their data for patients over the age of 50 years, the rate of tardive dyskinesia becomes higher among females (50.5%) than among males (45.7%). Those authors also briefly described a similar survey of 97 patients with psychoses in an outpatient clinic who had a tardive dyskinesia rate of only 4%; those were "good-outcome schizophrenics" with shorter durations of illness (2–10 years).

In summary, the more meticulous German studies found tardive dyskinesia prevalence rates between 17% and 34%. The prevalence rate of 34% found by Hippius and Lange (1970), high for such an early study, may partly be attributable to their inclusion of very minor movements.

Interestingly, Degkwitz et al. (1967a) found the prevalence of dyskinesia in one Düsseldorf clinic to be particularly low, although no figures were quoted. That finding was attributed to the influence of the medical director, who had insisted that neuroleptic dosage not exceed the neuroleptic "threshold" (Haase, 1980), that is, the therapeutic window between the occurrence of fine changes in handwriting (micrographia) and more marked neurological involvement. Because of increasing interest in low-dosage treatment, the neuroleptic-threshold concept has been revived in the United States (McEvoy, 1986), and Haase's work has been reviewed (Bitter, Volavka, & Scheurer, 1991).

Switzerland. Using their own rating scale for abnormal movements that incorporates severity grading and division by body region, Fleischhauer et al. (1985) surveyed 646 inpatients. Of the 608 inpatients examined, 29.8% of males and 32.9% of females had dyskinesia. Those authors found increasing age to be associated with higher rates of tardive dyskinesia. The same group of investigators (Kocher et al., 1986), in a 1-year follow-up study of the patients with dyskinesia, found reductions in severity: Whereas 22% of patients had been graded as having severe tardive dyskinesia on the first examination, only 8% were graded as severe at follow-up.

Austria

Miller et al. (1995) reported a 10-year follow-up study. The Skale für abnormal unwill kurliche Bewegungen (SKAUB) (Seeler & Kulhanek, 1980) was used. The investigators stated that it is a German equivalent of AIMS. There were 861 patients examined in 1982, with 270 still in hospital 10 years later. The prevalence rate for tardive dyskinesia was 3.2% in 1982 and 12.7% in 1992. The average daily dose of CPZE in 1982 and 1992 for men and women was between 140 and 170 mg. The major risk factor was found to be advanced age. In 1992, in the follow-up, the diagnoses were schizophrenia 40.2%, mental retardation 49.6%, and "other diagnoses" 10.2%. The low prevalence rate found in that study is surprising.

Great Britain and Ireland

From the 1960s up to the present, tardive dyskinesia has been a subject of continuing interest to psychiatrists in Great Britain and Ireland.

Evans (1965), a specialist in internal medicine, reported 4 cases of persistent dyskinesia in nonpsychotic patients on small dosages of trifluoperazine. Hunter, Earl, and Janz (1964a) reported gross facial dyskinesia, associated with dementia, in 3 leucotomized schizophrenic patients treated with phenothiazines. In passing, they commented that 7% of the leucotomized patients in their hospital had such facial movements. Hunter et al. (1964b) then surveyed 450 inpatients and found a dyskinesia rate of zero among 200 males and a 5% rate among 250 females, "most of whom had been given phenothazines

Table 21.1. *Prevalence studies, British Isles*

Investigators	Neuroleptic-treated patients				Patients not treated with neuroleptics			
	Both sexes	% with dyskinesia	Females only	% with dyskinesia	Both sexes	% with dyskinesia	Females only	% with dyskinesia
Hunter et al. (1964b)[a]	450	2.9	250	5.2	—	—	—	—
Demars (1966)[b]	372	7.0	205	8.8	117	6.8	—	—
Pryce & Edwards (1966)	—	—	121	23.1	—	—	—	—
Jones & Hunter (1969)	82	20.7	69	23.2	45	2.2	21	0
Kennedy et al. (1971)	63	41.3	31	58.0	—	—	—	—
Brandon et al. (1971)	625	24.5	361	30.5	285	19.3	123	9
Famuyiwa et al. (1979)	50	34.0	24	41.6	—	—	—	—
McCreadie et al. (1982)	117	31.0	?	?	—	—	—	—
Owens et al. (1982)	364	~63.0[d]	?	?	47	53.2	?	?
Waddington & Youssef (1985)	68	41.0	46	43.4	—	—	—	—
Waddington & Youssef (1986)[c]	51	16.0	19	~70[d] (>55 yr)	—	—	—	—

Note: These studies involved patients with functional psychoses, with the exceptions of the studies of Pryce and Edwards (1966), Jones and Hunter (1969), and Brandon et al. (1971), which included patients with organic diagnoses. Studies were conducted on inpatients, except for the McCreadie et al. (1982) study (conducted on both inpatients and outpatients), and the Waddington and Youssef studies (1985, 1986) (conducted on outpatients).
[a] Severe cases only.
[b] Mild cases excluded.
[c] AIMS score of 2 or more.
[d] Approximate figures are derived from authors' bar graphs.

288

at one time or another." Whereas all the dyskinetic patients were over 55 years of age and had received neuroleptics, 6 had had bilateral standard leucotomies. All were "demented" in terms of marked intellectual deterioration, as distinct from a schizophrenic-defect state. No other study has reported such a number of patients with clinically gross organic brain syndrome in association with dyskinesia and schizophrenia.

Over the two decades beginning in 1964, several studies of hospital inpatients (Table 21.1) were conducted in the United Kingdom. The early studies reported findings similar to those from other countries and helped establish basic markers for dyskinesia in psychiatric patients. Thus, dyskinesia was characterized as being more common among females than among males (Hunter, Earl, & Thornicroft, 1964b; Demars, 1966; Jones & Hunter, 1969; Brandon, McClelland, & Protheroe, 1971) and as increasing with age (Brandon et al., 1971; Owens, Johnstone, & Frith, 1982). Brain damage, as distinct from organic brain syndrome, was found to be associated significantly with tardive dyskinesia by both Edwards (1970) and Famuyiwa et al. (1979); the latter, however, found that impaired psychological functioning by dyskinetic patients was linked with cortical atrophy or dilated ventricles, as seen on brain scans. Owens (1985) reported that brain scans showed that those patients with severe dyskinesia had significantly larger ventricles. Apart from the study by Hunter et al. (1964b), no association between organic treatments (ECT, leucotomy, insulin coma) and dyskinesia has been demonstrated. Moreover, even when specifically looking for such linkage, most investigators have found no significant association between high neuroleptic dosages and dyskinesia, the exception being Pryce and Edwards (1966), who reported that high phenothiazine dosages were associated with dyskinesia. In contrast, Kennedy, Hershon, and McGuire (1971) found a low-dosage association with dyskinesia.

Two surveys (Demars, 1966; Brandon et al., 1971) found dyskinesia to be no more common among patients treated with neuroleptics than among those not so treated. Owens et al. (1982) reported the prevalences of abnormal movements to be very high (but not significantly different) among neuroleptic-treated and non-neuroleptic-treated populations. However, those investigators later reported significant differences in age-restricted subgroups (Crow et al., 1982; Owens, 1985).

Waddington and colleagues in Ireland, who have published extensive studies of tardive dyskinesia and chronic schizophrenia, have found tardive dyskinesia to be particularly common among patients with late-onset illness, as well as among elderly females, and to be associated with cognitive impairment. Their two studies (Waddington & Youssef, 1985, 1986) shown in

Table 21.1 were conducted on inpatient and outpatient cohorts of schizophrenics who met the Feighner diagnostic criteria (Feighner et al., 1972).

In a 3-year study of 99 patients (58 outpatients, 41 inpatients) receiving
antipsychotic medication, Barnes et al. (1983) found the point prevalence for
tardive dyskinesia to have increased from 39% to 47% during the follow-up
period. Of the original 39 patients with tardive dyskinesia, 25 were
unchanged, and 14 had gone into remission. A further 22 patients had developed the condition. Those authors noted that younger patients, under 50 years
of age, were more likely to go into remission. They also found that patients
receiving more than 1,000 mg/day (CPZE) were unlikely to develop tardive
dyskinesia, attributing that to the suppression of dyskinesia (covert dyskinesia).

Hunt and Silverstone (1991) studied 69 patients with bipolar affective
disorder consecutively admitted. All but one had been on neuroleptic treatment. The prevalence rate for tardive dyskinesia was 19%, and dyskinetic
patients were found to be significantly impaired, as compared with those
without dyskinesia, on a test of cognitive function. The prevalence increased
with age, age of onset, and number of past episodes. Such findings mirror
those found in schizophrenic patients.

Robinson and McCreadie (1986) reported on a 3.5-year follow-up study of
tardive dyskinesia among all schizophrenic patients (130) in the Nithsdale
area of Scotland, 17% of whom were in hospital. They used the AIMS,
having decided that for tardive dyskinesia to be diagnosed there would have to
be a rating of at least "mild" on the global item. After prevalence rates
reached 31% in 1981, 27% in 1982, and 30% in 1984, those authors suggested that the prevalence had reached a plateau, which was later confirmed
by the prevalence rate for the sample of 29% in 1989 (McCreadie et al.,
1992). Those authors emphasized that only 8% of patients showed persistent
dyskinesia, that is to say, dyskinesia present in all examinations. This confirms how tardive dyskinesia can fluctuate in severity and prevalence over
time. They found that worsening of dyskinesia over time was more common
in younger patients. That survey, with its high percentages of outpatients and
of patients with short durations of schizophrenia, might have been expected to
yield a low prevalence rate, as compared with long-term patients in the other
two follow-up studies (Barnes et al., 1983; McClelland et al., 1991).

A follow-up study in Newcastle, England (McClelland et al., 1991),
involving 99 females in an inpatient hospital survey (Brandon et al., 1971),
reported an increase in the prevalence rate from 18.4% to 46.5% over 16
years – a substantial increase, even allowing for age. Only 1 of 8 schizo-

phrenic patients who had never received neuroleptics developed mild dyskinesia. Moreover, 6 of the 14 patients with initial dyskinesia became dyskinesia-free by the time of follow-up. In addition, 48 patients remained free of dyskinesia in the follow-up period, but 37 patients developed tardive dyskinesia, 35 of whom had a mild form. Those authors found the neuroleptic items – "total duration," "increasing amounts," "total amount of neuroleptics" – to be significantly associated with the development of tardive dyskinesia. That study also showed, in common with others, that schizoaffective and affective patients had higher prevalences of tardive dyskinesia than did the schizophrenic cohort.

In summary, the Barnes and the McClelland studies point to a high plateau of about 45%, a figure similar to that found in an American study by Bell and Smith (1978). Moreover, the three follow-up British studies cited here confirm the fluctuating nature of tardive dyskinesia, indicating that the outlook can be good, rather than one of deterioration.

Conclusion

Research on tardive dyskinesia in different European countries has been patchy, with some countries making substantial contributions, and others providing little or no information. Precise comparisons between countries with regard to prevalence rates and risk factors are therefore impossible. Moreover, the use of different methods and research standards makes it unwise to draw general conclusions or to generate hypotheses. A true comparison of prevalence rates can be achieved only after we have standard rating scales and agreement on diagnostic criteria. Also needed is agreement on the methods of examination, perhaps including videotape recordings that could be rated by observers in different countries.

Nevertheless, there are indications that when the neuroleptic dosage is low, the prevalence rate will also be low. Furthermore, one can say that the more careful the study, the higher will be the prevalences of dyskinesia found among both neuroleptic-treated and non-neuroleptic-treated patients.

Because the point-prevalence studies discussed in this chapter had such variations in methods and findings, no conclusion can be drawn as to whether or not, as argued by Jeste and Wyatt (1982b), the prevalence of tardive dyskinesia is increasing. However, three follow-up studies (Barnes et al., 1983; Gardos et al., 1988; McClelland et al., 1991) consistently suggest increasing prevalence with continuation of antipsychotic medication, to a plateau of about 40%.

Acknowledgments

We thank Ms. Pamela McClelland for her help in the literature search, as well as for translations from French, Russian, and Spanish. We also thank Ms. Sarah Miller for translations from the German. Dr. Marc Domken gave unstintingly of his time in providing French textbooks and discussing French psychiatric concepts.

References

Altamura, A. C., Cavallaro, R., & Regazzetti, M. G. (1990). Prevalence and risk factors for tardive dyskinesia: a study in an Italian population of chronic schizophrenics. *Eur. Arch. Psychiatry Clin. Neurosci.* 240:9–12.

Appleton, W. S. (1982). Fourth psychoactive drug usage guide. *J. Clin. Psychiatry* 43:12–27.

Barnes, T. R. E., Kidger, T., & Gore, S. M. (1983). Tardive dyskinesia: a 3-year follow-up study. *Psychol. Med.* 13:71–81.

Bell, R. C. H., & Smith, R. C. (1978). Tardive dyskinesia: characterization and prevalences in a state-wide system. *J. Clin. Psychiatry* 39:39–47.

Bitter, I., Volavka, J., & Scheurer, J. (1991). The concept of the neuroleptic threshold: an update. *J. Clin. Psychopharmacol.* 11:28–32.

Bourgeois, M. (1988). Les dyskinésies tardives des neuroleptiques en France. *Encephale* 14:195–201.

Bourgeois, M., Boueilh, P., Peyre, C., & Gauthier-Bernard, F. (1977). Les dyskinésies tardives des neuroleptiques. Enquête complémentaire chez 1480 malades d'hôpital psychiatrique. *Ann. Med. Psychol. (Paris)* 1:660–79.

Bourgeois, M., Boueilh, P., & Tignol, J. (1980a). Dyskinésies tardives des neuroleptiques: enquête chez 270 veillards. *Encephale* 4:37–9.

Bourgeois, M., Boueilh, P., Tignol, J., & Yesavage, J. (1980b). Spontaneous dyskinesia versus neuroleptic-induced dystonias in 270 elderly subjects. *J. Nerv. Ment. Dis.* 168:177–8.

Bourgeois, M., Grau, C., & Arretche-Berthelot, N. (1976). Les dyskinésies tardives des neuroleptiques. Enquête sur 1660 malades d'hôpital psychiatrique. *Ann. Med. Psychol. (Paris)* 1:734–46.

Brandon, S., McClelland, H. A., & Protheroe, C. (1971). A study of facial dyskinesia in a mental hospital population. *Br. J. Psychiatry* 118:171–84.

Cavallaro, R., Regazzetti, M. G., Mundo, E., Brancato, V., & Smeraldi, E. (1993). Tardive dyskinesia outcomes: clinical and pharmacological correlates of remission and persistence. *Neuropsychopharmacology* 8:233–9.

Chatterjee, A., Chakos, M., Koreen, A., Geisler, S., Sheitman, B., Woerner, M., Kane, J. M., Alvir, J., & Lieberman, J. A. (1995). Relevance and clinical correlates of extra-pyramidal signs and spontaneous dyskinesia in never-medicated schizophrenic patients. *Am. J. Psychiatry* 152:1724–9.

Chiu, H., Shum, P., Lau, J., Lam, L., & Lee, S. (1992). Prevalence of tardive dyskinesia, tardive dystonia and respiratory dyskinesia among Chinese psychiatric patients in Hong Kong. *Am. J. Psychiatry* 149:1081–5.

Crow, T. J., Cross, A. J., Johnstone, E. C., Owen, F., Owens, D. G. C., & Waddington, J. L. (1982). Abnormal involuntary movements in schizophrenia:

Are they related to its disease process or its treatment? Are they associated with changes in dopamine receptors? *J. Clin. Psychopharmacol.* 2:336–40.

Degkwitz, R., Binsack, K. F., Herkert, H., Luxenburger, O., & Wenzel, W. (1967a). Zum problem der persistierenden extrapyramidalen Hyperkinesen nach langfristiger Anwendung von Neuroleptika. *Nervenarzt* 38:170–4.

Degkwitz, R., & Wenzel, W. (1967b). Persistent extrapyramidal side effects after long-term application of neuroleptics. In *Neuropsychopharmacology*, ed. H. Brill et al., pp. 608–15. International congress series no. 129. Amsterdam: Excerpta Medica.

Delwaide, P. J., & Desseilles, M. (1977). Spontaneous buccolinguofacial dyskinesia in the elderly. *Acta Neurol. Scand.* 56:256–62.

Deniker, P. (1960). Experimental neurological syndromes and the new drug therapies in psychiatry. *Compr. Psychiatry* 1:92–102.

Demars, J. C. A. (1966). Neuromuscular effects of long-term phenothiazine medication, electroconvulsive therapy and leucotomy. *J. Nerv. Ment. Dis.* 143:73–9.

Doongaji, D. R., Jeste, D. V., Jape, N. M., Sheth, A. S., Apte, J. S., Vahia, V. N., Desai, A. B., Vahora, S. A., Thatte, S., Vevaina, T., & Bharadwaj, J. (1982). Tardive dyskinesia in India: a prevalence study. *J. Clin. Psychopharmacol.* 2:341–4.

Eckmann, F. (1968). Zur Problematik von Dauerschaden nach neuroleptischer Langzeitbehandlung. *Therapie der Gegenwart* 107:316–23.

Edwards, H. (1970). The significance of brain damage in persistent oral dyskinesia. *Br. J. Psychiatry* 116:271–5.

Eldridge, R. (1970). The torsion dystonias: literature review and genetic and clinical studies. *Neurology* 20:1–78.

Evans, J. H. (1965). Persistent oral dyskinesia in treatment with phenothiazine derivatives. *Lancet* 1:458–60.

Famuyiwa, O. O., Eccleston, D., Donaldson, A. A., & Garside, R. F. (1979). Tardive dyskinesia and dementia. *Br. J. Psychiatry* 135:500–4.

Fanget, F., Henry, E., & Aimard, G. (1986). Incidence des dyskinésies tardives sous traitment neuroleptique. *Presse Med.* 15:2147–50.

Faurbye, A., Rasch, P.-J., Bender Petersen, P., Brandborg, G., & Pakkenberg, H. (1964). Neurological symptoms in pharmacotherapy of psychoses. *Acta Psychiatr. Scand.* 40:10–27.

Feighner, J. P., Robins, E., Guze, S. B., Woodruff, R. A., Winokur, G., & Munoz, R. (1972). Diagnostic criteria for use in psychiatric research. *Arch. Gen. Psychiatry* 26:57–63.

Fenton, W. S., Wyatt, R. J., McGlashan, T. J. (1994). Risk factors for spontaneous dyskinesias in schizophrenia. *Arch. Gen. Psychiatry* 51:643–50.

Fleischhauer, J., Kocher, R., Hobi, V., & Gilsdorf, U. (1985). Prevalence of tardive dyskinesia in a clinic population. In *Dyskinesia – Research and Treatment*, ed. D. E. Casey et al., pp. 162–72. Berlin: Springer-Verlag.

Flugel, F. (1956). Therapeutique par médication neuroleptique obtenue en réalisant systematiquement des états parkinsoniformes. *Encephale* 45: 790–2.

Fombonne, E., Mousson, F., Dassonville, B., Bost, P.-J., Jaeger, M., Roques, N., & Swain, G. (1989). Etude des préscriptions de médicaments psychotropes dan un hôpital psychiatrique français. *Rev. Epidemiol. Sante Publique* 37:29–36.

Gardos, G., Casey, D. E., Cole, J. O., Peréneyi, A., Koosis, E., Arato, M., Samson, J. A., & Conley, C. (1994). Ten year outcome of tardive dyskinesia. *Am. J. Psychiatry* 151:836–41.

Gardos, G., Perényi, A., Cole, J. O., Samu, I., Kocsis, E., & Casey, D. E. (1988). Seven-year follow-up of tardive dyskinesia in Hungarian out-patients. *Neuropsychopharmacology* 1:169–72.

Gardos, G., Samu, I., Kallos, M., & Cole, J. O. (1980). Absence of severe tardive dyskinesia in Hungarian schizophrenic out-patients. *Psychopharmacology* 71:29–34.

Gibson, A. C. (1978). Depot injections and tardive dyskinesia. *Br. J. Psychiatry* 132:361–5.

Gomez-Feria Prieto, I. (1989). Epidmiolgia y factores de riesgo en la diskinesia tardia. *Ann. Psiquiatria (Madrid)* 5:154–60.

Grimes, J.-D., Hessan, M. N., & Preston, D. N. (1982). Adverse neuralgic effects of metoclopramide. *Can. Med. Assoc. J.* 120:23–5.

Grimsson, A., Idanpaan-Heikkila, J., Lunde, P. K. M., Olafsson, O., & Westerholm, B. (1979). The utilisation of psychotropic drugs in Finland, Iceland, Norway and Sweden. In *Studies in Drug Utilisation*, WHO regional publications series no. 8. Copenhagen: World Health Organization.

Haase, H.-J. (1980). Dosierung der Neuroleptika. *Munchener Medizinische Wochenschrift* 122:1808–13.

Heinrich, K., Wegener, I., & Bender, H.-J. (1968). Spate extrapyramidale Hyperkinesen bei neuroleptischer Langzeittherapie. *Pharmakopsychiatr. Neuropsychopharmakol.* 1:169–95.

Hippius, H. Von, & Lange, J. (1970). Zur Problematik der spaten extrapyramidalen Hyperkinesen nach langfristiger neuroleptischer Therapie. *Arzneimittelforschung* 20:888–90.

Hoff, V. H., & Hoffmann, G. (1967). Das persistierende extrapyramidale Syndrom bei Neuroleptikatherapie. *Wien. Med. Wochenschr.* 117:14–17.

Hunt, N., & Silverstone, T. (1991). Tardive dyskinesia in bipolar affective disorder: a catchment area study. *Int. Clin. Psychopharmacol.* 6:45–50.

Hunter, R., Earl, C. J., & Janz, D. (1964a). A syndrome of abnormal movements and dementia in leucotomized patients treated with phenothiazines. *J. Neurol. Neurosurg. Psychiatry* 27:219–23.

Hunter, R., Earl, C. J., & Thornicroft, S. (1964b). An apparently irreversible syndrome of abnormal movements following phenothiazine medication. *Proc. R. Soc. Med.* 57:758–62.

Jeste, D. V., & Wyatt, R. J. (1982a). *Understanding and Treating Tardive Dyskinesia.* New York: Guilford Press.

Jeste, D. V., & Wyatt, R. J. (1982b). Changing epidemiology of tardive dyskinesia: an overview. *Am. J. Psychiatry* 138:297–308.

Johnson, D. A. W., Ludlow, J. M., Street, K., & Taylor, R. D. W. (1987). Double blind comparison of half-dose and standard-dose flupenthixol decanoate in the maintenance treatment of stabilised outpatients with schizophrenia. *Br. J. Psychiatry* 151:634–8.

Jolley, A. G., Hirsch, S. R., McRink, A., & Manchanda, R. (1989). Trial of brief intermittent neuroleptic prophylaxis for selected schizophrenic out-patients: clinical outcome at one year. *Br. Med. J.* 298:985–90.

Jones, M., & Hunter, R. (1969). Abnormal movements in chronic psychiatric illness. In *Psychotropic Drugs and Dysfunctions of the Basal Ganglia*, ed. G. E. Gardner & R. Gardner, Jr., pp. 53–9. U.S. Public Health Service publication no. 1938. Washington, DC: U.S. Government Printing Office.

Jus, A., Villeneuve, J., Gautier, J., Jus, K., Villeneuve, C., Pires, P., & Villeneuve, R. (1978). Deanol, lithium and placebo in the treatment of tardive dyskinesia. *Neuropsychobiology* 4:140–9.

Kane, J. M., & Smith, J. M. (1982). Tardive dyskinesia: prevalence and risk factors. *Arch. Gen. Psychiatry* 39:473–81.

Kane, J. M., Weinhold, P., Kinan, B., Wegner, J., & Leader, M. (1982). Prevalence of abnormal involuntary movements ("spontaneous dyskinesias") in the normal elderly. *Psychopharmacology* 77:105–8.

Katabia, M., Traube, M., & Marsden, C. D. (1978). Extra-pyramidal effects of metoclopramide. *Lancet* 2:1254–5.

Kennedy, P. F., Hershon, H. I., & McGuire, R. J. (1971). Extrapyramidal disorders after prolonged phenothiazine. *Br. J. Psychiatry* 118:509–18.

Kocher, R., Fleischhauer, J., Hobi, V., & Gilsdorf, U. (1986). Dyskinesien in einer klinischeen Population: Ergebnisse einer Nachuntersuchung im Vergleich. *Schweizer Arch. Neurol. Neurochirurg. Psychiatr.* 137:63–78.

Koller, W. C. (1982). Edentulous orodyskinesia. *Ann. Neurol.* 13:97–9.

Lavy, S., Melamed, E., & Penchas, S. (1978). Tardive dyskinesia associated with metoclopramide. *Br. Med. J.* 1:77–8.

Lerner, V. E. (1988). Tardive dyskinesia (review of the literature). *Zh. Nevropatol. Psikhiatr. (Moskva)* 88:124–32.

McClelland, H. A., Metcalfe, A. V., Kerr, T. A., Dutta, D., & Watson, P. (1991). Facial dyskinesia: a 16-year follow-up study. *Br. J. Psychiatry* 158–691–6.

McCreadie, R. G., Barron, E. T., & Winslow, G. J. (1982). The Nithsdale survey. II. Abnormal movements. *Br. J. Psychiatry* 140:587–90.

McCreadie, R. G., & Ohaeri, J. (1994). Movement disorders in never and minimally-treated Nigerian schizophrenic patients. *Br. J. Psychiatry* 164:184–9.

McCreadie, R. G., Robertson, L. J., & Wiles, D. H. (1992). The Nithsdale schizophrenia survey. IX. Akathisia, Parkinsonism, tardive dyskinesia and plasma neuroleptic levels. *Br. J. Psychiatry* 161:793–9.

McCreadie, R. G., Thara, R., Kamath, S., Padmarathy, R., Latha, S., Mathrubootham, N., & Menon, M. S. (1996). Abnormal movements in never-medicated Indian patients with schizophrenia. *Br. J. Psychiatry* 168:221–6.

McEvoy, J. P. (1986). The neuroleptic threshold as a marker of minimum effective neuroleptic dose. *Comp. Psychiatry* 27:327–35.

Maurel, H., Ruel, M., & Kabare, A. (1966). Les dyskinésies prolongées induites par les médicaments neuroleptiques. In *IVe Congrès Mondial de Psychiatrie,* pp. 2258–9. Amsterdam: Excerpta Medica.

Miller, C. H., Simian, I., Oberbauer, H., Schwitzer, J., Barnas, C., Kulhanek, F., Baissel, K. E., Meise, U., Hinterhuber, H., & Fleischhacker, W. W. (1995). Tardive dyskinesia prevalence rates during a ten year follow-up. *J. Nerv. Ment. Dis.* 183:404–7.

Morgenstern, H., Glazer, W. M., Niedzweicki, D., & Noorjah, P. (1987). The impact of neuroleptic medication on tardive dyskinesia: a meta-analysis of published studies. *Am. J. Public Health* 77:717–24.

Muscettola, G., Pampallona, S., Barbato, G., Casiello, M., & Bollini, P. (1993). Persistent tardive dyskinesia: demographic and pharmacological risk factors. *Acta Psychiatr. Scand.* 87:29–36.

Myrianthopoulos, N. C., Kurland, A. A., & Kurland, T. (1962). Hereditary predisposition in drug-induced parkinsonism. *Arch. Neurol.* 6:19–23.

Ogita, K., Yagi, G., & Itoh, H. (1975). Comparative analysis of persistent dyskinesias of long-term usage with neuroleptics in France and Japan. *Folia Psychiatrica et Neurologica* 29:315–20.
Owens, D. G. C. (1985). Involuntary disorders of movements in chronic schizophrenia. In *Dyskinesia – Research and Treatment*, ed. D. E. Casey et al., pp. 79–87. Berlin: Springer-Verlag.
Owens, D. G. C., Johnstone, E. C., & Frith, C. D. (1982). Spontaneous involuntary disorders of movement. *Arch. Gen. Psychiatry* 39:452–61.
Perényi, A., & Arato, M. (1980). Tardive dyskinesia on Hungarian psychiatric wards. *Psychosomatics* 21:904–9.
Perris, C., Predrag, D., Jacobssorg, L., Paulsson, P., Rapp, W., & Froberg, H. (1979). Tardive dyskinesia treated with neuroleptics. *Br. J. Psychiatry* 135:509–14.
Pryce, I.-G., & Edwards, H. (1966). Persistent oral dyskinesia in female mental hospital patients. *Br. J. Psychiatry* 112:983–7.
Reardon, G. T., Rifkin, A., Schwartz, A., Myerson, A., & Siris, S. G. (1989). Changing patterns of neuroleptic dosage over a decade. *Am. J. Psychiatry* 146:726–9.
Robinson, A. D. T., & McCreadie, R. G. (1986). The Nithsdale schizophrenic survey. V. Follow-up of tardive dyskinesia at three and a half years. *Br. J. Psychiatry* 149:621–3.
Schmidt, L. G., Niemeyer, R., & Muller-Oerlinghausen, B. (1983). Drug prescribing pattern of a psychiatric university hospital in Germany. *Pharmacopsychiatria* 16:35–42.
Schonecker, M. (1957). Ein eigentumliches Syndrom im oralem Bereich bei Megaphen Applikation. *Nervenarzt.* 28:35.
Schooler, N. R., & Kane, J. M. (1982). Research diagnoses for tardive dyskinesia. *Arch. Gen. Psychiatry* 39:486–7.
Seeler, W., & Kulhanek, F. (1980). *Späte extrapyramidale* Hyperkinesien. München: Schwarzeck Verlag.
Sigwald, J., Bouttier, D., Raymondeaud, C., & Piot, C. (1959). Quatre cas de dyskinésie facio-bucco-linguo-mastricatrice à évolution prolongée secondaire à un traitement par les neuroleptiques. *Rev. Neurol.* 100:751–5.
Sramek, J., Roy, S., Ahrens, T., Pinanong, P., Cutler, N. R., & Pi, E. (1991). Prevalence of tardive dyskinesia among three ethnic groups of chronic psychiatric patients. *Hosp. Commun. Psychiatry* 42:590–2.
Tan, C. H., & Tay, L. K. (1991). Tardive dyskinesia in elderly psychiatric patients in Singapore. *Aust. N.Z. J. Psychiatry* 25:119–22.
Ticehurst, S. B. (1990). Is spontaneous orofacial dyskinesia an artifact due to incomplete drug history? *J. Geriatr. Psychiatry Neurol.* 3:208–11.
Topiar, A., & Kanczucka, A. (1975). Dosage of neuroleptic drugs for schizophrenic patients. (analysis of hospital cases in the psychiatric hospital during 1969–1973). *Activitas Nervosa Superior (Praha)* 17:203–4.
Uhrbrand, L., & Faurbye, A. (1960). Reversible and irreversible dyskinesia after treatment with perphenazine, chlorpromazine, reserpine and electroconvulsive therapy. *Psychopharmacologia* 1:408–18.
Varela Guzman, M., Tapia Villanueva, L., & La Roche Olsen, P. (1984). Prevalencia de discinesia tardia en pacientes psiquiatricos cronicos hospitalizados. *Actas Luso Esp. Neurol. Psiquiatr. Cienc. Afines* 12:259–66.
Waddington, J. L. (1989). Schizophrenia, affective psychoses, and other disorders treated with neuroleptic drugs: the enigma of tardive dyskinesia, its neuro-

biological determinants, and the conflict of paradigms. *Int. Rev. Neurobiol.* 31:297–353.

Waddington, J. L., & Youssef, H. A. (1985). Late onset involuntary movements in chronic schizophrenia: age-related vulnerability to "tardive" dyskinesia independent of extent of neuroleptic medication. *Ir. Med. J.* 78:143–6.

Waddington, J., & Youssef, H. (1986). Involuntary movements and cognitive dysfunction in late onset schizophrenic out-patients. *Ir. Med. J.* 79:347–50.

Waddington, J., & Youssef, H. (1988). The expression of schizophrenia, affective disorder and vulnerability to tardive dyskinesia in an extensive pedigree. *Br. J. Psychiatry* 153:176–81.

Weinhold, P., Wegner, J., & Kane, J. (1981). Familial occurrence of tardive dyskinesia. *J. Clin. Psychiatry* 42:165–6.

Wiholm, B.-E., Mortimar, O., Boethius, G., & Häggström, J. E. (1984). Tardive dyskinesia associated with metoclopramide. *Br. Med. J.* 288:545–7.

Woerner, M. G., Kane, J. M., Lieberman, J. A., Alvir, J., Bergmann, K. J., Borenstein, M., Schooler, N. R., Mukherjee, S., Rotrosen, J., Morton, R., & Basavaraju, N. (1991). The prevalence of tardive dyskinesia. *J. Clin. Psychopharmacol.* 11:34–42.

Yassa, R. L., & Ananth, J. (1981). Familial tardive dyskinesia. *Am. J. Psychiatry* 138:1618–19.

Yassa, R. L., & Nair, V. (1989). Mild tardive dyskinesia: an 8-year follow-up study. *Acta Psychiatr. Scand.* 81:139–40.

Youssef, H., Lyster, G., & Youssef, F. (1989). Familial psychosis and vulnerability to tardive dyskinesia. *Int. Clin. Psychopharmacol.* 4:323–8.

22

Role of Ethnicity in the Development of Tardive Dyskinesia

JONATHAN P. LACRO, Pharm.D., and
DILIP V. JESTE, M.D.

Since the first published report of tardive dyskinesia (Schonecker, 1957), numerous investigators have contributed to our understanding of the epidemiology and risk factors associated with this condition. In terms of numbers, such reports have noted that tardive dyskinesia is present at any given time in approximately 24% of patients treated with neuroleptics (Jeste & Caligiuri, 1993). As for risk factors, investigators have repeatedly associated older age with increased risk for tardive dyskinesia. Other reported factors, although less consistently associated with increased risk for tardive dyskinesia, include female gender, a psychiatric diagnosis involving affective features, early extrapyramidal symptoms, organic brain damage, and higher dosages and longer durations of neuroleptic treatment (Kane et al., 1992). Although considerable progress has been made in recent years through studies that have provided better estimates of the incidence of tardive dyskinesia and more meaningful data concerning the risk factors for tardive dyskinesia, relatively few have focused on the role of ethnicity as a risk factor (Pi, Gutierrez, & Gray, 1993).

In this chapter, we briefly review the relationship between ethnicity and tardive dyskinesia and present findings from our own study. We look at ethnicity vis-à-vis the presence of tardive dyskinesia, diagnosis of psychosis, neuroleptic dosage, and pharmacogenetics; we examine ethnic differences in terms of pharmacokinetics and pharmacodynamics; we look at a prospective study of the incidence of neuroleptic-induced tardive dyskinesia; and, finally, we offer suggestions for future research.

Ethnicity and Tardive Dyskinesia

There is limited evidence of differences in the prevalence of tardive dyskinesia among ethnic groups. Yassa and Jeste (1992), in a recent review of 76 selected studies of the prevalence of tardive dyskinesia published through 1989, with a combined total of 39,187 patients, found prevalence rates ranging from 3% to 62% (average 24.2%). That review, looking for potential cultural/environmental differences, grouped the reports according to their origin in one of four continents: North America, Europe, Africa, and Asia. It was reported that patients from Asia seemed to have a lower prevalence of tardive dyskinesia (16.6%) than did those from North America (27.6%), Europe (21.5%), and Africa (25.5%). Although that review acknowledged the problems of grouping studies from different countries into single continental collections, several reasons were suggested for the differences in the reported rates of prevalence, including ethnicity and variations in practices of prescribing neuroleptics.

Several other reports in the literature have supported the notion of decreased prevalences of tardive dyskinesia in Asian countries. For example, Ko et al. (1989), in an investigation of the prevalence of tardive dyskinesia at the Shanghai Psychiatric Hospital, in the People's Republic of China, found that only 73 (8.4%) of the 866 neuroleptic-treated schizophrenic patients examined had been diagnosed as having tardive dyskinesia. Those authors suggested that the low prevalence rate might be related to the use of relatively low dosages of neuroleptics: The mean ($\pm$SD) daily neuroleptic dose for the entire patient sample had been 311.3 $\pm$ 254 mg, chlorpromazine equivalent (CPZE). A study by Chiu et al. (1992) surveyed 917 Chinese inpatients in Hong Kong and also found a relatively low prevalence (9.3%) of tardive dyskinesia, although the mean ($\pm$SD) daily neuroleptic dose (CPZE) of 876.3 $\pm$ 853.1 mg was twice that reported for the population studied by Ko et al. (1989).

Other investigators, however, have reported contrary findings with regard to any decreased prevalence of tardive dyskinesia among Asian populations. Binder et al. (1987), in an examination of 126 randomly selected patients from six psychiatric hospitals in Tokyo and Osaka, Japan, found that 20.6% had at least mild tardive dyskinesia. Pi et al. (1990, 1993), in a multinational tardive dyskinesia study of Asians in China (Beijing, Yanji, and Hong Kong), Korea (Seoul), and Japan (Tottori), found an overall prevalence of 17.2%. Subsequent multiple-logistic-regression analysis revealed that the odds of being diagnosed as having tardive dyskinesia were 1.9–2.9 times greater for patients outside Beijing, as compared with those inside Beijing. Although Beijing's 8.2% prevalence rate for tardive dyskinesia resembled the rates in both the Shanghai (Ko et al., 1989) and Hong Kong (Chiu et al., 1992) studies, the prevalences of tardive dyskinesia were found to be 15.8% for the Koreans in Seoul, 20.3% for the Koreans in Yanji, 19.4% for the Chinese in

Hong Kong, and 18.6% for the Chinese in Yanji. Given the significant differences in the prevalences of tardive dyskinesia among those different sites with the same ethnic groups (e.g., Koreans in Korea and Koreans in China), as well as the similarities in the prevalences of tardive dyskinesia between different ethnic groups at the same site (Chinese and Korean patients in Yanji, China), those authors concluded that environmental factors might be more important predictors of the risk for tardive dyskinesia than are racial and genetic factors.

Contradictory findings were reported in two multiethnicity studies conducted in the United States. Sramek et al. (1991), in a survey of 491 long-term psychiatric patients at a large state psychiatric hospital in California, found no significant differences in the prevalence of tardive dyskinesia among three ethnic groups: African-Americans (17%), Caucasians (18.9%), and Hispanics (15.2%). On the other hand, Morgenstern and Glazer (1993) reported that nonwhite patients (mostly African-Americans) were nearly twice as likely to develop tardive dyskinesia as were Caucasian patients. Each of those multiethnicity studies used a single site for selection of patients.

Were there ethnic differences in the prevalences of tardive dyskinesia in the studies just discussed? It is not clear that the suggestion of a lower risk among Asians and a higher risk among African-Americans is indeed valid. In future tardive dyskinesia studies, investigators should control for the possible effects of race.

Ethnicity and Diagnosis of Psychosis

In any investigation of the relationship between ethnicity and diagnosis, the question arises whether or not non-Caucasian patients are discriminated against during the diagnosis of psychotic disorders. Several issues warrant consideration. The first concerns the rates of use of mental-health services. For example, some reports indicate that Mexican-Americans use mental-health services proportionately less than Anglos (Hough et al., 1987), that Asians tend not to seek psychiatric treatment until illness becomes severe (Sue & Sue, 1987), and that African-Americans living in the United States do not use mental-health services at the same rate as Caucasians for similar psychiatric problems (Neighbors, 1985). Clearly, epidemiologic studies of psychotic disorders should take into account the discrepancies attributed to underuse or overuse of mental-health services.

The second issue relates to possible racial discrimination. Lindsey and Paul (1989) have contended that African-American patients are overrepresented among admissions to public institutions and that such a pattern is related to their lower socioeconomic status and to institutional racial bias. For example, Dunn and Fahy (1990), in a study of black versus white or Afro-Caribbean versus Caucasian patients admitted to a psychiatric hospital under police escort, found that the former were more likely to receive a diagnosis of schizophrenia and drug-induced psychosis than were the latter. In addition, studies using standardized diagnostic instruments have identified Afro-Caribbean patients as having higher rates of schizophrenia than the general population (Harrison et al., 1988).

The whole issue of psychiatric diagnosis is critical to investigations of tardive dyskinesia. One concern is whether or not, because psychotic diagnoses have been associated with higher medication usage (Flaskerud & Hu, 1992), neuroleptics are being administered more frequently to the African-American population than to the Caucasian population. Such increased exposure to neuroleptics presumably would increase the former group's risk for development of tardive dyskinesia.

Ethnicity and Neuroleptic Dosage

Strickland et al. (1991), in a recent review of neuroleptic use in the African-American population, stated that "black patients tend to receive substantially higher doses of neuroleptics." Those authors attributed that pattern, at least partially, to clinical biases and misdiagnoses. Adams, Dworkin, and Rosenberg (1984), in an examination of pharmacologic treatment and ethnicity, started with the premise that the data for Hispanics would be found to differ from those for Anglos and African-Americans. Using clinical data from 980 ambulatory patients treated with oral neuroleptics at five public mental-health clinics in Houston, those authors attempted to determine whether or not the amounts of neuroleptics prescribed differed by ethnic group. They converted the prescribed neuroleptic doses to CPZE values and found that the mean ($\pm$SD) daily dose of antipsychotic medication given to African-Americans (539.19 $\pm$ 830.46 mg) was somewhat higher than those given to Hispanics (430.17 $\pm$ 616.82 mg) and to Anglos (431.17 $\pm$ 611.17 mg). However, using ANOVA techniques, they found that ethnicity was not a significant main effect; the only significant main effect was diagnosis. In other words, considerably higher proportions of African-Americans were being diagnosed as having schizophrenia, as compared with Hispanics and Anglos. Similarly, Sramek et al. (1991) found no significant differences in the daily neuroleptic doses prescribed to African-Americans (2,173 $\pm$ 1,954 mg), Hispanics (1,785 $\pm$ 1,708), and Caucasians (1,701 $\pm$ 1,721) in their multiethnicity prevalence study described earlier in this chapter.

Whereas some clinical investigators have suggested that Asian patients generally respond to substantially lower dosages of neuroleptics than do Caucasians (Lin & Finder, 1983), others have not found that to be the case (Sramek, Sayles, & Simpson, 1986). Lin and Finder (1983) compared neuroleptic dosages for 26 patients (13 Asian and 13 Caucasian) matched for age, gender, diagnosis, and time of discharge. Neuroleptic dosages were converted to CPZE units for comparison and were corrected for weight, using 68 kg as the standard. Significant differences in both the maximum and stabilized CPZE doses (1,066 and 827 mg/day for the Asian group, and 2,205 and 1,568 mg/day for the Caucasians) were found. However, Sramek et al. (1986), using similar methods in a retrospective chart review of 30 Asian and 30 matched Caucasian patients, failed to replicate those findings. Only small, statistically nonsignificant differences between Asians and Caucasians were found, whether for maximum neuroleptic dose (1,314 mg versus 1,421 mg) or stabilized dose (726 mg versus 966 mg).

In general, the data reported have been inconsistent with respect to side effects and neuroleptic dosing for Hispanic and Native American populations. The reader is referred to Mendoza et al. (1991) for a review of that literature.

Clinical biases and misdiagnoses can only partially solve the controversy surrounding ethnicity and neuroleptic dosage, whether prescribed or required. Some discrepancies, however, may be related to pharmacogenetics, pharmacokinetics, and pharmacodynamics. For example, some dramatic ethnic differences in responses to drugs have been reported in the literature (Kalow, 1990), and increasing numbers of investigators are designing pharmacokinetic and pharmacodynamic studies to explore the biological mechanisms that might be responsible for such differences. Many such studies have involved Asian versus Caucasian comparisons. In the following two sections, we briefly review the roles of ethnicity in pharmacogenetics, pharmacokinetics, and pharmacodynamics.

Ethnicity and Pharmacogenetics

Drug-metabolizing enzymes are of paramount importance in drug disposition. The cytochrome P-450 isozyme P450IID6 debrisoquine hydroxylase has been shown to be responsible for the metabolism of several neuroleptic medications, including chlorpromazine, perphenazine, thioridazine, and the metabolite of haloperidol (reduced haloperidol) (Eichelbaum & Gross, 1990; Llerena et al., 1992). Thus, genetically determined differences in the activity of this enzyme will influence drug dispositions (plasma concentrations) and therefore responses (therapeutic, as well as adverse) in patients treated with neuroleptic medications.

During routine pharmacokinetic studies, Mahgoub et al. (1977) discovered the polymorphic oxidative metabolism of debrisoquine. They found that certain individuals were unable to metabolize debrisoquine in the same manner as others. Those individuals accumulated excessively high plasma concentrations of the parent compound and therefore experienced more side effects. Familial studies demonstrated that impairment of the ability to metabolize debrisoquine is inherited in a Mendelian manner, as an autosomal-recessive trait (Price Evans et al., 1980). The prevalence of poor metabolizers and extensive metabolizers of debrisoquine has since been investigated, using a number of probe drugs and various ethnic groups (Eichelbaum & Gross, 1990). In particular, probe drugs such as antipyrine, debrisoquine, sparteine, dextromethorphan, and mephenytoin have been used over the past decade to study the polymorphism of the cytochrome P-450 isozyme P450IID6 debrisoquine hydroxylase.

The proportion of poor metabolizers of debrisoquine has been found to be extremely low (0–0.7%) among the Japanese (Nakamura et al., 1985; Horai et al., 1989) and the Chinese (Lou et al., 1987; Horai et al., 1989). Among different Caucasian populations, some 6–10% are poor metabolizers. Because such studies have yielded conflicting data, the clinical significance of this enzyme deficiency in the field of psychopharmacology is still largely unexplored.

Two factors determine the clinical importance of the rate of metabolism. First, is the medication under investigation actually metabolized by debrisoquine hydroxylase? Second, is the activity of the medication dependent on active metabolites? Answers to those questions will reveal whether or not poor metabolizers accumulate higher plasma concentrations of parent neuroleptic compounds. In the case of haloperidol, reduction of the benzylic ketone group of haloperidol forms the metabolite called "reduced haloperidol" (Froemming et al., 1989). Several investigators have reported quite substantial in vivo and in vitro conversions of the metabolite (reduced haloperidol) back to the parent compound (haloperidol) (Jann, Lam, & Chang, 1990; Chang, Lin, & Jann, 1991). Thus, reduced haloperidol can act as a pro-drug or reservoir of haloperidol. But the reoxidation of reduced haloperidol to haloperidol is mediated, at least partly, by debrisoquine hydroxylase (Tyndale, Kalow, & Inaba, 1991). Thus, decreased reconversion of the metabolite back to the parent compound would be expected with poor metabolizers.

Ethnic Differences in Pharmacokinetics and Pharmacodynamics

A number of the pharmacokinetic and pharmacodynamic studies of ethnicity and neuroleptics have compared Asian and Caucasian groups. Lin et al. (1988) demonstrated clear-cut pharmacokinetic and pharmacodynamic differences between Asians (foreign and American-born) and Caucasians in terms of plasma concentrations of haloperidol, as well as haloperidol-induced increases in plasma concentrations of prolactin. On two separate days they randomly administered haloperidol (either 1.0 mg orally or 0.5 mg intramuscularly) to physically healthy, normal volunteers. Analysis revealed significantly higher mean serum concentrations of haloperidol and prolactin in the Asians after either an oral or an intramuscular dose of haloperidol. Given that those findings remained statistically significant after controlling for body surface area, they represent a pharmacokinetic difference. Also, after differences in plasma concentrations of haloperidol were accounted for, the prolactin response was found to be significantly greater in the Asians – potentially representing increased sensitivity of the tuberoinfundibular dopamine system to pituitary dopamine-receptor blockade.

Lin et al. (1989) systematically examined these issues, using 13 Caucasian and 16 Asian schizophrenic patients. During the initial fixed-dosage phase (0.15 mg per kilogram of body weight per day), the difference in the average haloperidol concentrations did not reach statistical significance. The Asians, however, had significantly higher ratings for extrapyramidal symptoms. During the variable-dosage phase (clinically adjusted according to the patient's clinical condition), the serum concentrations of haloperidol were lower in the Asians than in the Caucasians, although the side-effect profiles were strikingly similar. That later work of Lin et al. (1989) thus confirms the increased-sensitivity phenomenon and argues against a pharmacokinetic difference in the pharmacology of neuroleptics in Asians and Caucasians. The limitations of neuroleptic plasma concentrations need to be kept in mind, however, when interpreting pharmacokinetic studies (Marder, Davis, & Janicak, 1993).

Our Study of the Risk for Tardive Dyskinesia Among Patients Over Age 45

For some time we have been studying the incidence of tardive dyskinesia and the risk factors for tardive dyskinesia among psychiatric outpatients over the age of 45 years. Our overall results from earlier data analyses have already been published (Harris et al., 1992; Jeste & Caligiuri, 1993; Jeste et al., 1993;

Lacro et al., 1994; Jest et al., 1995). We therefore report here on a comparative study of Caucasian and non-Caucasian patients (a majority being African-Americans) in terms of risk for tardive dyskinesia, cumulative neuroleptic exposure, and average neuroleptic dosage.

Methods

The patients were enrolled in this study early in the course of their neuroleptic treatment (70% had experienced less than 90 days of lifetime treatment with neuroleptics when they entered the study). Patients were treated with the lowest effective dosages of neuroleptics (commonly haloperidol or thioridazine). All patients received comprehensive psychiatric, neurological, medical, and neuropsychological evaluations at study entry. In addition, they were assessed for psychopathology, cognitive impairment, and movement disorders at study entry, at 1 month, at 3 months, and every 3 months thereafter. The diagnosis of tardive dyskinesia was based on the criteria of Schooler and Kane (1982), except that the minimum duration of neuroleptic treatment was 1 month instead of 3 months. Details of the evaluation and treatment have been described elsewhere (Harris et al., 1992; Jeste & Caligiuri, 1993; Jeste et al., 1993; Lacro et al., 1994).

Results

Of the 266 patients we have studied to date, 81.5% have been men, and 81.9% have been Caucasian. The mean age for our patients was 66 years (SD = 12 years). The cumulative proportion developing tardive dyskinesia after 12 months of study and treatment (i.e., the total number of patients who manifested tardive dyskinesia for the first time during the 12-month study period) was 26.1% (95% confidence interval, 19.3–32.9%), using actuarial life-tables analysis (Cutler & Ederer, 1958). To assess the role of ethnicity in our study subjects, we compared data for Caucasians and non-Caucasians (52% African-Americans, 31% Hispanics, 17% others) (Table 22.1). The groups were similar in terms of psychopathologic severity at baseline, as measured by the Brief Psychiatric Rating Scale (BPRS) (Overall & Gorham, 1962) and the Hamilton Rating Scale for Depression (HAM-D) (Hamilton, 1967), and were given similar neuroleptic treatments (cumulative exposure and daily dose during study observation). The differences in age and diagnosis, based on the criteria of the *Diagnostic and Statistical Manual of Mental Disorders,* third edition, revised (DSM-III-R) (American Psychiatric Association, 1987), showed a nonsignificant trend ($p < .10$). The cumulative inci-

Table 22.1. *Comparisons of Caucasians and non-Caucasians*

Variable	Caucasians (N = 217)	Non-Caucasians (N = 48)	p
Age (years)	66.1 ± 12.2	62.6 ± 10.6	.064
Gender (% male)	80.2%	87.5%	NS
Education (years)	12.5 ± 3.3	11.9 ± 3.6	NS
Diagnosis			.0757
Schizophrenia	18.9%	33.3%	
Mood disorder	23.5%	10.4%	
Other nonorganic	15.2%	20.8%	
Alzheimer's disease	25.3%	23.1%	
Other organic	17.1%	16.7%	
BPRS at study entry	32.7 ± 8.9	35.2 ± 10.2	NS
HAM-D at study entry	10.6 ± 10.5	13.7 ± 11.5	NS
ADRS at study entry	18.8 ± 2.5	19.0 ± 2.4	NS
AIMS (sum of items 1–7) at study entry	1.0 ± 1.2	1.3 ± 1.5	NS
MMSE at study entry	24.2 ± 6.5	24.0 ± 7.1	NS
Mean neuroleptic dosage (mg/day, CPZE)	111.5 ± 351.2	86.5 ± 152.6	NS
Cumulative proportion of patients developing tardive dyskinesia by 12 months	23.2%	36.8%	NS

Unpaired Student's t-tests were used to detect significant group differences in terms of age, education, HAM-D, BPRS, ADRS, AIMS, and MMSE. Chi-square tests were used to detect significant differences in gender and diagnosis between the groups. An Actuarial Life Tables analysis was performed to detect differences in the cumulative proportion of patients developing TD in both groups. Mann-Whitney U-tests were performed to detect significant differences in neuroleptic exposure between the two groups. All the statistical tests were two-tailed.
BPRS = Brief Psychiatric Rating Scale (Overall and Gorham 1962).
Ham-D = Hamilton Rating Scale for Depression (Hamilton 1967).
ADRS = Rockland Dyskinesia Rating Scale (Simpson et al. 1979).
AIMS = Abnormal Involuntary Movement Scale (National Institute of Mental Health 1975).
MMSE = Mini-Mental State Examination (Folstein et al. 1975).
NS = Not significant.

dence of tardive dyskinesia was higher among the non-Caucasians (36.8%) than among the Caucasians (23.2%), although the difference failed to reach statistical significance.

Discussion

The nonsignificantly higher risk for tardive dyskinesia among non-Caucasians could not be explained by the differences in amounts of neuroleptics prescribed. Despite their higher percentage of schizophrenia diagnoses, the non-

Caucasians did not receive greater dosages of neuroleptics. We acknowledge the main limitations of our study: unequally proportioned groups (Caucasians versus non-Caucasians) and the grouping of African-Americans, Hispanics, Asians, and other ethnic groups into a single cluster. More appropriate studies of the role of ethnicity in determining the risk for tardive dyskinesia will require larger numbers of patients from the various minority ethnic groups.

Suggestions for Future Research

Ethnicity appears to represent an important variable that may contribute to variations in drug responses, including the propensity to develop tardive dyskinesia. In order to accurately assess its contribution to the risk for tardive dyskinesia, investigators should address the influence of ethnicity in terms of psychiatric diagnosis, prescribed neuroleptic dosages, pharmacogenetics, pharmacokinetics, and pharmacodynamics.

Patients who receive diagnoses of psychotic disorders presumably will receive more extensive neuroleptic treatment. We therefore recommend using well-defined criteria, such as those of the DSM-IV. We also suggest standardization of treatment paradigms so as to minimize the potential for ethnically biased prescription practices. For example, study designs involving a fixed neuroleptic dosage may, in some circumstances, be preferable to flexible dosage paradigms. We recommend considering the use of well-defined treatment strategies, directed toward the use of the lowest effective dosage of the neuroleptic. We also suggest the use of data on plasma concentrations of neuroleptics for assessing possible ethnic differences in pharmacogenetics and pharmacokinetics. We recommend that neurobiological measures such as receptor sensitivity be identified for use as pharmacodynamic markers, after controlling for the previously mentioned factors. Finally, we believe that a diagnosis of tardive dyskinesia should be based on objective and reliable criteria.

Acknowledgments

This work was supported in part by National Institute of Mental Health grants MH43693, MH45131, and MH49671-01 and by the Department of Veterans Affairs.

References

Adams, G. L., Dworkin, R. J., & Rosenberg, S. D. (1984). Diagnosis and pharmacotherapy issues in the care of Hispanics in the public sector. *Am. J. Psychiatry* 141:970–4.

American Psychiatric Association (1987). *Diagnostic and Statistical Manual of Mental Disorders,* 3rd ed., revised. Washington, DC: American Psychiatric Association.

Binder, R. L., Kazamatsuri, H., Nishimura, T., & McNiel, D. E. (1987). Tardive dyskinesia and neuroleptic-induced parkinsonism in Japan. *Am. J. Psychiatry* 144:1494–6.

Chang, W. H., Lin, K. S., & Jann, M. W. (1991). Interconversions between haloperidol and reduced haloperidol in schizophrenic patients and guinea pigs. *J. Clin. Psychopharmacol.* 11:99–105.

Chiu, H., Shum, P., Lau, J., Lam, L., & Lee, S. (1992). Prevalence of tardive dyskinesia, tardive dystonia, and respiratory dyskinesia among Chinese psychiatric patients in Hong Kong. *Am. J. Psychiatry* 149:1081–5.

Cutler, S. J., & Ederer, F. (1958). Maximum utilization of the life table method in analyzing survival. *J. Chronic Dis.* 8:669–712.

Dunn, J., & Fahy, T. A. (1990). Police admissions to a psychiatric hospital: demographic and clinical differences between ethnic groups. *Br. J. Psychiatry* 156:373–8.

Eichelbaum, M., & Gross, A. S. (1990). The genetic polymorphism of debrisoquine/sparteine clinical aspects. *Pharmacol. Ther.* 46:377–95.

Flaskerud, J. H., & Hu, L. (1992). Racial/ethnic identity and amount and type of psychiatric treatment. *Am. J. Psychiatry* 149:379–84.

Folstein, M. F., Folstein, S. E., & McHugh, P. R. (1975). Mini-Mental State: a practical method for grading the cognitive state of patients for the clinician. *J. Psychiatr. Res.* 12:189–98.

Froemming, J. H., Lam, Y. W. F., Jann, M. W., & Davis, C. M. (1989). Pharmacokinetics of haloperidol. *Clin. Pharmacokinet.* 17:396–423.

Hamilton, M. (1967). Development of a rating scale for primary depressive illness. *Br. J. Soc. Clin. Psychol.* 6:278–96.

Harris, M. J., Panton, D., Caligiuri, M. P., Krull, A. J., Tran-Johnson, T. K., & Jeste, D. V. (1992). High incidence of tardive dyskinesia in older outpatients on low doses of neuroleptics. *Psychopharmacol. Bull.* 28:87–92.

Harrison, G., Owens, D., Holton, A., Neilson, D., & Boot, D. (1988). A prospective study of severe mental disorder in Afro-Caribbean patients. *Psychol. Med.* 18:643–57.

Horai, Y., Nakano, M., Ishizaki, T., Ishikawa, K., Zhou, B., Liao, C., & Zhang, L. (1989). Metoprolol and mephenytoin oxidation polymorphisms in Far Eastern Oriental subjects: Japanese versus mainland Chinese. *Clin. Pharmacol. Ther.* 46:198–207.

Hough, R. L., Landsverk, J. A., Karno, M., Burnam, A., Timbers, D. M., Escobar, J. I., & Regier, D. A. (1987). Utilization of health and mental health services by Los Angeles Mexican-Americans and non-Hispanic whites. *Arch. Gen. Psychiatry* 44:702–9.

Jann, M. W., Lam, Y. W. F., & Chang, W. H. (1990). Reversible metabolism of haloperidol and reduced haloperidol in Chinese schizophrenic patients. *Psychopharmacology (Berlin)* 101:107–11.

Jeste, D. V., & Caligiuri, M. P. (1993). Tardive dyskinesia. *Schizophr. Bull.* 19:303–15.

Jeste, D. V., Lacro, J. P., Gilbert, P. L., Kline, J., & Kline, N. (1993). Treatment of late-life schizophrenia with neuroleptics. *Schizophr. Bull.* 19:817–30.

Jeste, D. V., Caligiuri, M. P., Paulsen, J. S., Heaton, R. K., Lacro, J. P., Harris, M. J., Bailey, A., Fell, R. L., & McAdams, L. A. (1995). Risk of tardive dyskenesia in older patients: A prospective longitudinal study of 266 outpatients. *Arch. Gen. Psychiatry* 52:756-765.

Kalow, W. (1990). Pharmacogenetics: past and future. *Life Sci.* 47:1385–97.

Kane, J. M., Jeste, D. V., Barnes, T. R. E., Casey, D. E., Cole, J. O., Davis, J. M., Gualtieri, C. T., Schooler, N. R., Sprague, R. L., & Wettstein, R. M. (1992). *Tardive Dyskinesia: A Task Force Report of the American Psychiatric Association.* Washington, DC: American Psychiatric Association.

Ko, G. N., Zhang, L. O., Yan, W. W., Zhang, M. D., Bucher, D., Xia, Z. Y., Wyatt, R. J., & Jeste, D. V. (1989). The Shanghai 800: prevalence of tardive dyskinesia in a Chinese psychiatric hospital. *Am. J. Psychiatry* 146:387–9.

Lacro, J. P., Gilbert, P. L., Paulsen, J. S., Fell, R., Bailey, A., Juels, C., Caligiuri, M. P., McAdams, L. A., Harris, M. J., & Jeste, D. V. (1994). Early course of new-onset tardive dyskinesia in older patients. *Psychopharmacol. Bull.* 30:187–91.

Lin, K., & Finder, E. (1983). Neuroleptic dosage for Asians. *Am. J. Psychiatry* 140:490–1.

Lin, K., Poland, R. E., Lau, J. K., & Rubin, R. T. (1988). Haloperidol and prolactin concentrations in Asians and Caucasians. *J. Clin. Psychopharmacol.* 8:195–201.

Lin, K., Poland, R. E., Nuccio, I., Matsuda, K., Hathuc, N., Su, T., & Fu, P. (1989). A longitudinal assessment of haloperidol doses and serum concentrations in Asian and Caucasian schizophrenic patients. *Am. J. Psychiatry* 146:1307–11.

Lindsey, K. P., & Paul, G. L. (1989). Involuntary commitments to public mental institutions: issues involving the overrepresentation of blacks and assessment of relevant functioning. *Psychol. Bull.* 106:171–83.

Llerena, A., Dahl, M.-L., Ekqvist, B., & Bertilsson, L. (1992). Genetic factors in the metabolism of haloperidol. *Clin. Neuropharmacol. (Suppl. 1)* 15:84–5.

Lou, Y., Yink, L., Bertilsson, L., & Sjöqvist, F. (1987). Low frequency of slow debrisoquine hydroxylation in a native Chinese population. *Clin. Pharmacol.* 15:443–50.

Mahgoub, A., Idle, J. R., Dring, L. G., Lancaster, R., & Smith, R. L. (1977). Polymorphic hydroxylation of debrisoquine in man. *Lancet* 2:584–6.

Marder, S. R., Davis, J. M., & Janicak, P. G. (1993). *Clinical Use of Neuroleptic Plasma Levels.* Washington, DC: American Psychiatric Press.

Mendoza, R., Smith, M. W., Poland, R. E., Lin, K., & Strickland, T. L. (1991). Ethnic psychopharmacology: the Hispanic and Native American perspective. *Psychopharmacol. Bull.* 27:449–61.

Morgenstern, H., & Glazer, W. M. (1993). Identifying risk factors for tardive dyskinesia among long-term outpatients maintained with neuroleptic medications. *Arch. Gen. Psychiatry* 50:723–33.

Nakamura, K., Goto, F., Ray, W. A., McAllister, C. B., Jacqz, E., Wilkinson, G. R., & Branch, R. A. (1985). Interethnic differences in generic polymorphism of debrisoquine and mephenytoin hydroxylation between Japanese and Caucasian population. *Clin. Pharmacol. Ther.* 38:402–8.

National Institute of Mental Health (1975). Abnormal Involuntary Movement Scale (AIMS). *Early Clin. Drug Eval. Unit Intercom.* 4:3–6.

Neighbors, H. W. (1985). Seeking professional help for personal problems: black Americans' use of health and mental health services. *Community Ment. Health J.* 21:156–66.

Overall, J. E., & Gorham, D. R. (1962). The brief psychiatric rating scale. *Psychol. Rep.* 10:799–812.

Pi, E. H., Gray, G. E., Lee, D. G., Ji, Z., Weng, Y., Kim, C. K., Kim, Y. S., Leung, T. M., Kishimoto, A., & Wu, C. (1990). Tardive dyskinesia in Asians:

a multinational study. Presented at the 143rd annual meeting of American Psychiatric Association, New York.

Pi, E. H., Gutierrez, M. A., & Gray, G. E. (1993). Tardive dyskinesia: cross-cultural perspectives. In *Psychopharmacology and Psychobiology of Ethnicity,* ed. K. Lin, R. E. Poland, and G. Nakasaki, pp. 153–67. Washington, DC: American Psychiatric Press.

Price Evans, D. A., Mahgoub, A., Sloan, T. P., Idle, J. R., & Smith, R. L. (1980). A family and population study of the genetic polymorphism of debrisoquine oxidation in a white British population. *J. Med. Genet.* 17:102–5.

Schonecker, M. (1957). Ein eigentumliches Syndrom im oralen Bereich bei Megaphen Applikation. *Nervenarzt* 28:35.

Schooler, N. R., & Kane, J. M. (1982). Research diagnoses for tardive dyskinesia. *Arch. Gen. Psychiatry* 39:486–7.

Simpson, G. M., Lee, J. H., Zoubok, B., & Gardos, G. (1979). A rating scale for tardive dyskinesia. *Psychopharmacology (Berlin)* 64:171–9.

Sramek, J., Roy, S., Ahrens, T., Pinanong, P., Cutler, N. R., & Pi, E. (1991). Prevalence of tardive dyskinesia among three ethnic groups of chronic psychiatric patients. *Hosp. Community Psychiatry* 42:590–2.

Sramek, J. J., Sayles, M. A., & Simpson, G. M. (1986). Neuroleptic dosage for Asians: a failure to replicate. *Am. J. Psychiatry* 143:535–6.

Strickland, T. L., Ranganath, V., Lin, K., Poland, R. E., Mendoza, R., & Smith, M. W. (1991). Psychopharmacologic considerations in the treatment of black American populations. *Psychopharmacol. Bull.* 27:441–8.

Sue, D., & Sue, S. (1987). Cultural factors in the clinical assessment of Asian Americans. *J. Consult. Clin. Psychol.* 55:479–87.

Tyndale, R. F., Kalow, W., & Inaba, T. (1991). Oxidation of reduced haloperidol to haloperidol: involvement of human P450IID6 (sparteine/debrisoquine monooxygenase). *Br. J. Clin. Pharmacol.* 31:655–60.

Yassa, R., & Jeste, D. V. (1992). Gender differences in tardive dyskinesia: a critical review of the literature. *Schizophr. Bull.* 18:701–15.

23

Tardive Dyskinesia in Children and Adolescents

MARK MAGULAC, M.D.

The prevalences of neuroleptic-induced tardive dyskinesia reported in studies of children and adolescents have matched or exceeded the prevalences reported in studies of adults (McAndrew, Case, & Treffert, 1972; Polizos et al., 1973; Engelhardt, Polizos, & Waizer, 1974; Paulson, Rizvi, & Crane, 1975; Polizos & Engelhardt, 1978; Frank & Djavadi, 1980; Jeste & Wyatt, 1981; Gualtieri et al., 1982, 1984, 1986; Kane et al., 1984; Campbell et al., 1988, 1990; Meiselas et al., 1989; Locascio et al., 1991). Those studies used a variety of disease definitions, research methods, and pediatric populations at risk for tardive dyskinesia. The comparative analysis of the literature presented in this chapter attempts to organize that heterogeneity and establish a range for the prevalence of tardive dyskinesia, as well as the more transient withdrawal dyskinesia.

Diagnosing tardive dyskinesia in children is a complicated matter. Highly variable neuroleptic exposures will have preceded the onset of tardive dyskinesia in children and adolescents (Campbell et al., 1983a). The symptoms of tardive dyskinesia will vary in frequency, severity, and anatomic distribution (Engelhardt et al., 1974; Simpson et al., 1979; Perry et al., 1985; Gualtieri et al., 1986). The use of maintenance neuroleptic treatment will make recognition of tardive dyskinesia more difficult by reducing its symptoms. At times, even indisputable cases of tardive dyskinesia may not be recognized clinically (Weidon et al., 1987), and patients may grossly underreport their symptoms (Alexopoulos, 1979). Furthermore, there are various definitions for tardive dyskinesia that require different durations of symptom persistence (Quitkin et al., 1977; Jeste et al., 1979; Malone et al., 1991). All of these variables have led to several different diagnostic descriptions for tardive dyskinesia, making comparisons between studies difficult. Still, comparative analysis is important, because prolonged impairments can result from tardive dyskinesia that presents in childhood or adolescence. Follow-up studies of children and adolescents with tardive dyskinesia (Paulson et al., 1975; Gualtieri et al., 1986) have shown that less than half of the diagnosed cases will resolve in the first 3–4 years following cessation of neuroleptic treatment.

These difficulties in characterizing tardive dyskinesia have created controversy as to the prevalence of tardive dyskinesia among children and adolescents and the appropriate indications for use of neuroleptics (Weiner, 1982; Singer, 1986). Silverstein and Johnston (1987) surveyed 410 members of the Child Neurology Society for their opinions concerning the risks of using neuroleptic drugs. They found that most (40%) of the respondents had told the involved families that the risks from neuroleptic treatment were unknown, 30% had told the families that the risk for developing tardive dyskinesia was 1–10%, and the rest had given other responses. Establishment of a standard of care for the use of neuroleptics in children must await a consensus on the rate of occurrence of tardive dyskinesia in this age group. Tardive dyskinesia's complicated diagnostic puzzle and its potential for impairing children and adolescents have motivated research articles and historical reviews of the literature (Gualtieri & Hawk, 1980; Campbell et al., 1983a). But the diagnostic and methodological differences in the prior research studies have necessitated a comparative analysis such as this present report, with its further consideration of the prevalences of tardive dyskinesia and withdrawal dyskinesia.

Design of This Review

The scarcity of published information about tardive dyskinesia in children and adolescents might well lead one to believe that it is infrequent. Indeed, using a Medline computerized search and the *Index Medicus* for publications within the past 20 years, I found only half a dozen articles on tardive dyskinesia in this age group, although cross-references subsequently provided more citations. In all, I found 15 investigations of the incidence and prevalence of tardive dyskinesia in this age group, in addition to 12 case reports describing 25 separate cases, as well as one inconclusive study of the neurochemistry of tardive dyskinesia in children. This review includes the pertinent published data on the rating scales used in the research papers, reviews, book chapters, letters, and communications examined.

Methodological Issues

My investigation yielded a number of critical methodological issues:

1. Among populations of children exposed to neuroleptic medication, some may have preexisting movement disorders that will present methodological

problems during assessment for tardive dyskinesia. Autistic children are characterized in the *Diagnostic and Statistical Manual of Mental Disorders,* fourth edition (American Psychiatric Association, 1995) as having "stereotyped body movements [such as] hand flicking or twisting, spinning, headbanging and complex whole body movements." Such stereotypies must be distinguished from the varied motor symptoms of tardive dyskinesia.

The stereotypies most frequently observed prior to neuroleptic treatment in a prospective study of autistic children by Campbell et al. (1988) were biting, chewing, putting tongue in cheek, and moving the tongue in and out. Because tardive dyskinesia is predominantly expressed by the buccolingual masticatory muscles, it can be obscured by such stereotypies or even mistaken for them (Meiselas et al., 1989). In the study by Campbell et al. (1988) a change in severity or topography of preexisting stereotypies was interpreted as a drug-induced change, and no control group of autistic children without neuroleptic exposure was used.

The roles of autism and mental retardation in assessment for tardive dyskinesia and as risk factors for tardive dyskinesia were illustrated in a study of 120 youths by Frank and Djavadi (1980). When that heterogeneous population was considered as a whole, 8.3% had tardive dyskinesia while on neuroleptics. However, when only the autistic and mentally retarded individuals were analyzed, a 55% prevalence of tardive dyskinesia was identified during neuroleptic treatment. That increased prevalence is unexplained and must await new assessment procedures, more complete treatment histories, and identification of risk factors inherent to autism and mental retardation.

2. Neuroleptic medications suppress stereotypies (Campbell, Anderson, & Cohen, 1982; Campbell et al., 1988), but stereotypies can reappear when a placebo is substituted for the neuroleptic. Observing patients for tardive dyskinesia can therefore be confusing during the period of drug withdrawal, inasmuch as both stereotypies and tardive dyskinesia may emerge.

Cohen et al. (1980), in a study of the behavioral effects of haloperidol in 10 autistic children with a mean age of 4.7 years (2.1–7.0 years), reported that stereotypies were suppressed by haloperidol and that they reemerged when haloperidol was withdrawn. That study indicated greater suppression of stereotypies with haloperidol in older children than in younger children, even though the older children had more severe symptoms prior to treatment. Those authors hypothesized that younger children experienced more rebound stereotypies, on the basis of the shorter half-life of haloperidol in younger subjects (3–7 hours), and that was believed to be responsible for their apparent refractoriness.

3. Apart from displaying stereotypies, children with moderate or severe

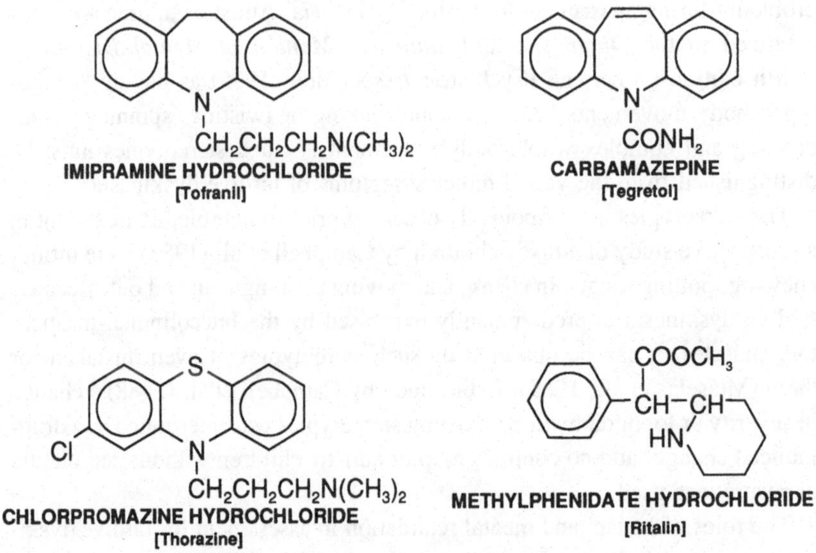

Figure 23.1. Chemical structures of some psychotropic drugs.

mental retardation may not understand or may not be motivated to comply with the simple commands involved in examinations such as the Abnormal Involuntary Movement Scale (AIMS) (Guy, 1976). Nonetheless, Gualtieri et al. (1986) have used that instrument extensively with such patients and have reported an interrater reliability of .83.

4. The use of other psychotropic medications during the period of neuroleptic treatment raises methodological concerns. The motor side effects of nonneuroleptic psychotropic drugs have been reported, especially those of antidepressants (Cooperative Study 1973; Dekret et al., 1977; Lippman, Moskovitz, & O'Tuama, 1977a; Lippman et al., 1977b; Riddle, Leckman, & Hardin, 1988; Spencer et al., 1993), anticonvulsants (Chadwick, Reynolds, & Marsden, 1976; Chalhub, Devivo, & Volpe, 1976; Joyce & Gunderson, 1980; Bimpong-Buta & Froescher, 1982; Gualtieri & Evans, 1984), and stimulants (Denckla, Bemporad, & Mackay, 1976; Lowe et al., 1982; El-Defrawi & Greenhill, 1984; Sallee et al., 1989; Barkley et al., 1990). Similarities in the structures of these psychothropic drugs are apparent, despite their varied applications (Figure 23.1).

Should all neuroleptics be considered equivalent, despite their different affinities for dopamine-receptor populations and other psychoactive receptor sites? Engelhardt et al. (1974) argued that their data from studies in children implicated the high-potency neuroleptics in creating abnormal movements. However, when those same data are converted to chlorpromazine equivalents, no distinction between neuroleptic drugs remains. Reports concerning the use of atypical neuroleptics in children and adolescents have yet to be published.

5. Prevalence estimates are affected by the nonuniform definitions used in the various studies (Table 23.1). The nomenclature of Jeste et al. (1979) is used throughout this review. Those investigators preferred to use the term "withdrawal dyskinesia" for symptoms seen during the month after drug discontinuation, when oral neuroleptics are still being cleared from the body. In addition, they used the descriptions "reversible" and "persistent" tardive dyskinesia to describe symptom durations that were shorter or longer than 3 months, regardless of neuroleptic use. Thus, Jeste et al. (1979) identified three outcome categories: withdrawal dyskinesia, reversible tardive dyskinesia, and persistent tardive dyskinesia. Schooler and Kane (1982) also required a duration of at least 3 months for the designation of persistent tardive dyskinesia. Their desire to modify the criteria for diagnosis of tardive dyskinesia to reflect current patterns of neuroleptic use and to reflect the duration of symptoms led them to devise six separate outcome categories. The criteria of Gualtieri et al. (1986) stipulated 4 months as the minimum duration for tardive dyskinesia; they called dyskinesias with shorter courses "withdrawal dyskinesias." Campbell et al. (1988) defined withdrawal dyskinesias as dyskinesias that appeared after discontinuation of neuroleptic treatment; they equated tardive dyskinesia with abnormal movements of any duration that appeared during a child's treatment with neuroleptics.

6. The longer it takes to diagnose tardive dyskinesia, the greater the ambiguity that will surround this condition, and the lower will be its reported prevalence. Indeed, when patients are unable to tolerate drug withdrawal, the subsequent reinstitution of neuroleptic treatment may take place during that time interval that is critical in the differential diagnosis of dyskinesias. Moreover, subsequent diagnosis of withdrawal dyskinesia or tardive dyskinesia will be impossible after neuroleptics are reinstituted. Ambiguity is inevitable, because if symptoms resolve, then the two possible explanations – that the resolution was due to the progression of time, or was due to the return to neuroleptic treatment – are equally likely.

7. The symptoms of tardive dyskinesia are rated subjectively. Indeed, the examiners' expertise in using the various rating scales and their interest in either stereotypies or tardive dyskinesia can both influence the reliability of symptom ratings (Lane et al., 1985). Although interrater reliability is the usual concern in regard to subjective bias, Bergen et al. (1984) questioned

Table 23.1. *Nomenclature for dyskinesias apparent after neuroleptic discontinuation*

Study	Months off neuroleptics				
	0	1	2	3	4
Schooler & Kane (1982)	Withdrawal TD[a]			→Persistent TD	→
Campbell et al. (1982, 1983a,b, 1988)	Withdrawal dyskinesia				→
Gualtieri et al. (1982, 1984, 1986)	Withdrawal dyskinesia			→TD	→
Polizos & Engelhardt (1978), Polizos et al. (1973)	WES[b]	→No observations			

[a]Tardive dyskinesia.
[b]Withdrawal-emergent syndrome.

316

intrarater reproducibility as well in their study of video-recorded patients rated via the AIMS; when the evaluators rated a given tape in different sessions, intrarater variability was found to exceed interrater variability. In that study, both of those intraclass correlation coefficients were high ($r \leq .90$), making the distinction less crucial.

8. Subjective reports of distress due to the symptoms of tardive dyskinesia are unreliable and highly variable. Alexopoulos (1979) noted that about half of schizophrenic patients with tardive dyskinesia denied awareness of their abnormal movements. Although such nonidentification is likely to reduce casual estimates of prevalence, formal research on tardive dyskinesia would be much less affected.

9. The symptoms of tardive dyskinesia can vary in severity and distribution within a given patient. Indeed, voluntary, brief suppression of tardive dyskinesia is possible. Its symptoms usually are increased by anxiety and lessened by relaxation and disappear altogether during sleep. Simpson et al. (1979) proposed using videotaped evaluations to reduce the variability of observations by raters. Videotapes might tend to reduce evaluators' sensitivity to dyskinesias by creating thresholds of auditory and visual perceptions. However, regardless of the nature of the rating session – whether in vivo or using video – determining a patient's most characteristic degree of symptoms remains problematic.

10. The multiple withdrawals from neuroleptics needed to detect the incidence of tardive dyskinesia in longitudinal studies may increase the risk for tardive dyskinesia (Jeste et al., 1979). If that is the case, only prospective studies will be confounded by the increased risk for tardive dyskinesia resulting from the repeated drug-free observations used to determine the incidence of tardive dyskinesia (Campbell et al., 1988).

11. The prevalence of dyskinesias developing spontaneously in the pediatric population has not been well established. Therefore, the lack of control groups in the published studies of tardive dyskinesia in children and adolescents is not a trivial matter. Their absence may mean that raters feel certain that every patient is at risk, an attitude that may affect their assessments and hence the research findings.

12. Finally, tardive dyskinesia in children and adolescents is itself in the process of being validated as a syndrome (Golden, Campbell, & Perry, 1987). To date, there are not pathognomonic physical signs of tardive dyskinesia. No assessment instrument can demonstrate the presence of tardive dyskinesia on the basis of its rating system. Additionally, no psychiatric subpopulation of children or adolescents can be used to define tardive dyskinesia without it being defined in other groups as well.

Definition and Diagnosis of Tardive Dyskinesia

Tardive dyskinesia is a disorder of abnormal involuntary movements associated with exposure to neuroleptic drugs. Although oral dyskinesias are characteristic, tardive dyskinesia often involves the extremities as well as the axial muscles. The classic (Uhrbrand & Faurbye, 1960) perioral symptoms of tardive dyskinesia result from excessive involuntary movements in the buccolingual and masticatory muscles. The buccal muscles may produce sucking, smacking, or puckering. The tongue muscles may cause lateral excursions, protrusions, licking, panting, and even fly-catching movements. The masticatory muscles may open the mouth or produce chewing movements.

Movements of the extremities in patients with tardive dyskinesia characteristically are of two types: rapid and jerky (choreiform), or slow, complex, and serpentine (athetoid). The lack of predictability of movement or rhythm in these dyskinesias distinguishes them from tremors. Ballistic, rolling, and tic-like disruptions of movements (Moros & Yahr, 1984) are also associated with tardive dyskinesia, although less commonly than with chorea and athetosis.

Truncal and diaphragmatic movements are also seen in patients with tardive dyskinesia. Neck, shoulder, and hip muscles may involuntarily rock, twist, or flex the patient.

The fact that the distribution and severity of the symptoms of tardive dyskinesia are variable can be exploited for diagnostic purposes. Repetitive voluntary movements such as walking or finger-tapping may amplify tardive dyskinesia symptoms and help to identify the syndrome. Assessment is impaired, however, by the tendency for anxiety to increase the symptoms of tardive dyskinesia and for relaxation to decrease them. Voluntary suppression of symptoms may impair assessment as well. For that reason, Munetz and Benjamin (1988) and Simpson et al. (1979) have recommended that one first observe a patient's movements when the patient is unaware of scrutiny.

Schooler and Kane (1982) have defined persistence and severity criteria for use in assessments of tardive dyskinesia. A minimum of 3 months of exposure to neuroleptics is a prerequisite. They have also proposed that a diagnosis of tardive dyskinesia should require involvement of two body regions with mild symptoms, or else moderate severity in one area. In their diagnostic system, persistent tardive dyskinesia is defined as having a duration of more than 3 months.

Risk Factors for Tardive Dyskinesia

A prospective study of young adults (age 28 ± 10 years) by Kane et al. (1984) suggested five risk factors for tardive dyskinesia: (1) a long duration of antipsychotic treatment, (2) concurrent use of antiparkinson medications, (3) older age, (4) a long psychiatric history, and (5) prior affective symptoms, as evidenced by administration of lithium or electroconvulsive treatment. The only risk factor proved to be associated with the development of tardive dyskinesia in children is the log of the total lifetime dose of antipsychotic medications (Gualtieri et al., 1986).

Campbell's group investigated a continuous haloperidol regimen versus one that delivered medicine for 5 days, and then placebo for 2 days. No difference in the incidence of tardive dyskinesia resulted from that interrupted schedule. Because no mention was made of a discrepancy in average daily dose between groups, it must be assumed that the interrupted-schedule patients received only about 70% of the dosage that the continuous-regimen patients were given. Thus, that prospective study implicates treatment duration, as much as total lifetime exposure, as a risk factor for tardive dyskinesia.

In their regression analysis of the variables that might be associated with the development of moderate or severe tardive dyskinesia, Gualtieri et al. (1986) pinpointed three independent variables: total lifetime exposure (log dose), IQ, and age at which neuroleptic treatment began ($r^2 = .65$). When treatment duration was added to the analysis, the variance did not increase appreciably ($r^2 = .68$), because total lifetime antipsychotic exposure was highly correlated to treatment duration.

Low IQ has been reported to be statistically related to moderate and severe forms of tardive dyskinesia (Gualtieri et al., 1984, 1986). That may have been an artifact of more intensive and more prolonged treatment with antipsychotics in that population. Alternatively, prematurity, encephalopathies, and head trauma may link low IQ to brain damage, which is a putative risk factor for tardive dyskinesia in adults.

The age at which subjects begin antipsychotic treatment has not yet been firmly correlated with increased risk for tardive dyskinesia. Gualtieri et al. (1986) observed that withdrawal dyskinesia was more common in younger subjects (mean age 15.7 years) and that tardive dyskinesia was more likely in older subjects (mean age 27.3 years). Increasing age, total lifetime neuroleptic dose, and duration of neuroleptic treatment were predictors of tardive dyskinesia in that study. Younger subjects had lower mean lifetime exposures to chlorpromazine equivalents (CPZE) of neuroleptic drugs (<14 years, 125 g CPZE; 14–20 years, 452 g CPZE; >20 years, 2,278 g CPZE) and longer mean durations of treatment (<14 years, a mean of 37 months; 14–20 years, a mean of 74 months; >20 years, a mean of 172 months). To date, because the total lifetime exposure to neuroleptics and the duration of treatment are the most highly correlated risk factors for development of tardive dyskinesia, and both covary with age, the unique risk conferred by age is unknown.

Gender was identified as a risk factor by Gualtieri et al. (1984) in a multiple-regression analysis. Although *p* values were not reported, female patients on higher doses were at even greater risk. In the study by Paulson et al. (1975), among 103 mentally retarded patients at risk and living in an institution, 15 females and 6 males developed tardive dyskinesia. Unfortunately, no gender distribution was given for the group as a whole. As for the patients of Campbell et al. (1988), the fact that the 20% who were female developed 40% of the tardive dyskinesia that was detected was not statistically significant (*p* = .42).

The development of extrapyramidal symptoms (EPS) in children has received some study, as has the presence of EPS as a possible predisposition to develop tardive dyskinesia. When Polizos et al. (1973) examined patients with EPS, they found that 52% developed withdrawal dyskinesia, and 48% did not. Those proportions reflect the prevalence of withdrawal dyskinesia in the population as a whole, however, and do not implicate EPS as a risk factor.

Symptoms of Tardive Dyskinesia

As the signs of tardive dyskinesia evolve, neuroleptics suppress their expression, and that is the paradox of the pharmacology of tardive dyskinesia. In the Campbell et al. (1982, 1983a,b, 1988, 1990) prospective study of neuroleptic-related dyskinesias in autistic children, less than half of the patients with tardive dyskinesia were identified while on maintenance antipsychotic medications. In the remainder, tardive dyskinesia did not become apparent until after drugs were discontinued. Similarly, the cross-sectional study by Gualtieri et al. (1984) identified only one-quarter of the tardive dyskinesia prevalence in that population during maintenance treatment; it was only after withdrawal of neuroleptics that the full prevalence was identified. Gualtieri et al. (1984) asserted that the onset of tardive dyskinesia while on maintenance neuroleptic treatment carries a poorer prognosis than does onset after neuroleptic medication is discontinued. According to the literature, tardive dyskinesia symptoms in children and adolescents have characteristically been in the buccolingual and masticatory areas. Use of the AIMS has permitted direct comparison of the reports from the past decade (Table 23.2).

This concordance of symptom topography contrasts sharply with the findings in studies published more than 10 years ago. For example, in the study by McAndrew et al. (1972), all of the patients with tardive dyskinesia had upper-extremity involvement, and 60% had orofacial symptoms. And Engelhardt et al. (1974) and Polizos et al. (1973) reported that the 82% of their patients who developed withdrawal-emergent symptoms were classified as having "ataxia,

Table 23.2. *Distribution of neuroleptic-induced dyskinesias in children (percentage of patients with dyskinesias in a given region)*

Study	Orofacial	Extremity	Truncal
Campbell et al. (1988)	83	45	29
Gualtieri et al. (1986)	78	26	21
Gualtieri et al. (1984)	87	33	27
Polizos & Engelhardt (1978)	17	86	0
McAndrew et al. (1972)	60	100	0

which was always jointly present with involuntary movements." Only 17% of that population exhibited orofacial symptoms.

Epidemiology

Because the modal age for onset of psychotic disorders is in adolescence or young adulthood, there have been fewer studies of the effects of neuroleptic treatment in children. Still, important data on the incidence and prevalence of tardive dyskinesia among children has been gained by studying the effects of neuroleptics in autistic and mentally retarded children.

Incidence

Almost one-third of autistic children will show a movement disorder when exposed to a mean haloperidol dose less than 1 g, according to Campbell et al. (1983a,b) and Perry et al. (1985), who conducted prospective studies of dyskinesias. In the summation of all those studies (Perry et al., 1985), it was reported that 82 children (2.3–8.2 years old, for a mean of 5 years) with autism were treated with haloperidol for a mean of 18.1 months (0.84–78.48 months). The mean dosage of haloperidol was 1.67 mg daily (0.25–10.5 mg daily); the mean lifetime total dose was $707 \pm 1,197$ mg. In that study, "tardive dyskinesia" was used according to the Schooler and Kane (1982) severity criteria to describe dyskinesia appearing during maintenance treatment, and "withdrawal dyskinesia" was used to describe dyskinesia that became apparent after neuroleptic discontinuation, regardless of its duration. Either tardive dyskinesia or withdrawal dyskinesia developed in 29% of patients. Onset during maintenance neuroleptic treatment was observed in 20% of patients with dyskinesias. The remainder of the dyskinesias presented, on average, 14.4 days after drug discontinuation (mode, 6.0 days; range, 4–34 days). The tardive dyskinesia and withdrawal dyskinesia symptoms continued for 1–32 weeks. Although an increased risk for females was suggested by the data, statistical significance was not reached. The durations of exposure to haloperidol for patients who developed tardive dyskinesia and withdrawal dyskinesia had ranged from 0.15 to 3.47 years.

Prevalence

Measuring the prevalence of tardive dyskinesia is complicated by the paradox that neuroleptic drugs suppress dyskinetic symptoms and the large proportion of children receiving neuroleptics who require ongoing treatment. Abrupt discontinuation of neuroleptics has been the predominant method used in studies of tardive dyskinesia in children. Well-documented studies of tardive dyskinesia in patients who continue on maintenance neuroleptic treatment (Gualtieri et al., 1982; Campbell et al., 1983a, 1988; Perry et al., 1985; Richardson & Haugland, 1991) generally have reported lower incidences of tardive dyskinesia than those reported after abrupt discontinuation of neuroleptics (Table 23.3). Frank and Djavadi (1980), who studied 120 adolescents, and Paulson et al. (1975), who studied 103 children, reported tardive dyskinesia prevalences of 18% and 20%, respectively, during neuroleptic treatment. Only one study has measured both maintenance-onset tardive dyskinesia and tardive dyskinesia that met the Schooler and Kane (1982) criteria for duration after cessation of neuroleptic treatment (Gualtieri et al., 1982). In that study, the patients who had persistent tardive dyskinesia while not taking neuroleptics were five times as numerous as those who had tardive dyskinesia with (and had onset while on) maintenance neuroleptic treatment. Richardson and Haugland (1991) identified 41 children at risk for tardive dyskinesia because of exposure to neuroleptics for 3 months or longer (Schooler & Kane, 1982). Of those 41 children, 5 (12%) met the criteria for tardive dyskinesia while being treated with neuroleptics. Follow-up was used to confirm the diagnosis of tardive dyskinesia, but the course of the disease was not systematically studied.

Gualtieri et al. (1986) studied a mentally retarded group of adolescents and young adults (29 males, 9 females; mean age 19.4 ± 10.3 years) who were treated with various neuroleptics for behavioral disorders associated with low IQ. Their mean daily dose was 225 ± 27 mg (CPZE). Those young patients had been treated with neuroleptics continuously for at least the preceding 6 months and had a mean duration of treatment of 8.1 ± 5.8 years. Their mean total lifetime dose was 1,012 ± 82,132 g (CPZE). Incidentally, those data represent a geographic subset of the patients reported by Gualtieri et al.

(1982). Their neuroleptics were discontinued, and they were observed for the emergence of tardive dyskinesia and withdrawal dyskinesia. If withdrawal dyskinesia persisted for more than 16 weeks after neuroleptic discontinuation, or if tardive dyskinesia was apparent during maintenance neuroleptic treatment, tardive dyskinesia was diagnosed.

Withdrawal dyskinesias were identified in 26% of that population, and persistent tardive dyskinesia occurred in an additional 34%. When a 3-year follow-up study of the tardive dyskinesia cases was conducted, 9 of the 13 index patients were available for reexamination. In 4 patients, tardive dyskinesia had remitted within the first year; in the other 5 patients tardive dyskinesia had persisted.

Gualtieri et al. (1984) also studied the prevalence of tardive dyskinesia in a separate population of 41 children and adolescents (mean age 12.8 ± 4.5 years) treated with various neuroleptics for a mean duration of 49 ± 36 months for the behavioral problems associated with their mental retardation. A mean daily dose of 128 ± 88 mg (CPZE) and a mean total lifetime dose of 235 ± 338 g (CPZE) were reported. After discontinuance of neuroleptics, withdrawal dyskinesia and tardive dyskinesia were observed. The diagnostic criteria were the same as in those researchers' other studies, allowing direct comparison with the population described earlier (Gualtieri et al., 1986). A 7% prevalence of tardive dyskinesia was reported. Although an additional 7% of the study population developed either tardive dyskinesia or withdrawal dyskinesia, that segment was not included in the analysis because neuroleptics were restarted for behavioral problems before the course of dyskinesia could be adequately observed and typed. In an additional 22% of that pediatric population, withdrawal dyskinesia was diagnosed, bringing the total of tardive dyskinesia and withdrawal dyskinesia to 37%.

In the study by McAndrew et al. (1972), neuroleptic treatment was discontinued for 74 children and adolescents with behavioral or psychotic disorders. Tardive dyskinesia was diagnosed in 14% of that population. Symptoms persisted for periods of 3–12 months. When compared with a group consisting of patients who had not developed tardive dyskinesia symptoms after discontinuation of drugs, those with tardive dyskinesia had significant ($p \leq .001$) increases in mean duration of drug intake, median daily dose at discontinuation, and median total drug intake, using a CPZE comparison.

Course

In a mentally retarded population undergoing long-term treatment with antipsychotics, Gualtieri et al. (1986) diagnosed 13 cases of tardive dyskinesia following withdrawal of antipsychotic treatment. In 4 patients, the tardive

Table 23.3. Comparison of three dyskinesia outcome categories

Study	N	Mean lifetime dose CPZE (g)	Rating scale	TD:[a] dyskinesias while on neuroleptics (%)	WD:[b] dyskinesias during first month off neuroleptics (%)	TD: dyskinesias persisting >4 months after neuroleptics withdrawn (%)
McAndrew et al. (1972) Heterogeneous children and adolescents	125	Unknown	None	8		
Polizos et al. (1973) Schizophrenic children	34	Unknown	None		41[c]	
Paulson et al. (1975) Mentally retarded adolescents	103	Unknown	None	20		
Engelhardt et al. (1974)[d] Autistic children	47	Unknown	None		48[c]	
Winsberg et al. (1978) Heterogeneous children and adolescents	11	Unknown	None		46[c]	
Polizos & Englehardt (1978)[d,e] Childhood schizophrenia with autistic features	95	Unknown	None		52	
Frank & Djavadi (1980) Heterogeneous adolescents	120	Unknown	None	18.3		
Frank & Djavadi (1980)[f] Autistic and mentally retarded adolescents	33	Unknown	None	55		
Gualtieri et al. (1982) Mentally retarded adolescents and young adults	95	1,047	AIMS	7	68	33

324

Campbell et al. (1983b)[g] Autistic and mentally retarded children	36	Unknown	AIMS	8	24	
Gualtieri et al. (1984) Mentally retarded children and adolescents	41	236	AIMS	22–29[h]	7–15[h]	
Perry et al. (1985)[g] Autistic and mentally retarded children	58	Unknown	AIMS	7	16	
Gualtieri et al. (1986)[i] Mentally retarded adolescents and young adults	38	1,012	AIMS		60	34
Campbell et al. (1988)[g] Autistic and mentally retarded children	82	71	AIMS	6.1	29	
Richardson & Hougland (1991) Heterogeneous adolescents	41	Unknown	AIMS	12		

[a] Tardive dyskinesia.
[b] Withdrawal dyskinesia.
[c] Described "withdrawal-emergent syndrome" as only outcome.
[d] Subjects in these studies participated in an average of three measured and analyzed outcomes.
[e] This analysis included the 47 subjects of Engelhardt et al. (1974).
[f] This analysis was of a subset ($n = 120$) from the study of Frank and Djavadi (1980), separated to contrast the risks for autistic and mentally retarded individuals and the risks for other psychiatrically affected youths.
[g] These populations had subjects in common; as subjects were added for prospective study, subsequent reports were published.
[h] Seven percent of this population had dyskinesias that could not be typed because of resumption of neuroleptic treatment.
[i] This analysis was of a subset of the patients of Gualtieri et al. (1982).

dyskinesia resolved within the first year off medications; each of them had initially been rated as having tardive dyskinesia of mild severity. Another 5 patients, initially rated as having severe symptoms still had mild-to-moderate tardive dyskinesia after 3 years. The remaining cases were equivocal: Three patients had resumed taking neuroleptics and were free of dyskinesia, and 1 patient had developed stereotypies and peculiar mannerisms that precluded assessment.

Paulson et al. (1975), in an examination of 103 institutionalized mentally retarded children between 11 and 16 years of age, identified maintenance-onset tardive dyskinesia in 20% of those patients, using two observers and blind ratings. Those patients were followed for 4 years. Drug histories were sketchy: In one case, the precipitating phenothiazine treatment had gone on "for a long period of time"; subsequent treatment had been intermittent, as required for continuing psychiatric symptoms. Unfortunately, the 4-year evaluation did not track the patients' subsequent neuroleptic status. After the 4 years of following the 21 patients with tardive dyskinesia, 4 patients had become worse, 5 patients were unchanged, 5 patients had improved, and 6 patients had been lost to follow-up.

In both series, half of the patients known to have tardive dyskinesia continued to have tardive dyskinesia after 3–4 years. One-quarter of the patients seen at follow-up had experienced resolution of their tardive dyskinesia in less than 4 years. Symptom intensity varied directly with symptom duration in those populations.

Effects of Using Different Neuroleptics

Polizos and Engelhardt (1978) studied 53 autistic and psychotic children (mean age 8.8 years) who had been treated for 3–24 months with neuroleptics at dosages "comparable to those for adults." Earlier publications by Polizos et al. (1973) and Engelhardt et al. (1974) had described subpopulations of that group of patients. Polizos and Engelhardt coined the phrase withdrawal-emergent syndrome (WES) to describe the mild oral dyskinesias and choreoathetoid movements precipitated by abrupt neuroleptic withdrawal in 51% of their patient population. Tardive dyskinesia was not an outcome measure in that study. The study design called for the majority of children to resume neuroleptic treatment within 1 week of drug withdrawal. A methodological flaw in that research was the participation of a given child in more than one outcome event.

Polizos and Engelhardt (1978) reported that the children on high-potency neuroleptics developed WES at twice the rate seen in those on low-potency drugs. Although they did not mention it, their data show that twice as many CPZEs were delivered to patients on high-potency drugs. That absence of dosage equivalence between high- and low-potency neuroleptics should have tempered their interpretation that high-potency neuroleptics pose greater risks for dyskinesias.

Nondyskinetic Symptoms Following Neuroleptic Withdrawal

Withdrawal dyskinesias can be accompanied by physiological symptoms – nausea, vomiting, weight loss, and diaphoresis (Gualtieri et al., 1986). Some researchers (Davis & Rosenberg, 1977; Gualtieri & Guimond, 1981; Bogomolny, Erenberg, & Rothner, 1982; Schroeder & Gualtieri, 1985; Bruun, 1988) have attempted to measure the behavioral withdrawal symptoms that have emerged during the development of withdrawal dyskinesia. They have reported that the hyperactivity, aggression, agitation, emotional lability, and tantrums often observed at the time of neuroleptic discontinuation may resolve spontaneously within 3 months after the withdrawal.

Gualtieri et al. (1986) suggested that the hypothesized behavioral withdrawal syndrome would be particularly relevant when it could be distinguished from the initial indications for neuroleptic treatment. For example, if withdrawal symptoms were in contrast to the patient's initial symptoms, or began within 2 weeks of neuroleptic discontinuation, or if withdrawal dyskinesia, nausea, vomiting, and diaphoresis were present, relapse would be considered a less probable explanation than would nondyskinetic symptoms of neuroleptic withdrawal. In such cases, Gualtieri et al. (1986) proposed environmental control of the behavioral symptoms for up to 3 months before resuming neuroleptic treatment.

Biology

Blockade of dopamine receptors in the basal ganglia, especially the nigrostriatum, likely accounts for the acute extrapyramidal and parkinsonian side effects of antipsychotic agents. Although blockade of dopamine receptors in the limbic system and cortical forebrain is the basis postulated for the effects of antipsychotic drugs, the evidence that tardive dyskinesia is a catecholamine-hyperfunction syndrome is compelling. Tardive dyskinesia symptoms are exacerbated by administration of L-dopa or a dopaminergic agonist such as bromocryptine. The suppression of tardive dyskinesia by neuroleptics and, conversely, the phenomena of withdrawal-emergent dyskinesias argue for the hyperfunctioning of catecholamine systems in patients with tardive dyskinesia.

The paradox is apparent: Neuroleptic drugs reduce brain dopamine activity, whereas tardive dyskinesia is evidence of increased dopamine activity. The hypothesis of dopamine-receptor disuse supersensitivity, along with inhibitory presynaptic autoreceptors, or the failure of a negative-feedback loop from the striatum to the substantia nigra, will usually be invoked by way of explanations. Neuroleptic-treated animals experience a proliferation of postsynaptic dopamine receptors. However, in animal models, supersensitivity to dopamine agonists does not persist beyond a few weeks after exposure to the antagonist. Thus, this mechanism may be more closely related to withdrawal dyskinesia than to tardive dyskinesia.

The case history of a pre-school-age boy treated with methylphenidate for attention-deficit hyperactivity disorder (ADHD) and thioridazine for the iatrogenic insomnia (Husain, Chapel, & Malek-Ahmadi, 1980) may be relevant to the dopamine-supersensitivity hypothesis. In that case, no symptoms of tardive dyskinesia appeared when his mother discontinued both the methylphenidate and the thioridazine. The next day, the mother reinstated only the boy's methylphenidate. Two days later the boy was restless, ataxic, and uncoordinated. He was walking on his toes, rotating his lower extremities inward, and showing orobuccal movements that included his tongue. It should be noted that the patient had had none of those symptoms prior to the thioridazine treatment for his methylphenidate-induced insomnia. One explanation for the movement disorder might be a proliferation of dopamine receptors postsynaptically or an increase in their efficiency resulting from the neuroleptic exposure, which would have increased the magnitude of the dopaminergic effects of the methylphenidate.

The presence of presynaptic inhibitory autoreceptors on the dopaminergic neurons and their ability to reduce the cell's firing rate are well known. Low doses of L-dopa, apomorphine, and bromocryptine have been used in attempts to reduce the firing of the dopaminergic cell – thus reducing tardive dyskinesia – but with inconsistent success.

One neurochemical study of withdrawal dyskinesia in children (Winsberg et al., 1978), using CSF data, has been reported. In that study, probenecid was used to minimize the high variability in the rates at which the major metabolites of dopamine and serotonin (homovanillic acid and 5-hydroxyindoleacetic acid, respectively) are transported out of the CSF. Eleven children who received between 6 months and 3 years of antipsychotic treatment for diagnoses of autism, mental deficiency, or minimal brain dysfunction had CSF drawn while on maintenance treatment and then drawn again 3–4 weeks after discontinuation of the drug. Although 5 patients developed withdrawal dyskinesia, the CSF accumulations of 5-hydroxyindoleacetic acid and homovanillic acid did not differentiate the two groups. Limitations of the probenecid technique prohibited the use of a drug-free group for comparison. However, for those who developed withdrawal dyskinesia, the decrement in 5-hydroxyindoleacetic acid was statistically significant between the drug-maintenance and drug-withdrawal states. Hence, those authors postulated that long-term treatment with antipsychotics may affect serotonin metabolism in children.

Treatment

The treatment of tardive dyskinesia in children has not been systematically studied, beyond discontinuation or reduction of neuroleptic dosages. However, some case reports have described positive outcomes resulting from other management approaches (Kumar, 1976; Caine, Margolin, & Brown, 1978; McLean & Casey, 1978; Fann et al., 1980; Gualtieri et al., 1980; Mizrahi, Holtzman, & Tharp, 1980; Petty & Spar, 1980; American Psychiatric Association, 1980; Caine & Polinsky, 1981).

As described by Caine and Polinsky (1981), a 16-year-old boy with Gilles de la Tourette's disorder experienced repetitive episodes of buccolingual masticatory tardive dyskinesia when challenged with haloperidol. His socially disabling coprolalia required such treatment, despite those dyskinesias. Lecithin (13–20% phosphatidylcholine) was given at a dosage of 18 g daily. A major phospholipid, lecithin contains choline, a methyl-group donor and a precursor of the neurotransmitter acetylcholine. Although that treatment succeeded in markedly reducing his dyskinetic movements, the patient balked at routinely swallowing the 15 large capsules required. Instead, he chose a less satisfying way of suppressing his symptoms: reducing his haloperidol dosage to half that taken previously. The dosage did not lead to unacceptable dyskinetic symptoms, and it modified his Tourette symptoms.

Jacobson, Baldessarini, and Manschreck (1974) reported the case of an 18-year-old schizophrenic male with a history of 2 years of hospitalization. He had been receiving low dosages of chlorpromazine (50 mg daily) and trihexyphenidyl (4 mg daily). Haloperidol (4 mg daily) was substituted for his chlorpromazine. He received no psychotropic medications other than haloperidol for the next 17 months, at which time it was abruptly discontinued. Within 1 week he developed facial grimacing and severe choreiform movements of the extremities. Daily doses of amantadine (100 mg), benztropine (4 mg), and diazepam (10 mg) were tried in succession for several days or weeks, but the dyskinetic symptoms remained. Eleven weeks after the onset, reserpine (0.5 mg daily) was given; a gradual improvement in neurological status was noted. However, on the basis of that report the role of reserpine in the suppression of symptoms cannot be differentiated from the possibility of dyskinetic symptoms subsiding with time.

The best-substantiated risk factor for tardive dyskinesia in pediatric populations is the cumulative exposure to neuroleptic drugs. Prevention of tardive dyskinesia is therefore based on reducing the use of neuroleptics. The mentally retarded patients studied by Gualtieri et al. (1984) were evaluated for tardive dyskinesia on the basis of their reactions following neuroleptic discontinuation; many of those patients benefited from drug withdrawal simply because they did not need further neuroleptic treatment. Of the 41 patients withdrawn from treatment, only 12 required resumption of psychotropic drugs. A short-term follow-up showed that 51% of the patients continued without medications, and 29% required ongoing neuroleptic medications. Thus, the effort to determine the presence of tardive dyskinesia by means of neuroleptic withdrawal can foster prevention in the form of dosage reduction or discontinuation.

Rating Scales

The AIMS (Guy, 1976) was developed by the Psychopharmacology Research Branch of the National Institute of Mental Health (NIMH) to rate adults with dyskinesias resulting from use of neuroleptic drugs. The 5-point severity scale is applied for observations of seven mutually exclusive body regions: the muscles of facial expression, the lips and perioral area, the jaw, the tongue, the upper extremities, the lower extremities, and the trunk. Three additional ratings – severity of abnormal movements, resulting incapacitation, and patients' reports of distress – are included as global judgments. The global ratings allow characterization of symptoms in terms of intensity, frequency, and the proportion of time they are present. Ratings for dental health and the use of dentures are included on the AIMS to differentiate oral dyskinesias caused by tooth loss or gum disease (Koller, 1982), rather than neuroleptic exposure. Gualtieri et al. (1982, 1984, 1986) and Gualtieri and Evans (1984) have used the AIMS to rate dyskinesias in mentally retarded children from 3 to 21 years of age. In their studies, interrater reliability was .83 for various pairings of a child psychiatrist, an adult psychiatrist, and a child neurologist. Validity was established via blind reviews carried out by two psychiatrists and two neurologists not involved in the original rating process. Campbell and Palij (1985), Lane et al. (1985), and Munetz and Benjamin (1988) have all published revisions of the AIMS, giving it more scoring conventions. Those researchers did not reduce a patient's severity score when the patient demonstrated dyskinesia only during motor activation, such as when walking or alternately opposing fingers. The form of administration of the AIMS is undergoing redefinition as well. Campbell (1985a), for example, published a protocol for videotaping AIMS interviews. Munetz and Benjamin (1988) expanded the AIMS examination procedure so as to clarify its content and purpose, thus increasing interrater reliability. Both Munetz and Benjamin (1988) and Schooler, as cited by Campbell and Palij (1985), recommended the removal of shoes and socks to improve observations of toe dyskinesias.

The AIMS instrument provides data on raters as well as on the subjects rated. Lane et al. (1985), who contrasted the findings of two experienced raters and two inexperienced raters in their assessments of 33 patients with tardive dyskinesia, found that the experienced raters showed better interrater reliability (.86) than did the inexperienced raters (.59–.67) on the total AIMS score. Bergen et al. (1984) found increased intrarater variability by using videotapes of mild tardive dyskinesia symptoms reevaluated after 6 weeks. However, the actual intrarater variability (Pearson correlation coefficient + .94) reduced the methodological concerns over that phenomenon.

Sprague et al. (1984) developed the Dyskinesia Identification System– Coldwater (DIS-Co), which rates abnormal movements in the mentally retarded using assessments, on a 5-point severity scale, of 34 observations in 10 body regions. Reliability, as measured by repeated testing, was reported to be .77; interrater reliability was .78. The DIS-Co was not administered to a strictly pediatric population in arriving at those statistics; only 13% of the reported data came from subjects under 20 years old.

The Tardive Dyskinesia Rating Scale (TDRS) developed by Simpson et al. (1979) rates 36 items on a 6-point severity scale. Gardos, Cole, and LaBrie (1977) found the TDRS to have an interrater reliability of .90 when patients were assessed simultaneously, and .80 when independent ratings were made. Simpson et al. (1979) also designed an Abbreviated Dyskinesia Scale (ADS) for dyskinesia screening and the less comprehensive needs of follow-up assessments. The ADS had a total-score interrater reliability of .97 when used for the 26 patients initially studied (Simpson et al., 1979). Perry et al. (1985) used the ADS with children and reported an interrater reliability of .7–.9; they also reported an interinstrument reliability of .7–.9 with the AIMS.

The Timed Stereotypies Rating Scale (TSRS) (Campbell 1985a,b) of the NIMH Children's Psychopharmacology Unit was developed in an attempt to distinguish between tardive dyskinesia and the rebound stereotypies that can emerge at the time of neuroleptic discontinuation. Perry et al. (1985), using the TSRS to assess a population of autistic children withdrawn from halo-peridol, reported an interrater reliability of .7–.9. Interinstrument reliability with the AIMS and ADS, when applied to stereotypies, was also .7–.9.

However, use of the AIMS and ADS for populations with stereotypies is a divergence from their original design, which was for use in and validation in patients with neuroleptic-induced dyskinesias. Although these various dyskinesia rating scales may produce reliable measurements of stereotypies or tardive dyskinesia in populations at particular risk for one or the other, they are poor at discriminating between the two.

Discussion

Determination of the prevalence of withdrawal dyskinesia or tardive dyskinesia in children and adolescents is a difficult methodological task. The most recent and most methodologically sophisticated studies have been conducted among autistic and mentally retarded patients suffering from movement disorders that are difficult to discriminate from tardive dyskinesia. A control group matched for age and pathology would be helpful for estimating the number of dyskinesias that will develop in a population.

The nomenclature used in the studies that have contributed to our present understanding of tardive dyskinesia in children and adolescents is not uniform, although comparable aspects can be found. The adverse effects of neuroleptic drugs on motor behavior can be described in terms of two outcomes: withdrawal dyskinesia and tardive dyskinesia. They describe the same abnormal involuntary motor syndrome. "Withdrawal dyskinesia" describes the higher prevalence of dyskinesias noted during the initial month – after neuroleptics have been discontinued and are being cleared from the body. "Tardive dyskinesia" describes identical dyskinesias (often associated with higher total lifetime exposures to neuroleptic drugs) that persist for longer than 3 months after neuroleptic discontinuation, or for any duration during maintenance treatment with neuroleptics.

The AIMS has been used to identify withdrawal dyskinesia and tardive dyskinesia in studies of children and adolescents, and acceptable interrater reliability has been reported. Although less widely used, the ADS scale has matched the AIMS in terms of interrater reliability, while concurring with its diagnostic findings. More scales such as the TSRS are needed for the difficult task of differentiating between stereotypies and tardive dyskinesia.

Conclusion

Because certain diagnostic categories are associated with movement disorders, control groups matched for psychopathology will be necessary in future studies, and prevalence rates must be interpreted cautiously. Thus far, there have been no studies of normative or unmedicated psychiatric populations that could be used to determine the rate of dyskinesia that is not attributable to psychopharmacology. Mindful of the foregoing caveat, the prevalences of tardive dyskinesia in the studies of children and adolescents reviewed here were reported to be between 8% and 34%. Higher prevalences of dyskinesias were apparent during the first month after discontinuation of neuroleptics, as reflected by combined prevalences for tardive dyskinesia and withdrawal dyskinesia between 8% and 60%. The only clearly established risk factor for tardive dyskinesia among children and adolescents was the total lifetime neuroleptic exposure; higher daily doses and longer duration of treatment were found to covary. Female gender and low IQ, although they showed trends toward becoming accepted as risk factors, have not yet been established as significant. Age effects have not yet been identified, because of their covariance with the total lifetime neuroleptic dose, a substantial risk factor for the development of tardive dyskinesia.

References

Alexopoulos, G. (1979). Lack of complaints in schizophrenics with tardive dyskinesia. *J. Nerv. Ment. Dis.* 167:125–7.

American Psychiatric Association (1980). Tardive dyskinesia ESCA: summary of a task force report on the late neurological effects of antipsychotic drugs. *Am. J. Psychiatry* 137:1163–71.

American Psychiatric Association (1987). *Diagnostic and Statistical Manual of Mental Disorders,* 4th ed. Washington, DC: American Psychiatric Association.

Barkley, R. A., McMurray, M. B., Edelbrock, C. S., & Robbins, K. (1990). Side effects of methylphenidate in children with attention deficit hyperactivity disorder: a systemic, placebo-controlled evaluation. *Pediatrics* 86:184–92.

Bergen, J., Griffiths, D., Rey, J., & Beumont, P. J. (1984). Tardive dyskinesia: fluctuating patient or fluctuating rater? *Br. J. Psychiatry* 144:498–502.

Bimpong-Buta, K., & Froescher, W. (1982). Carbamazepine-induced choreoathetoid dyskinesias. *J. Neurol. Neurosurg. Psychiatry* 45:560.

Bogomolny, A., Erenberg, G., & Rothner, A. (1982). *Gilles de la Tourette Syndrome,* ed. A. Friedhoff & T. Chase. New York: Raven Press.

Boston Collaborative Drug Surveillance Program (1973). Drug-induced extrapyramidal symptoms. *J. Am. Med. Assoc.* 224:889–91.

Bruun, R. (1988). Subtle and underrecognized side effects of neuroleptic treatment in children with Tourette's disorder. *Am. J. Psychiatry* 145: 621–4.

Caine, E. D., Margolin, D. I., & Brown, G. L. (1978). Gilles de la Tourette's syndrome, tardive dyskinesia, and psychosis in an adolescent. *Am. J. Psychiatry* 135:241–3.

Caine, E. D., & Polinsky, R. (1981). Tardive dyskinesia in persons with Gilles de la Tourette's disease. *Arch. Neurol.* 38:471–2.

Campbell, M. (1985a). Protocol for rating drug-related AIMS, stereotypies and CPRS assessments. *Psychopharmacol. Bull.* 21:1081.

Campbell, M. (1985b). Timed stereotypies rating scale. *Psychopharmacol. Bull.* 21:1082.

Campbell, M., Adams, P., Perry, R., Spencer, E. K., & Overall, J. E. (1988). Tardive and withdrawal dyskinesia in autistic children: a prospective study. *Psychopharmacol. Bull.* 24:251–5.

Campbell, M., Anderson, L. T., & Cohen, I. L. (1982). Haloperidol in autistic children: effects on learning, behavior, and abnormal involuntary movements. *Psychopharmacol. Bull.* 18:110–12.

Campbell, M., Grega, D. M., Green, W. H., & Bennett, N. G. (1983a). Neuroleptic induced dyskinesias in children. *Clin. Neuropharmacol.* 6:207–22.

Campbell, M., Locascio, J. J., Milagros, C. C., Spencer, E. K., Malone, R. P., Kafantaris, V., & Overall, J. E. (1990). Stereotypes and tardive dyskinesia: abnormal movements in autistic children. *Psychopharmacol. Bull.* 26:103–8.

Campbell, M., & Palij, M. (1985). Measurement of side effects including tardive dyskinesia. *Psychopharmacol. Bull.* 21:1063–82.

Campbell, M., Perry, R., Bennett, W. G., Small, A. M., Green, W. H., Grega, D. G., Schwartz, V., & Anderson, L. (1983b). Long-term therapeutic efficacy and drug-related abnormal movements: a prospective study of haloperidol in autistic children. *Psychopharmacol. Bull.* 19:80–3.

Chadwick, D., Reynolds, E. H., & Marsden, C. D. (1976). Anticonvulsant-induced dyskinesias: a comparison with dyskinesias induced by neuroleptics. *J. Neurol. Neurosurg. Psychiatry* 39:1210–18.

Chalhub, E., Devivo, D., & Volpe, J. (1976). Phenytoin induced dystonia and choreoathetosis in two retarded epileptic children. *Neurology* 26:494.

Cohen, I. L., Campbell, M., Posner, D., Small, A., Triebel, D., & Anderson, L. T. (1980). Behavioral effects of haloperidol in young autistic children: an objective analysis using a within-subjects reversal design. *J. Am. Acad. Child Psychiatry* 19:665–77.

Davis, K. L., & Rosenberg, G. S. (1977). Is there a limbic system equivalent of tardive dyskinesia? *Biol. Psychiatry* 14:699–703.

Dekret, J. J., Maany, I., Ramsey, T. A., & Mendels, J. (1977). A case of oral dyskinesia associated with imipramine treatment. *Am. J. Psychiatry* 134:1297–8.

Denckla, M. B., Bemporad, J. R., & Mackay, M. C. (1976). Tics following methylphenidate administration. *J. Am. Med. Assoc.* 235:1349–51.

El-Defrawi, M. H., & Greenhill, L. I. (1984). Substituting stimulants in treating behavior disorders. *Am. J. Psychiatry* 141:610.

Engelhardt, D. M., Polizos, P., & Waizer, J. (1974). CNS consequences of psychotropic drug withdrawal in autistic children: a follow-up report. *Psychopharmacol. Bull.* 11:6–7.

Fann, W., Smith, J., Davis, J., & Domino, E. (1980). *Tardive Dyskinesia: Research and Treatment.* New York: Spectrum Publications.

Frank, S. M., & Djavadi, N. A. (1980). Tardive dyskinesia in children and adolescents. Presented at the annual meeting of the American Psychiatric Association.

Gardos, G., Cole, J. O., & LaBrie, R. (1977). The assessment of tardive dyskinesia. *Arch. Gen. Psychiatry* 34:1206–12.

Golden, R., Campbell, M., & Perry, R. (1987). Taxometric method for diagnosis of tardive dyskinesia. *J. Psychiatr. Res.* 21:233–41.

Gualtieri, C. T., Barnhill, J., McGimsey, J., & Schell, D. (1980). Tardive dyskinesia and other movement disorders in children treated with psychoactive drugs. *J. Am. Acad. Child Psychiatry* 19:491–510.

Gualtieri, C. T., Breuning, S. E., Schroeder, S. R., & Quade, D. (1982). The assessment of tardive dyskinesia. *Arch. Gen. Psychiatry* 34:1206–12.

Gualtieri, C. T., & Evans, R. (1984). Carbamazepime induced tics. *Dev. Med. Child Neurol.* 26:546–8.

Gualtieri, C. T., & Guimond, M. (1981). Tardive dyskinesia and the behavioral consequences of chronic neuroleptic treatment. *Dev. Med. Child Neurol.* 23:255–9.

Gualtieri, C. T., & Hawk, B. (1980). Tardive dyskinesia and other drug induced movement disorders among handicapped children and youth. *J. Appl. Res. Ment. Retardation* 1:55–69.

Gualtieri, C. T., Quade, D., Hicks, R. E., Mayo, J. P., & Schroeder, S. R. (1984). Tardive dyskinesia and other clinical consequences of neuroleptic treatment in children and adolescents. *Am. J. Psychiatry* 141:20–3.

Gualtieri, C. T., Schroeder, S. R., Hicks, R. E., & Quade, D. (1986). Tardive dyskinesia in young mentally retarded individuals. *Arch. Gen. Psychiatry* 43:335–40.

Guy, W. (ed.) (1976). *ECDEU Assessment Manual for Psychopharmacology.* Washington, DC: U.S. Department of Health, Education, and Welfare.

Husain, A., Chapel, J., & Malek-Ahmadi, P. (1980). Methylphenidate, neuroleptics and dyskinesia-dystonia. *Can. J. Psychiatry* 25:254–8.

Jacobson, G., Baldessarini, R., & Manschreck, T. (1974). Tardive and withdrawal dyskinesia associated with haloperidol. *Am. J. Psychiatry* 131:910–13.

Jeste, D. V., Potkin, S. G., Sinha, S., Feder, S., & Wyatt, R. J. (1979). Tardive dyskinesia – reversible and persistent. *Arch. Gen. Psychiatry* 36:585–90.

Jeste, D. V., & Wyatt, R. J. (1981). The changing epidemiology of tardive dyskinesia: an overview. *Am. J. Psychiatry* 138:297–309.

Joyce, R. P., & Gunderson, C. H. (1980). Carbamazepine-induced orofacial dyskinesia. *Neurology* 30:1333–4.

Kane, J. M., Woerner, M., Weinhold, P., Wegner, J., & Kinen, B. (1984). Incidence of tardive dyskinesia: five-year data from a prospective study. *Psychopharmacol. Bull.* 20:387–9.

Koller, W. D. (1982). Edentulous orodyskinesia. *Ann. Neurol.* 13:97–9.

Kumar, B. (1976). Treatment of tardive dyskinesia with deanol. *Am. J. Psychiatry* 133:978.

Lane, R. D., Glazer, W. M., Hansen, T. F., Berman, W. H., & Kramer, S. I. (1985). Assessment of tardive dyskinesia using the Abnormal Involuntary Movement Scale. *J. Nerv. Ment. Dis.* 173:353–7.

Lippman, S., Moskovitz, R., & O'Tuama, L. (1977a). Tricyclic-induced myoclonus. *Am. J. Psychiatry* 134:90–1.

Lippman, S., Tucker, D., Wagemaker, H., & Schulte, T. (1977b). A second report of tricyclic-induced myoclonus. *Am. J. Psychiatry* 134:585–6.

Locascio, J. L., Malone, R. P., Small, A. M., Kafantaris, V., Ernst, M., Lynch, N. S., Overall, J. E., & Campbell, M. (1991). Factors related to haloperidol response and dyskinesias in autistic children. *Psychopharmacol. Bull.* 27:119–26.

Lowe, T. L., Cohen, D. J., Detlor, J., Kremenitzer, M. W., & Shaywitz, B. A. (1982). Stimulant medications precipitate Tourette's syndrome. *J. Am. Med. Assoc.* 247:1729–31.

McAndrew, J. B., Case, Q., & Treffert, D. A. (1972). Effects of prolonged phenothiazine intake on psychotic and other hospitalized children. *J. Autism Child. Schizophrenia* 2:75–91.

McLean, P., & Casey, O. O. (1978). Tardive dyskinesia in an adolescent. *Am. J. Psychiatry* 135:969–71.

Malone, R. P., Ernst, M., Godfrey, K. A., Locascio, J. J., & Campbell, M. (1991). Repeated episodes of neuroleptic-related dyskinesias in autistic children. *Psychopharmacol. Bull.* 27:113–17.

Meiselas, K. D., Spencer, E. K., Oberfield, R., Peselow, E., Angrist, B., & Campbell, M. (1989). Differentiation of stereotypes from neuroleptic-related dyskinesias in autistic children. *J. Clin. Psychopharmacol.* 9:207–9.

Mizrahi, E., Holtzman, D., & Tharp, B. (1980). Haloperidol induced tardive dyskinesia in a child with Gilles de la Tourette's disease. *Arch. Neurol.* 37:780.

Moros, D., & Yahr, M. (1984). Movement disorders in the psychiatric patient. *Hosp. Community Psychiatry* 35:377–83.

Munetz, M., & Benjamin, S. (1988). How to examine patients using the Abnormal Involuntary Movement Scale. *Hosp. Community Psychiatry* 39:1172–7.

Paulson, G. W., Rizvi, C. A., & Crane, G. E. (1975). Tardive dyskinesia as a possible sequel of long-term therapy with phenothiazines. *Clin. Pediatr. (Philadelphia)* 14:953–5.

Perry, R., Campbell, M., Green, W. H., Small, A. M., Dietrill, M. L., Meiselas, K., Golden, R. R., & Deitsch, S. I. (1985). Neuroleptic related dyskinesias in autistic children: a prospective study. *Psychopharmacol. Bull.* 21:140–3.

Petty, L., & Spar, C. (1980). Haloperidol induced tardive dyskinesia in a 10-year-old girl. *Am. J. Psychiatry* 137:745–6.

Polizos, P., & Engelhardt, D. (1978). Dyskinetic phenomena in children treated with psychotropic medications. *Psychopharmacol. Bull.* 14:65–8.

Polizos, P., Engelhardt, D. M., Hoffman, S. P., & Waizer, J. (1973). Neurological consequences of psychotropic drug withdrawal in schizophrenic children. *J. Autism Child. Schizophrenia* 3:247–53.

Quitkin, F., Rifkin, R., Gouchfeld, L., & Klein, D. F. (1977). Tardive dyskinesia: Are first signs reversible? *Am. J. Psychiatry* 134:84–7.

Richardson, M. A., & Haugland, G. (1991). Neuroleptic use, parkinsonian symptoms, tardive dyskinesia and associated factors in child and adolescent psychiatric patients. *Am. J. Psychiatry* 148:1322–8.

Riddle, M., Leckman, J., & Hardin, M. (1988). Fluoxetine treatment of obsessions and compulsions in patients with Tourette syndrome. *Am. J. Psychiatry* 145:1173–4.

Sallee, F. R., Stiller, R. L., Perel, J. M., & Everett, G. (1989). Pemoline-induced abnormal involuntary movements. *J. Clin. Psychopharmacol.* 9:125–9.

Schooler, N. R., & Kane, J. M. (1982). Research diagnoses for tardive dyskinesia. *Arch. Gen. Psychiatry* 39:486–7.

Schroeder, S., & Gualtieri, C. (1985). Behavioral interactions induced by chronic neuroleptic therapy in persons with mental retardation. *Psychopharmacol. Bull.* 21:310–15.

Silverstein, F., & Johnston, M. (1987). Risks of neuroleptic drugs in children. *J. Child Neurol.* 2:41–3.

Simpson, G. M., Lee, J. H., Zoubok, B., & Gardos, G. (1979). A rating scale for tardive dyskinesia. *Psychopharmacology* 64:171–9.

Singer, H. S. (1986). Tardive dyskinesia: a concern for the pediatrician. *Pediatrics* 77:553–6.

Spencer, T., Biederman, J., Steingard, R., & Wilens, T. (1993). Bupropion exacerbates tics in children with attention-deficit hyperactivity disorder and Tourette's syndrome. *J. Am. Acad. Child Adolesc. Psychiatry* 32:211–14.

Sprague, R. L., Kalachnik, J. E., Bruenig, S. E., Davis, V. J., Ullman, R. K., Ferguson, D. G., & Hoffner, B. A. (1984). The Dyskinesia Identification System–Coldwater (DIS-Co): a tardive dyskinesia rating scale for the developmentally disabled. *Psychopharmacol. Bull.* 20:329–38.

Uhrbrand, L., & Faurbye, A. (1960). Reversible and irreversible dyskinesia after treatment with perphenazine, chlorpromazine, reserpine and ECT therapy. *Psychopharmacology* 1:408–18.

Weidon, P. J., Mann, J. J., Naas, G., Mattson, M., & Frances, A. (1987). Clinical non-recognition of neuroleptic induced movement disorders: a cautionary study. *Am. J. Psychiatry* 144:1148–53.

Weiner, J. M. (1982). Psychotropic drug therapy in children and adolescents. *Psychosomatics* 23:488–95.

Winsberg, B., Hurwic, M., Sverd, J., & Klutch, A. (1978). Neurochemistry of withdrawal emergent symptoms in children. *Psychopharmacology* 56:157–61.

Part VI

Other Neuroleptic-Induced Movement
Disorders

24

Drug-Induced Parkinsonism

THOMAS E. HANSEN, M.D., and
WILLIAM F. HOFFMAN, Ph.D., M.D.

Descriptions of drug-induced parkinsonism (DIP) began to appear early in the decade that followed the introduction of antipsychotic medications (Lehmann & Hanrahan, 1954; Hall, Jackson, & Swain, 1956; Deniker, 1960; Kruse, 1960; Goldman, 1961; McGeer et al., 1961; Ayd, 1961; Simpson et al., 1964). DIP is one of the most common side effects of antipsychotic medications. Although other syndromes may have received more attention, because of their apparent irreversibility or because of novelty of presentation, DIP probably causes the greatest morbidity. This chapter will review the typical clinical presentation, differential diagnosis, epidemiology, evaluation, pathophysiology, and treatment for this major iatrogenic problem.

Clinical Presentation

Description of the Syndrome

All the cardinal signs of idiopathic Parkinson's disease (IPD) occur in DIP (Hall et al., 1956; Lader, 1970; Goetz & Klawans, 1981; Rajput, 1984; Casey, 1991; Friedman, 1992). Although some authors have used the term "pseudoparkinsonism" to describe DIP, given that DIP and IPD appear to have the same symptoms and basic biochemical mechanism, that term is no longer favored. The signs of DIP can be grouped into five categories: bradykinesia, rigidity, tremor, loss of postural reflexes, and a miscellaneous category. This grouping of specific motor signs is somewhat arbitrary, for the causes of the signs cannot always be determined, and the groups are not entirely independent.

Bradykinesia. Bradykinesia is a syndrome of reduced movement, including decreased spontaneous adjusting movements, reduction of facial expression,

341

slowing of voluntary movements, rapid fatigue of repetitive movements (such as finger-tapping or rapid alternating movements), difficulty in executing sequential actions, and loss of associated movements such as arm swing while walking. The terms "akinesia" and "hypokinesia" have been used both as synonyms for bradykinesia and as differential descriptors of the bradykinetic syndrome. Thus, akinesia, although sometimes described as if distinct from DIP, should be considered part of the spectrum of bradykinesia (Ayd, 1961; Rifkin, Quitkin, & Klein, 1975; Van Putten, May, & Wilkins, 1980; Goetz & Klawans, 1981).

Rigidity. "Rigidity" refers to increased muscle tone, with or without cog-wheeling, with a paratonic or "lead-pipe" consistency. The severity of the rigidity, which is the same in both agonist and antagonist muscles, affects distal, proximal, and axial musculature. The severity can be increased by movement (or immobilization) of the contralateral limb, or by intense affect.

Tremor. Although a variety of tremors can be seen in parkinsonian patients, the tremor typical of both IPD and DIP is a resting tremor with a frequency of 3–6 Hz. When present in the hands, the rhythmic contractions of the partially flexed fingers are reminiscent of a nineteenth-century pharmacist shaping pills ("pill-rolling tremor"). However, any body part can be affected, including the lips and tongue. The rabbit syndrome (Villeneuve, 1972; Jus, Villeneuve, & Jus, 1972; Jus et al., 1973; Villeneuve, Jus, & Jus, 1973; Todd et al., 1983; Yassa & Lal, 1986; Deshmukh, Joshi, & Agarwal, 1990; Decina, Caracci, & Scapicchio, 1990b; Fornazzari et al., 1991) appears to be a perioral variant of a parkinsonian tremor.

Posture and Gait. Parkinsonian patients have characteristic changes in gait, posture, and postural reflexes. Patients may experience either retropulsion (tendency to fall backward) or propulsion (tendency to fall forward). The festinating gait of patients with parkinsonism (i.e., walking with short, shuf-fling steps at an increasing rate) appears to be a consequence of propulsion. The flexed posture (bent forward at the hips) commonly seen in patients with parkinsonism contributes to postural instability and festination. The fixed, flexed posture of the arms and the lack of arm swing result from both rigidity and decomposition of motor activity.

Other Signs. Seborrheic dermatitis (Hall et al., 1956; Binder & Jonelis, 1984), hypophonia (soft and monotonous speech), micrographia (Ayd, 1983), hypersalivation, and hypomimia (lack of facial expression) also occur in patients with DIP. Hypersalivation, hypophonia, and hypomimia may be secondary to pharyngeal, laryngeal, and facial bradykinesias, respectively. Similarly, micrographia is likely secondary to the effects of bradykinesia and rigidity of the arms and hands.

Comparison with IPD

Although all the symptoms of IPD occur in patients with DIP, their comparative frequencies may differ. Hausner (1983) suggested that prominent tremor is less common in patients with DIP, especially younger patients. Rozzini, Missale, and Gadola (1985) compared IPD (30 cases) to DIP (39 cases) in nursing-home residents and found that rigidity was relatively more common in those with DIP. Specifically, rigidity and tremor occurred at the same frequency in IPD patients, whereas rigidity was more common than tremor in DIP patients. That finding was partially replicated in a similar study (Stephen & Williamson, 1984) in which comparable prevalence rates for tremor (40%) and bradykinesia (80%) were found for 48 DIP and 47 IPD patients seen in a geriatric medical clinic. Rigidity was more common in the DIP patients (86% vs. 72%; $p < .05$).

As discussed later in the section on pathophysiology, there are good reasons to expect differences between IPD and DIP. The typical neuroleptics block primarily the dopamine D_2 receptors, which modulate the indirect thalamocortical–basal-ganglia pathway. Patients with IPD suffer losses of striatal D_1 and D_2 activation secondary to global loss of nigrostriatal dopaminergic projections. It is not yet known, from either human or animal studies, whether or not selective D_2 antagonists or mixed D_1/D_2 antagonists (atypical neuroleptics) will produce syndromes that are qualitatively different from IPD.

Asymmetric signs often occur in IPD (Weiner & Lang, 1989a). Although some authors (Hausner, 1983; Weiner & Lang, 1989b) have suggested that laterality of signs distinguished DIP from IPD, empirical analyses have demonstrated that DIP can also show asymmetric presentation in 10–75% of patients (Rudenko & Lepakhin, 1979; Myslobodsky, Holden, & Sandler, 1984; Tomer et al., 1987; Hardie & Lees, 1988; Caligiuri, Bracha, & Lohr, 1989; Caligiuri et al., 1991). Although the symptoms tend to occur on the right side, studies have differed in their estimations of the prevalence and side of laterality. For example, in a retrospective review of videotapes of right-handed antipsychotic-treated inpatients (97 serial exams from 25 patients), we found that bradykinesia tended to occur on the left, and tremor on the right (unpublished data). Some of the inconsistency in the literature on DIP laterality may have derived from investigations that studied only one type of symptom or included symptoms that canceled each other. The rate of laterality (left or right side predominant) in our study varied by symptom, ranging from 5% (lower-extremity bradykinesia) to 80% (upper-extremity tremor) of all examinations.

Time Course

Studies in which patients were carefully examined early in the course of treatment have shown that the onset of DIP can occur within the first week of antipsychotic treatment (McGeer et al., 1961; Simpson et al., 1964; Angus & Simpson, 1970; Crowley et al., 1978; McEvoy, Stiller, & Farr, 1986). However, additional cases and/or worsening of symptoms can occur over periods of weeks (Simpson et al., 1964) or months (Ayd, 1961) after initiation of medication. The reports of the earliest occurrences included observations of initial handwriting changes or subtle rigidity and hypokinesia in studies whose aim was to determine the minimal effective dosages for antipsychotics (the neuroleptic-threshold dosage) (Alpert et al., 1978; McEvoy, 1986; McEvoy et al., 1986; McEvoy, Hogarty, & Steingard, 1991). Even though Ayd (1961) reported that DIP was the last of the acute extrapyramidal syndromes (EPSs) to occur, inspection of his data indicates that some cases occurred within 1 week. In a more recent review, Ayd (1983) concluded that all EPS types seem to be occurring earlier than they once did, presumably because of the increasing use of more-potent antipsychotics.

Some clinicians have deferred treatment for DIP, expecting tolerance to occur. However, short- and long-term follow-up studies and investigations of withdrawal of antiparkinson medication indicate that tolerance should not be expected in most cases. For instance, no evidence for tolerance was seen when the severity of EPSs was observed over 6 weeks (Simpson et al., 1970) or 3 months of treatment (Kruse, 1960). When antiparkinson drugs have been withdrawn, DIP has emerged or been exacerbated in anywhere from 10% to more than 50% of patients (McGeer et al, 1961; Klett & Caffey, 1972; Manos, Gkiouzepas, & Logothetis, 1981; Caradoc-Davies et al., 1986; Wada, Koshino, & Yamaguchi, 1987; Wilson, Primrose, & Smith, 1987; Comaty et al., 1990). The variations in the rates reported in those studies can be attributed to differing degrees of DIP before neuroleptics were prescribed (some patients had been given prophylactic treatment), as well as to inconsistent sensitivities of the examinations and the variable periods during which patients were not taking antiparkinsonian agents. Also, the increasing risk for DIP and IPD with increasing age may effectively offset any reduction in symptoms expected from tolerance over the long term. For instance, among 33 patients followed for 3–11 years, parkinsonism increased by 9% despite reductions in antipsychotic dosages, and it increased by 20–30% among patients on stable or increased antipsychotic dosages (Casey et al., 1986).

DIP can persist long after the offending antipsychotic agent has been discontinued. Early studies indicated that the syndrome typically persisted for 10–60 days after drug withdrawal (Ayd, 1961; Demars, 1966). More recent investigations have extended that range, particularly in the elderly. Stephen and Williamson (1984) found that although the mean time to resolution of DIP was 7 weeks in a series of 48 elderly patients (mean age 76 years), 1 patient took 36 weeks to recover. In another study, 4 of 20 patients still had DIP after 3.5 months without medication (Simpson et al., 1964), and Crane (1971) reported that in 5 of 12 patients the syndrome persisted for 6 months to 2 years after cessation of neuroleptics. Individual case reports have also shown that in some cases DIP can persist for up to several years (Klawans, Bergen, & Bruyn, 1973; Sahoo, Mitra, & Mohanty, 1975; Aronson, 1985; Friedman, Max, & Swift, 1987; Wilson & Smith, 1987).

When DIP persists, it may be that subclinical IPD has been unmasked by antipsychotic treatment, though it would be difficult to confirm or refute that hypothesis. In one report of nonpersistent DIP, neuropathologic changes consistent with IPD were seen at autopsy (Rajput et al., 1982). Exacerbated subclinical IPD has also been demonstrated in patients in whom DIP had resolved, but who subsequently developed parkinsonism months or years later, while not taking antipsychotics (Goetz, 1983; Wilson & Primrose, 1986; Wilson et al., 1987). Cases that persist following minimal antipsychotic exposure (Aronson, 1985), or are of extreme duration, and/or progress without antipsychotics (Sahoo et al., 1975; Friedman et al., 1987) are likely to represent unmasked IPD.

Differential Diagnosis

The complete differential diagnosis for DIP is much the same as that for IPD. Table 24.1, using data from Stern (1988), Weiner and Lang (1989c), and other sources (Adler, Stern, & Brooks, 1989), lists possible causes of parkinsonism other than IPD and DIP. Clearly, in patients treated with neuroleptics, parkinsonian symptoms most likely reflect DIP. The principal issues that must be addressed in arriving at a diagnosis of DIP in younger psychiatric patients include (1) avoiding confusion with the motoric abnormalities associated with certain psychiatric disorders for which antipsychotic medications were originally prescribed and (2) differentiating between parkinsonism and other drug-

Table 24.1. *Differential diagnosis for parkinsonism (excluding Parkinson's disease and antipsychotic-induced DIP)*

Infectious causes	Post-encephalitis
	Neurosyphilis
	Creutzfeldt-Jakob disease
	Abscess
Vascular causes	Post-infarction or lacunar state
Toxic causes	MPTP
	Manganese
	Carbon disulfide
	Cyanide
	Carbon monoxide
Drug-induced causes	Metoclopramide
	Reserpine
	Ca-channel blockers
	Antiemetics (e.g., prochlorperazine)
	Tetrabenazine and α-methyldopa
	Miscellaneous
Metabolic causes	Wilson's disease
	Hallervorden-Spatz disease
	Hypoparathyroidism
	Hepatocerebral degeneration
Structural causes	Brain tumors
	Hydrocephalus
	Head trauma
Degenerative causes	Progressive supranuclear palsy
	Multiple-system atrophy
	Spinocerebellar-nigral degeneration
	Corticonigral degeneration with neuronal achromasia
	Parkinson-dementia (or Guam) complex
	Parkinsonism with amyotrophy
	Senile-gait apraxia
	Alzheimer's disease

induced EPSs. In elderly patients treated with antipsychotics, the differential diagnosis must be broadened, especially when parkinsonism appears after many years of neuroleptic treatment. In this population, IPD, degenerative neurological disorders, other neuroleptic-induced EPSs, and motoric changes associated with aging occur with increasing frequency. Finally, clinicians should be aware that drugs other than antipsychotics can cause parkinsonism.

Psychiatric Syndromes

Co-occurrences of depression, negative symptoms of schizophrenia, and DIP can confound the assessment of each of these syndromes (Rifkin et al., 1975;

Van Putten & May, 1978; Van Putten et al., 1980; Craig et al., 1985; Hoffman, Labs, & Casey, 1987; Prosser et al., 1987; Weiden et al., 1987; Sandyk & Kay, 1990; Hansen et al., 1992b). Patients with DIP will have reduced facial expression, will be less active (slowed down), and may have reduced verbal output (low volume and slow speech). Often it is difficult to distinguish this set of symptoms from the psychomotor retardation, apathy, and constricted affect seen in patients with depression, or from the flat affect, poverty of speech, and apathy characterizing the negative symptoms of schizophrenia. To some extent, this is an issue of overlapping assessment criteria that can be addressed by developing more discriminative scales. However, Prosser et al. (1987) conducted a comparison of tremor and negative symptoms and still found a positive correlation. That suggests either that the two syndromes were related in terms of shared underlying pathophysiology or that the relationship existed because attempts to treat poorly responsive negative symptoms with antipsychotics had caused DIP. The possibility that the syndromes share a common underlying abnormality is supported by neuroradiologic, neurochemical, neuroanatomic, and clinical findings (Hoffman et al., 1987; Sandyk & Kay, 1990; Alexander, Crutcher, & DeLong, 1990) and may accord with recent hypotheses about the role of hypodopaminergic function in causing some symptoms of schizophrenia (Csernansky, Murphy, & Faustman, 1991; Davis et al., 1991). Some authors (Rifkin et al., 1975; Van Putten & May, 1978) believe that if akinetic symptoms improve with antipsychotic dosage reduction or treatment with anticholinergic medication, DIP should be considered causative. This problem can also be addressed through examination of the responses to antipsychotic treatment. In one study (Crowley et al., 1978), pretreatment rigidity and akinesia did not predict vulnerability to DIP, and actually improved in catatonic patients treated with trifluoperazine, leading those authors to conclude that motor symptoms (perhaps negative symptoms) in untreated schizophrenics do not reflect extrapyramidal abnormalities.

Catatonia is an additional psychiatric disorder to be considered in the differential diagnosis of DIP. Gelenberg and Mandel (1977) reviewed cases from the literature and described a series of 8 patients who had catatonic symptoms (waxy flexibility, posturing, mutism) while taking antipsychotics. The symptoms coexisted with DIP, and the patients improved following neuroleptic withdrawal and institution of antiparkinsonism treatment (amantadine was preferred to anticholinergics). Although this syndrome could simply be an extreme example of DIP, it is more likely another form of psychosis that shares an underlying abnormality with DIP.

Although a differential diagnosis involving negative symptoms, depression, and DIP may be difficult, proper clinical assessment is the first and most important step in the process. The clinician should conduct a focused neurological examination of any patient under consideration for antipsychotic phar-macotherapy. Use of a standard rating scale to evaluate extrapyramidal symp-toms is helpful, as discussed later in the section on evaluation. Nonetheless, regularly repeated examinations after initiation of drug treatment will provide the best indicators of increases in parkinsonian symptoms. The clinician must be aware that symptoms that appear to be "psychiatric" may be the conse-quences of antipsychotic drugs in patients treated for long periods. For those patients who were not drug-free for their baseline examinations, an empiric attempt at dosage reduction or treatment with anticholinergics is the obvious next step, as discussed later in the section on treatment.

Other Neuroleptic-Drug-Induced Movement Disorders

Other neuroleptic-drug-induced movement disorders can confound the diag-nosis of DIP. This can occur when a patient has signs in a part of the body where they would not be expected, when two disorders coexist, or when the DIP signs are integral parts of another syndrome (as in the neuroleptic malig-nant syndrome). Also, clinicians may misidentify oral tremors (rabbit syn-drome) as tardive dyskinesia if they are unaware that tremors can affect all body parts. Also, rapid lower-extremity movements caused by akathisia can be difficult to distinguish from tremor. When faced with coexisting disorders that feature seemingly opposed pathologic conditions, as with DIP and tardive dyskinesia, clinicians may be tempted to ascribe all abnormalities to one disorder. However, tardive dyskinesia and DIP clearly can coexist (Rich-ardson & Craig, 1982; Caligiuri et al., 1991; Hansen et al., 1992c) and sometimes can affect the same body area simultaneously.

The neuroleptic malignant syndrome (NMS) consists of fever, rigidity, autonomic dysfunction, alterations in consciousness, and often elevated serum concentrations of creatine phosphokinase (CPK) (Pearlman, 1986; Pope, Keck, & McElroy, 1986; Kellam, 1987; Addonizio, Susman, & Roth, 1987; Rosebush & Stewart, 1989; Lazarus, Mann, & Caroff, 1989). The presence of parkinsonian signs suggests that dopaminergic hypofunction may contribute to the abnormalities of this relatively rare, but potentially lethal, disorder. In fact, the additional signs and symptoms suggest pathologic pro-cesses more extensive than those associated with DIP. However, Levinson and Simpson (1986) have suggested that many cases of NMS simply reflect severe extrapyramidal symptoms and that the fever and other signs can be accounted for by co-morbid medical conditions, central medication effects, or peripheral muscle contractions. Regardless of whether one accepts NMS as a disorder distinct from DIP or considers it to be DIP complicated by hetero-geneous medical conditions, the potential lethality of the process demands that some distinction be made and that appropriate interventions be taken. Indeed, NMS requires immediate discontinuation of antipsychotic medication and avoidance of anticholinergics (because of impaired temperature regulation and confusion) (Lazarus et al., 1989) – approaches not required for treatment of DIP.

Parkinsonism Caused by Drugs Other Than Standard Antipsychotics

A number of medications not generally considered to be antipsychotic drugs can cause DIP. One is reserpine, used as an antipsychotic in the past, but now primarily used to treat hypertension. Others include tetrabenazine (unavailable in the United States) and the antihypertensive α-methyldopa, both of which deplete central catecholamines and warrant special mention because of their occasional use for treatment of tardive dyskinesia. Antiemetics and metoclopramide are particularly important causes of unrecognized DIP, because of their frequent use in nonpsychiatric patients (Grimes, 1981, 1982; Grimes, Hassan, & Preston, 1982; Indo & Ando, 1982; Stephen & Williamson, 1984; Sirota et al., 1986; Wilson & Smith, 1987; Ganzini et al., 1993). Miscellaneous other drugs should also be considered as possible sources of or contributors to DIP. Among these are flunarizine and cinnarizine (Chouza et al., 1986; Micheli et al., 1987), nifedipine (Singh, 1987), phenelzine (Teusink, Alexopoulos, & Shamoian, 1984; Gillman & Sandyk, 1986), high-dosage diazepam (Suranyi-Cadotte et al., 1985), zimelidine (Ansseau et al., 1985), and amiodarone (Lombard, Sarsfield, & Keogh, 1986), all of which have been reported to cause or exacerbate DIP.

The parkinsonian syndrome caused by MPTP (1-methyl-4-phenyl-1,2,5,6-tetrahydropyridine) (Langston & Ballard, 1983; Burns et al., 1985; Snyder & D'Amato, 1986; Jenner, 1989) might be considered a version of DIP as well. However, like the drugs just described, MPTP obviously is not used as an antipsychotic. Further, MPTP acts, after metabolism to MPP$^+$ (1-methyl-4-phenylpyridine), as a cellular neurotoxin that destroys nigral dopaminergic neurons (Snyder & D'Amato, 1986; Jenner, 1989). Interestingly, cognitive deficits comparable to those seen in patients with idiopathic parkinsonism are also seen in patients with MPTP-induced parkinsonism (Stern & Langston, 1985; Stern et al., 1990).

Epidemiology

Prevalence and Incidence of DIP

Investigators have reported a wide range of occurrence rates for DIP, both the rates of appearance of new cases (incidence) and the cross-sectional frequen-

Table 24.2. *Occurrences of drug-induced parkinsonism*

Study	Sample size	Number affected	Occurrence rate (%)	Comment
Ayd (1961)	3,775	581	15.4	—
Goldman (1961)	5,275	1,981	37.6	Cases required change in treatment
Demars (1966)	371	32·	8.7	—
Lehmann et al. (1970)	350	255	72.8	Used rating scale
Crane (1974)	669	82	12.3	Used rating scale; minimal DIP in 159 additional patients
Korczyn & Goldberg (1976)	66	40	61	Used rating scale; included mild and more severe cases (12 were "more obvious")
Jose et al. (1979)	76	34	44.7	Used rating scale; case threshold not given; depot medications
Binder & Levy (1981)	80	25	31.2	Combined data from three racial groups
Tune & Coyle (1981)	76	27	35.5	Used rating scale; all treated with anticholinergics
McCreadie et al. (1982)	117	31	26.5	Used rating scale; 20% off medications; corrected rate same
Moleman et al. (1982)	98	38	38.8	Included in Moleman et al. (1986) (not counted in total)
Ayd (1983)	5,000	660	13.2	Included uncited cases from literature (not counted in total)
Luchins et al. (1983)	20	8	40.0	Cases defined by use of antiparkinson agents
El-Defrawi & Craig (1984)	27	8	29.6	Used rating scale
Moleman et al. (1986)	230	100	43.5	Low threshold for diagnosis; haloperidol only medication
Hoffman et al. (1987)[a]	21	16	76.2	Used rating scale; older patients only; mostly males
Kucharski et al. (1987)	331	89	26.8	Used rating scale
Wagner et al. (1988)	322	88	27.3	—

Table 24.2. (*cont.*)

Study	Sample size	Number affected	Occurrence rate (%)	Comment
Decina et al. (1990a)	130	35	26.9	Used rating scale
Grohmann et al. (1990)	754	129	17.1	German ADR[b] study
Keepers & Casey (1991)	62	18	29.0	Chart review; in subsequent treatment, 37% had DIP
Richardson et al. (1991)	61	21	34.4	Used rating scale; children and adolescents
Ganzini et al. (1991a)	17	12	70.6	Used rating scale; very elderly sample; premorbid parkinsonism confounded rate
Sandyk & Kay (1991)	35	17	48.6	Used rating scale
Hansen et al. (1992a)	101	26	25.7	Used rating scale; mostly males

[a]A study (Hoffman et al., 1991) of the same patients found no change in frequency of DIP.
[b]ADR, adverse drug reaction.

cies of DIP in various populations (prevalence). Table 24.2 lists studies that have reported the number of patients in the base population and either the frequency of DIP or the number of cases found. The overall rate of occurrence was 28.2%, with 3,630 cases identified among 12,886 patients at risk. Two samples were excluded from the totals – one because the author indicated that he had collected some of his data from the literature, and the other because the cases were described in a larger subsequent report. DIP was reported to have occurred at rates that varied from 10% to 75% of patients in the various studies. Interestingly, methodological differences (such as use of standardized rates and years of study) did not readily explain the variation in rates. Other variables such as the length of the observation period (e.g., prevalence vs. incidence) and various risk factors in the study population may have contributed to the wide range of occurrences reported.

Risk Factors for DIP

A number of variables can influence the occurrence and/or severity of DIP. Possible risk factors include age, gender, pharmacologic variables, concurrent use of lithium, coarse brain disease, acquired immune-deficiency syndrome (AIDS), smoking, family history of EPS, race, and histocompatibility antigen (HLA) type.

Age. Age is a well-established risk factor for DIP. In six studies that examined the age dependence of DIP, it was concluded that the disorder is more common in older patients (Ayd, 1961, 1983; Demars, 1966; Crane, 1974; Jose et al., 1979; Rajput, 1984; Hansen et al., 1988). We, too, found the highest rates of DIP in reports of older patients (Hoffman et al., 1987; Ganzini et al., 1991b). The elderly are more vulnerable even though they often receive lower dosages of less potent neuroleptics. Some investigators, however, have not found an age relationship in their studies (Korczyn & Goldberg, 1976; McCreadie, Barron, & Winslow, 1982; Luchins, Jackman, & Meltzer, 1983), although the covariates that influence DIP rates may not have been controlled in two of those studies (Korczyn & Goldberg, 1976; McCreadie et al., 1982). In a third study, the patients were all quite young (27 years for DIP vs. 29 years for non-DIP). One group actually found DIP to be more common in younger patients (Moleman, Schmitz, & Ladee, 1982; Moleman et al., 1986). Their patients included a range of ages, and they controlled for other variables by using multiple-regression analysis. Keepers, Clappison, and Casey (1983) found that DIP was most common in two age groups (10–19-year-olds and 50–59-year-olds). Perhaps age is associated with opposing influences on DIP. Older patients, for example, may become more vulnerable to DIP because of the age-related reduction in nigrostriatal dopaminergic projections or, less commonly, the development of IPD (Rozzini et al., 1985). Young patients, on the other hand, may have increased vulnerability based on some other factor.

There is little information on the epidemiology of DIP in child and adolescent populations. One study (Richardson, Haugland, & Craig, 1991) reported that the overall prevalence of DIP among young patients was 34%. Although that rate is somewhat higher than the average shown in Table 24.2, it is substantially lower than that seen in geriatric settings. Another report examined childhood schizophrenic patients with autistic features and found EPS (primarily DIP) rates ranging from zero to 40%, depending on the antipsychotic drug studied (Engelhardt & Polizos, 1978). The data presented in the latter report do not allow for calculation of an overall rate for the 95 patients.

Gender. Female gender has been considered a DIP risk factor since the earliest studies (Ayd, 1960, 1961), in which women were found to be affected two to three times as often as men. Other reports have concurred that women are at greater risk for DIP (Demars, 1966; Sheppard & Merlis, 1967; Crane, 1974; Korczyn & Goldberg, 1976; Ayd, 1983; Luchins et al., 1983), although the increase in risk has not always been significant or independent of covariates. Only one study has concluded that males are more often affected (Wagner, Wolf, & Ulmar, 1988). Several, however, have reported no difference in the rate of DIP between the genders (Lehmann, Ban, & Saxena, 1970; McCreadie et al., 1982; Moleman et al., 1986). To further investigate this issue, we determined the numbers of males and females affected and the numbers at risk in the studies from which such data could be extracted (Ayd, 1961; Demars, 1966; Sheppard & Merlis, 1967; Lehmann et al., 1970; Luchins et al., 1983; Moleman et al., 1986). Of the 7,574 men and 8,122 women at risk, 755 (10%) men and 1,433 (18%) women had DIP. The prevalence of DIP among females was significantly greater than that among males ($\chi^2 = 79.9$, df $= 1$, $p < .001$)

Pharmacologic Variables. A variety of pharmacologic factors can influence rates of DIP. Higher potency antipsychotics consistently cause higher rates of DIP (Ayd, 1961; Sheppard & Merlis, 1967; Gollomp et al., 1983; Grohmann, Koch, & Schmidt, 1990), an association that may occur with atypical neuroleptics (Seeman, 1990). Clozapine, a low-potency neuroleptic, does not cause DIP and may actually have antiparkinsonian activity (Casey, 1989). Other atypical neuroleptics could turn out to be more potent than clozapine and still cause low rates of extrapyramidal symptoms (Seeman, 1990). For instance, risperidone, an antipsychotic with both antiserotonergic and antidopaminergic activities, causes fewer extrapyramidal symptoms than do comparable doses of haloperidol (Casey & Hansen, 1995).

Unlike potency, antipsychotic dosage has not consistently been found to correlate with either the prevalence or severity of DIP (Goldman, 1961; Demars, 1966; Richardson et al., 1991). Moleman et al. (1986) found the intuitively expected increased rate of DIP with increased dosage of haloperidol, and we (Hansen et al., 1988) found recent use of antipsychotics (an indirect measure of dosage) to be associated with the presence of DIP on admission to an inpatient psychiatry unit. Perhaps the absence of a robust dose–response relationship reflects poor correlation between blood concentrations and extrapyramidal symptoms. Witness the six studies in which blood concentrations of neuroleptics were positively and significantly correlated with the severity and prevalence of extrapyramidal symptoms (Itoh et al., 1981; Hansen, Larsen, & Vestergard, 1981; Hansen, Larsen, & Gulmann, 1982; Aoba et al., 1985; Hansen & Larsen, 1985; Krska et al., 1986). However, in five other studies, no such correlation was found (Calil et al., 1979; Tune & Coyle, 1980; Van Putten et al., 1980; Escobar, Barron, & Kiriakos, 1983; Gaffney & Tune, 1985). Perhaps variations in the dosages of concomitant anticholinergic medications across the various studies can explain some of this disparity. In the only study in which both antipsychotic and anticholinergic concentrations were measured, the latter significantly influenced the severity of DIP, but the former did not (Tune & Coyle, 1981).

Other Factors. Other medications have been implicated as DIP risk factors. For instance, case reports have suggested that lithium can cause or exacerbate DIP (Khaitan & Laha, 1985; Addonizio, 1985; Sachdev, 1986). In one study, a high prevalence of DIP was found among patients on lithium and antipsychotics (Perényi, Rihmer, & Banki, 1983b); in another, DIP was exacerbated in 10 antipsychotic-treated patients when lithium was added to their medication regimen (Feinstein, Ron, & Wessely, 1990).

Although the influence of cigarette smoking on the expression of DIP has been examined, there is no consensus as to its effect. Whereas two studies concluded that smoking reduces the risk for DIP (Decina et al., 1990a; Goff, Henderson, & Amico, 1992), two others did not (Yassa et al., 1987; Wagner et al., 1988). In the first of the former studies (Decina et al., 1990a), gender affected the outcome, with male smokers having lower mean DIP scores and a lower conditional probability of being classified as having DIP on the basis of a log linear-regression equation. In the second study (Goff et al., 1992), the mean parkinsonism score was significantly lower for schizophrenics who were currently smoking, as compared with nonsmoking patients, even though the smokers received a higher mean antipsychotic dosage. However, because the parkinsonism scores were low and the number of cases of DIP was not reported, one cannot say that the frequency of DIP was lower among the smokers. A third study (Wagner et al., 1988) showed no significant difference in frequency of smoking between patients with DIP (55%) and matched controls without DIP (58%). A fourth study failed to show a relationship between smoking and DIP, but those authors had examined only a small sample of DIP patients (Yassa et al., 1987). One might expect to find that smoking would provide a protective effect against DIP, for smoking can reduce serum concentrations of neuroleptics (Ereshefsky et al., 1985) (higher dosages given to smoking patients, however, can offset this effect). Smoking may also more directly affect the risk for DIP, perhaps by modulating dopaminergic neurotransmission, inasmuch as smoking seems to have an overall protective effect against IPD (Baron, 1986).

Coarse or diffuse brain disease may contribute to DIP vulnerability as well, in the form of "organic damage" (Korczyn & Goldberg, 1976) or lobotomies (Holden, Itil, & Keskiner, 1969), or as reflected in increased ventricular brain ratios (Luchins et al., 1983; Hoffman et al., 1987; Fayen et al., 1988; Sandyk & Kay, 1991). Also, case reports indicate that patients with AIDS may be especially vulnerable to EPSs, including DIP (Edelstein & Knight, 1987; Swenson et al., 1989). Judging from the frequent neuropsychiatric findings, including movement disorders, in AIDS patients (Nath, Jankovic, & Pettigrew, 1987), human immunodeficiency virus (HIV) infection of the basal ganglia may be causing that increase in vulnerability.

Finally, genetic factors can influence DIP. One study (Metzer et al., 1989) showed an increased prevalence of the antigen HLA-B44 in patients with DIP (55%), as compared with patients without DIP (13%). Although that finding was highly statistically significant, its clinical significance is unclear. Perhaps some patient characteristic that serves as a risk factor is coded for by a gene close to the HLA locus. Alternatively, the HLA antigens may directly affect neurotransmission through their influence on cell surface interactions, as suggested by an HLA study that was prompted by the possibility of a genetic predisposition to DIP (Metzer et al., 1989). Case studies of DIP probands have occasionally noted that family members have had either IPD or DIP (Aronson, 1985). One research group has published two studies that suggest an inherited component of risk for DIP patients, with DIP patients being more likely than controls to have family members with parkinsonism (Myrianthopoulos, Kurland, & Kurland, 1962; Myrianthopoulos, Waldrop, & Vincent, 1967). Also, race may influence the overall occurrence of extrapyramidal symptoms, perhaps in part by affecting neuroleptic concentrations achieved for a given dosage of medicine (Lin et al., 1988). Few studies, however, have specifically examined differential rates of DIP between races. In one study, the rates of DIP were comparable for Asians and Caucasians (40% vs. 35%), but lower for blacks (15%).

Even within a group of patients at risk for DIP, not all are affected. This suggests that additional unknown or idiosyncratic factors must be important. Not surprisingly, the best predictor for future episodes of DIP is a history of DIP during prior treatment. Using data from two episodes of treatment, Keepers and Casey (1991) found that previous history regarding DIP correctly predicted the recurrence of DIP or the absence of DIP in 76% of 62 patients. Perhaps more detailed biochemical or laboratory tests will identify the individual characteristics associated with this idiosyncratic vulnerability. Patients who have alterations in the excretion or metabolism of dopamine during or prior to antipsychotic treatment may be at increased risk (Crowley et al., 1978; Bowers, 1985), as may patients with low concentrations of calcium (El-Defrawi & Craig, 1984).

DIP and Risk for Tardive Dyskinesia

The relationship between DIP and tardive dyskinesia is more complex than was predicted by the model in which the syndromes represented opposing dopaminergic states. First, the two disorders often coexist (Gerlach, 1977; Richardson & Craig, 1982; Oyebode & McClelland, 1986; Jankovic & Casabona, 1987; Sramek, Potkin, & Hahn, 1988; Hansen et al., 1988, 1992c; Wirshing et al., 1989). Furthermore, within-patient correlations between the disorders have been found to range from positive to negative (Hansen et al., 1992c). Still, when neuroleptics are suddenly withdrawn from patients who have been treated for long periods, the expected reciprocal decrease in DIP and increase in tardive dyskinesia are observed (Hoffman et al., 1987, 1992). When a transition from DIP to tardive dyskinesia is seen during a reduction in antipsychotic treatment (Crane, 1972), there is a high probability that the sequence reflects a common neurobiological process in the basal ganglia. An alternative hypothesis is that co-occurrence of the two movement disorders reveals that a patient's circuitry connecting cortex, basal ganglia, and thalamus has a general vulnerability to the effects of neuroleptics. In that case, DIP (the more acute disorder) may appear to create greater risk for tardive dyskinesia. Indeed, one prospective study of the incidence of tardive dyskinesia indicated that DIP early in the course of treatment is a risk factor for later hyperkinesia (Kane, Woerner, & Lieberman, 1988).

Although many of the established risk factors for DIP are similar to those for tardive dyskinesia, two of the risk factors for tardive dyskinesia apparently do not affect the occurrence of DIP. First, no difference in handedness between patients with and without DIP was found in a study that showed right-handed patients at greater risk for tardive dyskinesia (Brown et al., 1992). Second, although diabetes mellitus increases the risk for tardive dyskinesia (Ganzini et al., 1991a), it does not affect DIP (Ganzini et al., 1993).

Evaluation

Clinical Evaluation

If clinicians are to evaluate patients properly for the presence of DIP, they must (1) be alert for the possible presence of DIP and (2) perform the focused neurological examination necessary to identify symptoms of EPSs. Studies have shown, however, that psychiatric residents may fail to record observations of DIP in as many as 50% of symptomatic cases (Weiden et al., 1987; Hansen et al., 1992a). It appears that the residents' performance improves, however, after specific training in this aspect of psychopharmacology (Dixon et al., 1989). In our experience, it appears that medical students and residents have learned to use a screening neurological examination that focuses on localization of motor abnormalities, rather than on detection of extrapyramidal signs. We thus recommend that physicians take particular care to examine patients for all signs of DIP during physical examinations and while monitoring responses to antipsychotic medications. This will require that they observe each patient at rest for tremor and choreiform movements, that they note normal adjusting movements throughout the examination period, that they ask the patient to do a simple, repetitive task as quickly as possible (e.g., rapid alternating hand movements, hand-tapping, or finger-tapping), that they check muscle tone for rigidity (noting cogwheeling, if present), and that they observe the patient's arm swing, speed, stride length, and turns while walking. If the patient seems unsteady, postural stability can be assessed. Some clinicians also evaluate the glabellar tap, though we do not find this particularly useful. These procedures should add only 5–10 minutes to a physical examination or medication check-up. The results of the examination, whether indications of DIP are present or not, should be recorded in the patient's medical record.

The need for additional clinical examination will be influenced by the patient's history and physical examination. Some examination of brain structure probably is indicated for most patients with movement disorders. For instance, we found a surprising number of patients (6 of 21) with focal brain loss (presumably from unrecognized strokes) in a computed tomography (CT) study of schizophrenic patients more than 55 years of age (Hoffman et al., 1987).

Rating Scales

Researchers need to measure DIP objectively, and clinicians may want to do so. We believe that the use of rating scales, a number of which exist for rating DIP, can facilitate the performance and recording of a thorough examination. Unfortunately, no scale is entirely satisfactory. Probably the one most often used is the Simpson-Angus Rating Scale for Extrapyramidal Side Effects (Simpson et al., 1964, 1970), also called the Neurologic Rating Scale (NRS). Although it measures the common clinical signs of parkinsonism with anchor points on a 5-point (0–4) scale, it emphasizes rigidity and does not evaluate bradykinesia and facial immobility. These limitations and the need for adaptations for special circumstances have led investigators to create several forms of the NRS.

The St. Hans Rating Scale for Extrapyramidal Side Effects (SHS), developed by Jes Gerlach at the St. Hans Hospital in Roskilde, Denmark, although less well known in the United States than abroad, offers advantages over the NRS (Gardos et al., 1987). For one thing, all EPSs (DIP, tardive dyskinesia, akathisia, and dystonia) can be rated on the same form, but recorded in separate sections. All the key DIP symptoms (facial expression, bradykinesia, rigidity, tremor, arm swing, posture, gait, and salivation) are rated on a 7-point (0–6) scale. This permits the rater to distinguish severity ratings that fall between mild and moderate, and between moderate and severe, which is an improvement over other scales that use 0–3 or 0–4 scaling. The SHS, limited by a lack of descriptive anchor points, does not allow the investigator to rate more than one aspect of each key symptom.

Studies of IPD have used the Webster Scale (Webster, 1968) and, more recently the Unified Rating Scale (URS) for parkinsonism (Stern, 1988). The 18 items of the URS are scored on a 5-point (0–4) scale, and each level has anchor points. The URS is a complete and relatively well balanced instrument, but considerable time is required to complete it. The anchor points, moreover, are skewed to the more severe end of the spectrum.

Other scales are used less often. The Targeting Abnormal Kinetic Effects (TAKE) scale (Wojcik et al., 1980), which has the advantage of including some miscellaneous signs (drooling and seborrhea), suffers from its incorporation of akathisia. The Smith-TRIMS scale (Smith et al., 1983), which mixes tardive dyskinesia and DIP signs on the same scale, is infrequently used. Mindham (1976) and Chouinard et al. (1980) have developed scales for use with their own protocols. The DiMascio Extrapyramidal Symptom Rating Scale (DiMascio et al., 1976), although it covers a number of useful symptom areas, has anchor points of questionable validity (e.g., "cogwheeling" is used to define more severe rigidity, and "akinesia" seems to rate only gait).

After rating 288 patients with three rating scales (NRS, SHS, URS), we performed a principal-components analysis of the nonredundant items and found a four-factor varimax solution that accounted for 68% of the variance (Keepers, Hansen, & Casey, 1988). The structure of the solution is shown in Table 24.3. This analysis allows us to avoid purely arbitrary placement of items into symptom groups. For instance, for the question whether reduced arm swing should be considered primarily bradykinesia, rigidity, or loss of postural reflexes, the principal-components solution suggests that it is more

Table 24.3. *Structure of parkinsonian subscales
derived from principal-components analysis*

Scale	Bradykinesia	Rigidity	Gait	Tremor
SHS	Facial expression Bradykinesia	Rigidity	Gait Posture Arm swing	Tremor
NRS		Wrist Elbow Shoulder Arm dropping		

URS	Finger-tapping
	Rapid alternating
	    movements
	Rapid successive
	    movements
		Neck
		Leg
			Rapid leg
			    movements
				Postural tremor
				Upper extremity
				Facial tremor
				Lower extremity

closely related to items specifically associated with posture and gait. The components analysis, in tandem with an assessment of interrater reliability, has enabled us to identify items that form the irreducible minimum for an accurate research assessment of DIP. These have been incorporated into a new rating scale for acute extrapyramidal symptoms (the Casey-Portland EPS scale), currently in preparation for publication.

Measurement of DIP symptoms with various recording devices (instrumentation measurement) provides a potentially useful alternative to clinical ratings. It is beyond the scope of this chapter to describe the great variety of tools used, including accelerometers, ultrasound, strain gauges, photodetectors, electromagnetic systems, blink counters, electromyographs, and others (Draper & Johns, 1964; Collins, Lee, & Tyrer, 1979; Marsden & Schachter, 1981; May, Lee, & Bacon, 1983; Bathien, Koutlidis, & Rondot, 1984; Andersen, 1986; May, 1987; Teravainen et al., 1989; Caligiuri et al., 1989). Although such methods can be quite sensitive, they do not allow a comprehensive view of the entire DIP syndrome.

Pathophysiology

For many years, clinicians have wondered whether or not the occurrence of DIP is a necessary event prior to a clinical response to antipsychotics (Simpson et al., 1964; Bishop, Gallant, & Sykes, 1965; Gerken, Wetzel, & Benkert, 1991). Indeed, the term "neuroleptic" literally means "to grip the nerve." The pathophysiology of DIP presumably involves D_2 dopamine-receptor blockade (Marsden & Jenner, 1980). Because effectiveness of the D_2-receptor blockade is the single best predictor of antipsychotic activity for typical drugs, some relationship between DIP and an antipsychotic response might reasonably be expected. However, the discovery of drugs that act as antipsychotics with low dopamine-antagonist activity (e.g., clozapine) suggests that DIP is not necessarily coupled to a clinical response (Bishop et al., 1965; Gerken et al., 1991).

Several groups have examined the use of DIP as a marker for adequate brain concentrations of antipsychotic medications. That has led to studies of changes in handwriting to guide selection of an antipsychotic dosage (Simpson et al., 1970; Angus & Simpson, 1970), as well as efforts to use the first subtle manifestations of DIP to determine the "neuroleptic-threshold dosage" (Alpert et al., 1978; McEvoy, 1986; McEvoy et al., 1986, 1991). Although that approach to establishing minimum effective dosages has not proved an easy alternative to standard clinical practice, it does suggest that DIP provides a crude index of the effects of brain neuroleptic concentrations on the motor system. Recent positron-emission tomographic data have substantiated that concept (Farde et al., 1992). Patients with acute EPSs (primarily DIP and akathisia) were found to have higher D_2 dopamine-receptor occupancy than other patients. The threshold for causing DIP fell between blockade of 74% and blockade of 82% of D_2 receptors. Because patients showed good clinical responses (and did not have DIP) at even lower D_2-receptor occupancy, that study (Farde et al., 1992) provides more evidence that DIP is not necessarily linked to clinical response.

Our current understanding of the structure and connectivity of the basal ganglia, cortex, and thalamus offers a model for understanding the complex relationship between DIP and clinical response. Several investigators, most notably Alexander and colleagues, have described multiple parallel loops connecting cortex, basal ganglia, and thalamus (Figure 24.1) (Nauta, 1986; Alexander, DeLong, & Strick, 1986; Alexander et al., 1990). Although the pathways are anatomically and functionally separate, it is not known if they are pharmacologically distinct. It is hypothesized that the parallel anatomic circuits subserve parallel functions. Thus, the motor loop is involved in planning and targeting motor behavior, the prefrontal loop is involved in working memory and related cognitive processes, and the limbic circuit is part of an affective and motivational subsystem (Alexander et al., 1990; Goldman-Rakic, 1990; Smith & Bolam, 1990). If, as has been proposed, the limbic (Buchsbaum, 1990; Csernansky et al., 1991) and prefrontal (Goldman-Rakic, 1990; Robbins, 1990) circuits compose the primary anatomic substrate for psychotic symptoms, the differing sensitivities to dopaminergic blockade in

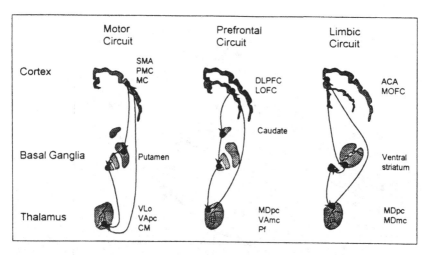

Figure 24.1. Multiple parallel circuits connecting cortex, basal ganglia, and thalamus. The specificity of projections is maintained throughout each pathway. SMA, supplementary motor area; PMC, premotor cortex; MC, motor cortex; DLPFC, dorsolateral prefrontal cortex; LOFC, lateral orbitofrontal cortex; ACA, anterior cingulate area; MOFC, medial orbitofrontal cortex; VLo, nucleus ventrolateralis pars oralis; VApc, nucleus ventroanterior pars parvocellularis; CM, nucleus centromedianus; MDpc, nucleus mediodorsalis pars parvocellularis; VAmc, nucleus ventroanterior pars magnocellularis; Pf, nucleus parafascicularis; MDmc, nucleus mediocorsalis pars magnocellularis.

these circuits relative to the motor circuit could lead to either correlation or dissociation of abnormalities in their respective functional domains. Clearly, high-potency medications, which block most of the dopamine receptors in the striatum (Farde et al., 1992), are more likely to produce both DIP and an antipsychotic effect. Lower-potency drugs, such as clozapine, that block fewer receptors have the potential to affect the corticostriatal circuits differentially.

In addition to the anatomic parallelism, there is an additional level of pharmacologic and functional parallelism within each circuit linking cortex, basal ganglia, and thalamus (Alexander et al., 1990; DeLong, 1990). Figures 24.2–24.4 illustrate this parallelism in a normal individual and in patients with IPD and DIP. The figures provide a simplified model of the true system and omit several feedback loops and inputs from other brain regions. The central features of the model emphasize that (1) the projection of cortex to striatum is phasic and excitatory, (2) the influence of the globus pallidus on the thalamus is tonic and inhibitory, and (3) the thalamocortical output is phasic and excitatory. The two parallel circuits originating in the striatum phasically increase or decrease thalamic inhibition. Cortical stimulation of the

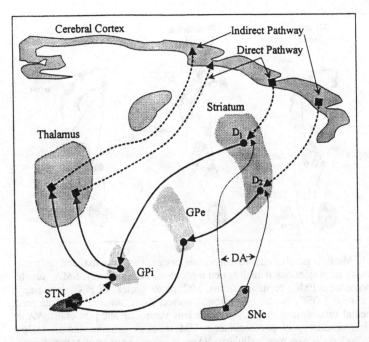

Figure 24.2. Circuitry linking cortex, basal ganglia, and thalamus. Activation of the indirect pathway (through the subthalamic nucleus) by excitatory input from the cortex results in thalamic (and hence cortical) inhibition. Activation of the direct pathway by excitatory corticostriatal fibers results in thalamic (and cortical) disinhibition. Note that in the normal brain, stimulation of both D_1 and D_2 receptors results in thalamic activation. Identifications of neurotransmitters other than dopamine are omitted for simplicity. Dashed lines and solid lines indicate excitatory and inhibitory projections, respectively. DA, dopamine; GPe, globus pallidus externa; GPi, globus pallidus pars interna; STN, subthalamic nucleus; SNc, substantia nigra pars compacta. (Adapted from Alexander et al., 1990.)

direct pathway results in an increase in thalamic output, whereas stimulation of the indirect pathway causes a corresponding decrease (Figure 24.2). The direct and indirect pathways differ in their modes of dopaminergic modulation (Graybiel, 1990; Alexander et al., 1990). Striatal neurons in the direct circuit express D_1 receptors and are stimulated by nigrostriatal dopaminergic input. Striatal neurons in the indirect circuit, on the other hand, express D_2 receptors and are inhibited by dopamine. The net result of nigrostriatal dopaminergic release is thalamic disinhibition, with resultant increases in motoric output and cortical arousal. Loss of nigral dopaminergic cells in patients with IPD (Figure 24.3) results in excessive thalamic inhibition due to net overactivity in

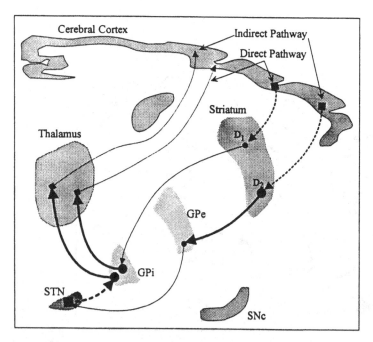

Figure 24.3. Circuitry linking cortex, basal ganglia, and thalamus in a patient with idiopathic Parkinson's disease. Loss of dopaminergic cells in SNc results in net thalamic (and hence cortical) inhibition due to net overactivity of the indirect pathway. Dashed lines and solid lines indicate excitatory and inhibitory projections, respectively. Thicknesses of arrows correspond to relative neuronal activities. GPe, globus pallidus externa; GPi, globus pallidus pars interna; STN, subthalamic nucleus; SNc, substantia nigra pars compacta. (Adapted from Alexander et al., 1990.)

the indirect circuit (DeLong, 1990). DIP (Figure 24.4) results from treatment with D_2-receptor antagonists. This results in a loss of D_2-mediated modulation of striatal-projection neurons and subsequent increased thalamic inhibition in the indirect channel. The D_1-modulated direct pathway, however, is less affected in patients with DIP, inasmuch as typical neuroleptics are weak D_1 antagonists. Thus, under circumstances in which the indirect loop is disabled but the direct loop is still functioning – specifically, patients treated with highly selective D_2 antagonists (e.g., raclopride) and younger patients without baseline loss of dopaminergic projections – DIP may be less severe than the idiopathic disorder or of different character than the idiopathic disorder. Clozapine may exert its unique spectrum of activity because (1) it is, overall, a weak dopamine antagonist, (2) it is slightly more active at the D_1 site than at the D_2 site, and (3) it is a potent anticholinergic and antiserotonergic agent.

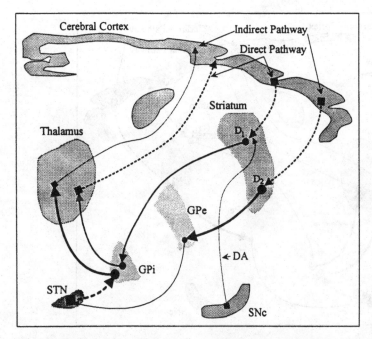

Figure 24.4. Circuitry linking cortex, basal ganglia, and thalamus in a patient with neuroleptic-induced DIP. Treatment with typical neuroleptics results in blockade of the D_2 input to the indirect pathway, but leaves the D_1-modulated indirect pathway intact. Dashed lines and solid lines indicate excitatory and inhibitory projections, respectively. Thicknesses of arrows correspond to relative neuronal activities. DA, dopamine, GPe, globus pallidus externa; GPi, globus pallidus pars interna; STN, subthalamic nucleus; SNc, substantia nigra pars compacta.

Treatment

Treatment strategies for DIP can include changing the dosage or type of antipsychotic and/or introducing another medication to treat the side effect. Centrally acting anticholinergic medications (benztropine, trihexyphenidyl, diphenhydramine, procyclidine, and biperiden) are most commonly used to treat DIP. In addition, amantadine, dopamine agonists (e.g., bromocriptine), electroconvulsive treatment, and a variety of other medications have been reported to reduce the severity of DIP.

The literature describing the use of anticholinergic agents, both for prophylaxis and as acute treatment for DIP, has been summarized in several reviews (McEvoy, 1983; Keepers & Casey, 1986). The usual daily doses are as follows: benztropine, 1–6 mg; trihexyphenidyl, 5–15 mg; diphenhydramine,

25–100 mg; procyclidine, 5–30 mg; biperiden, 2–10 mg. Most studies have concluded that anticholinergics have antiparkinsonian effects for DIP, although their benefit for prophylaxis is less well supported (Keepers & Casey, 1986). For instance, Keepers et al. (1983) reported that 10% of their patients receiving anticholinergic prophylaxis developed dystonia, as compared with almost 40% of patients who did not receive prophylaxis; the comparable difference for DIP was about 15% versus 30%, still significant, but less dramatic than for dystonia. Although it is clear that anticholinergic drugs have antiparkinsonian effects, the extent of their efficacy may be limited; moreover, they are associated with additional side effects. In our experience, it is unusual for DIP to resolve entirely with the addition of anticholinergic medications.

The potential toxic effects of anticholinergic medications can vary from an uncomfortable dry mouth and blurred vision to potentially dangerous urinary retention, severe constipation, and even frank delirium (McEvoy, 1983). Memory impairment should also be considered a toxic effect of the use of anticholinergics, even at standard or low dosages (benztropine equivalents of 1–4 mg daily). Short-term memory deficits have been reported for normal subjects (McEvoy et al., 1987b; Gelenberg et al., 1989) as well as for patients (Tune et al., 1982; Perlick et al., 1986; Fayen et al., 1988; Strauss et al., 1990). Although one study did not reveal a memory abnormality, it was a cross-sectional study in which the authors believed that variances in patients' performances caused by psychotic symptoms and other factors prevented observation of an anticholinergic amnestic effect (Katz et al., 1985).

Additional concerns regarding the use of anticholinergics include possible antagonism of antipsychotic effects and the potential for abuse. Anticholinergics may reduce blood concentrations of some antipsychotic agents (Simpson et al., 1980; Bamrah et al., 1986). Alternatively, anticholinergic drugs may reduce antipsychotic effects via dopaminergic activity, as suggested for benztropine (Modell, Tandon, & Beresford, 1989). The potential for abuse of anticholinergics to achieve euphoric effects has been documented (Dilsaver, 1988), with a suggestion that this side effect might have utility in treating the negative symptoms of schizophrenia (Fisch, 1987).

Given these problems with anticholinergic medications, the attempt to find other modes of treatment for DIP is not surprising. Many medications have been tried, with varying results, including ritanserin (Bersani et al., 1990), valproic acid (Friis, Christensen, & Gerlach, 1983), piracetam (Kabes et al., 1982), mianserin (Korsgaard & Friis, 1986), adrenergic antagonists (Kulik & Wilbur, 1980; Chaudhry, Radonjic, & Waters, 1982; Chaturvedi, 1987, L-deprenyl (Perényi, Bagdy, & Arato, 1983a), and pyridoxine (Sandyk &

Pardeshi, 1990). Amantadine, a putative partial dopamine agonist, is probably the most commonly prescribed alternative to anticholinergics for treatment of DIP. Many studies have documented fewer side effects with amantadine than with other drugs, especially less memory impairment (McEvoy et al., 1987b; Fayen et al., 1988; Gelenberg et al., 1989). Nevertheless, although amantadine clearly reduces parkinsonian symptoms (Kelly et al., 1974; Fann & Lake, 1976; Pacifici et al., 1976), the lingering concern that it is not as efficacious as anticholinergic medications (Kelly et al., 1974; McEvoy, McCue, & Freter, 1987a) has kept it a second-line agent in the management of DIP. Dopamine agonists such as L-dopa and bromocriptine have also been used to treat patients with extrapyramidal symptoms (Shoulson, 1983; Chouinard et al., 1987; Perovich et al., 1989). For most clinicians, the anticipated exacerbation of psychosis and/or reduction of antipsychotic efficacy have limited the use of these medications to complicated cases (Shoulson, 1983), although one study reported that bromocriptine can be safely used in clinically stable patients if they are receiving antipsychotic agents (Perovich et al., 1989).

Coexisting DIP and tardive dyskinesia have long been considered to present a clinical dilemma: Treatment that alleviates one disorder may exacerbate the other. However, we have found that these disorders do not necessarily have an inverse relationship (Hansen et al., 1992c). Moreover, Wirshing et al. (1989) found that tardive dyskinesia patients with coexisting DIP tremors showed reductions of tremors without exacerbation of tardive dyskinesia during anticholinergic treatment. Accordingly, we advise clinicians to intervene to reduce the most problematic of the two disorders and to carefully observe the effect of the intervention on the other syndrome.

Electroconvulsive treatment (ECT) can be a useful modality for treating selected cases of DIP. Reductions in symptoms with ECT have been seen in patients with idiopathic parkinsonism (Faber & Trimble, 1991; Rasmussen & Abrams, 1991) and in patients with DIP (Goswami et al., 1989; Hermesh et al., 1992). Although ECT is generally a safe procedure (Weiner et al., 1990), some risk is involved; it is unlikely, therefore, that uncomplicated DIP will ever be a primary indication for ECT. ECT should be considered as a possible treatment for patients with delusional depression who develop marked DIP or who have had serious problems with DIP in the past.

Our recommendations for managing DIP are summarized in Figure 24.5. Prevention of DIP by using the lowest effective dosage (or using a lower-potency drug) is the first step, especially for patients with a prior history of severe DIP. If DIP develops, the antipsychotic dosage should be reduced. If a patient's psychosis is too severe, or if the DIP is intolerable, treatment with an

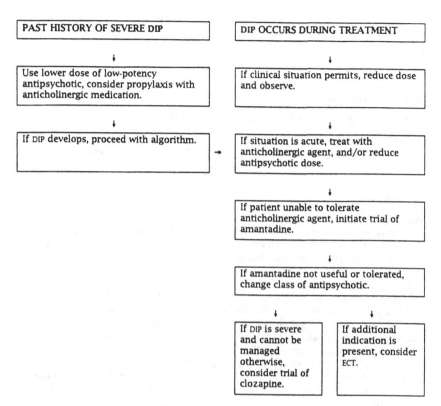

PAST HISTORY OF SEVERE DIP

↓

Use lower dose of low-potency antipsychotic, consider propylaxis with anticholinergic medication.

↓

If DIP develops, proceed with algorithm.

→

DIP OCCURS DURING TREATMENT

↓

If clinical situation permits, reduce dose and observe.

↓

If situation is acute, treat with anticholinergic agent, and/or reduce antipsychotic dose.

↓

If patient unable to tolerate anticholinergic agent, initiate trial of amantadine.

↓

If amantadine not useful or tolerated, change class of antipsychotic.

↓ ↓

If DIP is severe and cannot be managed otherwise, consider trial of clozapine.	If additional indication is present, consider ECT.

Figure 24.5. Managing DIP.

anticholinergic agent should be initiated. If the anticholinergic side effects are intolerable, amantadine can be considered as an alternative. Changing to a different class of antipsychotic should also be considered at this point. If a patient's psychosis and severe DIP cannot otherwise be managed, clozapine may be considered. Although ECT will be useful occasionally, it most likely will be for patients with additional indications, such as delusional depression or refractory mania.

Conclusion

This chapter has reviewed the clinical presentation, differential diagnosis, epidemiology, evaluation, pathophysiology, and treatment for DIP. This disorder occurs commonly, creating substantial morbidity for patients treated with antipsychotic drugs. Through study of DIP, much has been learned about both IPD and the mechanisms of action of antipsychotic medications. Future developments based on this knowledge are likely to improve our understanding of brain mechanisms and allow development of less toxic antipsychotic agents.

Acknowledgments

This work was supported by funding from the U.S. Department of Veterans Affairs Research Service (T. E. Hansen and W. F. Hoffman) and by National Institute of Mental Health grant R29-MH43586-05 (W. F. Hoffman).

References

Addonizio, G. (1985). Rapid induction of extrapyramidal side effects with combined use of lithium and neuroleptics. *J. Clin. Psychopharmacol.* 5:296–8.

Addonizio, G., Roth, S. D., Stokes, P. E., & Stoll, P. M. (1989). Increased extrapyramidal symptoms with addition of lithium to neuroleptics. *J. Nerv. Ment. Dis.* 176:682–5.

Addonizio, G., Susman, V. L., & Roth, S. D. (1987). Neuroleptic malignant syndrome: review and analysis of 115 cases. *Biol. Psychiatry* 22:1004–20.

Adler, C. H., Stern, M. B., & Brooks, M. L. (1989). Parkinsonism secondary to bilateral striatal fungal abscesses. *Mov. Disord.* 4:333–7.

Alexander, G. E., Crutcher, M. D., & DeLong, M. R. (1990). Basal ganglia–thalamocortical circuits: parallel substrates for motor, oculomotor, "prefrontal" and "limbic" functions. *Prog. Brain Res.* 85:119–46.

Alexander, G. E., DeLong, M. R., & Strick, P. L. (1986). Parallel organization of functionally segregated circuits linking basal ganglia and cortex. *Annu. Rev. Neurosci.* 9:357–81.

Alpert, M., Diamond, F., Weisenfreund, J., Taleporos, E., & Friedhoff, A. J. (1978). The neuroleptic hypothesis: study of the covariation of extrapyramidal and therapeutic drug effects. *Br. J. Psychiatry* 133:169–75.

Andersen, O. T. (1986). A system for quantitative assessment of dyscoordination and tremor. *Acta Neurol. Scand.* 73:291–4.

Angus, J. W. S., & Simpson, G. M. (1970). Handwriting changes and response to drugs: a controlled study. *Acta Psychiatr. Scand. (Suppl.)* 212:28–37.

Ansseau, M., Reynolds, C. F., III, Kupfer, D. J., Doumont, A., Geenen, V., Dresse, A. E., & Juorio, A. V. (1985). Extrapyramidal signs following zimelidine overdose. *J. Clin. Psychopharmacol.* 5:347–9.

Aoba, A., Kakita, Y., Yamaguchi, N., Shido, M., Tsuneizumi, T., Shibata, M., Kitani, K., & Hasegawa, K. (1985). Absence of age effect on plasma haloperidol neuroleptic levels in psychiatric patients. *J. Gerontol.* 40:303–8.

Aronson, T. A. (1985). Persistent drug-induced parkinsonism. *Biol. Psychiatry* 20:795–8.

Ayd, F. J., Jr. (1960). Drug-induced extrapyramidal reactions: their clinical manifestations and treatment with Akineton. *Psychosomatics* 1:143–50.

Ayd, F. J., Jr. (1961). A survey of drug-induced extrapyramidal reactions. *J. Am. Med. Assoc.* 175:1054–60.

Ayd, F. J., Jr. (1983). Early-onset neuroleptic-induced extrapyramidal reactions: a second survey, 1961–1981. In *Neuroleptics: Neurochemical, Behavioral and*

Clinical Perspectives, ed. J. T. Coyle & S. J. Enna, pp. 75–92. New York: Raven Press.

Bamrah, J. S., Kumar, V., Krska, J., & Soni, S. D. (1986). Interactions between procyclidine and neuroleptic drugs. Some pharmacological and clinical aspects. *Br. J. Psychiatry* 149:726–33.

Baron, J. A. (1986). Cigarette smoking and Parkinson's disease. *Neurology* 36:1490–6.

Bateman, D. N., Darling, W. M., Boys, R., & Rawlins, M. D. (1989). Extrapyramidal reactions to metoclopramide and prochlorperazine. *Q. J. Med.* 71:307–11.

Bathien, N., Koutlidis, R. M., & Rondot, P. (1984). EMG patterns in abnormal involuntary movements induced by neuroleptics. *J. Neurol. Neurosurg. Psychiatry* 47:1002–8.

Bersani, G., Grispini, A., Marini, S., Pasini, A., Valducci, M., & Ciani, N. (1990). 5-HT$_2$ antagonist ritanserin in neuroleptic-induced parkinsonism: a double-blind comparison with orphenadrine and placebo. *Clin. Neuropharmacol.* 13:500–6.

Binder, R. L., & Jonelis, F. J. (1984). Seborrheic dermatitis: a newly reported side effect of neuroleptics. *J. Clin. Psychiatry* 45:125–6.

Binder, R. L., & Levy, R. (1981). Extrapyramidal reactions in Asians. *Am. J. Psychiatry* 138:1243–4.

Bishop, M. P., Gallant, D. M., & Sykes, T. F. (1965). Extrapyramidal side effects and therapeutic response. *Arch. Gen. Psychiatry* 13:155–62.

Bowers, M. B., Jr. (1985). Cerebrospinal fluid homovanillic acid and hypokinetic side effects of neuroleptics. *Psychopharmacology (Berlin)* 85:184–6.

Brown, K. W., White, T., Anderson, F., & McGilp, R. (1992). Handedness as a risk factor for neuroleptic-induced movement disorders. *Biol. Psychiatry* 31:746–8.

Buchsbaum, M. S. (1990). The frontal lobes, basal ganglia, and temporal lobes as sites for schizophrenia. *Schizophr. Bull.* 16:379–89.

Burns, R. S., LeWitt, P. A., Ebert, M. H., Pakkenberg, H., & Kopin, I. J. (1985). The clinical syndrome of striatal dopamine deficiency: parkinsonism induced by 1-methyl-4-phenyl-1,2,3,6-tetrahydropyridine (MPTP). *N. Engl. J. Med.* 312:1418–21.

Caligiuri, M. P., Bracha, H. S., & Lohr, J. B. (1989). Asymmetry of neuroleptic-induced rigidity: development of quantitative methods and clinical correlates. *Psychiatry Res.* 30:275–84.

Caligiuri, M. P., Lohr, J. B., Bracha, H. S., & Jeste, D. V. (1991). Clinical and instrumental assessment of neuroleptic-induced parkinsonism in patients with tardive dyskinesia. *Biol. Psychiatry* 29:139–48.

Calil, H. M., Avery, D. H., Hollister, L. E., Creese, I., & Snyder, S. H. (1979). Serum levels of neuroleptics measured by dopamine radioreceptor assay and some clinical observations. *Psychiatry Res.* 1:39–44.

Caradoc-Davies, G., Menkes, D. B., Clarkson, H. O., & Mullen, P. E. (1986). A study of the need for anticholinergic medication in patients treated with long-term antipsychotics. *Aust. N.Z. J. Psychiatry* 20:225–32.

Casey, D. E. (1989). Clozapine: neuroleptic-induced EPS and tardive dyskinesia. *Psychopharmacology (Berlin)* 99:S47–53.

Casey, D. E. (1991). Neuroleptic drug-induced extrapyramidal syndromes and tardive dyskinesia. *Schizophr. Res.* 4:109–20.

Casey, D. E., & Hansen, T. (1995). Schizophrenia psychopharmacology: risperidone and clozapine. *Psychiatr. Clin. North Am.: Ann. Drug Ther.* 2:119–49.

Casey, D. E., Povlsen, U. J., Meidahl, B., & Gerlach, J. (1986). Neuroleptic-induced tardive dyskinesia and parkinsonism: changes during several years of continuing treatment. *Psychopharmacol. Bull.* 22:250–3.

Chaturvedi, S. K. (1987). Metoprolol in the treatment of neuroleptic-induced tremor: case report. *J. Clin. Psychiatry* 48:378.

Chaudhry, R., Radonjic, D., & Waters, B. (1982). Efficacy of propranolol in a patient with tardive dyskinesia and extrapyramidal syndrome. *Am. J. Psychiatry* 139:674–76.

Chouinard, G., Annable, L., Mercier, P., & Turnier, L. (1987). Long-term effects of L-dopa and procyclidine on neuroleptic-induced extrapyramidal and schizophrenic symptoms. *Psychopharmacol. Bull.* 23:221–6.

Chouinard, G., Ross-Chouinard, A., Annable, L., & Jones, B. D. (1980). Extrapyramidal symptom rating scale. *Can. J. Neurol. Sci.* 7:233.

Chouza, C., Caamano, J. L., Aljanati, R., Scaramelli, A., De Medina, O., & Romero, S. (1986). Parkinsonism, tardive dyskinesia, akathisia, depression induced by flunarizine. *Lancet* 1:1303–4.

Collins, P., Lee, I., & Tyrer, P. (1979). Finger tremor and extrapyramidal side effects of neuroleptic drugs. *Br. J. Psychiatry* 134:488–93.

Comaty, J. E., Janicak, P. G., Rajaratnam, J., Sharma, R. P., Baker, D., & Davis, J. M. (1990). Is maintenance antiparkinsonian treatment necessary? *Psychopharmacol. Bull.* 26:267–70.

Craig, T. J., Richardson, M. A., Pass, R., & Bregman, Z. (1985). Measurement of mood and affect in schizophrenic inpatients. *Am. J. Psychiatry* 142:1272–7.

Crane, G. E. (1971). Persistence of neurological symptoms due to neuroleptic drugs. *Am. J. Psychiatry* 127: 1407–10.

Crane, G. E. (1972). Pseudoparkinsonism and tardive dyskinesia. *Arch. Neurol.* 27:426–30.

Crane, G. E. (1974). Factors predisposing to drug-induced neurologic effects. In *The Phenothiazines and Structurally Related Drugs*, ed. C. J. Carr & E. Usdin, pp. 269–79. New York: Raven Press.

Crowley, T. J., Hoehn, M. M., Rutledge, C. O., Stallings, M. A., Heaton, R. K., Sundell, S., & Stilson, D. (1978). Dopamine excretion and vulnerability to drug-induced parkinsonism: schizophrenic patients. *Arch. Gen. Psychiatry* 35:97–104.

Csernansky, J. G., Murphy, G. M., & Faustman, W. O. (1991). Limbic/mesolimbic connections and the pathogenesis of schizophrenia. *Biol. Psychiatry* 30:383–400.

Davis, K. L., Kahn, R. S., Ko, G., & Davidson, M. (1991). Dopamine in schizophrenia: a review and reconceptualization. *Am. J. Psychiatry* 148:1474–86.

Decina, P., Caracci, G., Sandik, R., Berman, W., Mukherjee, S., & Scapicchio, P. (1990a). Cigarette smoking and neuroleptic-induced parkinsonism. *Biol. Psychiatry* 28:502–8.

Decina, P., Caracci, G., & Scapicchio, P. L. (1990b). The rabbit syndrome (letter). *Mov. Disord.* 5:263.

DeLong, M. R. (1990). Primate models of movement disorders of basal ganglia origin. *Trends Neurosci.* 13:281–5.

Demars, J.-P. C. A. (1966). Neuromuscular effects of long-term phenothiazine medication, electroconvulsive therapy and leucotomy. *J. Nerv. Ment. Dis.* 143:73–9.

Deniker, P. (1960). Experimental neurological syndromes and the new drug therapies in psychiatry. *Compr. Psychiatry* 1:92–102.

Deshmukh, D. K., Joshi, V. S., & Agarwal, M. R. (1990). Rabbit syndrome – a rare complication of long-term neuroleptic medication. *Br. J. Psychiatry* 157:293.

Dilsaver, S. C. (1988). Antimuscarinic agents as substance of abuse: a review. *J. Clin. Psychopharmacol.* 8:14–22.

DiMascio, A., Bernardo, D. L., Greenblatt, D. J., & Marder, J. E. (1976). A controlled trial of amantadine in drug-induced extrapyramidal disorders. *Arch. Gen. Psychiatry* 33:599–602.

Dixon, L., Weiden, P. J., Frances, A. J., & Rapkin, B. (1989). Management of neuroleptic-induced movement disorders: effects of physician training. *Am. J. Psychiatry* 146:104–6.

Draper, I. T., & Johns, R. J. (1964). The disordered movement in parkinsonism and the effects of drug treatment. *Bull. Johns Hopkins Hosp.* 115:465–80.

Edelstein, H., & Knight, R. T. (1987). Severe parkinsonism in two AIDS patients taking prochlorperazine. *Lancet* 2:341–2.

El-Defrawi, M. H., & Craig, T. J. (1984). Neuroleptics, extrapyramidal symptoms, and serum-calcium levels. *Compr. Psychiatry* 25:539–45.

Engelhardt, D. M., & Polizos, P. (1978). Adverse effects of pharmacotherapy in childhood psychosis. In *Psychopharmacology: A Generation of Progress,* ed. M. A. Lipton, A. DiMascio, & K. F. Killam, pp. 1463–9. New York: Raven Press.

Ereshefsky, L., Jann, M. W., Saklad, S. R., Davis, C. M., Richards, A. L., & Burch, N. R. (1985). Effects of smoking on fluphenazine clearance in psychiatric inpatients. *Biol. Psychiatry* 20:329–52.

Escobar, J. I., Barron, A., & Kiriakos, R. (1983). Serum levels of fluphenazine: effect of dosage and route of administration, and relation to side effects and clinical response. *Psychopharmacol. Bull.* 19:131–4.

Faber, R., & Trimble, M. R. (1991). Electroconvulsive therapy in Parkinson's disease and other movement disorders. *Mov. Disord.* 6:293–303.

Fann, W. E., & Lake, C. R. (1976). Amantadine versus trihexyphenidyl in the treatment of neuroleptic-induced parkinsonism. *Am. J. Psychiatry* 133:940–3.

Farde, L., Nordstrom, A.-L., Wiesel, F.-A., Pauli, S., Halldin, C., & Sedvall, G. (1992). Positron emission tomographic analysis of central D_1 and D_2 dopamine receptor occupancy in patients treated with classical neuroleptics and clozapine: relation to extrapyramidal side effects. *Arch. Gen. Psychiatry* 49:538–44.

Fayen, M., Goldman, M. B., Moulthrop, M. A., & Luchins, D. J. (1988). Differential memory function with dopaminergic versus anticholinergic treatment of drug-induced extrapyramidal symptoms. *Am. J. Psychiatry* 145:483–6.

Feinstein, A., Ron, M., & Wessely, S. (1990). Disappearing brain lesions, psychosis and epilepsy: a report of two cases. *J. Neurol. Neurosurg. Psychiatry* 53:244–6.

Fisch, R. Z. (1987). Trihexyphenidyl abuse: therapeutic implications for negative symptoms of schizophrenia? *Acta Psychiatr. Scand.* 75:91–4.

Fornazzari, L., Ichise, M., Remington, G., & Smith, I. (1991). Rabbit syndrome, antidepressant use, and cerebral perfusion SPECT scan findings. *J. Psychiatry Neurosci.* 16:227–9.

Friedman, J. H. (1992). Drug-induced parkinsonism. In *Drug-induced Movement*

Disorders, ed. A. E. Lang & W. J. Weiner, pp. 41–83. Mt. Kisco, NY: Futura Publishing.

Friedman, J. H., Max, J., & Swift, R. (1987). Idiopathic Parkinson's disease in a chronic schizophrenic patient: long-term treatment with clozapine and L-dopa. *Clin. Neuropharmacol.* 10:470–5.

Friis, T., Christensen, T. R., & Gerlach, J. (1983). Sodium valproate and biperiden in neuroleptic-induced akathisia, parkinsonism and hyperkinesia. *Acta Psychiatr. Scand.* 67:178–87.

Gaffney, G. R., & Tune, L. E. (1985). Serum neuroleptic levels and extrapyramidal side effects in patients treated with amoxapine. *J. Clin. Psychiatry* 46:428–9.

Ganzini, L., Casey, D. E., Hoffman, W. F., & McCall, A. L. (1993). The prevalence of metoclopramide-induced tardive dyskinesia and acute extrapyramidal movement disorders. *Arch. Intern. Med.* 153:1469–75.

Ganzini, L., Heintz, R. T., Hoffman, W. F., & Casey, D. E. (1991a). The prevalence of tardive dyskinesia in neuroleptic-treated diabetics. A controlled study. *Arch. Gen. Psychiatry* 48:259–63.

Ganzini, L., Heintz, R., Hoffman, W. F., Keepers, G. A., & Casey, D. E. (1991b). Acute extrapyramidal syndromes in neuroleptic-treated elders: a pilot study. *J. Geriatr. Psychiatry Neurol.* 4:222–2.

Gardos, G., Cole, J. O., Schniebolk, S., & Salomon, M. (1987). Comparison of severe and mild tardive dyskinesia: implications for etiology. *J. Clin. Psychiatry* 48:359–62.

Gelenberg, A. J., & Mandel, M. R. (1977). Catatonic reactions to high-potency neuroleptic drugs. *Arch. Gen. Psychiatry* 34:947–50.

Gelenberg, A. J., Van Putten, T., Lavori, P. W., Wojcik, J. D., Falk, W. E., Marder, S., Galvin-Nadeau, M., Spring, B., Mohs, R. C., & Brotman, A. W. (1989). Anticholinergic effects on memory: benztropine versus amantadine. *J. Clin. Pharmacol.* 9:180–5.

Gerken, A., Wetzel, H., & Benkert, O. (1991). Extrapyramidal symptoms and their relationship to clinical efficacy under perphenazine treatment: a controlled prospective handwriting-test study in 22 acutely ill schizophrenic patients. *Pharmacopsychiatry* 24:132–7.

Gerlach, J. (1977). The relationship between parkinsonism and tardive dyskinesia. *Am. J. Psychiatry* 134:781–4.

Gillman, M. A., & Sandyk, R. (1986). Parkinsonism induced by a monoamine oxidase inhibitor. *Postgrad. Med. J.* 62:235–6.

Goetz, C. G. (1983). Drug-induced parkinsonism and idiopathic Parkinson's disease. *Arch. Neurol.* 40:325–6.

Goetz, C. G., & Klawans, H. L. (1981). Drug-induced extrapyramidal disorders – a neuropsychiatric interface. *J. Clin. Psychopharmacol.* 1:297–303.

Goff, D. C., Henderson, D. C., & Amico, E. (1992). Cigarette smoking in schizophrenia: relationship to psychopathology and medication side effects. *Am. J. Psychiatry* 149:1189–94.

Goldman, D. (1961). Parkinsonism and related phenomena from administration of drugs: their production and control under clinical conditions and possible relation to therapeutic effect. *Rev. Can. Biol.* 20:549–60.

Goldman-Rakic, P. S. (1990). Cellular and circuit basis of working memory in prefrontal cortex of nonhuman primates. *Prog. Brain Res.* 85:325–35.

Gollomp, S. M., Fahn, S., Burke, R. E., Reches, A., & Ilson, J. (1983). Therapeutic trials in Meige syndrome. *Adv. Neurol.* 37:207–13.

Goswami, U., Dutta, S., Kuruvilla, K., Papp, E., & Perényi, A. (1989). Electro-convulsive therapy in neuroleptic-induced parkinsonism. *Biol. Psychiatry* 26:234–8.

Graybiel, A. M. (1990). Neurotransmitters and neuromodulators in the basal ganglia. *Trends Neurosci.* 13:244–54.

Grimes, J. D. (1981). Parkinsonism and tardive dyskinesia associated with long-term metoclopramide therapy (letter). *N. Engl. J. Med.* 305:1417.

Grimes, J. D. (1982). Drug-induced parkinsonism and tardive dyskinesia in nonpsychiatric patients. *Can. Med. Assoc. J.* 126:468.

Grimes, J. D., Hassan, M. N., & Preston, D. N. (1982). Adverse neurologic effects of metoclopramide. *Can. Med. Assoc. J.* 126:23–5.

Grohmann, R., Koch, R., & Schmidt, L. G. (1990). Extrapyramidal symptoms in neuroleptic recipients. *Agents Actions (Suppl.)* 29:71–82.

Hall, R. A., Jackson, R. B., & Swain, J. M. (1956). Neurotoxic reactions resulting from chlorpromazine administration. *J. Am. Med. Assoc.* 161:214–18.

Hansen, L. B., & Larsen, N. E. (1985). Therapeutic advantages of monitoring plasma concentrations of perphenazine in clinical practice. *Psychopharmacology (Berlin)* 87:16–19.

Hansen, L. B., Larsen, N. E., & Gulmann, N. (1982). Dose–response relationships of perphenazine in the treatment of acute psychoses. *Psychopharmacology (Berlin)* 78:112–15.

Hansen, L. B., Larsen, N., & Vestergard, P. (1981). Plasma levels of perphenazine (Trilafon) related to development of extrapyramidal side effects. *Psychopharmacology (Berlin)* 74:306–9.

Hansen, T. E., Brown, W. L., Weigel, R. M., & Casey, D. E. (1988). Risk factors for drug-induced parkinsonism in tardive dyskinesia patients. *J. Clin. Psychiatry* 49:139–41.

Hansen, T. E., Brown, W. L., Weigel, R. M., & Casey, D. E. (1992a). Under-recognition of tardive dyskinesia and drug-induced parkinsonism by psychiatric residents. *Gen. Hosp. Psychiatry* 14:340–4.

Hansen, T. E., Hoffman, W. F., Keepers, G. A., & Casey, D. E. (1992b). Influence of affective disorders on tardive dyskinesia and drug-induced parkinsonism. In *Proceedings of the 7th International Catecholamine Symposium.* Amsterdam.

Hansen, T. E., Weigel, R. M., Brown, W. L., Hoffman, W. F., & Casey, D. E. (1992c). A longitudinal study of correlations among tardive dyskinesia, drug-induced parkinsonism, and psychosis. *J. Neuropsychiatry* 4:29–35.

Hardie, R. J., & Lees, A. J. (1988). Neuroleptic-induced Parkinson's syndrome: clinical features and results of treatment with levodopa. *J. Neurol. Neurosurg. Psychiatry* 51:850–4.

Hausner, R. S. (1983). Neuroleptic-induced parkinsonism and Parkinson's disease: differential diagnosis and treatment. *J. Clin. Psychiatry* 44:13–16.

Hermesh, H., Aizenberg, D., Friedberg, G., Lapidot, M., & Munitz, H. (1992). Electroconvulsive therapy for persistent neuroleptic-induced akathisia and parkinsonism: a case report. *Biol. Psychiatry* 31:407–11.

Hoffman, W. F., Ballard, L. C., Fenn, D. S., Keepers, G. A., Hansen, T. E., & Casey, D. E. (1992). Short-term neuroleptic withdrawal in schizophrenia. *Clin. Neuropharmacol. (Suppl. 1, part B)* 15:264B.

Hoffman, W. F., Ballard, L., Turner, E. H., & Casey, D. E. (1991). Three-year follow-up of older schizophrenics: extrapyramidal syndromes, psychiatric symptoms, and ventricular brain ratio. *Biol. Psychiatry* 30:913–26.

Hoffman, W. F., Labs, S. M., & Casey, D. E. (1987). Neuroleptic-induced parkinsonism in older schizophrenics. *Biol. Psychiatry* 22:427–39.

Holden, J. M., Itil, T. M., & Keskiner, A. (1969). The treatment of lobotomized schizophrenic patients with butaperazine. *Curr. Ther. Res. Clin. Exp.* 11:418–28.

Hunter, R., Earl, C. J., & Thornicroft, S. (1964). An apparently irreversible syndrome of abnormal movements following phenothiazine medication. *Proc. R. Soc. Med.* 57:758–62.

Indo, T., & Ando, K. (1982). Metoclopramide-induced parkinsonism: clinical characteristics of ten cases. *Arch. Neurol.* 39:494–6.

Itoh, H., Yagi, G., Ohtsuka, N., Iwamura, K., & Ichikawa, K. (1981). Serum level of haloperidol and its clinical significance. *Prog. Neuropsychopharmacol.* 4:171–83.

Jankovic, J., & Casabona, J. (1987). Coexistent tardive dyskinesia and parkinsonism. *Clin. Neuropharmacol.* 10:511–21.

Jenner, P. (1989). MPTP-induced parkinsonism: the relevance to idiopathic Parkinson's disease. In *Disorders of Movement: Clinical, Pharmacological and Physiological Aspects*, ed. N. P. Quinn & P. G. Jenner, pp. 157–75. London: Academic Press.

Jose, C., Mallya, A., Mehta, D., & Evenson, R. (1979). Iatrogenic morbidity in patients taking depot fluphenazine. *Am. J. Psychiatry* 136:976–7.

Jus, K., Jus, A., Villeneuve, A., & Villeneuve, R. (1973). Influence of concentration and motor performance on tardive dyskinesia and rabbit syndrome: polygraphic studies. *Can. Psychiatr. Assoc. J.* 18:327–30.

Jus, K., Villeneuve, A., & Jus, A. (1972). Tardive dyskinesia and the rabbit syndrome during wakefulness and sleep (letter). *Am. J. Psychiatry* 129:765.

Kabes, J., Sikora, J., Pisvejc, J., Hanzlicek, L., & Skondia, V. (1982). Effect of piracetam on extrapyramidal side effects induced by neuroleptic drugs. *Int. Pharmacopsychiatry* 17:185–92.

Kane, J. M., Woerner, M., & Lieberman, J. (1988). Tardive dyskinesia: prevalence, incidence, and risk factors. *J. Clin. Psychopharmacol.* 8:52S–6S.

Katz, I. R., Greenberg, W. H., Barr, G. A., Garbarino, C., Buckley, P., & Smith, D. (1985). Screening for cognitive toxicity of anticholinergic drugs. *J. Clin. Psychiatry* 46:323–6.

Keepers, G. A., & Casey, D. E. (1986). Clinical management of acute neuroleptic-induced extrapyramidal syndromes. In *Current Psychiatric Therapies*, ed. J. H. Masserman, pp. 139–57. New York: Grune & Stratton.

Keepers, G. A., & Casey, D. E. (1991). Use of neuroleptic-induced extrapyramidal symptoms to predict future vulnerability to side effects. *Am. J. Psychiatry* 148:85–9.

Keepers, G. A., Clappison, V. J., & Casey, D. E. (1983). Initial anticholinergic prophylaxis for neuroleptic-induced extrapyramidal syndromes. *Arch. Gen. Psychiatry* 40:1113–17.

Keepers, G. A., Hansen, T. E., & Casey, D. E. (1988). Differences in rating scales for the measurement of neuroleptic-induced parkinsonism. In *Proceedings of the Society of Biological Psychiatry*. Montreal.

Kellam, A. M. P. (1987). The neuroleptic malignant syndrome, so-called. A survey of the world literature. *Br. J. Psychiatry* 150:752–9.

Kelly, J. T., Zimmermann, R. L., Abuzzahab, F. S., & Schiele, B. C. (1974). A double-blind study of amantadine hydrochloride versus benztropine mesylate in drug-induced parkinsonism. *Pharmacology* 12:65–73.

Khaitan, A. K., & Laha, H. (1985). Lithium induced extrapyramidal syndrome. *J. Indian Med. Assoc.* 83:319.

Klawans, H. L., Bergen, D., & Bruyn, G. W. (1973). Prolonged drug-induced parkinsonism. *Confinia Neurologica* 35:368–77.

Klett, C. J., & Caffey, E., Jr. (1972). Evaluating the long-term need for antiparkinson drugs by chronic schizophrenics. *Arch. Gen. Psychiatry* 26:374–9.

Korczyn, A. D., & Goldberg, G. J. (1976). Extrapyramidal effects of neuroleptics. *J. Neurol. Neurosurg. Psychiatry* 39:866–9.

Korsgaard, S., & Friis, T. (1986). Effects of mianserin in neuroleptic-induced parkinsonism. *Psychopharmacology (Berlin)* 88:109–11.

Krska, J., Sampath, G., Shah, A., & Soni, S. D. (1986). Radio receptor assay of serum neuroleptic levels in psychiatric patients. *Br. J. Psychiatry* 148:187–93.

Kruse, W. (1960). Treatment of drug-induced extrapyramidal symptoms: a comparative study of three antiparkinson agents. *Dis. Nerv. Syst.* 21:79–81.

Kucharski, L. T., Wagner, R. L., & Friedman, J. H. (1987). An investigation of the coexistence of abnormal involuntary movements, parkinsonism, and akathisia in chronic psychiatric inpatients. *Psychopharmcol. Bull.* 23:215–17.

Kulik, F. A., & Wilbur, R. (1980). Propranolol for tardive dyskinesia and extrapyramidal side effects (psuedoparkinsonism) from neuroleptics. *Psychopharmacol. Bull.* 16:18–19.

Lader, M. H., (1970). Drug-induced extrapyramidal syndromes. *J. R. Coll. Physicians (London)* 5:87–98.

Langston, J. W., & Ballard, P. (1983). Chronic parkinsonism in humans due to a product of meperidine-analog synthesis. *Science* 219:979–80.

Lazarus, A., Mann, S. C., & Caroff, S. N. (1989). The neuroleptic malignant syndrome. In *The Neuroleptic Malignant Syndrome and Related Conditions*, ed. J. H. Gold, pp. 3–56. Washington, DC: American Psychiatric Press.

Lehmann, H. E., Ban, T. A., & Saxena, B. M. (1970). A survey of extrapyramidal manifestations in the inpatient population of a psychiatric hospital. *Laval. Med.* 41:909–16.

Lehmann, H. E., & Hanrahan, G. E. (1954). Chlorpromazine: new inhibiting agent for psychomotor excitement and manic states. *Arch. Neurol. Psychiatry* 71:227–37.

Levinson, D. F., & Simpson, G. M. (1986). Neuroleptic-induced extrapyramidal symptoms with fever: heterogeneity of the "neuroleptic malignant syndrome." *Psychiatry* 43:839–48.

Lin, K.-M., Poland, R. E., Lau, J. K., & Rubin, R. T. (1988). Haloperidol and prolactin concentrations in Asians and Caucasians. *J. Clin. Psychopharmacol.* 8:195–201.

Lombard, M., Sarsfield, P., & Keogh, J. A. B. (1986). Adverse neurological response to amiodarone. *Ir. Med. J.* 79:71–2.

Luchins, D. J., Jackman, H., & Meltzer, H. Y. (1983). Lateral ventricular size and drug-induced parkinsonism. *Psychiatry Res.* 9:9–16.

McCreadie, R. G., Barron, E. T., & Winslow, G. S. (1982). The Nithsdale schizophrenia survey. II: Abnormal movements. *Br. J. Psychiatry* 140:587–90.

McEvoy, J. P. (1983). The clinical use of anticholinergic drugs as treatment for extrapyramidal side effects of neuroleptic drugs. *J. Clin. Psychopharmacol.* 3:288–302.

McEvoy, J. P. (1986). The neuroleptic threshold as a marker of minimum effective neuroleptic dose. *Compr. Psychiatry* 27:327–35.

McEvoy, J. P., Hogarty, G. E., & Steingard, S. (1991). Optimal dose of neuroleptic in acute schizophrenia: a controlled study of the neuroleptic threshold and higher haloperidol dose. *Arch. Gen. Psychiatry* 48:739–45.

McEvoy, J. P., McCue, M., & Freter, S. (1987a). Replacement of chronically administered anticholinergic drugs by amantadine in outpatient management of chronic schizophrenia. *Clin. Ther.* 9:429–33.

McEvoy, J. P., McCue, M., Spring, B., Mohs, R. C., Lavori, P. W., & Farr, R. M. (1987b). Effects of amantadine and trihexyphenidyl on memory in elderly normal volunteers. *Am. J. Psychiatry* 144:573–7.

McEvoy, J. P., Stiller, R. L., & Farr, R. (1986). Plasma haloperidol levels drawn at neuroleptic threshold doses: a pilot study. *J. Clin. Psychopharmacol.* 6:133–8.

McGeer, P. L., Boulding, J. E., Gibson, W. C., & Foulkes, R. G. (1961). Drug-induced extrapyramidal reactions: treatment with diphenhydramine hydrochloride and dihydroxyphenylalanine. *J. Am. Med. Assoc.* 177:665–70.

Manos, N., Gkiouzepas, J., & Logotethis, J. (1981). The need for continuous use of antiparkinsonian medication with chronic schizophrenic patients receiving long-term neuroleptic therapy. *Am. J. Psychiatry* 138:184–8.

Marsden, C. D., & Jenner, P. (1980). The pathophysiology of extrapyramidal side-effects of neuroleptic drugs. *Psychol. Med.* 10:55–72.

Marsden, C. D., & Schachter, M. (1981). Assessment of extrapyramidal disorders. *Br. J. Clin. Pharmacol.* 11:129–51.

May, P. R. A. (1987). Measurement of extrapyramidal symptoms and involuntary movements by electronic instruments. *Psychopharmacol. Bull.* 23:187–8.

May, P. R. A., Lee, M. A., & Bacon, R. C. (1983). Quantitative assessment of neuroleptic-induced extrapyramidal symptoms: clinical and nonclinical approaches. *Clin. Neuropharmacol.* 6:S35–51.

Metzer, W. S., Newton, J. E. O., Steele, R. W., Claybrook, M., Paige, S. R., McMillan, D. E., & Hays, S. (1989). HLA antigens in drug-induced parkinsonism. *Mov. Disord.* 4:121–8.

Micheli, F., Pardal, M. F., Gatto, M., Torres, M., Paradiso, G., Parera, I. C., & Giannaula, R. (1987). Flunarizine- and cinnarizine-induced extrapyramidal reactions. *Neurology* 37:881–4.

Mindham, R. H. S. (1976). Assessment of drug-induced extrapyramidal reactions and of drugs given for their control. *Br. J. Clin. Pharmacol. (Suppl. 2)* 3:395–400.

Modell, J. G., Tandon, R., & Beresford, T. P. (1989). Dopaminergic activity of the antimuscarinic antiparkinsonian agents. *J. Clin. Psychopharmacol.* 9:347–51.

Moleman, P., Janzen, G., von Bargen, B. A., Kappers, E. J., Pepplinkhuizen, L., & Schmitz, P. I. M. (1986). Relationship between age and incidence of parkinsonism in psychiatric patients treated with haloperidol. *Am. J. Psychiatry* 143:232–4.

Moleman, P., Schmitz, P. I. M., & Ladee, G. A. (1982). Extrapyramidal side effects and oral haloperidol: an analysis of explanatory patient and treatment characteristics. *J. Clin. Psychiatry* 43:492–6.

Myrianthopoulos, N. C., Kurland, A. A., & Kurland, L. T. (1962). Hereditary predisposition in drug-induced parkinsonism. *Arch. Neurol.* 6:5–9.

Myrianthopoulos, N. C., Waldrop, F. N., & Vincent, B. L. (1967). A repeat study of hereditary predisposition to drug-induced parkinsonism. *Prog. Neurogene.* 175:486–91.

Myslobodsky, M. S., Holden, T., & Sandler, R. (1984). Asymmetry of abnormal involuntary movements: a prevalence study. *Biol. Psychiatry* 19:623–8.

Nath, A., Jankovic, J., & Pettigrew, L. C. (1987). Movement disorders and AIDS. *Neurology* 37:37–41.

Nauta, W. J. H. (1986). Circuitous connections linking cerebral cortex, limbic system, and corpus striatum. In *The Limbic System: Functional Organization and Clinical Disorders,* ed. B. K. Doane & K. F. Livingston, pp. 43–54. New York: Raven Press.

Oyebode, F., & McClelland, H. (1986). Tardive dyskinesia and parkinsonism. *Br. J. Psychiatry* 149:122–3.

Pacifici, G. M., Nardini, M., Ferrari, P., Latini, R., Fieschi, C., & Morselli, P. L. (1976). Effect of amantadine on drug-induced parkinsonism: relationship between plasma levels and effect. *Br. J. Clin. Pharmacol.* 3:883–9.

Pearlman, C. A. (1986). Neuroleptic malignant syndrome: a review of the literature. *J. Clin. Psychopharmacol.* 6:257–73.

Perényi, A., Bagdy, G., & Arato, M. (1983a). An early phase II trial with L-deprenyl for the treatment of neuroleptic-induced parkinsonism. *Pharmacopsychiatria* 16:143–6.

Perényi, A., Rihmer, Z., & Banki, C. M. (1983b). Parkinsonian systems with lithium, lithium-neuroleptic, and lithium-antidepressant treatment. *J. Affect. Disord.* 5:171–7.

Perlick, D., Stastny, P., Katz, I., Mayer, M., & Mattis, S. (1986). Memory deficits and anticholinergic levels in chronic schizophrenia. *Am. J. Psychiatry* 143:230–2.

Perovich, R. M., Lieberman, J. A., Fleischhacker, W. W., & Alvir, J. (1989). The behavioral toxicity of bromocriptine in patients with psychiatric illness. *J. Clin. Psychopharmacol.* 9:417–22.

Pope, H. G., Keck, P. E., & McElroy, S. L. (1986). Frequency and presentation of neuroleptic malignant syndrome in a large psychiatric hospital. *Am. J. Psychiatry* 143:1227–33.

Prosser, E. S., Csernansky, J. G., Kaplan, J., Thiemann, S., Backer, T. J., & Hollister, L. E. (1987). Depression, parkinsonian symptoms, and negative symptoms in schizophrenics treated with neuroleptics. *J. Nerv. Ment. Dis.* 175:100–5.

Rajput, A. H. (1984). Drug-induced parkinsonism in the elderly. *Geriatric Med. Today* 3:99–107.

Rajput, A. H., Rozdilsky, B., Hornykiewicz, O., Shannak, K., Lee, T., & Seeman, P. (1982). Reversible drug-induced parkinsonism: clinicopathologic study of two cases. *Arch. Neurol.* 39:644–6.

Rasmussen, K., & Abrams, R. (1991). Treatment of Parkinson's disease with electroconvulsive therapy. *Psychiatr. Clin. North Am.* 14:925–3.

Richardson, M. A., & Craig, T. J. (1982). The coexistence of parkinsonism-like symptoms and tardive dyskinesia. *Am. J. Psychiatry* 139:341–3.

Richardson, M. A., Haugland, G., & Craig, T. J. (1991). Neuroleptic use, parkinsonian symptoms, tardive dyskinesia, and associated factors in child and adolescent psychiatric patients. *Am. J. Psychiatry* 148:1322–8.

Rifkin, A., Quitkin, F., & Klein, D. F. (1975). Akinesia: a poorly recognized drug-induced extrapyramidal behavior disorder. *Arch. Gen. Psychiatry* 32:672–4.

Robbins, T. W. (1990). The case for frontostriatal dysfunction in schizophrenia. *Schizophr. Bull.* 16:391–402.

Rosebush, P., & Stewart, T. (1989). A prospective analysis of 24 episodes of neuroleptic malignant syndrome. *Am. J. Psychiatry* 146:717–25.

Rozzini, R., Missale, C., & Gadola, M. (1985). Drug-induced parkinsonism. *Lancet* 1:113.

Rudenko, G. M., & Lepakhin, V. K. (1979). The major tranquilizers. *Side Eff. Drugs Annu.* 3:39–58.

Sachdev, P. S. (1986). Lithium potentiation of neuroleptic-related extrapyramidal side effects. *Am. J. Psychiatry* 143:942.

Sahoo, R. N., Mitra, G. C., & Mohanty, P. C. (1975). Irreversible drug induced parkinsonism. *J. Assoc. Physicians India* 23:529–30.

Sandyk, R., & Kay, S. R. (1990). The relationship of negative schizophrenia to parkinsonism. *Int. J. Neurosci.* 55:1–59.

Sandyk, R., & Kay, S. R. (1991). Neuroradiological covariates of drug-induced parkinsonism and tardive dyskinesia in schizophrenia. *Int. J. Neurosci.* 58:7–53.

Sandyk, R., & Pardeshi, R. (1990). Pyridoxine improves drug-induced parkinsonism and psychosis in a schizophrenic patient. *Int. J. Neurosci.* 52:225–32.

Seeman, P. (1990). Atypical neuroleptics: role of multiple receptors, endogenous dopamine, and receptor linkage. *Acta Psychiatr. Scand.* 82:14–20.

Sheppard, C., & Merlis, S. (1967). Drug-induced extrapyramidal symptoms: their incidence and treatment. *Am. J. Psychiatry* 123:886–9.

Shoulson, I. (1983). Carbidopa/levodopa therapy of coexistent drug-induced parkinsonism and tardive dyskinesia. *Adv. Neurol.* 37:259–66.

Simpson, G. M., Amuso, D., Blair, J. H., & Farkas, T. (1964). Phenothiazine-produced extra-pyramidal system disturbance. *Arch. Gen. Psychiatry* 10:199–208.

Simpson, G. M., Cooper, T. B., Bark, N., Sud, I., & Lee, J. H. (1980). Effect of antiparkinsonian medication on plasma levels of chlorpromazine. *Arch. Gen. Psychiatry* 37:205–8.

Simpson, G. M., Krakow, L., Mattke, D., & St. Phard, G. (1970). A controlled comparison of the treatment of schizophrenic patients when treated according to the neuroleptic threshold or by clinical judgment. *Acta Psychiatr. Scand.* (*Suppl.*) 212:38–43.

Singh, I. (1987). Prolonged oculogyric crisis on addition of nifedipine to neuroleptic medication regime. *Br. J. Psychiatry* 150:127–8.

Sirota, R. A., Kimmel, P. L., Trichtinger, M. D., Diamond, B. F., Stein, H. D., & Yudis, M. (1986). Metoclopramide-induced parkinsonism in hemodialysis patients: report of two cases. *Arch. Intern. Med.* 146:2070–1.

Smith, A. D., & Bolam, J. P. (1990). The neural network of the basal ganglia as revealed by the study of synaptic connections of identified neurones. *Trends Neurosci.* 13:259–65.

Smith, R. C., Allen, R., Gordon, J., & Wolff, J. (1983). A rating scale for tardive dyskinesia and parkinsonian symptoms. *Psychopharmacol. Bull.* 19:266–76.

Snyder, S. H., & D'Amato, R. J. (1986). MPTP: a neurotoxin relevant to the pathophysiology of Parkinson's disease. *Neurology* 36:250–8.

Sramek, J., Potkin, S., & Hahn, R. (1988). Neuroleptic plasma concentrations and clinical response: in search of a therapeutic window. *Drug Intell. Clin. Pharm.* 22:373–80.

Stephen, P. J., & Williamson, J. (1984). Drug-induced parkinsonism in the elderly. *Lancet* 2:1082–3.

Stern, M. B. (1988). The clinical characteristics of Parkinson's disease and parkinsonian syndromes: diagnosis and assessment. In *The Comprehensive Manage-*

ment of Parkinson's Disease, ed. M. B. Stern & H. I. Hurtig, pp. 3–50. New York: PMA Publishing.

Stern, Y., & Langston, J. W. (1985). Intellectual changes in patients with MPTP-induced parkinsonism. *Neurology* 35:1506–9.

Stern, Y., Tetrud, J. W., Martin, W. R. W., Kutner, S. J., & Langston, J. W. (1990). Cognitive change following MPTP exposure. *Neurology* 40:261–4.

Strauss, M. E., Reynolds, K. S., Jayaram, G., & Tune, L. E. (1990). Effects of anticholinergic medication on memory in schizophrenia. *Schizophr. Res.* 3:127–9.

Suranyi-Cadotte, B. E., Nestoros, J. N., Nair, N. P. V., Lal, S., & Gauthier, S. (1985). Parkinsonism induced by high doses of diazepam. *Biol. Psychiatry* 20:455–7.

Swenson, J. R., Erman, M., Labelle, J., & Dimsdale, J. E. (1989). Extrapyramidal reactions. Neuropsychiatric mimics in patients with AIDS. *Gen. Hosp. Psychiatry* 11:248–53.

Teravainen, H., Tsui, J. K. C., Mak, E., & Calne, D. B. (1989). Optimal indices for testing parkinsonian rigidity. *Can. J. Neurol. Sci.* 16:180–3.

Teusink, J. P., Alexopoulos, G. S., & Shamoian, C. A. (1984). Parkinsonian side effects induced by a monoamine oxidase inhibitor. *Am. J. Psychiatry* 141:118–19.

Todd, R., Lippmann, S., Manshadi, M., & Chang, A. (1983). Recognition and treatment of rabbit syndrome, an uncommon complication of neuroleptic therapies. *Am. J. Psychiatry* 140:1519–20.

Tomer, R., Mintz, M., Kempler, S., & Sigal, M. (1987). Lateralized neuroleptic-induced side effects are associated with asymmetric visual evoked potentials. *Psychiatry Res.* 22:311–18.

Tune, L., & Coyle, J. T. (1980). Serum levels of anticholinergic drugs in treatment of acute extrapyramidal side effects. *Arch. Gen. Psychiatry* 37:293–7.

Tune, L., & Coyle, J. T. (1981). Acute extrapyramidal side effects: serum levels of neuroleptics and anticholinergics. *Psychopharmacology (Berlin)* 75:9–15.

Tune, L. E., Strauss, M. E., Lew, M. F., Breitlinger, E., & Coyle, J. T. (1982). Serum levels of anticholinergic drugs and impaired recent memory in chronic schizophrenic patients. *Am. J. Psychiatry* 139:1460–2.

Van Putten, T., & May, P. R. A. (1978). "Akinetic depression" in schizophrenia. *Arch. Gen. Psychiatry* 35:1101–7.

Van Putten, T., May, P. R. A., & Wilkins, J. N. (1980). Importance of akinesia: plasma chlorpromazine and prolactin levels. *Am. J. Psychiatry* 137:1446–8.

Villeneuve, A. (1972). The rabbit syndrome: a peculiar extrapyramidal reaction. *Can. Psychiatr. Assoc. J.* 17:SS69–72.

Villeneuve, A., Jus, K., & Jus, A. (1973). Polygraphic studies of tardive dyskinesia and of the rabbit syndrome during different stages of sleep. *Biol. Psychiatry* 6:259–74.

Wada, Y., Koshino, Y., & Yamaguchi, N. (1987). Biperiden withdrawal in schizophrenic inpatients receiving long-term antipsychotic medication. *Clin. Neuropharmacol.* 10:370–5.

Wagner, B., Wolf, G. K., & Ulmar, G. (1988). Does smoking reduce the risk of neuroleptic parkinsonoids? *Pharmacopsychiatry* 21:302–3.

Webster, D. D. (1968). Critical analysis of the disability in Parkinson's disease. *Mod. Treat.* 5:2582.

Weiden, P. J., Mann, J. J., Haas, G., Mattson, M., & Frances, A. (1987). Clinical nonrecognition of drug-induced movement disorders: a cautionary study. *Am. J. Psychiatry* 144:1148–53.

Weiner, R. D., Fink, M., Hammersley, D. W., Small, I. F., Moench, L. A., & Sackeim, H. (1990). *The Practice of Electroconvulsive Therapy: Recommendations for Treatment, Training, and Privileging.* Washington, DC: American Psychiatric Association.

Weiner, W. J., & Lang, A. E. (1989a). Drug-induced movement disorders (not including tardive dyskinesia). In *Movement Disorders: A Comprehensive Survey,* pp. 599–644. Mount Kisco, NY: Futura Publishing.

Weiner, W. J., & Lang, A. E. (1989b). Parkinson's disease. In *Movement Disorders: A Comprehensive Survey,* p. 24. Mount Kisco, NY: Futura Publishing.

Weiner, W. J., & Lang, A. E. (1989c). Parkinson's disease. In *Movement Disorders: A Comprehensive Survey,* p. 49. Mount Kisco, NY: Futura Publishing.

Wilson, J. A., & Primrose, W. R. (1986). Drug induced parkinsonism. *Br. Med. J.* 293:957.

Wilson, J. A., Primrose, W. R., & Smith, R. G. (1987). Prognosis of drug-induced Parkinson's disease. *Lancet* 1:443–4.

Wilson, J. A., & Smith, R. G. (1987). Relation between elderly and AIDS patients with drug-induced Parkinson's disease. *Lancet* 2:686.

Wirshing, W. C., Freidenberg, D. L., Cummings, J. L., & Bartzokis, G. (1989). Effects of anticholinergic agents on patients with tardive dyskinesia and concomitant drug-induced parkinsonism. *J. Clin. Psychopharmacol.* 9:407–11.

Wojcik, J. D., Gelenberg, A. J., LaBrie, R. A., & Mieske, M. (1980). Prevalence of tardive dyskinesia in an outpatient population. *Compr. Psychiatry* 21:370–80.

Yassa, R., & Lal, S. (1986). Prevalence of the rabbit syndrome. *Am. J. Psychiatry* 143:656–67.

Yassa, R., Lal, S., Korpassy, A., & Ally, J. (1987). Nicotine exposure and tardive dyskinesia. *Biol. Psychiatry* 22:67–72.

25

Clinical Aspects of Neuroleptic-Induced Dystonia

GEORGE A. KEEPERS, M.D.,
and LINDA GANZINI, M.D.

Acute dystonia, a common and distressing side effect of antipsychotic medication, can complicate the care of neuroleptic-treated patients in several ways. First, dystonia can cause significant morbidity and is occasionally lethal. Second, after experiencing a dystonic reaction, many patients have refused subsequent treatment with antipsychotic drugs; some have even left hospitals prematurely. Third, clinicians sometimes fail to recognize acute dystonia or misdiagnose acute dystonia, resulting in greatly increased morbidity and delays in treatment.

Treatment of dystonic reactions with parenteral anticholinergic agents is highly effective. But prophylactic administration of anticholinergic agents, although effective in preventing dystonias, has been controversial. Unfortunately, anticholinergics are not benign and can produce serious side effects. Thus, blanket prescription of anticholinergics for all patients is ill-advised. Accurate knowledge concerning clinical manifestations, risk factors, and proper management of acute dystonia can lead to rational clinical strategies for these complications.

Clinical Manifestations of Acute Dystonia

Dystonia is an involuntary muscular contraction that results in peculiar, slow movements and may progress to a fixed abnormal posture. The muscle groups affected can include those of the neck (torticollis or retrocollis), jaw (trismus), extraocular muscles (oculogyric crisis), tongue, larynx and pharynx, trunk, and limbs. Among adults, the neck and face are most often involved; among children, trunk and extremity dystonias are common (Ayd, 1961; Chiles, 1978).

Dystonia frequently begins with the patient's awareness of an abnormal feeling, increased muscle tension, muscle cramping, and/or pain due to the

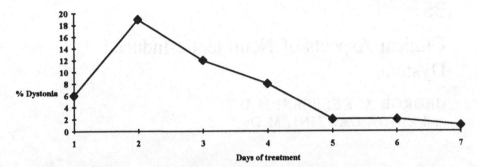

Figure 25.1. Percentage of patients with dystonia during antipsychotic treatment. (Adapted from Keepers et al., 1983.)

tonic muscular contraction in the affected part. In some patients, the spasm progresses within minutes to produce a severe, prolonged muscle contraction with fixed abnormal posture. Sometimes, however, these symptoms are intermittent, disappearing for a few hours or even a day, and then reappearing. Functional disturbances such as dysarthria and dysphagia may be the only manifestations when symptoms are mild. In some cases these symptoms will worsen, eventually producing classic dystonias with lengthy muscle spasms that result in fixed, aberrant positions. Although the muscle spasm is involuntary, patients can partially and briefly overcome the contractions. If untreated, dystonias can persist for days.

Dystonia usually occurs during the first few days of treatment with antipsychotic drugs. As shown in Figure 25.1, 90% of dystonic reactions will occur within the first 4 days of treatment with antipsychotics. Rarely, these extrapyramidal side effects (EPS) will occur after prolonged use of antipsychotics (Gardos, 1981). This usually happens when the neuroleptic dosage is changed or an anticholinergic agent is withdrawn (Rifkin et al., 1978; Manos & Gkiouzepas, 1981; Jellinek, Gardos, & Cole, 1981).

Because other conditions can sometimes be mistaken for acute neuroleptic-induced dystonia, physicians should know the differential diagnosis (Table 25.1). The majority of these conditions are neurological disorders in which neural degeneration produces a secondary dystonia (Calne & Lang, 1988; Marsden, 1988). These syndromes include several illnesses with known enzymatic defects, such as Wilson's disease and glutaric acidemia. Several neurodegenerative disorders of unclear origin, such as Hallervorden-Spatz disease and Fahr's disease, which respectively lead to iron and calcium deposition in the brain, can also cause dystonia. A number of such conditions (e.g., Huntington's disease) will produce characteristic findings when patients are examined with computed tomography (CT) or magnetic-resonance imag-

Table 25.1. *Drugs, toxins, injuries, and conditions associated with dystonia*

Drugs
  Anticonvulsants
  D_2-receptor antagonists (antipsychotic drugs)
  Ergots
  Levodopa
Toxins
  Manganese, carbon monoxide, carbon disulfide, methanol
Cerebral injury
  Anoxia
  Brain tumor
  Brain-stem lesions
  Cerebrovascular injury
  Cervical-cord injury
  Encephalitis
  Wasp-sting encephalopathy
  Head trauma
  Multiple sclerosis
  Perinatal injury
  Peripheral nerve injury
  Reye's syndrome
  Thalamotomy
Hereditary neurological conditions
  Ataxia-telangiectasia
  Dystonic lipidosis
  Familial basal-ganglia calcification
  Familial dystonia with visual loss
  Glutaric acidemia
  GM_1 and GM_2 gangliosidosis
  Hallervorden-Spatz disease
  Hartnup's disease
  Hexosaminidase A and B deficiency
  Homocystinuria
  Huntington's disease
  Intraneuronal inclusion disease
  Joseph's disease
  Juvenile neuronal ceroid-lipofuscinosis
  Leigh's syndrome
  Lesch-Nyhan syndrome
  Metachromatic leucodystrophy
  Methylmalonic aciduria
  Neuroacanthocytosis
  Olivopontocerebellar atrophy
  Progressive pallidal degeneration
  Rett's syndrome
  Triosephosphate isomerase deficiency
  Wilson's disease
Idiopathic dystonia, heritable and sporadic
Dystonia associated with parkinsonism
Psychogenic dystonia

ing (MRI) of the brain. Anoxia and a variety of toxins and infections can result in dystonic syndromes as well. In some cases, however, dystonia occurs without other neurological or systemic symptoms, and that is called *idiopathic* or *torsion dystonia.* Many such cases are hereditary. Autosomal-dominant, autosomal-recessive, and X-linked recessive forms occur.

Prolonged treatment with antipsychotic drugs can produce a late-appearing syndrome known as *tardive dystonia,* which is similar to tardive dyskinesia in its course and possibly in its causation. Tardive dystonia occurs in 1–2% of neuroleptic-treated patients (Yassa, Nair, & Dimitry, 1986). Unlike acute dystonia, the syndrome does not improve with neuroleptic withdrawal, and anticholinergics are rarely effective (Kang, Burke, & Fahn, 1986). Tardive dystonia, which can develop after a few weeks of treatment with antipsychotics, can be very disabling and difficult to treat.

Physicians can distinguish these conditions from acute dystonia by examining patients for dystonic symptoms before treatment with antipsychotic drugs. The neurological evaluation should be carefully recorded. The muscles should be tested for strength, tone, and bulk; any involuntary movements should be noted.

Even severe, acute dystonic symptoms have sometimes been characterized as psychological in origin (Cavenar, Hammett, & Maltsies, 1979); the most common misdiagnoses include malingering, conversion disorder, and "resistance" to treatment. These mistakes are more likely to occur with patients in whom the severity of dystonia waxes and wanes, as well as with patients who are able to overcome the contractions voluntarily. These errors are particularly problematic because they can lead caretakers to ignore or even to seclude and restrain a patient who responds to painful dystonia with agitation, verbal outbursts, or violence. Occasionally, patients will begin to seek excess amounts of anticholinergics for their psychotropic effects and may imitate dystonia to procure these drugs (Rubenstein, 1978; Saran, 1986). Trihexyphenidyl (Artane) and procyclidine (Kemadrin) are more frequently used for such abuse than other anticholinergics. Differences in muscarinic receptors M_1 and M_2 vis-à-vis anticholinergic drugs may account for the differing propensities to abuse (Avissar & Schreiber, 1989). Examination of a patient for characteristic tonic, involuntary muscle contraction will allow one to distinguish between imitation and real dystonia.

There are several important clinical consequences of acute dystonia. Often the experience of dystonia is distressing and frightening for patients. Adverse outcomes can range from disruption of the therapeutic alliance to refusal to take antipsychotic medications and premature, ill-advised hospital discharge.

Other morbid consequences of dystonia include rhabdomylolysis (Cavanaugh & Finlayson, 1984), fractures, joint dislocations, dental fractures, and falls.

Acute dystonic reactions affecting the larynx or pharynx can be life-threatening and should be treated promptly; otherwise airway obstruction may occur (Flaherty & Lahmeyer, 1978; Mann, Cohen, & Boger, 1979; Noda et al., 1988). However, it is important to remember that other conditions besides dystonia can cause airway obstruction. The differential diagnosis includes anaphylaxis, foreign-body inhalation, and acute epiglottitis. Although some symptoms of anaphylaxis may respond to treatment with diphenhydramine, airway obstruction should be treated with adrenergic agents. Unfortunately, neither of the other two conditions will respond to pharmacologic treatments for dystonia.

Risk Factors for Acute Dystonia

The reported prevalence rates for dystonia have varied widely, ranging from 2.3% (Ayd, 1961) to 94% (Chiles, 1978; Ayers & Dawson, 1980). A number of factors can be involved in the disparate findings in the various studies, including differing patient characteristics, drug variables, and study design. In 1961, Ayd reported a rate of 2.3% among more than 3,000 patients treated with antipsychotic medications. Most surveys during the mid-1970s reported rates below 10% (DiMascio & Demirgian, 1970; Swett, 1975). After the late 1970s, however, with the increasing use of high-potency neuroleptics, depot forms, and high daily doses, rates reported in most studies were between 30% and 50% (Donlon & Stenson, 1976; Stern & Anderson, 1979). In a study of young patients receiving haloperidol, the incidence of dystonia was 94% (Chiles, 1978).

Patient Characteristics

Ayd's 1961 study of EPS showed that dystonia was more common among younger patients than among older patients. As shown in Figure 25.2, several investigators have since confirmed that finding, with a striking negative correlation between age and dystonia (Swett, 1975; Keepers & Casey, 1987). Among young adults, male gender may confer some added risk. Being of Indochinese origin may increase the risk for EPS as well (Binder & Levy, 1981), although that finding is disputed (Sramek, Sayles, & Simpson, 1986a).

Even within age and gender subgroups, individual vulnerability to EPS varies widely. Differences in dopamine metabolism or antipsychotic-

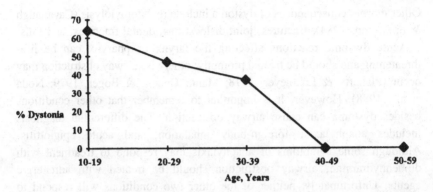

Figure 25.2. Relationship of age to dystonia. (Adapted from Keepers & Casey, 1987.)

drug metabolism may account for these differences in susceptibility (Chase, Schnur, & Gordon, 1970; Crowley et al., 1978; Cohen, Herschel, & Aoba, 1979). Recent retrospective work supports the hypothesis that individuals with a history of dystonia are at increased risk for future dystonic episodes (Keepers & Casey, 1987, 1991). Related experiments in nonhuman primates suggest that past episodes of EPS may increase the propensity for EPS upon reexposure to antipsychotic drugs (Casey, 1991).

Drug Variables

The balance of anticholinergic activity and antidopaminergic activity in each antipsychotic medication correlates with that drug's capacity to produce dystonia (Snyder, Greenberg, & Yamamura, 1974). High-potency drugs with little anticholinergic activity (e.g., haloperidol, trifluoperazine) produce more dystonia than do low-potency drugs, which are relatively more anticholinergic (e.g., chlorpromazine, thioridazine). Other pharmacologic properties of antipsychotic drugs, including their effects on norepinephrine and serotonin receptors, may influence EPS rates as well (Sayers et al., 1976; Keepers & Casey, 1986).

In general, low dosages of antipsychotic drugs produce fewer instances of EPS (Ayd, 1961, 1978). However, the dose–response curve for EPS may be U-shaped, because high dosages can be associated with low rates of EPS as well (Baldessarini, Cohen, & Teicher, 1989). Consider the case of haloperidol. Intravenous haloperidol has been used, without adverse effects, for treatment of acute psychosis (Carter, 1986) and delirium in patients with a variety of medical illnesses, including stroke and cardiac disease (Tesar, Murray, & Cassem, 1985). Anecdotally, it has been reported that dosages of haloperidol up to 600 mg/day have been administered without producing EPS (Tesar et al., 1985; Fernandez et al., 1988; Baldessarini et al., 1989). In a preliminary but blind study of EPS – 4 patients received intravenous haloperidol, and 6 patients received oral haloperidol – those on the intravenous drug experienced significantly ($p < .01$) less intense EPS (Menza et al., 1987). A subsequent investigation, in which 14 patients received intravenous haloperidol and benzodiazepine and 4 patients received intravenous haloperidol alone, also showed low rates of EPS (Kaneko et al., 1993). However, in a study in which 12 normal young men were rapidly administered intravenous haloperidol at 0.125 mg/kg, dystonic reactions occurred in 4 subjects (Magliozzi et al., 1985).

Studies of the relationship between serum concentrations of antipsychotics and the incidence of EPS have produced conflicting findings of both "no relationship" (Tune & Coyle, 1981) and a significant association (Hansen, Larsen, & Vestergard, 1981). The conflicting findings may have been due to failure to control for critical patient characteristics (age, gender, race), drug variables (potency, anticholinergic/dopamine blocking ratio), and syndromes (dystonia, drug-induced parkinsonism, akathisia).

Management of Acute Dystonia

Although EPS were at one time thought to be unavoidable concomitants for an effective antipsychotic drug, they are now recognized as reactions that interfere with successful treatment of psychiatric disorders (Chien & DiMascio, 1967; Greenblatt, Shader, & DiMascio, 1970). Studies have shown considerable adverse effects of EPS on behavior and the activities of daily living; in some cases, EPS appear to exacerbate the psychosis for which the drug is being prescribed. Even subtle EPS findings do not correlate with clinical improvement (Gerken, Wetzel, & Benkert, 1991). It is therefore inadvisable to leave EPS, especially those associated with dystonia, untreated. Three distinct strategies have been developed for clinical management of EPS during the initial phase of treatment with antipsychotic medications: (1) treatment of EPS after they emerge, (2) prescription of prophylactic anti-EPS drugs when neuroleptics are initiated (initial prophylaxis), and (3) treatment with low-dosage antipsychotic medication. In the last instance, dosages of antipsychotic drugs below the generally accepted range of 300–900 mg (chlorpromazine equivalents, CPZE) per day are recommended for acute exacerbations of schizophrenia.

Treatment

Two classes of drugs are used to treat dystonia that emerges during the course of neuroleptic treatment: anticholinergics such as benztropine, and benzodiazepines. Our review of studies of anticholinergic drugs for treatment of dystonia (Keepers & Casey, 1986) found three double-blind comparisons of benztropine with other agents and 18 open or single-blind evaluations of anticholinergics (Paulson, 1960; Smith & Miller, 1961; Medina, Kramer, & Kuland, 1962; Neu, DiMascio, & Demirgian, 1972; Chiles, 1978; Sinantios et al., 1978; Cavenar et al., 1979; Lee, 1979; Mann et al., 1979; Ott & Goeden, 1979; Ayers & Dawson, 1980; Gross, 1980; Wood & Water, 1980; Menuck, 1981). Almost 100% of the patients in those trials benefited from the anticholinergic medications. We have also found that administration of 25–50 mg of diphenhydramine (e.g., Benadryl) intramuscularly or 1–2 mg of benztropine intravenously or intramuscularly will terminate most dystonic reactions.

It seems that cases of severe dystonia that do not respond adequately to anticholinergic agents can be treated with benzodiazepines. However, despite reports that benzodiazepines have been used successfully for treatment of acute dystonia, there has been limited experimental confirmation of their efficacy (Gagrat, Hamilton, & Belmaker, 1978). Slow administration of 5–10 mg of diazepam (e.g., Valium) intravenously will terminate most dystonic reactions; however, patients should be observed for the possible complication of respiratory depression. With the exception of lorazepam (Ativan), diazepam and most other benzodiazepines should not be given intramuscularly, because they are erratically absorbed.

A few refractory cases of dystonia have been reported in patients with severe concurrent medical illnesses, such as hepatorenal failure or preexisting neurological disease (Wood & Water, 1980). Any failure of dystonia to respond to standard treatment should therefore prompt a search for underlying medical and neurological diseases.

Initial Prophylaxis

Only anticholinergic drugs have been extensively studied for initial prophylaxis. Because the early research findings were in conflict concerning the effectiveness of prophylaxis for acute dystonia, a controversy emerged concerning appropriate clinical practice. More recent studies and a meta-analysis of the resulting data, however, now support the prophylactic use of anticholinergics for dystonia.

A review by Keepers & Casey (1986) disclosed six older, single-blind or retrospective evaluations of the effectiveness of initial prophylaxis in preventing EPS (DiMascio & Demirgian, 1970; Bucci, 1971; Chien, DiMascio, & Cole, 1974; Idzorek, 1976; Swett et al., 1977; Stern & Anderson, 1979). The findings were in conflict, ranging from reports of prophylaxis having no effect at all to reports of very significant effects in which the no-prophylaxis group taking high-potency antipsychotics had 11-fold more dystonic symptoms than patients on prophylaxis. However, six recent studies focusing on the value of anticholinergic prophylaxis for dystonia have all supported the effectiveness of this approach (Keepers, Clappison, & Casey, 1983; Lake et al., 1986; Winslow et al., 1986; Manos, Lavrentiadis, & Gkiouzepas, 1986; Boyer, Honeycutt-Bakalar, & Lake, 1987).

A recent reanalysis of the data (Arana et al., 1988) from some of those studies has established the efficacy of anticholinergic prophylaxis for dystonia using high-potency agents. Those investigators included data from studies that had examined the point prevalence for dystonia among patients with and without anticholinergic prophylaxis. Nine studies were included in the overall analysis. The data were examined with particular regard to patients treated with high-potency antipsychotics such as haloperidol. Initial anticholinergic prophylaxis was found to be unequivocally effective in preventing dystonia. All the studies in which patients were treated with high-potency antipsychotics showed a reduced incidence of dystonia in prophylactically treated patients. Patients not given prophylaxis were more than five times as likely to have dystonic reactions.

Unfortunately, even therapeutic dosages of anticholinergic drugs can produce substantial impairments of memory for recent events (McEvoy, 1987; McEvoy et al., 1987; McEvoy & Freter, 1989). This significant morbidity and other side effects make it desirable to avoid prophylactic use of anticholinergics even for dystonia; except in those patients who will clearly benefit (McEvoy, 1983). Fortunately, as noted earlier in the section on risk factors, it is possible to predict which patients are most at risk for this syndrome. Anticholinergic prophylaxis can therefore be recommended for these groups. In contrast, one study found amantadine ineffective for EPS prophylaxis (Keepers et al., 1987). In that double-blind study of 72 patients, they compared amantadine with a placebo during the first week of treatment with antipsychotics. No differences in rates of dystonia were demonstrated for the two groups. Therefore, despite its superior side-effect profile, when compared with those for anticholinergics, amantadine cannot be recommended for dystonia prophylaxis.

Low-dosage Antipsychotics

Low dosages of antipsychotics are effective for many patients receiving long-term treatment for psychoses, and they probably reduce EPS morbidity in that setting (Kane et al., 1983; Schooler, 1991). In patients needing acute treatment, however, low-dosage antipsychotic treatment frequently is ineffective. A summary analysis of data from many studies has suggested that there is little difference between the dosage effective for acute treatment of psychoses and the dosage likely to produce EPS. For dystonia, especially, the highest incidences of EPS can occur at dosages in the middle of the therapeutic range (e.g., 400–600 mg/day, CPZE) (Baldessarini, et al., 1989). Thus, even when using a low-dosage strategy for treating psychosis, both treatment and prophylaxis for dystonia are required.

Conclusion

Knowledge of the clinical manifestations and differential diagnosis of dystonia is important in recognizing the syndrome and preventing adverse outcomes. A thorough knowledge of the risk factors for dystonia will allow the clinician to make rational decisions concerning the methods to be used to minimize dystonias and related complications. Patients at high risk for dystonia should receive initial prophylaxis unless definite contraindications are present. Patients at lower risk should be closely observed for manifestations of this side effect and treated early.

References

Arana, G. W., Goff, D. C., Baldessarini, R. J., & Keepers, G. A. (1988). Efficacy of anticholinergic prophylaxis for neuroleptic-induced acute dystonia. *Am. J. Psychiatry* 145:993–6.

Avissar, S., & Schreiber, G. (1989). Muscarinic receptor subclassification and G-proteins: significance for lithium action in affective disorders and for the treatment of the extrapyramidal side effects of neuroleptics. *Biol. Psychiatry* 26:113–30.

Ayd, F. J., Jr. (1961). A survey of drug-induced extrapyramidal reactions. *J. Am. Med. Assoc.* 175:1054–60.

Ayd, F. J., Jr. (1978). Intravenous haloperidol therapy. *Int. Drug Ther. News* 13:20–3.

Ayers, J. L., & Dawson, K. P. (1980). Acute dystonic reactions in childhood. *N.Z. Med. J.* 92:964–5.

Baldessarini, R. J., Cohen, B. M., & Teicher, M. H. (1989). The importance of dose in neuroleptic treatment. *Dir. Psychiatry* 6:1–8.

Binder, R. L., & Levy, R. (1981). Extrapyramidal reactions in Asians. *Am. J. Psychiatry* 138:1243–4.

Boyer, W. F., Honeycutt-Bakalar, N., & Lake, C. R. (1987). Anticholinergic prophylaxis of acute haloperidol-induced acute dystonic reactions. *J. Clin. Psychopharmacol.* 7:164–6.

Bucci, L. (1971). Combined intramuscular administration of depot fluphenazine and
benztropine mesylate in chronic schizophrenic patients. *Curr. Ther. Res.*
13:545–8.

Calne, D. B., & Lang, A. E. (1988). Secondary dystonia. In *Advances in Neurology. Vol. 50: Dystonia,* part 2, ed. S. Fahn, C. D. Marsden, & D. B. Calne,
pp. 9–33. New York: Raven Press.

Carter, J. G. (1986). Intravenous haloperidol in the treatment of acute psychosis
(letter). *Am. J. Psychiatry* 43:1316–17.

Casey, D. E. (1991). Serotonin and dopamine relationships in nonhuman primate
extrapyramidal syndromes. *J. Eur. Coll. Neuropsychopharmacol.* S15:351–
3.

Cavanaugh, J. J., & Finlayson, R. E. (1984). Rhabdomyolysis due to acute dystonic reaction to antipsychotic drugs. *J. Clin. Psychiatry* 45:356–7.

Cavenar, J. O., Jr., Hammett, E. B., & Maltsies, A. (1979). Misdiagnosis of
severe dystonia. *Psychosomatics* 20:209–10.

Chase, T. N., Schnur, J. A., & Gordon, E. K. (1970). Cerebrospinal fluid monoamine catabolites in drug-induced extrapyramidal disorders. *Neuropsychopharmacology* 9:256–68.

Chien, C. P., & DiMascio, A. (1967). Drug-induced extrapyramidal symptoms and
their relations to clinical efficacy. *Am. J. Psychiatry* 123:1490–8.

Chien, C., DiMascio, A., & Cole, J. O. (1974). Antiparkinsonian agents and depot
phenothiazine. *Am. J. Psychiatry* 131:86–90.

Chiles, J. A. (1978). Extrapyramidal reactions in adolescents treated with high-
potency antipsychotics. *Am. J. Psychiatry* 135:239–40.

Cohen, B. M., Herschel, M., & Aoba, A. (1979). Neuroleptic, antimuscarinic, and
antiadrenergic activity of chlorpromazine, thioridazine, and their metabolites.
Psychiatry Res. 1:199–208.

Crowley, T. J., Hoehn, M. M., Rutledge, C. O., Stallings, M. A., Heaton, R. K.,
Sundell, S., & Stilson, D. (1978). Dopamine excretion and vulnerability to
drug-induced parkinsonism: schizophrenic patients. *Arch. Gen. Psychiatry*
35:97–104.

DiMascio, A., & Demirgian, E. (1970). Antiparkinson drug overuse. *Psychosomatics* 11:596–601.

Donlon, P. T., & Stenson, R. L. (1976). Neuroleptic induced extrapyramidal symptoms. *Dis. Nerv. Syst.* 37:629–34.

Fernandez, F., Holmes, V. F., Adams, F., & Cavanaugh, J. J. (1988). Treatment of
severe, refractory agitation with a haloperidol drip. *J. Clin. Psychiatry* 49:239–
41.

Flaherty, J. A., & Lahmeyer, H. W. (1978). Laryngeal-pharyngeal dystonia as a
possible cause of asphyxia with haloperidol treatment. *Am. J. Psychiatry*
135:1414–15.

Gagrat, D., Hamilton, J., & Belmaker, R. H. (1978). Intravenous diazepam in the
treatment of neuroleptic-induced acute dystonia and akathisia. *Am. J. Psychiatry* 135:1232–3.

Gardos, G. (1981). Dystonic reaction during maintenance antipsychotic therapy.
Am. J. Psychiatry 138:114–15.

Gerken, A., Wetzel, H., & Benkert, O. (1991). Extrapyramidal symptoms and their
relationship to clinical efficacy under perphenazine treatment: a controlled pro-

spective handwriting-test study in 22 acutely ill schizophrenic patients. *Pharmacopsychiatry* 24:132–7.

Giron, L. T., Jr. (1987). Tardive dystonia after a short course of thioridazine. *J. Fam. Pract.* 24:405–6.

Greenblatt, D. J., Shader, R. I., & DiMascio, A. (1970). Extrapyramidal effects. In *Psychotropic Drug Side Effects: Clinical and Theoretical Perspectives,* ed. R. I. Shader & A. DiMascio, pp. 92–106. Baltimore: Williams & Wilkins.

Gross, M. L. P. (1980). Acute dystonia as idiosyncratic reaction to haloperidol. *Lancet* 2:479–80.

Hansen, L. B., Larsen, N., & Vestergard, P. (1981). Plasma levels of perphenazine (Trilafon) related to development of extrapyramidal side effects. *Psychopharmacology (Berlin)* 74:306–9.

Idzorek, S. (1976). Antiparkinsonian agents and fluphenazine decanoate. *Am. J. Psychiatry* 133:80–2.

Jellinek, T., Gardos, G., & Cole, J. O. (1981). Adverse effects of antiparkinson drug withdrawal. *Am. J. Psychiatry* 138:1567–71.

Kane, J. M., Rifkin, A., Woerner, M., Reardon, G., Sarantakus, S., Schneibel, D., & Ramos-Lorenzi, J. (1983). Low-dose neuroleptic treatment of outpatient schizophrenics. *Arch. Gen. Psychiatry* 40:893–6.

Kaneko, K., Yuasa, T., Miyatake, T., & Tsuji, S. (1993). Stereotyped hand clasping: an unusual tardive movement disorder. *Mov. Disord.* 8:230–1.

Kang, U. J., Burke, R. E., & Fahn, S. (1986). Natural history and treatment of tardive dystonia. *Mov. Disord.* 1:193–208.

Keepers, G. A., Brown, W. L., Clappison, V. J., & Casey, D. E. (1987). Amantadine treatment and prophylaxis of EPS. In *Proceedings of the American Psychiatric Association Annual Meeting,* vol. 45E, p. 96 (abstract).

Keepers, G. A., & Casey, D. E. (1986). Clinical management of acute neuroleptic-induced extrapyramidal syndromes. In *Current Psychiatric Therapies,* ed. J. H. Masserman, pp. 139–57. New York: Grune & Stratton.

Keepers, G. A., & Casey, D. E. (1987). Prediction of neuroleptic-induced dystonia. *J. Clin. Psychopharmacol.* 7:342–5.

Keepers, G. A., & Casey, D. E. (1991). Use of neuroleptic-induced extrapyramidal symptoms to predict future vulnerability in side effects. *Am. J. Psychiatry* 148:85–9.

Keepers, G. A., Clappison, V. J., & Casey, D. E. (1983). Initial anticholinergic prophylaxis for neuroleptic-induced extrapyramidal syndromes. *Arch. Gen. Psychiatry* 40:492–6.

Lake, C. R., Casey, D. E., McEvoy, J. P., Siris, S. G., Boyer, W. F., & Simpson, G. (1986). Anticholinergic prophylaxis in young adults treated with neuroleptic drugs. *Psychopharmacol. Bull.* 22:981–4.

Lee, A. (1979). Treatment of drug-induced dystonic reactions. *J. Am. Coll. Emergency Physicians* 8:453–7.

McEvoy, J. P. (1983). The clinical use of anticholinergic drugs as treatment for extrapyramidal side effects of neuroleptic drugs. *J. Clin. Psychopharmacol.* 3:288–302.

McEvoy, J. P. (1987). A double-blind crossover comparison of antiparkinson drug therapy: amantadine versus anticholinergics in 90 normal volunteers, with an emphasis on differential effects on memory function. *J. Clin. Psychiatry (Suppl.)* 48:20–3.

McEvoy, J. P., & Freter, S. (1989). The dose–response relationship for memory impairment by anticholinergic drugs. *Compr. Psychiatry* 30:135–8.

McEvoy, J. P., McCue, M., Spring, B., Mohs, R. C., Lavori, P. W., & Farr, R. M. (1987). Effects of amantadine and trihexyphenidyl on memory in elderly normal volunteers. *Am. J. Psychiatry* 144:573–7.

Magliozzi, J. R., Gillespie, H., Lombrozo, L., & Hollister, L. E. (1985). Mood alteration following oral and intravenous haloperidol and relationship to drug concentration in normal subjects. *J. Clin. Pharmacol.* 25:285–90.

Mann, S. C., Cohen, M. M., & Boger, W. P. (1979). The danger of laryngeal dystonia. *Am. J. Psychiatry* 136:1344–5.

Manos, N., & Gkiouzepas, J. (1981). Discontinuing antiparkinson medication in chronic schizophrenics: at what cost to the patient? *Acta Psychiatr. Scand.* 63:28–32.

Manos, N., Lavrentiadis, G., & Gkiouzepas, J. (1986). Evaluation of the need for prophylactic antiparkinsonian medication in psychotic patients treated with neuroleptics. *J. Clin. Psychiatry* 47:114–16.

Marsden, C. D. (1988). Investigation of dystonia. In *Advances in Neurology*, ed. S. Fahn, C. D. Marsden, & D. B. Calne, pp. 35–44. New York: Raven Press.

Medina, C., Kramer, M. D., & Kuland, A. A. (1962). Biperiden in the treatment of phenothiazine-induced extrapyramidal reactions. *J. Am. Med. Assoc.* 182:1127–9.

Menuck, M. (1981). Laryngeal-pharyngeal dystonia and haloperidol. *Am. J. Psychiatry* 138:394–5.

Menza, M. A., Murray, G. B., Holmes, V. F., & Rafuls, W. A. (1987). Decreased extrapyramidal symptoms with intravenous haloperidol. *J. Clin. Psychiatry* 48:278–80.

Menza, M. A., Murray, G. B., Holmes, V. F., & Rafuls, W. A. (1988). Controlled study of extrapyramidal reactions in the management of delirious, medically ill patients: intravenous haloperidol versus intravenous haloperidol plus benzodiazepines. *Heart Lung* 17:238–41.

Neu, C., DiMascio, A., & Demirgian, E. (1972). Antiparkinson medication in the treatment of extrapyramidal side effects: single or multiple daily doses. *Curr. Ther. Res.* 14:246–50.

Noda, S., Umezaki, H., Itoh, H., & Hiromatsuki, K. (1988). Orofacial dyskinesia in stupor and coma. *Neurology* 38:1331–2.

Ott, D. A., & Goeden, S. R. (1979). Treatment of acute phenothiazine reaction. *J. Am. Coll. Emergency Physicians* 8:471–2.

Paulson, G. (1960). Procyclidine for dystonia caused by phenothiazine derivatives. *Dis. Nerv. Syst.* 21:447–8.

Rifkin, A., Quitkin, F., Kane, J., Struve, F., & Klein, D. F. (1978). Are prophylactic antiparkinson drugs necessary? A controlled study of procyclidine withdrawal. *Arch. Gen. Psychiatry* 35:483–9.

Rubenstein, J. S. (1978). Abuse of antiparkinsonism drugs: feigning of extrapyramidal symptoms to obtain trihexyphenidyl. *J. Am. Med. Assoc.* 239:2365–6.

Saran, A. S. (1986). Use or abuse of antiparkinsonian drugs by psychiatric patients. *J. Clin. Psychiatry* 47:130–2.

Sayers, A. C., Burki, H. R., Ruch, W., & Asper, H. (1976). Anticholinergic properties of antipsychotic drugs and their relation to extrapyramidal side effects. *Psychopharmacology* 51:15–22.

Schooler, N. R. (1991). Maintenance medication for schizophrenia: strategies for dose reduction. *Schizophr. Bull.* 17:311–24.

Sinantios, C. A., Spyrides, P., Vlachos, P., & Papadatos, C. (1978). Acute halo-
peridol poisoning in children. *J. Pediatr.* 93:1038–9.
Smith, M. J., & Miller, M. M. (1961). Severe extrapyramidal reaction to per-
phenazine treated with diphenhydramine. *N. Engl. J. Med.* 264:396–7.
Snyder, S., Greenberg, D., & Yamamura, H. I. (1974). Antischizophrenic drugs
and brain cholinergic receptors. *Arch. Gen. Psychiatry* 31:58–61.
Sramek, J. J., Sayles, M. A., & Simpson, G. M. (1986a). Neuroleptic dosage for
Asians: a failure to replicate. *Am. J. Psychiatry* 143:535–6.
Sramek, J. J., Simpson, G. M., Morrison, R. L., & Heiser, J. F. (1986b). Anticholinergic agents for prophylaxis of neuroleptic-induced dystonic reactions: a
prospective study. *J. Clin. Psychiatry* 47:305–9.
Stern, T. A., & Anderson, W. H. (1979). Benztropine prophylaxis of dystonic reactions. *Psychopharmacology (Berlin)* 61:261–2.
Swett, C. (1975). Drug-induced dystonias. *Am. J. Psychiatry* 132:532–4.
Swett, C., Jr., Cole, J. O., Shapiro, S., & Slone, D. (1977). Extrapyramidal side
effects in chlorpromazine recipients: emergence according to benztropine prophylaxis. *Arch. Gen. Psychiatry* 34:942–3.
Tesar, G. E., Murray, G. B., & Cassem, N. H. (1985). Use of high-dose intravenous haloperidol in the treatment of agitated cardiac patients. *J. Clin. Psychopharmacol.* 5:344–7.
Tune, L., & Coyle, J. T. (1981). Acute extrapyramidal side effects: serum levels of
neuroleptics and anticholinergics. *Psychopharmacology (Berlin)* 75:9–15.
Waugh, W. H., & Metts, J. C. (1960). Severe extrapyramidal motor activity
induced by prochlorperazine: its relief by the intravenous injection of diph-
enhydramine. *N. Engl. J. Med.* 262:353–4.
Winslow, R. S., Stillner, V., Coons, D. J., & Robinson, M. W. (1986). Prevention
of acute dystonic reactions in patients beginning high-potency neuroleptics.
Am. J. Psychiatry 143:706–10.
Wood, G. M., & Water, A. K. (1980). Prolonged dystonic reaction to chlor-
promazine in myxoedema coma. *Postgrad. Med. J.* 56:192–3.
Yassa, R., Nair, V., & Dimitry, R. (1986). Prevalence of tardive dystonia. *Acta
Psychiatr. Scand.* 73:629–33.

26

Tardive Dystonia

PAUL GREENE, M.D.

Shortly after dopamine-receptor blocking agents began to be used for treatment of psychoses in the 1950s, a variety of movement disorders began to be described in the literature and to be attributed to the antipsychotic agents (Crane, 1973). Some of those movement disorders were difficult to treat, and they sometimes persisted after cessation of the antipsychotic treatment (Druckman, Seelinger, & Thulin, 1962). The resulting persistent syndrome, consisting of repetitive oral-buccal-lingual movements (chewing movements; lip puckering, sucking, or smacking; tongue protrusions; side-to-side jaw deviations), was referred to as *tardive dyskinesia,* and later as classic tardive dyskinesia (Fahn, 1985). The oral-buccal-lingual movements, sometimes accompanied by repetitive limb movements, were labeled "tardive" because they generally appeared only after prolonged treatment with antipsychotics (Faurbye et al., 1964), though there were some reports of persistent movements appearing soon after initiation of therapy (Angle & McIntire, 1968).

Beginning in 1962, a series of reports appeared describing persistent abnormal movements that resembled the symptoms of idiopathic dystonia and appeared after treatment with neuroleptics (Burke et al., 1982). According to the Scientific Advisory Board of the Dystonia Medical Research Foundation, dystonia is "a syndrome of sustained muscle contractions, frequently causing twisting and repetitive movements, or abnormal postures" (Fahn, 1988). The term *tardive dystonia,* analogous to *tardive dyskinesia,* was coined by Keegan and Rajput (1973). Burke et al. (1982) suggested specific criteria for the diagnosis of tardive dystonia: (1) the presence of chronic dystonia, (2) a history of exposure to a dopamine-receptor blocking agent (DRBA) concurrent with the onset of dystonia or preceding the dystonia by no more than 2 months, (3) exclusion of the known possible causes of secondary dystonia by appropriate clinical and laboratory evaluation, and (4) absence of a family history of dystonia. Subsequent studies have begun to diagnose tardive dystonia if the dystonia has appeared 3–6 months after exposure to a DRBA, for the actual delay in appearance of dystonia is unknown.

Kang, Burke, and Fahn (1986) argued that tardive dystonia should be considered distinct from classic tardive dyskinesia because (1) it has different phenomenologic manifestations, (2) patients with tardive dystonia are younger at onset, and lack the female predominance seen with tardive dyskinesia, and (3) the pharmacologic reactions involved are different (whereas tardive dystonia sometimes is alleviated by treatment with anticholinergics, tardive dyskinesia sometimes is exacerbated by anticholinergics). Since those reports, it has become clear, as well, that tardive dystonia and tardive dyskinesia differ in terms of prognosis: In general, tardive dystonia is more bothersome to patients (Gimenez-Roldan, Mateo, & Bartolome, 1985; Yassa, Nair, & Dimitry, 1986) and is less likely to remit than is tardive dyskinesia. Although the term "tardive dyskinesia" is sometimes used to refer to any movement disorder induced by a DRBA, I shall use the term "tardive dyskinesia" to refer specifically to the classic oral-buccal-lingual syndrome.

In their 1982 review, Burke and co-workers found 15 case reports of tardive dystonia in the literature and added 42 cases of their own; by 1990, at least 161 additional patients had been reported (Burke, 1992). Since then, at least 132 more patients have been described in the English literature (Table 26.1). I shall reexamine the epidemiology, etiology, and treatment of tardive dystonia in light of this expanded literature.

Phenomenology

There have been eight population-based studies of tardive dystonia (Owens, Johnstone, & Frith, 1982; Friedman, Kucharski, & Wagner, 1987; Yassa, Nair, & Iskandar, 1989; Gureje, 1989; Sachdev, 1989; Sethi, Hess, & Harp, 1990; Chiu et al., 1992; Raja, 1995). Sethi et al. (1990), in an atypical study (as explained later), found the most common sites for dystonic symptoms to be the upper extremities and jaw, present in 18 (67%) of their 27 patients. In most studies, the face and neck were the most common sites, and they were involved in at least 22 of about 23 patients – the total number of patients with tardive dystonia in the study by Owens et al. (1982) could only be estimated. In one series, the face, trunk, and limbs were equally involved (Raja, 1995). In three large referral series (Gimenez-Roldan et al., 1985; Kang et al., 1986; Wojcik et al., 1991), the neck and face were the most common sites of involvement, with 85 (87%) of 98 patients showing such involvement. The neck was involved in 87% of the patients, and the trunk in 41%, and only 14% had generalized dystonia. In the series of Kang et al. (1986), 9 (13%) of 67

Table 26.1. *Case reports of tardive dystonia since 1982*

Report	Number (male/female)	Mean age at onset of dystonia (years)
Luchins & Goldman (1985)	1/0	?
Sachdev (1989)	1/0	47
Kurata et al. (1989)	0/2	34, 48
Sethi et al. (1990)	26/1	?
Van Putten et al. (1990)	0/1	24
Sachdev (1991)	1/0	39
Wojcik et al. (1991)	21/11	34/40
Blake et al. (1991)	0/2	29, 46
Yazici et al. (1991)	0/2	23, 30
Sugawara et al. (1992)	1/0	26
Lieberman et al. (1991)	7 (?/?)	?
Chiu et al. (1992)	2/2	~36
Ferraz & Andrade (1992)	16 (?/?)	35.9
Gabellini et al. (1992)	0/1	47
Stip et al. (1992)	1/0	22
Micheli et al. (1993)	5/3	68.5
Lamberti & Bellnier (1993)	1/0	38
Sachdev (1993)	9/6	35.7
Abad & Ovsiew (1993)	1/0	?
Trugman et al. (1994)	1/0	25
Raja (1995)	5/3	?

patients had respiratory involvement, described as respiratory irregularities or grunting. In the series of Yassa et al. (1989), similar respiratory involvement was noted in 1 of 8 patients with tardive dystonia, as compared with 4 of 11 patients with severe tardive dyskinesia.

This distribution of symptoms is similar to but not identical with the distribution of symptoms in patients with idiopathic dystonia. Burke et al. (1982) observed that patients under 30 years of age with tardive dystonia were less likely to develop generalized dystonia than were young patients with idiopathic dystonia. They also observed that tardive dystonia was more likely to involve facial muscles early in the course of the syndrome, especially in younger patients. Whereas in their patients the mean age at onset of tardive dystonia affecting the upper or lower face was 34 years, patients with idiopathic facial dystonia at the same center had a mean age at onset of dystonia of 44 years ($p < .0003$ by t test) (R. E. Burke, unpublished data). In addition, 10 of 23 patients in their series with tardive facial dystonia (43%) were under the age of 29 years at onset, compared with 53 (11%) of 391 of patients with idiopathic facial dystonia at the same center ($p < .005$ using χ^2) (R. E. Burke, unpublished data).

The phenomenologic manifestations of idiopathic and tardive dystonic movements may be indistinguishable. Both idiopathic dystonia and tardive dystonia can be exacerbated by action and alleviated by "sensory tricks" (as torticollis can be relieved by gently touching the cheek with a finger). Tardive dystonia is commonly accompanied by other tardive movements. For example, tardive dyskinesia accompanied dystonia in 55–84% of patients in two large referral series (Kang et al., 1986; Wojcik et al., 1991), and akathisia (inner restlessness accompanied by fidgeting movements) accompanied dystonia in 21 (31%) of 67 patients in the series of Kang et al. (1986). Also, pure retrocollis, jerky supination of the upper extremities, and relief of symptoms with walking, may be more common in patients with tardive dystonia than in those with idiopathic dystonia; those observations, however, have not yet been corroborated in comparative studies (Kang et al., 1986).

Epidemiology and Risk Factors

Most estimates of the prevalence of tardive dystonia have ranged from 1% to 4%: 1% (Sachdev, 1991), 1.5% (Friedman et al., 1987), 1.5% Gureje, 1989), 1.6% (Yassa et al., 1990), 2% (Yassa et al., 1986), 2.7% (Owens et al., 1982; Raja, 1995). In the study by Yassa et al. (1986), patients under 50 years of age were significantly more likely (6 of 101, or 5.9%) to have dystonia than patients over age 50 (1 of 250, or 0.4%). In an attempt to detect patients with mild dystonia, Sethi et al. (1990) examined 125 young male psychotic inpatients (average age 45 years) and found 27 (22%) with dystonic symptoms. Many of those patients had mild symptoms (only 6 of 27 patients were aware of the dystonia), and 14 of 27 had focal dystonia of the upper extremities detected during the act of writing, a testing procedure generally not used in previous studies.

It is difficult to compare these estimates of the prevalence of tardive dystonia with the prevalence of tardive dyskinesia, which has been reported to vary from 0.5% to 51.6% (Kane & Smith, 1982). Some studies (Owens et al., 1982; Gureje, 1989; Sethi et al., 1990; Yassa et al., 1990; Chiu et al., 1992; Raja, 1995) have reported the prevalences of tardive dyskinesia and tardive dystonia in the same population, and the ratio of tardive dyskinesia to tardive dystonia has varied from about 4.9 : 1 (Owens et al., 1982) to 21 : 1 (Yassa et al., 1990). Such variation in the relative prevalances of the two disorders is expected, however. Indeed, the prevalence of tardive dyskinesia rises with age (Kane et al., 1986), whereas tardive dystonia is more prevalent among younger populations, as discussed later. The series of Sethi et al. (1990) was an exception; there, tardive dystonia was twice as common as tardive dyskinesia.

Most studies comparing tardive dyskinesia and tardive dystonia have found the mean age for patients with dystonia to be significantly lower than the age for patients with tardive dyskinesia (Gardos et al., 1987; Sethi et al., 1990; Yassa et al., 1990). In addition, referral series have found that the age for onset of dystonia in men tends to be lower than that for women (Gimenez-Roldan et al., 1985; Kang et al., 1986; Yadalam, Korn, & Simpson, 1990; Wojcik et al., 1991). In a survey of psychiatric inpatients (Yassa et al., 1986), the mean age at onset for 5 men was 29.4 years, compared with 57 years for 2 women ($p = .051$). Although many studies have reported male predominance (Burke et al., 1982; Gimenez-Roldan et al., 1985; Friedman et al., 1987; Gardos et al., 1987; Yassa et al., 1989, 1990), the differences have not always reached statistical significance, and subsequent studies (Kang et al., 1986; Miller & Jankovic, 1990) have reported equal numbers of men and women. There has been a suggestion, as well, that the mean duration of exposure to neuroleptics has been shorter for women with tardive dystonia than for men (Gimenez-Roldan et al., 1985; Wojcik et al., 1991). That was not true, however, in the series of Kang et al. (1986), who found no relationship between duration of exposure and either gender or age at onset of tardive dystonia.

Tardive dystonia has been reported with the use of almost every form of DRBA that penetrates the central nervous system (CNS): antipsychotics (phenothiazines, thioxanthenes, butyrophenones, the dibenzoxazepine loxapine, the indolone molindone, and the diphenylbutylpiperidine pimozide), the dibenzoxazepine antidepressant amoxapine (Kang et al., 1986), and antiemetics (promethazine, prochlorperazine, and metoclopramide) (Burke et al., 1982; Miller & Jankovic, 1990). Although the atypical neuroleptic clozapine and the dopamine depleter/dopamine-receptor blocker tetrabenazine both penetrate the CNS, neither has been convincingly linked to the development of tardive complications. However, both are often used in patients already exposed to another DRBA, thus complicating the interpretation of tardive symptoms that appear in such patients. There has been no controlled study concerning the impact of psychiatric diagnoses on the risk for developing tardive dystonia; all major diagnoses are represented, however, including schizophrenia, depression, anxiety, paranoid psychosis, bipolar disorder, schizoaffective disorder, and obsessive–compulsive disorder, as well as the less specific psychiatric indications such as aggressive behavior, mental retardation, and dementia (Burke et al., 1982; Yassa et al., 1986; Gardos et al., 1987). Small numbers of patients have developed dystonia after treatment with antiemetics for nausea or treatment with neuroleptics for movement disorders such as chorea or tics (Burke et al., 1982; Singh & Jankovic, 1988).

There is no evidence that medications administered concurrently with the DRBA either increase or decrease the risk for developing tardive dystonia, although this question has not been examined systematically. There has been no comparison of the risks for developing tardive dystonia in patients continuously treated with neuroleptics versus those with multiple separate exposures, although two reports (Gardos et al., 19897; Yassa et al., 1989) have noted that affected patients have tended to have had continuous neuroleptic exposure, with few drug-free periods. In addition, Burke et al. (1982) reported 3 patients whose tardive torticollis remitted after discontinuation of neuroleptics, but whose symptoms returned and were persistent after reexposure to neuroleptics.

It seems unlikely that a history of acute dystonic reactions is predictive of the development of tardive dystonia, because in the series of Burke et al. (1982), only 5 of 42 patients with tardive dystonia had a history of acute dystonic reactions. As noted earlier, other tardive symptoms often accompany tardive dystonia, but symptoms of tardive dyskinesia have preceded dystonia in only 6–16% of cases (Kang et al., 1986; Wojcik et al., 1991).

No clear relationship has been established between the prevalence or severity of tardive dystonia and the duration of exposure to neuroleptics. One population-based study (Sethi et al., 1990) found no correlation linking the prevalence of tardive dystonia with the duration of neuroleptic treatment; however, that study did include patients with extremely mild symptoms. In the referral series of Burke et al. (1982), no correlation was found between severity of dystonia and duration of exposure, although that population probably was biased toward inclusion of patients with more severe symptoms. In two referral studies (Kang et al., 1986; Wojcik et al., 1991), a trend was reported toward shorter exposures for patients whose dystonia decreased or remitted.

Several authors have commented on the appearance of tardive dystonia after relatively short exposures to DRBAs, as compared with the longer exposures leading to tardive dyskinesia (Kang et al., 1986; Gureje, 1989). Among the inpatient population of Yassa et al. (1990), although the exposures to neuroleptics that led to tardive dystonia (7.1 ± 4.8 years) were shorter than those (14.9 ± 8.6 years) that led to tardive dyskinesia, no attempt was made to correct for confounding variables such as age and gender.

Several reports have mentioned evidence of preexisting brain dysfunction in patients with tardive dystonia, such as mental retardation (Burke et al., 1982; Gimenez-Roldan et al., 1985; Friedman et al., 1987) and developmental abnormalities (Burke et al., 1982), as well as the effects of electroconvulsive treatment (ECT), insulin shock (Friedman et al., 1987), and extensive frontal leucotomy (Gimenez-Roldan et al., 1985). However, it is impossible to interpret those observations without knowing the prevalences of such abnormalities among patients with tardive dyskinesia and among the entire population of patients exposed to DRBAs.

Differential Diagnosis

The differential diagnosis of tardive dystonia must take account of the entire list of conditions associated with dystonia, most of which are rare and are associated with other neurological abnormalities (Calne & Lang, 1988). Wilson's disease must be considered, as it can be manifested in young patients as dystonia and psychiatric disturbances without other neurological abnormalities. Thus, serum ceruloplasmin determination and slit-lamp examination for Kayser-Fleischer rings are mandatory parts of the diagnosis, even when there is a clear history of DRBA exposure. Occasionally, when dystonia is the only neurological sign, the brain images from computed tomography (CT) or magnetic-resonance imaging (MRI) may show abnormal findings, as in some cases of delayed-onset dystonia after birth injury (Burke, Fahn, & Gold, 1980) or metachromatic leukodystrophy (Lang et al., 1985); therefore, some brain imaging is prudent. The procedures for diagnosis of dystonia in patients with other neurological abnormalities have been adequately discussed elsewhere (Marsden, 1988).

Idiopathic dystonia is not likely to be confused with tardive dystonia except in three specific situations. The first concerns patients who have a long history of dystonia, in whom it may be difficult to determine whether or not exposure to the DRBA preceded the onset of the dystonia and, if so, to determine the interval between the two events. The second concerns those patients treated for nonpsychiatric indications, such as nausea, who may fail to report prior DRBA exposure, especially if the dystonia appeared after the DRBA was withdrawn. Finally, if an individual with a family history of dystonia develops dystonia after DRBA exposure, the cause of the dystonia will be in question. Until the genes for idiopathic dystonia are identified (Ozelius et al., 1989), tardive dystonia can be diagnosed only if tardive dyskinesia or akathisia is present in addition to dystonia. In any case, a combination of dystonia and akathisia or repetitive oral-buccal-lingual movements should prompt a search for possible exposure to a DRBA (including some of the calcium-channel blockers, such as flunarizine, that are known to cause tardive dyskinesia) (Chouza et al., 1986). Because high-dosage anticholinergic medications used to treat dystonia can induce choreic movements, it may be necessary to withdraw the anticholinergic treatment if confirmation of a diagnosis of tardive dystonia is essential.

Prognosis

Burke et al. (1982) observed that tardive "dystonia was insidious in onset, progressive for months or years, and then persistent but static for years." With the exception of drug-free remissions (discussed later), most subsequent series (Gimenez-Roldan et al., 1985; Kang et al., 1986; Yassa et al., 1986; Gardos et al., 1987) have shown that same disease progression. Kang et al. (1986) found that the initial dystonic symptoms were focal in 61% of patients and that 85% of those eventually developed more widespread symptoms. Wojcik et al. (1991) reported decreases in symptoms in 15 of 29 patients followed for a mean period of 4.9 years, although 7 of those were drug-free, and 7 of the remaining 8 were on different dosages of neuroleptics.

Remissions of tardive dystonia sometimes occur. In one referral series, 5 (12%) of 42 drug-free patients experienced complete resolution of symptoms after drug-free periods ranging from 11 months to 5 years (Kang et al., 1986). In the population-based study of Yassa et al. (1986), 1 (20%) of 5 patients with tardive dystonia experienced remission (mean drug-free period, 2–3 years). That is considerably lower than the figure reported in the prospective study of Kane et al. (1986), who found a remission rate of 20–30% after 2 years of tardive dyskinesia.

Treatment

Kang et al. (1986) reviewed the results of treatment for 67 patients with tardive dystonia, 42 of whom were free of any DRBA. The most successful results were achieved with dopamine depleters, anticholinergics, or a combination of the two. Nineteen (63%) of 30 patients improved when given reserpine (2–9 mg/day) or the dopamine depleter/dopamine-receptor blocker tetrabenazine (12.5–250 mg/day). Adverse effects were common: 20–40% of patients had dosage-limiting side effects, including parkinsonism, hallucinations, depression, confusion, and lethargy. However, some patients who had side effects from one agent were able to tolerate the other. Only 3 of 11 patients with diagnoses of depression relapsed into depression when taking reserpine or tetrabenazine. Similarly, 18 (46.2%) of 39 patients improved when taking the anticholinergics trihexyphenidyl (10–32 mg/day) or ethopropazine (100–450 mg/day). Side effects included confusion, forgetfulness, gastrointestinal complaints, dry mouth, blurred vision, urinary retention, and, in 1 patient, psychosis. None of the 8 patients with diagnoses of schizophrenia experienced exacerbation of psychiatric symptoms while taking anticholinergics; only 1 of 10 patients suffered exacerbation of tardive dyskinesia. Although dopamine antagonists were able to suppress symptoms in 10 (77%) of 13 patients, it was observed that symptoms returned when the drugs were withdrawn. Overall, excluding remissions, 52% of patients responded to some treatment, but only 8 (13%) of 62 patients were sufficiently improved that it was deemed unnecessary to continue the search for additional treatment.

Although attempts at treatment have been described in many case reports, most have not adequately described the magnitudes and durations of benefits, the dosages, and the side effects. Response rates to the most commonly used agents are summarized in Table 26.2. The atypical neuroleptic clozapine was used successfully in 7 of 10 patients (Burke et al., 1982; Van Putten, Wirshing, & Marder, 1990; Wojcik et al., 1991; Blake et al., 1991; Lieberman et al., 1991; Lamberti & Bellnier, 1993; Trugman et al., 1994). Isolated trials have been described with deanol, choline, amantadine, physostigmine, lecithin, carbamazepine, lithium, propranolol, verapamil, clonidine (Nishikawa et al., 1984), and the cholecystokinin analogue ceruletide (Sugawara et al., 1992), as well as other agents. However, the occasional successes with those agents have not received wider confirmation, nor documentation by prospective trial. Similarly, reports of improvements after thalamotomy (Burke et al., 1982; Yadalam et al., 1990) and ECT (Kwentus, Schulz, & Hart, 1984; Adityanjee, Chan, & Subramaniam, 1990) remain anecdotal. Botulinum toxin injections, which are accepted therapy for idiopathic focal dystonia, may be of benefit to patients with severe dystonia in a particular body region, such as the jaw, eyelids, or neck (Stip et al., 1992). Furthermore, although reports of patients with bipolar disorder who improved during episodes of mania have been published (Weiner & Werner, 1982; Lal, Saxena, & Mohan, 1988; Yazici et al., 1991), that phenomenon is of only theoretical interest and is without therapeutic value at present.

Discussion

Burke et al. (1982) and Kang et al. (1986) attempted to establish tardive dystonia as an entity distinct from classic tardive dyskinesia. They also tried to confirm that dystonia is indeed caused by exposure to a DRBA and is not simply a coincidental occurrence of idiopathic dystonia (or misdiagnosed secondary dystonia). Although not yet proved, those tenets are well accepted today. The reported rates of prevalence of dystonia – between 1% and 4% (as

Table 26.2. Treatment of tardive dystonia

Report		Number improving/number not improving				
	Anticholinergic	Reserpine/ tetrabenazine	Benzodiazepine	Neuroleptic	Baclofen	Dopamine agonist
Glazer et al. (1983)	—	—	—	—	0/1	1/1
Luchins & Goldman (1985)	0/1	—	0/1	0/1	—	—
Quinn et al. (1985)	—	—	—	—	—	1/3
Wolf & Koller (1985)[a]	1/3	—	5/19	10/13	1/13	—
Kang et al. (1986)	18/39	19/30	—	—	—	—
Lang (1986)	3/5	—	—	—	—	—
Rosse et al. (1986)	—	—	—	—	1/1	—
Yassa et al. (1986)	—	0/1	0/1	—	1/3	0/1
Gardos et al. (1987)	3/6	0/3	4/9	—	0/3	—
Kurata et al. (1989)	1/1	—	1/1	—	—	—
Lieberman et al. (1989)	0/1	—	—	—	—	2/3
Adityanjee et al. (1990)	—	—	0/4	—	—	—
Yadalam et al. (1990)	2/4	1/3	—	—	0/2	—
Sachdev (1991)	1/1	—	—	—	—	—
Wojcik et al. (1991)	6/23	1/6	12/23	—	2/5	—
Sugawara et al. (1992)	0/1	—	—	2/4	—	—
Totals	35/85 (41%)	21/43 (49%)	22/58 (38%)	12/18 (67%)	5/28 (18%)	4/8 (50%)

well as an unusually high report of 22%) – among neuroleptic-treated populations are substantially higher than the published rate of 0.03% prevalence of
idiopathic dystonia among the general population (Nutt et al., 1988). The
prevalence of dystonic movements among an untreated psychiatric population
is unknown. Nonetheless, the temporal relationship between DRBA exposure
and the onset of dystonia, the common co-occurrences of classic tardive
dyskinesia or akathisia with dystonia, and the occasional evolution of acute,
DRBA-induced dystonia into persistent dystonia provide convincing evidence
that DRBA exposure can cause dystonia. Even in the absence of specific
markers for tardive dystonia and tardive dyskinesia, the differences in the
syndromes outlined by Kang et al. (1986) have been confirmed in subsequent
studies. Analyses of newer treatments, such as the use of clozapine, have led
to the conclusion that tardive dystonia and tardive dyskinesia are pharmacologically distinct (Lieberman et al., 1988). Novel attempts at a subclassification of tardive dyskinesia using computerized statistical methods
have also indicated that tardive dystonia is an entity distinct from tardive
dyskinesia (Inada et al., 1990).

The epidemiology of tardive dystonia remains poorly understood. Tardive
dystonia occurs in a younger population than tardive dyskinesia, and it likely
occurs at a younger age in men than in women. Other proposed gender and
age differences are not well established. Similarly, the relationships of tardive
dystonia to preexisting brain damage and other epidemiologic factors have not
been established. Once tardive dystonia develops, there is no way of predicting whether it will remain mild or become severe. Spontaneous remissions of
tardive dystonia have been well documented, but they have occurred less
frequently than in patients with tardive dyskinesia. The symptoms of tardive
dystonia are most common on the neck, face, and trunk (in about that order),
but occasionally can occur in any region of the body. Tardive dystonia is often
accompanied by tardive dyskinesia or akathisia, although isolated dystonia
also occurs as a tardive phenomenon and may be indistinguishable from
idiopathic dystonia.

Our ability to treat tardive dystonia has changed little since the review of
Kang et al. (1986). Dopamine depleters and dopamine-receptor blockers
remain the most effective agents. Depleters entail a high incidence of side
effects, including depression, thus limiting their usefulness; the use of a
DRBA probably forecloses the possibility of drug-free remission. Despite our
ignorance about the course of tardive dystonia, the most rational course of
action when tardive dystonia develops is to eliminate the DRBA, when
possible. If neuroleptics are required, atypical neuroleptics, like clozapine,
should be considered as alternatives to traditional neuroleptics.

References

Abad, V., & Ovsiew, F. (1993). Treatment of persistent myoclonic tardive dystonia with verapamil. *Br. J. Psychiatry* 162:554–6.

Adityanjee, J. S. D., Chan, T. M., & Subramaniam, M. (1990). Temporary remission of tardive dystonia following electroconvulsive therapy. *Br. J. Psychiatry* 156:443–5.

Angle, C. R., & McIntire, M. S. (1968). Persistent dystonia in a brain-damaged child after ingestion of phenothiazine. *Pediatr. Pharmacol. Ther.* 73:124–6.

Blake, L. M., Marks, R. C., Nierman, P., & Luchins, D. J. (1991). Clozapine and clonazepam in tardive dystonia. *J. Clin. Psychopharmacol.* 11:268–9.

Burke, R. E. (1992). Neuroleptic-induced tardive dyskinesia variants. In *Drug-induced Movement Disorders,* ed. A. E. Lang & W. J. Weiner, pp. 167–98. Mount Kisco, NY: Futura Publishing.

Burke, R. E., Fahn, S., & Gold, A. P. (1980). Delayed-onset dystonia in patients with "static" encephalopathy. *J. Neurol. Neurosurg. Psychiatry* 43:789–97.

Burke, R. E., Fahn, S., Jankovic, J., Marsden, C. D., Lang, A. E., Gollomp, S., & Illson, J. (1982). Tardive dystonia: late-onset and persistent dystonia caused by antipsychotic drugs. *Neurology* 32:1335–46.

Calne, D. B., & Lang, A. E. (1988). Secondary dystonia. In *Advances in Neurology. Vol. 50: Dystonia,* part 2, ed. S. Fahn, C. D. Marsden, & D. B. Calne, pp. 9–33. New York: Raven Press.

Chiu, H., Shum, P., Lau, J., Lam, L., & Lee, S. (1992). *Am. J. Psychiatry* 149:1081–5.

Chouza, C., Caamano, J. L., Alijanti, R., Scaramelli, A., De Medina, O., & Romero, S. (1986). Parkinsonism, tardive dyskinesia and depression induced by flunarizine. *Lancet* 1:1303–4.

Crane, G. E. (1973). Persistent dyskinesia. *Br. J. Psychiatry* 122:395–405.

Druckman, R., Seelinger, D., & Thulin, B. (1962). Chronic involuntary movements induced by phenothiazines. *J. Nerv. Ment. Dis.* 135:69–76.

Fahn, S. (1985). A therapeutic approach to tardive dyskinesia. *J. Clin. Psychiatry* 46:19–24.

Fahn, S. (1988). Concept and classification of dystonia. In *Advances in Neurology. Vol. 50: Dystonia,* part 2, ed. S. Fahn, C. D. Marsden, & D. B. Calne, pp. 1–8. New York: Raven Press.

Faurbye, A., Rasch, P. J., Petersen, P. B., Brandborg, G., & Pakkenberg, H. (1964). Neurological symptoms in pharmacotherapy of psychoses. *Acta Psychiatr. Scand.* 40:10–27.

Ferraz, H. B., & Andrade, L. A. F. (1992). Symptomatic dystonia: clinical profile of 46 Brazilian patients. *Can. J. Neurol. Sci.* 19:504–7.

Friedman, J. H., Kucharski, L. T., & Wagner, R. L. (1987). Tardive dystonia in a psychiatric hospital. *J. Neurol. Neurosurg. Psychiatry* 50:801–3.

Gabellini, A. S., Pezzoli, A., De Massis, P., & Sacquegna, T. (1992). Veralipride-induced tardive dystonia in a patient with bipolar psychosis. *Ital. J. Neurol. Sci.* 13:621–3.

Gardos, G., Cole, J. O., Salomon, M., & Schniebolk, S. (1987). Clinical forms of severe tardive dyskinesias. *Am. J. Psychiatry* 144:895–902.

Gimenez-Roldan, S., Mateo, D., & Bartolome, P. (1985). Tardive dystonia and severe dyskinesia. *Acta Psychiatr. Scand.* 71:488–94.

Glazer, W. M., Moore, D. C., Hansen, T. C., & Brenner, L. M. (1983). Meige syndrome and tardive dyskinesia. *Am. J. Psychiatry* 140:798–9.

Gureje, O. (1989). The significance of subtyping tardive dyskinesia: a study of prevalence and associated factors. *Psychol. Med.* 19:121–8.

Inada, T., Yagi, G., Kamijima, K., Ohnishi, K., Kamisada, M., Takamiya, M., Nakajima, S., & Rockhold, R. W. (1990). A statistical trial of subclassification for tardive dyskinesia. *Acta Psychiatr. Scand.* 82:404–7.

Kane, J. M., & Smith, J. (1982). Tardive dyskinesia: prevalence and risk factors 1959–1979. *Arch. Gen. Psychiatry* 39:473–81.

Kane, J. M., Woerner, M., Borenstein, M., Wegner, J., & Lieberman, J. (1986). Integrating incidence and prevalence of tardive dyskinesia. *Psychopharmacol. Bull.* 22:254–8.

Kang, U. J., Burke, R. E., & Fahn, S. (1986). Natural history and treatment of tardive dystonia. *Mov. Disord.* 1:193–208.

Keegan, D. L., & Rajput, A. H. (1973). Drug induced dystonia tarda: treatment of L-dopa. *Dis. Nerv. Syst.* 38:167–9.

Kurata, K., Yuasa, S., Kazukawa, S., Kurachi, M., & Fukuda, T. (1989). Meige's syndrome during long-term neuroleptic treatment. *Jpn. J. Psychiatry Neurol.* 43:627–31.

Kwentus, J. A., Schulz, S. C., & Hart, R. P. (1984). Tardive dystonia, catatonia, and electroconvulsive therapy. *J. Nerv. Ment. Dis.* 172:171–3.

Lal, K. P., Saxena, S., & Mohan, D. (1988). Tardive dystonia alternating with mania. *Biol. Psychiatry* 23:312–16.

Lamberti, J. S., & Bellnier, T. (1993). Clozapine and tardive dystonia. *J. Nerv. Ment. Dis.* 181:137–8.

Lang, A. E. (1986). High dose anticholinergic therapy in adult dystonia. *Can. J. Neurol. Sci.* 13:42–6.

Lang, A. E., Clarke, J. T. R., Resch, L., Strasberg, P., Skomorowski, M. A., & O'Connor, P. (1985). Progressive, longstanding "pure" dystonia – a new phenotype of juvenile metachromatic leukodystrophy. *Neurology (Suppl. 1)* 35:194.

Lieberman, J. A., Alvir, J., Mukherjee, S., & Kane, J. M. (1989). Treatment of tardive dyskinesia with bromocriptine. *Arch. Gen. Psychiatry* 46:908–13.

Lieberman, J. A., Alvir, J., Mukherjee, S., & Kane, J. M. (1991). The effects of clozapine on tardive dyskinesia. *Br. J. Psychiatry* 158:503–10.

Lieberman, J., Lesser, M., Johns, C., Pollack, S., Saltz, B., & Kane, J. (1988). Pharmacologic studies of tardive dyskinesia. *J. Clin. Psychopharmacol.* 8:57S–63.

Luchins, D. J., & Goldman, M. (1985). High-dose bromocriptine in a case of tardive dystonia. *Biol. Psychiatry* 20:179–81.

Marsden, C. D. (1988). Investigation of dystonia. In *Advances in Neurology. Vol. 50: Dystonia*, part 2, ed. S. Fahn, C. D. Marsden, & D. B. Calne, pp. 35–44. New York: Raven Press.

Micheli, F., Pardal, F., Gatto, M., Asconapé, J., Giannaula, R., & Parera, I. C. (1993). Bruxism secondary to chronic antidopaminergic drug exposure. *Clin. Neuropharmacol.* 16:315–23.

Miller, L. G., & Jankovic, J. (1990). Neurologic approach to drug-induced movement disorders: a study of 125 patients. *South. Med. J.* 83:525–32.

Nishikawa, T., Tanaka, M., Tsuda, A., Koga, I., & Uchida, Y. (1984). Clonidine therapy for tardive dystonia and related syndromes. *Clin. Neuropharmacol.* 7:239–45.

Nutt, J. G., Muenter, M. D., Aronson, A., Kurland, L. T., & Melton, I. J. (1988). Epidemiology of focal and generalized dystonia. *Mov. Disord.* 3:188–9.

Owens, D. G. C., Johnstone, E. C., & Frith, C. D. (1982). Spontaneous involuntary disorders of movement. *Arch. Gen. Psychiatry* 39:452–61.

Ozelius, L., Kramer, P. L., Moskowitz, C. B., Kwiatkowski, D. J., Brin, M. F., Bressman, S. B., Schuback, D. E., Falk, C. T., Risch, N., de Leon, D., Burke, R. E., Haines, J., Gusella, J. F., Fahn, S., & Breakefield, X. O. (1989). Human gene for torsion dystonia located on chromosome 9q32-34. *Neuron* 2:1427–34.

Quinn, N. P., Lang, A. E., Sheehy, M. P., & Marsden, C. D. (1985). Lisuride in dystonia. *Neurology* 35:766–9.

Raja, M. (1995). Tardive dystonia: prevalence, risk factors, and comparison with tardive dyskinesia in a population of 200 acute psychiatric inpatients. *Eur. Arch. Psychiatry Clin. Neurosci.* 245:145–51.

Rosse, R. B., Allen, A., & Lux, W. E. (1986). Baclofen treatment in a patient with tardive dystonia. *J. Clin. Psychiatry* 47:474–5.

Sachdev, P. (1989). Blinking-blepharospasm after long-term neuroleptic treatment. *Med. J. Aust.* 150:341–3.

Sachdev, P. (1991). The prevalence of tardive dystonia in patients with chronic schizophrenia. *Aust. N.Z. J. Psychiatry* 25:446–8.

Sachdev, P. (1993). Clinical characteristics of 15 patients with tardive dystonia. *Am. J. Psychiatry* 150:498–500.

Sethi, K. D., Hess, D. C., & Harp, R. J. (1990). Prevalence of dystonia in veterans on chronic antipsychotic therapy. *Mov. Disord.* 5:319–21.

Singh, S. K., & Jankovic, J. (1988). Tardive dystonia in Tourette's syndrome. *Mov. Disord.* 31:274–80.

Stip, E., Faughnan, M., Desjardin, I., & Labrecque, R. (1992). *Br. J. Psychiatry* 161:867–8.

Sugawara, M., Iizuka, H., Kawana, A., & Suzuki, J. (1992). Tardive dystonia and ceruletide effects: case report. *Prog. Neuropsychopharmacol. Biol. Psychiatry* 16:127–34.

Trugman, J. M., Leadbetter, R., Zalis, M. E., Burgdorf, R. O., & Wooten, G. F. (1994). Treatment of severe axial tardive dystonia with clozapine: case report and hypothesis. *Mov. Disord.* 9:441–6.

Van Putten, T., Wirshing, W., & Marder, S. (1990). Tardive Meige syndrome responsive to clozapine. *J. Clin. Psychopharmacol.* 10:381–2.

Weiner, W. J., & Werner, T. R. (1982). Mania-induced remission of tardive dyskinesia in manic–depressive illness. *Ann. Neurol.* 12:229–30.

Wojcik, J. D., Falk, W. E., Fink, J. S., Cole, J. O., & Gelenberg, A. J. (1991). A review of 32 cases of tardive dystonia. *Am. J. Psychiatry* 148:1055–9.

Wolf, M. E., & Koller, W. C. (1985). Tardive dystonia: treatment with trihexyphenidyl. *J. Clin. Psychopharmacol.* 5:247–8.

Yadalam, K. G., Korn, M. L., & Simpson, G. M. (1990). Tardive dystonia: four case histories. *J. Clin. Psychiatry* 51:17–20.

Yassa, R., Nair, V., & Dimitry, R. (1986). Prevalence of tardive dystonia. *Acta Psychiatr. Scand.* 73:629–33.

Yassa, R., Nair, V., & Iskandar, H. (1989). A comparison of severe tardive dystonia and severe tardive dyskinesia. *Acta Psychiatr. Scand.* 80:155–9.

Yassa, R., Nair, N. P. V., Iskandar, H., & Schwartz, G. (1990). Factors in the development of severe forms of tardive dyskinesia. *Am. J. Psychiatry* 147:1156–63.

Yazici, O., Kantemir, E., Tastaban, Y., Ocok, A., & Ozguroglu, M. (1991). Spontaneous improvement of tardive dystonia during mania. *Br. J. Psychiatry* 158:847–50.

27

Tardive Akathisia

ROBERT E. BURKE, M.D.

Akathisia has been aptly described by Stahl (1986) as "a stepchild of move-ment disorders and an orphan of psychiatry." In the past, many neurologists dealing with movement disorders considered akathisia not as any particular pattern of movement but rather as a subjective state characterized by a feeling of restlessness (Crane & Naranjo, 1971; Chase, 1972). Thus it was not con-sidered to be a movement disorder. On the other hand, because akathisia was not listed in either the diagnostic index or the symptom index of the *Diagnos-tic and Statistical Manual of Mental Disorders,* third edition, revised (DSM-III-R) (American Psychiatric Association, 1987), its status as an abnormal subjective state was ill-defined within psychiatry. Akathisia's uncertain status probably has contributed considerably to its neglect as an important and disabling neurological and psychiatric condition. Until recently, the persistent form of akathisia due to neuroleptics, referred to as *tardive akathisia,* has been particularly neglected. The early reports of classic oral-buccal-lingual tardive dyskinesia included clear descriptions of chronic motor restlessness: "[the] patient cannot stand still" (Uhrbrand & Faurbye, 1960); "inability to sit still" and "pacing the floor" (Kruse, 1960); "patients could not remain seated" (Hunter, Earl, & Thornicroft, 1964). In addition, the phenomenon of acute akathisia due to neuroleptics was clearly recognized shortly after the introduc-tion of those drugs; and it was considered one of the most common adverse effects of neuroleptics (Ayd, 1961). Only in later years, however, was late-onset, *persistent* akathisia due to neuroleptics actually reported, explicitly described as a distinct entity, and recognized as related to the other forms of tardive dyskinesia (Fahn, 1983; Braude & Barnes, 1983; Weiner & Luby, 1983; Barnes & Braude, 1984; Shearer, Bownes, & Curran, 1984).

Although it is difficult to understand why tardive akathisia went unrecog-nized for so many years, the reasons may be reflected in the difficulties faced today when studying the problem. For example, it is difficult to recognize and diagnose the disorder because of its characterization by a particular subjective state: an aversion to remaining still. Indeed, patients find it hard to describe, and doctors may find it difficult to document the disorder reliably. In addition, the subjective features of the disorder can merge with and be obscured by the subjective features of psychiatric illness. Second, the motor features of akathisia, as described later, are complex and variable. Not only do they not fall into many neurologists' conceptual categories of movement disorders, but also they merge with normal patterns of motor behavior, making recognition difficult. Finally, the fact that persistent akathisia can occur soon after the beginning of neuroleptic treatment makes it difficult to recognize as a disorder distinct from acute akathisia.

Whatever the reasons for the delay in the neurologists' recognition of tardive akathisia, the descriptions of large numbers of patients by Barnes and Braude (1985) and numerous other investigators (Walters et al., 1986; Gardos et al., 1987; Kucharski, Wagner, & Friedman, 1987; Dufresne & Wagner, 1988; Burke et al., 1989; Yassa & Bloom, 1990; Sachdev & Chee, 1990; Levin et al., 1992) have today accorded the disorder a firm conceptual basis. A consensus is growing that it exists as a distinct type of persistent movement disorder caused by neuroleptics.

Definition of Akathisia

To arrive at a consensus on the definition and concept of akathisia, we must consider the term's origins and precedents. Haskovec (1902, 1903) originally used the term to describe 2 patients (*un cas d'hystérie* and *un cas de névrasthénie*) who could not sit still. He coined the term "akathisie" from the Greek, meaning "not to sit." In today's psychiatric and neurological context, the diagnoses for those patients would be unclear. From Haskovec's description, however, those patients would seem to have had an irresistible urge to stand after sitting for any period of time. Subsequent use of the term by Sicard (1923) and Bing (1923) to refer to a similar phenomenon in patients with idiopathic or postencephalitic parkinsonism tended to link the condition with movement disorders due to organic neurological diseases. After the introduction of neuroleptics in the 1950s, the term became widely used to refer to the subjective motor restlessness associated with the use of those drugs. In that setting, the term was again used to refer to a disturbance with an organic basis – that of pharmacologic blockade of brain dopamine receptors. Thus, the major precedents for using the term have linked it with organic neurological disease, and movement disorders in particular.

In defining akathisia today, some investigators have taken the view that the disorder is strictly one of an abnormal subjective state, as mentioned earlier (Crane & Naranjo, 1971; Van Putten, May, & Marder, 1984). That point of view also implies that there is no characteristic movement disorder associated with akathisia – that, instead, the movements of these patients are varied, volitional responses to their state of subjective restlessness. However, we believe that subjective restlessness is necessary, but not sufficient, as a definition of akathisia. First, the subjective reporting of this so-called restlessness is not entirely specific. Witness the findings of Braude, Barnes, & Gore (1983) in a study of the clinical characteristics of akathisia – that subjective reports of "inner restlessness" were common not only to the group of patients with akathisia but also to a group of psychiatric patients with agitated depression and psychotic excitement, among other disorders. Second, the movements of akathisia are not random and nondescript, but rather characteristic and recognizable. Briefly, for they will be described in detail later, these movements are complex, stereotyped repetitive movements, such as rubbing the face with the hand, or crossing and uncrossing the legs. Such movements are characteristic among akathisia patients evaluated by independent investigators (Gibb & Lees, 1986; Burke et al., 1989). Moreover, although the movements are suppressible, they are accompanied by an irresistible urge; in that respect, they are not unlike tics. Clearly, given the characteristic appearance of the movements, the apparent irresistible urge to perform them, and the disability they cause, it is not unreasonable to consider them as a form of movement disorder, despite their resemblance to normal, volitional acts.

One must, nevertheless, consider whether or not the presence of such movements alone – either in the absence of an available subjective report or in the presence of a denial of subjective restlessness – is sufficient to make a diagnosis of akathisia. Certain authors who refer to these characteristic movements without associated subjective restlessness as "pseudoakathisia" (Barnes & Braude, 1985) have suggested that this pseudoakathisia may be a late stage in the evolution of chronic akathisia. Although it is tempting to think of such patients as having some minimal form of akathisia, I am reluctant to diagnose akathisia, especially in a research setting, in the absence of a subjective report of an aversion to being still. Too much is still unknown about the specificity of akathitic movements for them to be used as sufficient evidence for the diagnosis. For example, individuals with chronic psychoses, static encephalopathies, and autism are known to make complex, repetitive stereotyped movements, such as head bobbing, trunk flexion and extension, and lateral to-and-fro rocking movements, that may resemble those of akathisia. For our purposes, in the series of patients we have studied, both subjective and motor features of restlessness must be present for the diagnosis of akathisia.

Tardive Akathisia: Criteria for Diagnosis

In our studies, we use four criteria for a diagnosis of tardive akathisia. First, the patient must have akathisia, both as defined earlier – by the presence of subjective and motor features of restlessness – and as described in detail later.

Second, the akathisia must occur during neuroleptic treatment or within 3 months of discontinuing neuroleptic treatment. Although the 3-month interval is somewhat arbitrary, it attempts to take into account the observation that tardive akathisia, like other tardive disorders, may not appear until some time after the neuroleptics are withdrawn. Although these drugs cause these dyskinesias, they are, paradoxically, able to suppress them. Many neurologists dealing with movement disorders would be willing to attribute a movement disorder to a neuroleptic provided that it appeared within 3 months of discontinuation of the drug. Beyond that point, however, the causal relationship becomes more tenuous. Without an objective marker to prove that a particular movement disorder could arise 3 months or more after cessation of exposure to neuroleptics, it seems wisest to accept the admittedly arbitrary convention of the 3-month limit.

Third, to distinguish tardive akathisia from acute akathisia, the tardive akathisia must be persistent. We have proposed the criterion that it must last at least 1 month after discontinuation of neuroleptics. Note that although we refer to this disorder as *tardive* akathisia, it, like classic oral-buccal-lingual tardive dyskinesia and tardive dystonia, is not required to make its first appearance late in the course of treatment in order to qualify for this diagnosis. Figure 27.1 shows the correlation between the time of onset of persistent akathisia and the duration of treatment with dopamine antagonists. It can be seen that many patients develop this disorder soon after neuroleptic treatment is begun (about one-third of patients in our series developed it within the first year of exposure). Similar observations have been reported for classic oral-buccal-lingual tardive dyskinesia (Kane et al., 1986) and tardive dystonia (Kang, Burke, & Fahn, 1986). The critical difference between acute akathisia and tardive akathisia is the persistence of the latter following discontinuation of neuroleptic treatment. Barnes and Braude (1985) recognized that persistent akathisia can develop either early or late during neuroleptic treatment; they referred to the former as "acute persistent" akathisia, and the latter as "tardive" akathisia. We have chosen to lump these two designations together under the single term "tardive akathisia." One reason is that a smooth contin-

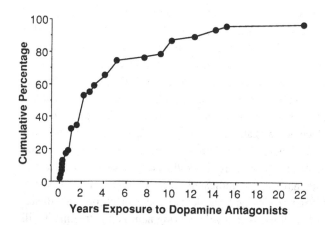

Figure 27.1. Relationship between the number of years of treatment with dopamine antagonists and the onset of tardive akathisia in our patients (*N* = 45). The number of years of exposure to dopamine antagonists is the time from a patient's first exposure to drugs to the occurrence of the tardive movement disorder, based on the patient's history. The occurrence of tardive akathisia is represented as a cumulative occurrence plot until the entire patient group (100%) is accounted for. Note the absence of a period of minimum safe exposure to dopamine antagonists, one free of the risk of inducing tardive akathisia; akathisia began to appear within the first few months of exposure. (From Burke et al., 1989, with permission.)

uum can be seen in the curve for cumulative occurrences (Figure 27.1). There is no apparent inflection point in the curve to indicate the presence of two separate disorders distinguished by time of onset. The second reason is that, in practical terms, both patients and physicians sometimes find it difficult to determine when akathisia began in relation to the initiation of neuroleptic treatment. An additional practical problem arises during diagnosis of tardive akathisia when a patient cannot, for psychiatric reasons, be taken off neuroleptic treatment in order to determine whether or not the akathisia would persist in its absence. In those circumstances, if it were possible to temporarily reduce the neuroleptic dosage, it might then be possible to determine whether or not akathisia would persist or even worsen – either of which would suggest a diagnosis of tardive akathisia.

Our fourth criterion for a diagnosis of tardive akathisia is that it must be determined that the patient has no other neurological illness that might cause akathisia, such as encephalitis or Parkinson's disease.

It is important to review briefly the evidence that persistent akathisia is due to neuroleptic treatment. For oral-buccal-lingual tardive dyskinesia, because a spontaneous (i.e., non-neuroleptic-induced) form of oral dyskinesia exists, it was necessary to obtain epidemiologic evidence indicating increased oral dyskinesia in association with the use of neuroleptics. Such evidence does exist (American Psychiatric Association, 1980). Although such evidence has not yet been sought for tardive akathisia, a causal relationship is difficult to deny, because spontaneous (non-neuroleptic-induced) akathisia is virtually nonexistent. Indeed, the vast majority of today's akathisia cases not attributable to obvious neurological disease, such as parkinsonism or encephalitis, are due to treatment with neuroleptic drugs. Second, no one today doubts that neuroleptics induce acute akathisia. Thus, the frequent observations that early-onset akathisia can persist as a chronic form support the belief that neuroleptics are capable of causing chronic akathisia. Moreover, observations of individual patients have often indicated a close temporal relationship between the use of neuroleptics and the development of chronic akathisia. Many chronic cases of akathisia that develop during neuroleptic treatment will gradually remit following discontinuation of the drugs. In addition, we have observed instances of patients in remission who, when reexposed to neuroleptics, have developed persistent akathisia a second time. Thus, these close temporal relationships suggest a causal role for neuroleptics in chronic akathisia. Finally, given the virtual certitude that classic oral-lingual tardive dyskinesia is due to neuroleptics, and given the frequent association of tardive akathisia with oral dyskinesia (90% of our cases), it is likely that tardive akathisia, too, is due to neuroleptics. Tardive akathisia is unique among the tardive disorders in that it rarely, if ever, occurs as a spontaneous idiopathic form, unlike oral dyskinesia and dystonia. Thus, patients with tardive akathisia are unlikely to manifest non-neuroleptic-induced movement disorders, whereas that phenomenon is a possibility in patient groups thought to have oral tardive dyskinesia or dystonia. On this basis, tardive akathisia is a particularly useful disorder for study.

Tardive Akathisia: Clinical Features

Patient Population

Because no prospective studies of tardive akathisia in representative psychiatric populations have been conducted, the available data regarding the frequency of the condition and patients' characteristics have been derived from point-prevalence and retrospective studies. In fact, though, tardive akathisia probably is not uncommon. In a study by Barnes and Braude (1985), for example, 28% of patients had chronic akathisia – that is, what we would consider tardive akathisia. That is similar to the findings of Schilkrut et al.

(1978), who reported the prevalence of late-onset akathisia to be 20% among their schizophrenic outpatients.

In our retrospective analysis of a group of 52 patients referred for neurological evaluation, the mean age at onset of tardive akathisia was 58.4 years (range 21–82 years). Whereas women outnumbered men by almost 2 to 1, men tended to have an earlier age of onset (54.1 years) than women (60.9 years). As previously reported for oral dyskinesia and tardive dystonia, various primary diagnoses are given to patients who develop tardive akathisia, including many nonpsychiatric conditions, as well as psychiatric conditions. In fact, in our series, 22% of patients had been treated with neuroleptics for nonpsychiatric indications, including nausea, esophagitis, pain, and dementia, and an additional 14% had been treated with these drugs for anxiety. Thus, more than one-third of our patients had been exposed to neuroleptics for secondary or even questionable indications. In addition, a large proportion of our patients (56%) had had primary diagnoses of affective disorder, either depression (47%) or manic–depressive illness (8%). This observation is of interest in light of data from prospective studies indicating that affective illness constitutes a risk factor for development of oral-lingual dyskinesia (Kane, Woerner, & Lieberman, 1988). Our observations, however, were made in neurological referral groups, and there may have been a selection bias. Further prospective studies in more representative patient groups are needed.

Like the other forms of tardive dyskinesia, tardive akathisia occurs after treatment with a variety of neuroleptics: all three classes of phenothiazines, butyrophenones, dibenzoxazepines, and metoclopramide (Burke et al., 1989). In our series of patients, tardive akathisia developed after a mean of 4.5 years of neuroleptic treatment. However, as stated earlier, about one-third developed persistent akathisia after only 1 year of treatment.

Subjective State

Patients with akathisia frequently find it difficult to describe their subjective discomfort; quite often they do not even spontaneously say they are "restless." They may complain of "jitteriness" or "a tortured sort of feeling," of feeling "fidgety," "nervous," "about to jump out of my skin," or "all revved up," and so on. Often it is helpful to ask patients what particular settings make them most uncomfortable, and how they relieve that discomfort. Patients with akathisia frequently will identify sitting as the most uncomfortable state, saying that they stand and pace to relieve the discomfort. It is also useful to ask open-ended questions about sitting: Does sitting make you uncomfortable? Are you able to sit through meals? If not, what do you do? It is valuable, as well, to ask open-ended questions about standing still: Are you able to tolerate standing in line? If not, what do you do? Usually, in their responses to these questions, patients with akathisia will communicate their aversion to being still, whether or not they spontaneously say they are "restless."

Coexisting psychiatric or neurological illness may have impaired the mental state of these patients, such that they find it difficult or impossible to define, clearly, their aversion to being still. To the extent that such patients can be interviewed, a critical aspect is to determine whether or not their agitation or anxiety is positional (i.e., is related to sitting or standing still) and whether or not they obtain some relief from movement. Interestingly, the majority of our patients with akathisia identified lying down as their most comfortable position. Again, this positional dependence relative to their subjective discomfort may be helpful in distinguishing akathisia from psychiatric causes of agitation.

A number of investigators have pointed out that severe akathisia can cause or be expressed as a number of abnormal behaviors or heightened emotional states: "acting out" (Siris, 1985), "disruptive" behavior (Kumar, 1979; Shen, 1981), aggressive behavior (Kechich, 1978), and fear (Van Putten, 1975). The subjective distress of akathisia, which can be agonizing, has been implicated in suicide attempts (Drake & Ehrlich, 1985). Clearly, clinicians must consider the possibility of underlying akathisia in the presence of any behavioral disturbance characterized by agitation. At the other end of the spectrum, patients with mild akathisia may simply be impatient, irritable, or unable to concentrate (Van Putten, 1975; Burke et al., 1989).

In summary, because its presentation can be diverse and subtle, clinicians must use detailed questioning to carefully delineate the subjective aversion to being still. In view of these observations, it remains an open question whether or not "pseudoakathisia" – that is, the movements of akathisia in the absence of subjective restlessness – actually exists. If pseudoakathisia does exist, its existence will require careful documentation, perhaps by way of an adequately detailed and structured interview that will take into account the variety and subtlety of the subjective features of akathisia.

Motor Features

In general, patients with akathisia perform frequent, repetitive movements. The movements are stereotyped in that they tend to be of the same pattern, repeated over and over. When asked, these patients often are able to suppress their movements, at least briefly. Commonly, though, they report an increasing urge to move as they sit still, accompanied by growing discomfort. Although in these respects the movements of akathisia are like those of tics, the phenomenology of tics differs from that of akathisia in several important respects. Tics typically occur in flurries or paroxysms of sudden, brief movements. In contrast, the movements of akathisia tend to be steadily ongoing and often rather slow. For example, a quite prolonged rubbing of the face or hair may occur. Second, patients with tics do not have the accompanying subjective state of restlessness; typically they are not averse to sitting in place or standing on line. Finally, whereas patients with tics may emit complex vocal sounds, such as barking, whistling, or coprolalia, patients with akathisia do not. Although they may moan or shout, patients with akathisia do not produce complex vocal utterances.

Our analysis of the movements made by patients with tardive akathisia showed that the legs were the most frequently affected body part (Table 27.1). For instance, as the patients sit, they may cross and uncross their legs, pump their legs up and down, or perform rapid abduction–adduction movements. When they stand, the most common leg movement involves marching in place.

Recognition of the characteristic arm movements of patients with akathisia can be helpful for diagnostic purposes. These patients often repeatedly use a hand to rub the lower face, mouth, or hair. Scratching the scalp is another typical movement. Some variations on these movements may occur; one

Table 27.1. *Frequencies of motor phenomena among patients with tardive akathisia*

Motor phenomenon	Patients affected (%)
Marching in place	58
Crossing/uncrossing legs	48
Trunk rocking	44
Respiratory grunting	29
Pumping legs up/down	25
Pacing	25
Shifting weight from foot to foot (standing)	25
Rising from chair	21
Moaning	19
Abducting/adducting legs	19
Face rubbing	10
Hair rubbing	8
Picking at clothes	8

Source: Adapted from Burke et al. (1989).

patient, for instance, repeatedly rubbed the brim of his hat. Other arm movements include repeated folding and unfolding of the arms, rubbing of the anterior surface of the thighs, and picking at clothes.

In our series of 52 patients, tardive akathisia was associated with either oral-lingual tardive dyskinesia or dystonia in all but 1 patient. Of these, 63% had oral dyskinesia, 8% had tardive dystonia, and 27% had both. The few patients with tardive akathisia and tardive dystonia had an earlier mean age of onset (39 years) than those with akathisia and oral dyskinesia (62.2 years).

Tardive Akathisia: Differential Diagnosis

For patients with movement disorders, the diagnostic process involves two steps: The first is to identify the clinical manifestations, that is, the type of movement disorder; the second is to determine the cause. For diagnosing akathisia, several types of movement disorders must be distinguished. As discussed earlier, tics can be similar to akathitic movements; they usually can be distinguished, however, on the basis of the previously mentioned features. Usually there is no difficulty in distinguishing between chorea and akathitic movements. The latter are complex movements, and the patterns are predictably repeated over and over; in other words, they are stereotyped. In contrast, choreic movements, random in their timing and location, consist of simple, primitive movements that are never so complex as, for instance, the stroking of the face that occurs with akathisia. In this regard, it is important to note that although the oral-buccal-lingual movements of classic tardive dyskinesia are frequently referred to as "choreic," they actually are not choreic in the strict meaning of the term. In fact, the predictable repetition of these patterns of movements, such as chewing, tongue popping, and lip smacking, makes them more similar to the stereotypies of akathisia than to true chorea. The movements of oral tardive dyskinesia are readily distinguished from those of akathisia, however, because of their restricted localization to the mouth and the absence of a subjective component of restlessness. In fact, most patients with oral dyskinesia are not troubled by the movements; subjectively, they are comfortable.

Many neurologists and psychiatrists confuse akathisia with Ekbom's "restless legs syndrome," the salient symptom of which is "peculiar creeping or crawling sensations most frequently localized to the lower leg" (Ekbom, 1960). However, akathisia is not typically associated with such sensory symptoms, and the disorder's subjective discomfort is not generally localized predominantly in the legs. In addition, the restless-leg syndrome usually is manifested most prominently when the patient lies down at night to sleep.

Akathisia, in contrast, is not typically nocturnal, and, as already stated, often the patient's most comfortable position is lying down.

In some circumstances it can be difficult to distinguish between akathisia and psychiatric conditions associated with agitation, especially when patients will not cooperate during an interview. When patients can be interviewed, the critical aspects of the subjective report to be noted in distinguishing between akathisia and psychiatric agitation are the aversion to being still and the relief provided by movement. If a patient cannot be interviewed, it may be possible to make a tentative diagnosis if the characteristic motor features of akathisia are observed, such as repeated rubbing of the face or hair with the hand. In the absence of a subjective report, however, only a tentative diagnosis can be made, even though in clinical practice that may be the only thing one has to guide therapeutic decisions. Finally, it should be remembered that many of the psychiatric conditions associated with agitation and the appearance of restlessness, such as anxiety or drug-withdrawal states, are acute and transient, whereas tardive akathisia is a persistent condition.

If the manifestations of akathisia can be identified and the disorder can be shown to be a chronic condition, two of our criteria for diagnosis will have been met. Then, if the condition is found to have developed during neuroleptic treatment, a diagnosis of tardive akathisia is certain. Indeed, today there are few other causes of chronic akathisia. Rarely, for instance, does encephalitis cause akathisia, although parkinsonism is not uncommonly associated with akathisia (Lang & Johnson, 1987). Nevertheless, given that both a postencephalitic state and parkinsonism usually can be identified on the basis of the patient's history and neurological examination, there should be no difficulty distinguishing between those conditions and tardive akathisia.

Tardive Akathisia: Clinical Course and Treatment

Our study of a series of tardive akathisia patients produced data concerning clinical course for 48 patients who continued to be monitored for a mean of 2.3 years. At follow-up, 32 (67%) of our patients continued to have akathisia, for a mean of 4.2 ± 0.6 years. Twenty-six of our patients had had their neuroleptics discontinued; in that group, akathisia persisted for a mean of 2.7 ± 0.4 years.

Sixteen patients (33%) did not have akathisia at follow-up. Three were in true remission; that is, their akathisia had remitted, and drugs for its treatment had been withdrawn, without recurrence of the disorder. One additional patient had gone into true remission, but was subsequently treated again with neuroleptics by other physicians and suffered a recurrence of akathisia. If we count that patient as having had a true remission, 8% of the patients in our series can be said to have experienced remission. The remaining 13 patients who did not have akathisia at follow-up were taking agents that suppressed it. Most of those patients ($n = 9$) were taking dopamine-depleting drugs such as tetrabenazine (TBZ) ($n = 4$) or reserpine ($n = 2$) or were taking dopamine-receptor antagonists ($n = 3$). One was taking alprazolam. A few ($n = 3$) were taking multiple drugs, and so a single effective agent, if any, could not be identified. The 16 patients without akathisia at follow-up had been younger than the other patients in the study when first exposed to neuroleptics; they had developed dyskinesia at an earlier age and had had their neuroleptics withdrawn at an earlier age as well.

The first step in managing a patient with tardive akathisia is to discontinue neuroleptics, if possible. Although that may not be feasible for many psychiatric patients, our experience with a group of patients referred for neurological reasons was that many of them, as mentioned earlier, were on neuroleptics for questionable reasons; their drugs could therefore be discontinued. A small percentage of patients (8% in our series) will eventually go into full remission. The next therapeutic step is to assess the degree of disability. If disability is minimal, it is reasonable to continue to monitor the patient without attempting pharmacologic treatment. In our experience, however, most patients with tardive akathisia have been significantly disabled and have required treatment.

Once the decision is made that treatment is necessary, we recommend treatment with dopamine-depleting drugs, such as reserpine. Unfortunately, TBZ, another effective dopamine depleter, is not available in the United States. As for the dopaminergic systems, the clinical pharmacologic picture for tardive akathisia is like that for classic oral dyskinesia: The patient is made better by dopamine antagonists or depleters, and is made worse by drugs that augment dopamine function, such as levodopa. In our experience, reserpine has often been an effective agent, and 13 of our 15 patients treated with it improved. More specifically, reserpine treatment produced either complete control ($n = 3$) or marked improvement ($n = 8$) in 73% of our patients. One patient in particular, who had experienced complete suppression of symptoms using reserpine, was able to be weaned from it and still remain in remission. Interestingly, none of our patients treated with TBZ could be weaned from that drug, although it did suppress symptoms in 58% of patients.

We tried a number of agents that had been reported to be beneficial for treating acute akathisia. Many β-adrenergic blockers, for example, have been reported to be effective for management of acute akathisia (Adler, Angrist, & Rotrosen, 1992). Two patients in our group were treated with propranolol at a mean maximum dose of 80 mg/day without benefit. Likewise, Levin et al. (1992) treated 3 patients with β-blockers and found no benefit. Nevertheless, Sachdev and Chee (1990), who reported extensively on the pharmacologic responses in a single patient with tardive akathisia, found that a single dose of propranolol produced benefits that lasted 4 hours. They did not, however, undertake long-term studies. Thus, although β-blockers clearly are effective in the management of acute akathisia, they remain unproven for tardive akathisia.

Opiates have also been reported to be effective in the management of acute akathisia (Walter et al., 1986). In our series of tardive akathisia patients, 12 were treated with various opiates. Two showed unsustained benefits. Subsequently, Walters and colleagues reported a similar experience with opiates in patients with tardive akathisia (Walters, Hening, & Chokroverty, 1990).

Anticholinergics have been used to treat acute neuroleptic-induced akathisia, but with mixed results (Adler et al., 1992). In our tardive akathisia patients, 10 were treated with anticholinergics; the majority did not improve.

Three of our patients treated with lorazepam benefited, and they all remained on the drug at follow-up. Two of those patients showed marked improvement. Yassa and Bloom (1990) reported a patient with akathisia who responded to a combination of lorazepam and procyclidine, an anticholinergic drug.

In practice, when we are able to discontinue a patient's neuroleptic medication, but the akathisia persists and is disabling, we first treat the patient with reserpine. We start with a single 0.25-mg dose each day, increasing it by 0.25 mg every 7 days, as tolerated, until suppression of akathisia is achieved. Among our patients, the mean maximum dosage is 5.0 mg/day. If orthostatic hypotension becomes a problem, we encourage the patient to increase salt intake; if the problem persists, we attempt to treat it with the mineralocorticoid fludrocortisone. If a patient develops severe depression while on reserpine, it should be discontinued. If the depression is mild, it may be possible to treat it with antidepressants while continuing reserpine. This combination of treatments will be worthwhile only if the reserpine is effectively suppressing the akathisia. TBZ may be less likely to induce depression; we have found it effective for certain patients who have not tolerated reserpine. Unfortunately, it is available only for investigational purposes and is not distributed within the United States.

If reserpine fails to produce benefit, I would recommend trying lorazepam. If lorazepam also fails, my next choice would be a trial of the atypical antipsychotic clozapine. A recent anecdotal report described excellent responses to clozapine in 3 patients with tardive akathisia who had otherwise been refractory to treatment (Levin et al., 1992). Those responses require further study and confirmation.

Acknowledgments

This work was supported in part by NINDS grant R29-NS26836 and by The Parkinson's Disease Foundation. I am grateful to Ms. Pat White for superb secretarial assistance.

References

Adler, L. A., Angrist, B., & Rotrosen, J. (1992). Acute neuroleptic-induced akathisia. In *Drug-induced Movement Disorders*, ed. A. E. Lang & W. J. Weiner, pp. 85–119. Mount Kisco, NY: Futura Publishing.

American Psychiatric Association (1980). *Tardive Dyskinesia: Report of the American Psychiatric Association Task Force on Late Neurological Effects of Antipsychotic Drugs.* Washington, DC: American Psychiatric Association.

American Psychiatric Association (1987). *Diagnostic and Statistical Manual of Mental Disorders,* 3rd ed., revised. Washington, DC: American Psychiatric Association.

Ayd, F. (1961). A survey of drug-induced extrapyramidal reactions. *J. Am. Med. Assoc.* 175:1054–60.

Barnes, T. R. E., & Braude, W. M. (1984). Persistent akathisia associated with early tardive dyskinesia. *Postgrad. Med. J.* 60:359–61.

Barnes, T. R. E., & Braude, W. M. (1985). Akathisia variants and tardive dyskinesia. *Arch. Gen. Psychiatry* 42:874–8.

Bing, R. (1923). Ueber einige Bemerkenswerte begleiterscheinunger der extrapyramidalen Rigiditat (Akathisie-Mikographic-Kinesia Paradoxa). *Schweiz. Med. Wochenschr.* 4:167–71.

Braude, W. M., & Barnes, T. R. E. (1983). Late-onset akathisia – an indicant of covert dyskinesia: two case reports. *Am. J. Psychiatry* 140:611–12.

Braude, W. M., Barnes, T. R. E., & Gore, S. (1983). Clinical characteristics of akathisia. A systematic investigation of acute psychiatric inpatient admissions. *Br. J. Psychiatry* 143:139–50.

Burke, R. E., Kang, U. K., Jankovic, J., Miller, L. G., & Fahn, S. (1989). Tardive akathisia: an analysis of clinical features and response to open therapeutic trials. *Mov. Disord.* 4:157–75.

Chase, T. N. (1972). Drug-induced extrapyramidal disorders. *Res. Publ. Assoc. Res. Nerv. Ment. Dis.* 50:448–71.

Crane, G. E., & Naranjo, E. R. (1971). Motor disorders induced by neuroleptics. *Arch. Gen. Psychiatry* 24:179–84.

Drake, R. E., & Ehrlich, J. (1985). Suicide attempts associated with akathisia. *Am. J. Psychiatry* 142:499–501.

Dufresne, R. L., & Wagner, R. L. (1988). Antipsychotic-withdrawal akathisia versus antipsychotic-induced akathisia: further evidence for the existence of tardive akathisia. *J. Clin. Psychiatry* 49:435–8.

Ekbom, K. A. (1960). Restless legs syndrome. *Neurology* 10:868–73.

Fahn, S. (1983). Long-term treatment of tardive dyskinesia with pre-synaptically acting dopamine-depleting agents. *Adv. Neurol.* 35:267–76.

Gardos, G., Cole, J. O., Salomon, M., & Schniebolk, S. (1987). Clinical forms of severe tardive dyskinesia. *Am. J. Psychiatry* 144:895–902.

Gibb, W. R. G., & Lees, A. J. (1986). The clinical phenomenon of akathisia. *J. Neurol. Neurosurg. Psychiatry* 49:861–6.

Haskovec, L. (1902). Akathisie. *Arch. Bohemes Med. Clin.* 3:193–200.

Haskovec, L. (1903). Nouvelles remarques sur l'akathisia. Nouvelle iconographie de la Salpetrière. *Clin. Maladies Système Nerv.* 16:287–96.

Hunter, R., Earl, C. J., & Thornicroft, S. (1964). An apparently irreversible syndrome of abnormal movements following phenothiazine medication. *Proc. R. Soc. Med.* 57:758–62.

Kane, J. M., Woerner, M., Borenstein, M., Wegner, J., & Lieberman, J. (1986). Integrating incidence and prevalence of tardive dyskinesia. *Psychopharmacol. Bull.* 22:254–8.

Kane, J., Woerner, M., & Lieberman, J. (1988). Tardive dyskinesia: prevalence, incidence, and risk factors. *J. Clin. Psychopharmacol.* 8:52s–6s.

Kang, U. J., Burke, R. E., & Fahn, S. (1986). Natural history and treatment of tardive dystonia. *Mov. Disord.* 1:193–208.

Kechich, W. A. (1978). Neuroleptics: violence as a manifestation of akathisia. *J. Am. Med. Assoc.* 240:2185.

Kruse, W. (1960). Persistent muscular restlessness after phenothiazine treatment: report of three cases. *Am. J. Psychiatry* 117:152–3.

Kucharski, L. T., Wagner, R. L., & Friedman, J. H. (1987). An investigation of the abnormal involuntary movements, parkinsonism, and akathisia in chronic psychiatric patients. *Psychopharmacol. Bull.* 23:215–17.

Kumar, B. (1979). An unusual case of akathisia. *Am. J. Psychiatry* 136:8.

Lang, A. E., & Johnson, K. (1987). Akathisia in idiopathic Parkinson's disease. *Neurology* 37:477–80.

Levin, H., Chengappa, R., Kambhampati, R. K., Mahdavi, N., & Ganguli, R. (1992). Should chronic treatment-refractory akathisia be an indication for the use of clozapine in schizophrenic patients? *J. Clin. Psychiatry* 53:248–51.

Sachdev, P., & Chee, K. (1990). Pharmacological characterization of tardive akathisia. *Biol. Psychiatry* 28:809–18.

Schilkrut, V. R., Duran, E., Haverbeck, C., Katz, I., & Vidal, P. (1978). Verlauf von psychopathologischen und extrapyramidalmotorischen Symptomen unter einer langzeit-neuroleptika Behandlung schizophrener Patienten. *Drug Res.* 28:1494–5.

Shearer, R. M., Bownes, I. T., & Curran, P. (1984). Tardive akathisia and agitated depression during metoclopramide therapy. *Acta Psychiatr. Scand.* 70:428–31.

Shen, W. W. (1981). Akathisia: an overlooked, distressing, but treatable condition. *J. Nerv. Ment. Dis.* 161:599–600.

Sicard, J. A. (1923). Akathisia and tasikinesia. *Presse Med.* 31:265–6.

Siris, S. (1985). Three cases of akathisia and "acting out." *Clin. Psychiatry* 46:395–7.

Stahl, S. M. (1986). Akathisia variants and tardive dyskinesia (letter). *Arch. Gen. Psychiatry* 43:1015.

Uhrbrand, L., & Faurbye, A. (1960). Reversible and irreversible dyskinesia after treatment with perphenazine, chlorpromazine, reserpine and electroconvulsive therapy. *Psychopharmacologia* 1:408–18.

Van Putten, T. (1975). The many faces of akathisia. *Comp. Psychiatry* 16:43–7.

Van Putten, T., May, P. R. A., & Marder, S. R. (1984). Akathisia with haloperidol and thiothixene. *Arch. Gen. Psychiatry* 41:1036–9.

Walters, A., Hening, W., Chokroverty, S., & Fahn, S. (1986). Opioid responsive-
     ness in patients with neuroleptic-induced akathisia. *Mov. Disord.* 1:119–28.
Walters, A., Hening, W., & Chokroverty, S. (1990). Tardive akathisia (Letter).
     Mov. Disord. 5:89–90.
Weiner, W. J., & Luby, E. D. (1983). Persistent akathisia following neuroleptic
     withdrawal. *Ann. Neurol.* 13:466–7.
Yassa, R., & Bloom, D. (1990). Lorazepam and anticholinergics in tardive
     akathisia. *Biol. Psychiatry* 27:457–67.

Part VII

Treatment of Tardive Dyskinesia

28

Development of Novel Antipsychotic Drugs with Reduced Extrapyramidal Side Effects

ALLAN Z. SAFFERMAN, M.D., JEFFREY A. LIEBERMAN, M.D., BRUCE J. KINON, M.D., DANIEL UMBRICHT, M.D., JEFFREY S. ARONOWITZ, M.D., and JOHN M. KANE, M.D.

The introduction of antipsychotic drugs such as chlorpromazine (CPZ) in the 1950s was a major advance in the treatment of schizophrenia and other psychotic disorders. Although CPZ and other typical antipsychotic drugs remain important, the limitations imposed by their adverse reactions and partial efficacy in a significant proportion of schizophrenic patients are widely recognized. The most prevalent and most troublesome adverse drug reactions associated with the typical antipsychotics are their acute and chronic extrapyramidal motor side effects (EPSEs). In contrast, the "atypical" antipsychotic drugs that have recently been marketed (e.g., clozapine, risperidone, and remoxipride) or that are in various stages of development are expected to entail significantly lower incidences of EPSEs and possibly offer greater therapeutic efficacy. This chapter focuses on how these new developments in antipsychotics will affect the incidence and severity of acute and chronic EPSEs.

Acute and Chronic EPSEs

The common acute EPSEs associated with typical antipsychotic treatment include drug-induced parkinsonism (characterized by tremor, rigidity, and bradykinesia), acute dystonic reactions, and akathisia (subjective and objective motor restlessness). Those side effects can lead to a wide range of deleterious clinical consequences: disruption of the doctor–patient therapeutic alliance; noncompliance with the prescribed treatment/medication (Van Putten, 1974; Kane, 1990); physical and emotional distress, resulting in a reduction in the overall quality of life and in poorer social and vocational functioning; behavioral toxicity (Van Putten & Marder, 1987), including "secondary" negative symptoms (Rifkin, Quitkin, & Klein, 1975; Van Putten & May,

1978) and cognitive impairment; cosmetic disfigurement, which can contribute to social isolation and stigmatization. In some cases, acute EPSEs go unrecognized (Weiden et al., 1987) and can lead to clinical deterioration and, in extreme cases, suicidal ideation or behavior. Estimates of the prevalences of acute EPSEs among patients taking typical antipsychotic drugs have varied from 2% to more than 90% (Ayd, 1961, 1983; Casey & Keepers, 1988; Kane, 1990); akathisia has been estimated to occur in as many as 75% of patients receiving typical antipsychotics (Adler et al., 1989). Studies generally have indicated that acute EPSEs, in one form or another, occur in the majority of patients treated with the typical antipsychotic drugs. A recent study of schizophrenic patients treated with typical antipsychotics during their first episode of psychosis reported that 62% of those patients suffered acute EPSEs within the initial 8 weeks of treatment (Chakos et al., 1992). Overall, acute EPSEs all too frequently present difficult clinical problems that complicate patient management.

Efforts to minimize acute EPSEs have included the use of prophylactic antiparkinsonian agents, treatment with low-potency antipsychotics rather than high-potency antipsychotics, and the use of low (Van Putten, Marder, & Mintz, 1990; Rifkin et al., 1991) or "threshold" (McEvoy, Hogarty, & Steingard, 1991) dosing strategies with antipsychotics. Akathisia may further respond to the addition of a benzodiazepine (Bartels et al., 1987) or a centrally acting β-adrenergic-receptor antagonist (Lipinski et al., 1984; Adler et al., 1989). Unfortunately, there are some patients in whom these strategies, alone or in combination, will not be able to eliminate acute EPSEs. For further reviews, see Fleischhacker, Roth, and Kane (1990), Casey (1991), Lavin and Rifkin (1992), and Barnes (1992).

Tardive dyskinesia is an abnormal involuntary movement disorder that results from ongoing treatment with typical antipsychotic drugs. Tardive dyskinesia, tardive dystonia, and other tardive variants are of great clinical concern because there is no consistently effective treatment for these movement disorders, which thus far have been irreversible in a significant number of patients. The prevalence of tardive dyskinesia is approximately 20% among patients at risk (Woerner et al., 1991). The incidence rate for tardive dyskinesia has been estimated to be 3–5% per year of exposure to antipsychotic drugs (Gerlach & Casey, 1988; Kane & Lieberman, 1993) and has not appeared to have diminished over at least the first few years of neuroleptic exposure (Kane & Lieberman, 1993). The risk for developing tardive dyskinesia is much greater among the elderly, with rates as high as 31% after 43 weeks of neuroleptic exposure (Saltz et al., 1991). Although tardive dysinesia is most often manifested as mild orobuccolingual movements and tends not to progress in severity (Richardson & Casey, 1988), some cases can worsen over time and involve one or more body areas in a severe and disabling manner. These severe cases often are of the tardive dystonic type, characterized by obvious disfiguring and painful muscle contractions. For further reviews, see Burke (1992) and Kane and Lieberman (1993).

The development of new antipsychotic drugs that would entail a reduced risk of producing acute or chronic EPSEs would represent a major improvement in the treatment of schizophrenia, even if they were to offer no significant increase in antipsychotic efficacy.

Mechanisms of Action of Antipsychotic Drugs and Induction of EPSEs

The typical antipsychotic drugs act as antagonists at dopamine D_2 receptors in the central nervous system (CNS) (Seeman et al., 1976). This property has been considered to play an essential role in mediating the therapeutic efficacy of these drugs and in determining the profiles of their adverse side effects (EPSEs, neuroendocrine abnormalities). Historically, it was believed that the antipsychotic benefit could not be separated from the liability of the EPSEs that accompanied treatment with the typical antipsychotic drugs (Delay, Deniker, & Hart, 1952). Over the past four decades, pharmaceutical companies have specifically sought to develop putative antipsychotic drugs based on a compound's ability to act as a dopamine D_2 antagonist and to produce catalepsy in rodents, an analogue of acute EPSEs in humans. That strategy is now considered to have been flawed (Baldessarini, 1985), for it tended to reinforce the development and use of drugs that caused significant EPSEs, but without improvements in therapeutic efficacy. More recently, the trend has been to seek putative antipsychotics whose dosages that will produce acute EPSEs will diverge greatly from the dosages that will have antipsychotic efficacy, such as members of the substituted-benzamide series of compounds (Ogren et al., 1990), or to seek putative antipsychotics whose therapeutic dosages will produce negligible acute extrapyramidal motor disturbances in rodents or humans, such as the prototype for the atypical antipsychotics: clozapine (Baldessarini & Frankenburg, 1991).

The development of clozapine (CLZ) has demonstrated that superior antipsychotic efficacy is an obtainable goal in new-drug development and that this property can be used to discriminate further between the newer atypical antipsychotics and the older typical antipsychotics. Despite its potentially lethal side effect of agranulocytosis, CLZ was eventually marketed because of its superior efficacy in patients with treatment-refractory schizophrenia, as well as its relatively low capacity to cause acute EPSEs at therapeutic dosages

(Kane et al., 1988; Pickar et al., 1992) during long-term treatment (Kane et al., 1993). These unique favorable properties of CLZ have sparked great interest in the development of atypical compounds that will not entail significant potential to cause blood dyscrasias and other undesirable side effects, such as grand mal seizures. Indeed, putative antipsychotic compounds are now screened to ensure that the dosages that are predicted to be therapeutic in humans will not cause catalepsy in rodents. Rather than being used only for treatment-refractory schizophrenia, it is hoped that such compounds will eventually become drugs of first choice for treatment of psychoses in general – which will be a significant therapeutic advance in clinical psychopharmacology.

The production of weak or negligible catalepsy in laboratory rats is currently the most sensitive laboratory measurement available to distinguish atypical antipsychotics from typical antipsychotics. CLZ is generally considered to cause no cataleptic effects (Burki et al., 1975). Although CLZ at rather high dosages can inhibit apomorphine- or amphetamine-induced stereotypies (Stille, Lauener, & Eichenberger, 1971; Ljungberg & Ungerstedt, 1978), at low dosages it can effectively inhibit the locomotor component of systemic dopamine agonists (Ljungberg & Ungerstedt, 1978; Mueller, 1993) or the locomotor hyperactivity induced by intra-accumbens application of dopamine (Costall & Naylor, 1976). Unlike the typical antipsychotics haloperidol (HAL) and CPZ, which are equipotent for antagonizing locomotor activity and stereotypies, CLZ may have a preferential limbic site of action.

In contrast to treatment with typical antipsychotics, acute treatment with CLZ in vitro can produce a relatively greater increase in dopamine turnover or metabolism in limbic structures than in the striatum (Anden & Stock, 1973; Bowers & Rozitis, 1974; Ackenheil, Blatt, & Lampart, 1974; Zivkovic et al., 1975; Bartholini, 1976; Crow et al., 1976; Waldmeier & Maitre, 1976; Westerink et al., 1977). In vivo studies, which may give a more accurate portrayal of functionally relevant dopamine release than of metabolism, have demonstrated that CLZ may have a preferential limbic site of action (Huff & Adams, 1980; Blaha & Lane, 1987; Lane & Blaha, 1987; Chen, Paredes, & Gardner, 1991). Those findings have led to speculation that regionally specific dopamine antagonism by antipsychotic drugs may differentially influence the antipsychotic effects and EPSEs of these drugs.

Acute administration of antipsychotic drugs has a profound effect on the activity of dopaminergic cells in both the A9 and A10 midbrain regions. Typical as well as atypical antipsychotics can activate nonfiring dopaminergic cells and can switch cells from firing in a spontaneous, irregular, single-spike mode to firing in a bursting mode, within which significantly more dopamine can be released (Bunney, 1992). Ongoing administration of typical anti-psychotics leads to inactivation of both A9 and A10 dopaminergic cells because of development of a persistent depolarized state termed "depolarization block" or "inactivation." In contrast, CLZ induces depolarization block only in A10 cells, implying that whereas A10 inactivation is associated with an antipsychotic effect, A9 inactivation may be associated with the development of EPSEs (White & Wang, 1983; Chiodo & Bunney, 1983, 1985; Skarsfeldt, 1988).

Studies of receptor binding measuring the in vivo displacement of [^{3}H]spiroperidol binding have demonstrated that the atypical antipsychotic drugs CLZ, thioridazine, sulpiride, and remoxipride have greater affinities for the D_2 receptor in certain limbic areas (usually, olfactory tubercle and septum) than in the striatum (Kohler et al., 1979, 1981; Ogren et al., 1984; Magnusson et al., 1986). Molecular cloning techniques have led to identification of two additional subtypes of the D_2 receptor, the D_3 and D_4 receptors, both of which appear to have a predominantly extrastriatal distribution that includes limbic structures. The atypical antipsychotic drugs CLZ and thioridazine and the substituted benzamides sulpiride, amisulpiride, and raclopride have greater relative affinities for the D_3 receptor than do the typical antipsychotics, although all antipsychotics have greater D_2 affinities than D_3 affinities (Sokoloff et al., 1990). CLZ and its congener, octoclothepin, have demonstrated approximately 10-fold greater affinities for the D_4 receptor than for the D_2 receptor; no other antipsychotic appears to approach that degree of selectivity (Van Tol et al., 1991). Biphasic displacement of binding to the substituted benzamide [^{3}H]YM-09151-2 by CLZ, thioridazine, and risperidone, but by no other antipsychotic, suggests that these three compounds may be able to discriminate an affinity state of the D_2 receptor not accessible to other D_2 antagonists and not characterized as D_3 or D_4 in nature (Assie, Sleight, & Koek, 1993).

In addition to its effects on a subset of D_2 receptors, CLZ has significant affinity for multiple neurotransmitter receptors, perhaps thereby contributing to its atypical functional profile. CLZ has a relatively low affinity for the D_2 receptor, as compared with the typical antipsychotic drugs. Moreover, its D_1 affinity does not necessarily distinguish it from other antipsychotics, except the butyrophenones and substituted benzamides, which have significantly lower D_1 affinities. CLZ is distinguished by having relatively high affinities for serotonin-2 (5-HT$_2$), α_1-adrenergic, α_2-adrenergic, and muscarinic acetylcholine (mACh) receptors, at least as compared with the high-potency phenothiazines and the butyrophenones (Snyder, Greenberg, & Yamamura, 1974; Richelson, 1984; Hyttel et al., 1985; Baldessarini & Frankenburg,

1991). Rates of binding to the 5-HT$_{1C}$ receptor do not appear to discriminate atypical from typical antipsychotics (Roth, Ciaranello, & Meltzer, 1992).

Studies in humans using positron-emission tomography (PET) have revealed that D$_2$-receptor occupancy in the brain is lowest with CLZ, as compared with other antipsychotics (Farde & Nordstrom, 1992); unlike most typical antipsychotics, CLZ produces D$_1$-receptor occupancy in the basal ganglia of significant magnitude (Farde et al., 1989, 1992; Farde & Nordstrom, 1992).

Discriminant-function analysis has been used to determine the relative contributions of D$_2$- and 5-HT$_2$-receptor affinities to the combined receptor affinities characteristic of atypical antipsychotics versus typical antipsychotics. Such analysis has indicated that a relatively low ratio of D$_2$ affinity to 5-HT$_2$ affinity, as determined through either in vitro (Meltzer, Matsubara, & Lee, 1989) or in vivo (Stockmeier et al., 1993) ligand binding, is most characteristic and predictive of an atypical profile.

Although the relative ratios of D$_2$: 5-HT$_2$-receptor binding affinities have long been considered important in the atypical mechanism of action, the actual extent of multiple neurotransmitter-receptor occupancy achieved during antipsychotic treatment may instead be crucial to determining the antipsychotic's functional profile. Through ex vivo quantitative autoradiography, investigators have demonstrated that CLZ doses (3.1 mg/kg) that will produce a low degree of D$_2$-receptor occupancy (25%) in rat or guinea pig striatal and limbic regions will also produce high degrees of 5-HT$_2$-receptor (65%), α$_1$-receptor (80%), and histamine-1-receptor (100%) occupancies and very low degrees of α$_2$-, ACh-, and 5-HT$_{1A}$-receptor occupancies. In contrast, HAL doses that will produce 25% D$_2$-receptor occupancy will not produce any other receptor occupancy, and risperidone at doses that will produce no more than 25% D$_2$-receptor occupancy will produce 60% 5-HT$_2$-receptor occupancy and less than 25% occupancy of other neurotransmitter receptors (Schotte et al., 1993). Those findings demonstrate that a low absolute value of D$_2$-receptor occupancy, together with a concomitant high degree of 5-HT$_2$-receptor (and possibly of α$_1$ and histamine-1, in the case of CLZ) occupancy, may contribute to an atypical antipsychotic profile.

Dopamine and 5-HT significantly influence each other's functioning. The interaction of 5-HT and dopamine can greatly affect the expression of catalepsy. The increased availability of 5-HT produced either by inhibitors of 5-HT reuptake (Waldmeier & Delini-Stula, 1979) or by the agonist quipazine (Balsara, Jadhav, & Chandorkar, 1979) can potentiate HAL-induced catalepsy. In contrast, lesions of the dorsal and medial raphe nuclei (Kostowski, Gumulka, & Czlonkowski, 1972; Costall et al., 1975), as well as 5-HT depletion caused by *p*-chlorophenylalanine (Gumulka, Kostowski, & Czlonkowski, 1973), can inhibit CPZ- and HAL-induced catalepsy. Neuroleptic-induced catalepsy in rodents (Riblet et al., 1982; McMillen, Scott, & Davanzo, 1988; Wadenberg, 1992), as well as dystonia in primates (Casey, 1992a), can be reversed by 5-HT$_{1A}$ agonists, possibly by an action at the 5-HT autoreceptor (Invernizzi, Cervo, & Samanin, 1988). The 5-HT$_2$ antagonists methysergide, cyproheptadine, and mesulergine (Maj et al., 1976; Balsara et al., 1979; Hicks, 1990) are able to reverse HAL-induced catalepsy, although those compounds are known to have activities at other serotonergic and nonserotonergic sites. The more selective 5-HT$_2$ antagonists ketanserin (Arnt, Hyttel, & Bach-Lauritsen, 1986) and ritanserin (Wadenberg, 1992) are unable to reverse the catalepsy induced by substituted benzamides (selective D$_2$ antagonists).

Clinically, 5-HT compounds have been shown in limited studies to reduce the motor symptoms of parkinsonism. In idiopathic Parkinson's disease, both the 5-HT agonist pizotifen (Friedman, 1978) and the 5-HT$_2$ antagonist ritanserin (Hildebrand & Delecluse, 1987; Auff et al., 1987) were able to reduce tremors. Ritanserin also reduced some symptoms of typical neuroleptic-induced parkinsonism (Bersani et al., 1986, 1990). Interestingly, L-dopa-induced dyskinesia was also reduced by ritanserin (Maertens de Noordhout & Delwaide, 1986; Meco et al., 1988). But neither neuroleptic-induced parkinsonism nor tardive dyskinesia was relieved by increasing the 5-HT activity through administration of citalopram, an inhibitor of 5-HT reuptake (Korsgaard et al., 1986).

A pathophysiological role for 5-HT in patients with schizophrenia has been inferred on the basis of several observations: the psychotomimetic effects of indole hallucinogens in normal individuals (Fischman, 1983); the exacerbation of schizophrenic symptoms caused by *m*-chlorophenylpiperazine challenge (Krystal et al., 1993); the significant 5-HT affinity seen with most effective antipsychotic drugs, and the reduction in 5-HT$_2$-receptor density in the frontal cortex in schizophrenics (Mita et al., 1986); the association of reduced central 5-HT metabolism, frontal cortical atrophy, and poor neuroleptic response in some schizophrenic patients (Breier et al., 1992). Use of the 5-HT$_2$ antagonist ritanserin alone has rather limited antipsychotic efficacy (Gelders, 1989), but when it has been used in a neuroleptic augmentation strategy, greater clinical efficacy has been demonstrated (Gelders et al., 1986; Awouters et al., 1988; Duinkerke et al., 1993). Neuroleptic augmentation with inhibitors of 5-HT reuptake has been found to reduce negative symptoms (Silver & Nassar, 1992).

Although the dopamine hypothesis of schizophrenia has enjoyed widespread acceptance, a noradrenergic contribution to this disease should also be considered (Antelman & Caggiula, 1977; Hornykiewicz, 1982; van Kammen et al., 1992). Antipsychotic treatment strategies using only an α_1 antagonist (Hommer et al., 1984), an α_2 agonist (Freedman et al., 1982), or a β antagonist (Lader, 1988) have shown only limited efficacy. Fluphenazine augmentation with the α_2 antagonist idazoxan has been reported (Litman et al., 1993). Although not as clinically effective as the use of CLZ, that strategy has produced an increase in the plasma concentration of norepinephrine (NE) intermediate between the concentrations found in patients receiving fluphenazine alone and those receiving CLZ alone. A clinical trial of neuroleptic augmentation with an α_1 antagonist has not been performed.

Acute CLZ treatment has been found to significantly increase NE turnover in rat brain (Bartholini, Keller, & Pletscher, 1973; Keller, Bartholini, & Pletscher, 1973). After long-term treatment of humans, CLZ, unlike the typical antipsychotics, produces marked increases in NE in cerebrospinal fluid (CSF) (Lieberman et al., 1991a) and in plasma (Pickar et al., 1992; Breier et al., 1993; Davidson et al., 1993); the increase in the plasma concentration of NE correlates with a decrease in schizophrenic symptoms (Breier et al., 1993).

The importance of the α_1-antagonist component in the profile of an atypical antipsychotic has been demonstrated by adding prazosin to ongoing HAL treatment for rats. In vivo determination of dopamine release has revealed that whereas that combined administration decreases basal dopamine release only in the nucleus accumbens, ongoing HAL treatment alone decreases basal dopamine release in the striatum as well as in the nucleus accumbens (Lane, Blaha, & Rivet, 1988).

The contribution of prominent α_1-antagonist activity to the profile of an atypical antipsychotic again becomes apparent with a long-term treatment paradigm. Augmentation of ongoing HAL treatment by addition of the α_1 antagonist prazosin, but not the α_2 antagonist idazoxan, was found to produce the selective pattern of an A10 depolarization block, with A9 sparing, that is characteristic of an atypical antipsychotic drug (Chiodo & Bunney, 1985).

Although the mACh-antagonist properties of CLZ contribute to its weak cataleptic effects, the anticholinergic component does not appear to be responsible for an atypical antipsychotic profile. In particular, the addition of atropine or trihexyphenidyl to HAL treatment did not produce a selective mesolimbic pattern of dopamine turnover (Westerink & Korf, 1975; Bartholini, Keller, & Pletscher, 1975). Neither did the addition of trihexyphenidyl or atropine to long-term treatment with the typical antipsychotic fluphenazine decanoate seem to prevent the up-regulation of striatal D_2 receptors seen after treatment with the typical antipsychotic alone (Boyson et al., 1988). Conversely, long-term treatment with CLZ does not produce any D_2-receptor increase.

Interestingly, augmentation of long-term HAL treatment with trihexyphenidyl has been reported to selectively drive only A10 cells into depolarization block (Chiodo & Bunney, 1985). Yet that same augmentation of treatment has not reproduced the pattern of selective mesolimbic-threshold reduction in an electrical-brain-stimulation–reward paradigm that characteristically develops after long-term CLZ treatment (Gardner, Walker, & Paredes, 1993). Despite those discrepant preclinical findings, clinical administration of CPZ plus benztropine during the course of a clinical trial has failed to mimic the superior antipsychotic efficacy of CLZ for treatment of antipsychotic-refractory schizophrenic patients (Kane et al., 1988), thus undermining the notion of an important contributory role for antimuscarinic activity in the atypical antipsychotic profile.

Decreased EPSEs with Atypical or Novel Antipsychotic Drugs

Mixed Atypical Compounds

Clozapine. It is generally established that the incidences of tremor, rigidity, and bradykinesia are considerably lower with CLZ treatment than with typical antipsychotics (Matz et al., 1974; Povlsen et al., 1985; Claghorn et al., 1987; Lindstrom, 1988; Kane et al., 1988; Casey, 1989; Lieberman & Safferman, 1992). Indeed, the observed rate for akathisia or rigidity has been approximately 3%. The benign EPSE profile of CLZ is further supported by the drug's failure to produce acute EPSEs in patients with a history of severe EPSEs while on typical antipsychotics (Small et al., 1987), as well as its failure to aggravate idiopathic Parkinson's disease when used to treat L-dopa-induced psychosis (Greene, Coté, & Fahn, 1993; Safferman et al., 1994).

Apparently CLZ does not produce acute dystonic reactions either, although in one report (Kastrup, Gastpar, & Schwartz, 1994) a 50-year-old developed that reaction after 6 weeks of CLZ treatment. A causal relationship between drug and symptoms is less than clear, however, for such reactions usually are observed in younger patients earlier in the course of antipsychotic treatment.

Some investigators have suggested that the incidence of CLZ-induced akathisia is similar to that seen with typical antipsychotics (Claghorn et al., 1987; Cohen et al., 1991). But Safferman et al. (1993) have disputed that and have provided further evidence suggesting that preexisting akathisia from prior exposure to typical antipsychotics may actually decrease after initiation of CLZ treatment and subsequent dosage escalation.

To date, there have been no documented cases of tardive dyskinesia directly attributable to CLZ. Kane et al. (1993) reported that 2 patients developed tardive dyskinesia after long-term treatment with CLZ. In addition, de Leon Moral & Camunas (1991) reported a case of jaw dyskinesia associated with CLZ treatment. However, it is impossible to be sure that CLZ produced tardive dyskinesia in those patients, because all 3 patients had histories of prior treatment with typical antipsychotic drugs. Only by prospectively treating antipsychotic-drug-naive patients with CLZ can a reliable risk for tardive dyskinesia due to CLZ be established. The clinical experience thus far indicates that the incidence of tardive dyskinesia probably would be significantly lower with CLZ treatment than with the typical antipsychotics. Interestingly, CLZ appears to have an antidyskinetic effect, particularly in patients with tardive dyskinesia (Lieberman et al., 1991b), that may represent a true ameliorative, rather than suppressive, effect (Tamminga, 1994).

Sertindole. Sertindole, currently under clinical investigation by Abbott Laboratories, is a substituted indole derivative that is predominantly a 5-HT_2 antagonist, with varying antagonist affinities at α_1, D_2, and D_1 receptors (Hyttel et al., 1992). Electrophysiological studies have demonstrated that the long-term administration of sertindole to rats produces selective depolarization inactivation of A10 neurons (Skarsfeldt, 1992), suggesting that in humans this drug might prove to be an effective atypical antipsychotic.

Grebb, Casey, and Tamminga (1993) reported that in a double-blind, placebo-controlled fixed-dosage trial (8, 12, or 20 mg/day for 4 weeks), schizophrenic patients receiving sertindole at 20 mg/day showed significant improvements in clinical outcome as measured by decreases in their scores on three scales: Positive and Negative Symptoms Scale (PANSS), Brief Psychiatric Rating Scale (BPRS), and Clinical Global Impression (CGI). Of particular interest, no difference in acute EPSEs was noted between the drug and placebo groups. Other clinically significant side effects found to be associated with sertindole include abnormal ejaculation, postural hypotension, dizziness, nasal congestion, and possibly minimal liver enzyme elevations and electrocardiogram changes. A double-blind phase-III study involving more than 500 schizophrenic patients at 40 sites is currently being conducted to compare different dosages of sertindole and HAL.

Seroquel. Seroquel (ICI 204,636), like CLZ, does not produce catalepsy and has a low propensity to induce dyskinesia in HAL-sensitized *Cebus* monkeys

(Migler, Warawa, & Malick, 1993). Seroquel induces selective depolarization inactivation of A10, but not A9, dopamine neurons after long-term administration (Goldstein et al., 1993). In vitro, Seroquel is an antagonist with a high affinity for the 5-HT$_2$ receptor, intermediate affinities for the α_1 and α_2 receptors, and weak affinities for the D$_2$ and D$_1$ receptors. In vivo studies of receptor binding also indicate greater 5-HT$_2$-receptor affinity compared with D$_2$ affinity, and virtually no D$_1$ affinity. In addition, ongoing administration (3 weeks) of Seroquel has failed to alter striatal dopamine turnover or to increase striatal D$_2$-receptor density (Saller & Salama, 1993). These preclinical findings suggest that Seroquel will produce few acute or chronic EPSEs in clinical use. An open-label trial with Seroquel involving patients (73 males, 32 females) with various DSM-III-R psychotic disorders (schizophrenia, delusional disorder, bipolar disorder, schizophreniform disorder, and schizoaffective disorder) was conducted over a 4-week period after a 2-day washout period (Fabre, 1993). Decreases of at least 30% from baseline BPRS scores were observed in 36% of the patients, with significant reductions seen as early as the first week of Seroquel treatment. Of particular interest was the significant decrease in acute EPSEs, as determined by Simpson-Angus ratings, after 28 days of treatment with a mean Seroquel dosage of almost 300 mg/day. No acute dystonic reactions were noted; tardive dyskinesia scores rated with the Abnormal Involuntary Movement Scale (AIMS) declined with treatment. The most common side effects from Seroquel encountered in that study were somnolence, agitation, dizziness, insomnia, tachycardia, and weight gain.

Olanzapine. Olanzapine is a potential atypical antipsychotic that is structurally similar to CLZ (Beasley et al., 1993). It has only weak cataleptic effects at clinically relevant doses. Olanzapine will pass for CLZ in setups where animals are trained to discriminate between CLZ and other compounds, thereby suggesting pharmacologic similarities between the two drugs. After long-term treatment, olanzapine produces depolarization inactivation of A10, but not A9, neurons. Its binding profile indicates greater receptor affinity for 5-HT$_2$ than for D$_2$ sites; it has significant affinities at multiple neurotransmitter receptors, including 5-HT$_{1C}$, D$_1$, mACh, α_1, and histamine-1 sites. Similar to CLZ, olanzapine displays greater affinity for the D$_4$ than for the D$_2$ dopamine-receptor subtype. Preliminary findings from a multicenter, fixed-range, dosage-ranging, placebo-controlled study involving more than 335 schizophrenic patients have indicated that olanzapine at a dosage range of 7.5–17.5 mg/day for 6 weeks significantly reduced BPRS total scores, to an extent comparable to that produced by HAL administered at 10–20 mg/day

(Beasley et al., 1993). Unlike HAL, olanzapine effectively reduced negative symptoms as well. Acute EPSEs were significantly reduced for olanzapine-treated patients, as compared with HAL-treated patients. It appears that olanzapine may fit the preclinical and clinical profile for an atypical anti-psychotic drug.

Serotonin Antagonists

Risperidone. Risperidone (RIS) is a benzisoxazole derivative synthesized by Janssen Pharmaceutica in 1984. Although RIS has relatively greater affinity as a 5-HT_2-receptor antagonist than as a D_2-receptor antagonist, its absolute affinities are quite high at both receptors (Janssen et al., 1988; Leysen et al., 1988). It is also an α_1, α_2, and histamine-1 antagonist and has essentially no antimuscarinic affinity.

RIS has been classified as an atypical antipsychotic because of its lower incidence of acute EPSEs as compared with typical antipsychotics (Livingston, 1994). The incidence of acute EPSEs during treatment with RIS appears to be dosage-related, with most symptoms emerging above a dosage threshold of approximately 10 mg/day. Double-blind studies, in general, have suggested that the incidences of acute EPSEs with RIS at dosages below 10 mg/day are significantly lower than those with HAL and are no different from those seen with placebos (Borison et al., 1992; Muller-Spahn, 1992; Marder, 1992; Ceskova & Svetska, 1993; Chouinard et al., 1993; Min et al., 1993). Double-blind studies have found RIS to be as good as or better than the typical antipsychotics for treatment of acute exacerbations of chronic schizophrenia (Borison et al., 1992; Muller-Spahn, 1992; Marder, 1992; Chouinard et al., 1993; Hoyberg et al., 1993). In a 28-day controlled comparison with CLZ at 400 mg/day, acutely ill schizophrenic patients tolerated RIS at 4 or 8 mg/day better than they did the CLZ (Heinrich et al., 1994). Although both drugs were found to be effective antipsychotics, more patients were withdrawn from the RIS treatment groups because of lack of efficacy than were withdrawn from the CLZ group.

There have been no published reports indicating that RIS causes tardive dyskinesia in otherwise neuroleptic-naive patients. However, because relatively few patients have received RIS for periods longer than 3 years, the true incidence is not yet known. In addition, even fewer patients have been treated solely with RIS throughout the entire course of illness. One might speculate that long-term RIS treatment at low dosages (4–8 mg/day) may entail a lower risk for tardive dyskinesia than does treatment with typical antipsychotics. Interestingly, RIS appears to have an antidyskinetic effect, greater than that of HAL, at dosages that do not produce acute EPSEs, suggesting that this reduced rate of tardive dyskinesia may not be purely suppression. One may further infer that the significant 5-HT$_2$ blockade seen with RIS treatment, alone or in combination with its D$_2$ blockade, may be an important factor in producing an antidyskinetic effect.

Specific D$_2$ Antagonists

Remoxipride. The substituted benzamides are selective D$_2$ antagonists. In addition to sulpiride (Harnryd et al., 1984), remoxipride appears to be an effective antipsychotic with a low EPSE profile. As noted previously, remoxipride has a preclinical profile that shows only weak cataleptic activity at dosages that effectively inhibit dopamine-agonist-induced locomotor hyperactivity and an affinity for extrastriatal dopamine D$_2$ receptors. In addition, long-term administration to rats can induce selective depolarization inactivation of A10, but not A9, neurons (Skarsfeldt, 1993). Those data suggest atypical antipsychotic activity in humans. In double-blind studies, remoxipride has demonstrated an antipsychotic efficacy comparable to those for the typical antipsychotic drugs (Chouinard, 1990; McCreadie et al., 1990; Lindstrom et al., 1990; Mendelwicz et al., 1990), but with consistently lower incidences of acute EPSEs. No reports have definitively attributed tardive dyskinesia to remoxipride. Given its favorable acute EPSE profile, one can speculate that this drug might be associated with reduced risk for development of tardive dyskinesia. That is unlikely to be accurately determined, however, now that the drug has been withdrawn from clinical use and its further development worldwide has ceased because of several reports of, and two deaths associated with, aplastic anemia (Philpott et al., 1993; Laidlaw, Snowden, & Brown, 1993).

It is unclear why a subgroup of the substituted benzamides, including raclopride and emonapride (Lewander, 1992), appear to induce significant EPSEs.

Specific D$_1$ Antagonists

Two specific antagonists of the dopamine D$_1$ receptor have been developed for clinical trials as putative atypical antipsychotic drugs: SCH 39166 (Schering-Plough) and NNC 756 (Novo Nordisk A/S). Preclinical studies have suggested that D_1 antagonists may have antipsychotic efficacies (Waddington, 1988; Chipkin et al., 1988; Andersen et al., 1992) and more favorable EPSE profiles than do typical antipsychotics (Gerlach & Hansen, 1993). In drug-naive monkeys, NNC 756 does not produce dystonia (Gerlach & Hansen, 1993), whereas the well-studied D_1 antagonist SCH 23390 induces dystonia and bradykinesia but to a somewhat lesser extent than does HAL (Casey, 1992b). In humans, though, SCH 23390 may induce akathisia, at least after intravenous administration (Farde, 1992). More clinical studies will be required before the antipsychotic efficacies of specific D_1 antagonists can be known.

Partial Dopamine Agonists and Selective Autoreceptor Agonists

Partial dopamine agonists are interesting compounds that have high affinities for the D_2 receptor and yet have limited intrinsic agonist effects (Coward et al., 1989). Their preclinical profile indicates an ability to block the behavioral stimulation of apomorphine or amphetamine, as would be expected of a dopamine-receptor antagonist; on the other hand, as partial agonists they are only weakly cataleptogenic, and they inhibit prolactin release and induce circling in rats with unilateral nigrostriatal lesions, as would be expected of a compound with some intrinsic dopamimetic activity and limited antagonist properties. Clinical application of these drugs would be most appropriate for a pathological process involving excessive dopaminergic activity, such as positive-symptom schizophrenia and hyperkinetic movement disorders, and also those presumably hypodopaminergic states possibly associated with negative-symptom schizophrenia. Partial dopamine agonists, including SDZ 208-911 and SDZ 208-912, terguride (Olbrich & Schanz, 1988), OPC-4392 (Gerbaldo et al., 1988), roxindole (Benkert, Wetzel, & Wiedemann, 1990), and B-HT 920 (Wiedemann, Benkert, & Holsboer, 1990), have shown varying degrees of therapeutic efficacy and low EPSE potentials in preliminary limited clinical trials.

Selective dopamine-autoreceptor agonists are compounds that possess greater affinity for the presynaptic autoreceptor than for the postsynaptic receptor. Agonist activity at the presynaptic receptor provides feedback inhibition of axon-terminal dopamine synthesis and release. These compounds may potentially provide an antipsychotic effect without producing the EPSEs associated with the more disruptive effects of potent dopamine antagonists. Also, (-)-3PPP, or preclamol (Hjorth et al., 1981; Tamminga et al., 1992), and U-66444B and U-68553B (Piercey et al., 1990) are in various stages of early clinical trials.

Glutamatergic Compounds

The neuronal link between cortical glutamatergic afferents to the basal ganglia and dopaminergic efferents from the midbrain may be involved in the pathophysiology of schizophrenia (Carlsson, 1988; Javitt & Zukin, 1990). Poor responses to typical neuroleptics as well as to CLZ (Friedman et al., 1991) have been associated with reductions in prefrontal cortical volume. Enhanced glutamatergic activity may inhibit subcortical dopaminergic nuclei and exert an antipsychotic effect. Only glycine and its pro-drug milacemide have been tested, in limited clinical trials, for their ability to enhance glutamate function. The results have not been encouraging (Rosse et al., 1989; Tamminga et al., 1990). Paradoxically, glycine antagonists of N-methyl-D-aspartic acid (NMDA) receptors appear to have selective inhibitory effects on the mesolimbic dopaminergic system and may offer an innovative antipsychotic strategy (Iversen, 1992). If a neurotoxic effect of excitatory amino acid neurotransmitters is found to be implicated in chronic schizophrenia, perhaps NMDA antagonists, including MK-801 and dextromethorphan, will be helpful in limiting the deterioration seen in this disease.

Gamma-Aminobutyric Acid (GABA) Active Compounds

GABA-mimetic compounds have not been found to be helpful in treating schizophrenia (Tamminga & Gerlach, 1987). And limited efficacy can be demonstrated with traditional benzodiazepine drugs (BDZs) (Arana et al., 1986). Unlike traditional BDZs, non-BDZ GABA agonists do not produce a ceiling response at the $GABA_A$ receptor; that may allow a desirable antipsychotic effect to emerge unobscured by deleterious GABA side effects. Bretazenil, a non-BDZ GABA agonist, has been found to produce a modest antipsychotic effect that approaches the efficacies of typical neuroleptics and may be particularly effective in resistant patients (Delini-Stula, Berdah-Tordjman, & Neumann, 1992).

Conclusion

The development of CLZ has heralded a new era in the treatment of schizophrenia. Antipsychotic treatment can be pursued without the problem of obligatory acute and chronic EPSEs. Moreover, clinical efficacy beyond that obtainable with typical antipsychotics is a realistic clinical goal. Today there is renewed interest in the development of other atypical or novel antipsychotics; no doubt this will soon change the manner in which schizophrenia and other psychoses are managed. Already this trend can be seen in the widespread use of risperidone and in the readiness of clinicians to use this drug as a first-line treatment for all forms of psychoses, without significant risk for acute EPSEs or possibly tardive dyskinesia. These new antipsychotic drugs also provide hope for increased antipsychotic efficacy. Studies specifically designed to demonstrate increased efficacy over typical antipsychotic treatment will be required to help guide the process of new-drug development, as well as to broaden our understanding of the pathophysiology of schizophrenia. Elimination of EPSEs and improvements in antipsychotic efficacy most likely will lead to rapid improvements in patient compliance with pharmacotherapy and favorable long-term clinical outcomes.

References

Ackenheil, M., Blatt, B., & Lampart, C. (1974). Biochemical changes in man and animal following clozapine treatment. *J. Pharmacol. (Paris) (Suppl. 2)* 5:1.

Adler, L. A., Angrist, B., Reiter, S., & Rotrosen, J. (1989). Neuroleptic-induced akathisia: a review. *Psychopharmacology* 97:1–11.

Anden, N. E., & Stock, G. (1973). Effect of clozapine on the turnover of dopamine in the corpus striatum and in the limbic system. *J. Pharm. Pharmacol.* 25:346–8.

Andersen, P. H., Gronvald, F., Hohlweg, R., Hansen, L., Guddal, E., Braestrup, C., & Nielsen, E. B. (1992). NNC-112, NNC-687 and NNC-756, new selective and highly potent dopamine D-1 receptor antagonists. *Eur. J. Pharmacol.* 219:45–52.

Antelman, S. M., & Caggiula, A. R. (1977). Norepinephrine–dopamine interactions and behavior. *Science* 195:646–53.

Arana, G. W., Ornsteen, M. L., Kanter, F., Friedman, H. L., Greenblatt, D. J., & Shader, R. I. (1986). The use of benzodiazepines for psychotic disorders: a literature review and preliminary clinical findings. *Psychopharmacol. Bull.* 22:77–87.

Arnt, J., Hyttel, J., & Bach-Lauritsen, T. (1986). Further studies of the mechanism behind scopolamine-induced reversal of antistereotypic and cataleptogenic effects of neuroleptics in rats. *Acta Pharmacol. Toxicol. (Copenhagen)* 59:319–24.

Assie, M. B., Sleight, A. J., & Koek, W. (1993). Biphasic displacement of [^{3}H]YM-09151-2 binding in the rat brain by thioridazine, risperidone and clozapine, but not by other antipsychotics. *Eur. J. Pharmacol.* 24:183–9.

Auff, E. Birkmayer, W., Brucke, T., Deecke, L., Emich, C., Goldenberg, G., Hirsch, E., Maly, J., Muller, C., Potzl, G., Riederer, P., Sofic, E., & Schnaberth, G. (1987). Ritanserin in the treatment of tremor-dominant Parkinson's disease: a preliminary study. *New Trends Clin. Neuropharmacol.* 1:149–58.

Awouters, F., Niemegeers, C. J. E., Megens, A. A. H. P., Meert, T. F., & Janssen, P. A. J. (1988). Pharmacological profile of ritanserin: a very specific central serotonin S2 antagonist. *Drug Devel. Res.* 15:61–73.

Ayd, F. J. (1961). A survey of drug-induced extrapyramidal reactions. *J. Am. Med. Assoc.* 175:1054–60.

Ayd, F. J. (1983). Early-onset neuroleptic-induced extrapyramidal reactions: a second survey, 1961–1981. In *Neuroleptics: Neurochemical, Behavioral, and Clinical Properties*, ed. J. T. Coyle & S. J. Enna, pp. 75–92. New York: Raven Press.

Baldessarini, R. J. (1985). Antipsychotic agents in chemotherapy. In *Psychiatry 1985*, pp. 14–92. Cambridge, MA: Harvard University Press.

Baldessarini, R. J., & Frankenburg, F. R. (1991). Clozapine. A novel antipsychotic agent. *N. Engl. J. Med.* 324:746–54.

Balsara, J. J., Jadhav, J. H., & Chandorkar, A. G. (1979). Effect of drugs influencing central serotonergic mechanisms on haloperidol-induced catalepsy. *Psychopharmacology (Berlin)* 62:67–9.

Barnes, T. R. E. (1992). Neuromuscular effects of neuroleptics: akathisia. In *Adverse Effects of Psychotropic Drugs*, ed. J. M. Kane & J. A. Lieberman, pp. 204–17. New York: Guilford Press.

Bartels, M., Heide, K., Mann, K., & Schied, H. W. (1987). Treatment of akathisia with lorazepam. An open clinical trial. *Pharmacopsychiatry* 20:51–3.

Bartholini, G. (1976). Differential effect of neuroleptic drugs on dopamine turnover in the extrapyramidal and limbic system. *J. Pharm. Pharmacol.* 28:429–33.

Bartholini, G., Keller, H. H., & Pletscher, A. (1973). Effect of neuroleptics on endogenous norepinephrine in rat brain. *Neuropharmacology* 12:751–6.

Bartholini, G., Keller, H. H., & Pletscher, A. (1975). Drug-induced changes of dopamine turnover in striatum and limbic system of the rat. *J. Pharm. Pharmacol.* 27:439–42.

Beasley, C. M., Tollesfson, G. D., Tye, N. D., & Moore, N. A. (1993). Olanzapine: a potential "atypical" antipsychotic agent. Presented at the 32nd annual meeting of the American College of Neuropsychopharmacology, Honolulu.

Benkert, O., Wetzel, H., & Wiedemann, K. (1990). Dopamine autoreceptor agonists in the treatment of positive and negative schizophrenia. In *Clinical Neuropharmacology: Proceedings from the 17th CINP Congress*, ed. I. Yamachita, M. Toru, & A. J. Coppen, pp. 178–9. New York: Raven Press.

Bersani, G., Grispini, A., Marini, S., Pasini, A., Valducci, M., & Ciani, N. (1986). Neuroleptic-induced extrapyramidal side effects: clinical perspectives with ritanserin (R-55667), a new selective 5-HT$_2$ receptor blocking agent. *Curr. Ther. Res.* 40:492–9.

Bersani, G., Grispini, A., Marini, S., Pasini, A., Valducci, M., & Ciani, N. (1990). 5-HT$_2$ antagonist ritanserin in neuroleptic-induced parkinsonism: a double-blind comparison with orphenadrine and placebo. *Clin. Neuropharmacol.* 13:500–6.

Blaha, C. D., & Lane, R. F. (1987). Chronic treatment with classical and atypical antipsychotic drugs differentially decreases dopamine release in striatum and nucleus accumbens in vivo. *Neurosci. Lett.* 78:199–204.

Borison, R. L., Pathiraja, A. P., Diamond, B. I., & Meibach, R. C. (1992). Risperidone: clinical safety and efficacy in schizophrenia. *Psychopharmacol. Bull.* 28:213–18.

Bowers, M. B., & Rozitis, A. (1974). Regional differences in homovanillic acid concentration after acute and chronic administration of antipsychotic drugs. *J. Pharm. Pharmacol.* 26:743–5.

Boyson, S. J., McGonigle, P., Luthin, G. R., Wolfe, B. B., & Molinoff, P. B. (1988). Effects of chronic administration of neuroleptic and anticholinergic agents on densities of D$_2$ dopamine and muscarinic cholinergic receptors in rat striatum. *J. Pharmacol. Exp. Ther.* 244:987–93.

Breier, A., Buchanan, R. W., Elkashef, A., Munson, R. C., Kirkpatrick, B., & Gellad, F. (1992). Brain morphology and schizophrenia. A magnetic resonance imaging study of limbic, prefrontal cortex, and caudate structures. *Arch. Gen. Psychiatry* 49:921–6.

Breier, A., Buchanan, R. W., Waltrip, R., II, Bryant, N. L., & Goldstein, D. S. (1993). Clozapine's superior efficacy is related to its noradrenergic properties (abstract). *Soc. Neurosci.* 19:856.

Bunney, B. S. (1992). Clozapine: a hypothesized mechanism for its unique clinical profile. *Br. J. Psychiatry (Suppl. 17)*, pp. 17–21.

Burke, R. E. (1992). Neuromuscular effects of neuroleptics: dystonia. In *Adverse Effects of Psychotropic Drugs*, ed. J. M. Kane & J. A. Lieberman, pp. 189–200. New York: Guilford Press.

Burki, H. R., Sayers, A. C., Ruch, W., & Asper, H. (1975). Clozapine and the dopamine hypothesis of schizophrenia, a critical appraisal. *Pharmacopsychiatry* 8:115–21.

Carlsson, A. (1988). The current status of the dopamine hypothesis of schizophrenia. *Neuropsychopharmacology* 1:179–86.

Casey, D. E. (1989). Clozapine: neuroleptic-induced EPS and tardive dyskinesia. *Psychopharmacology (Berlin)* 99:S47–53.

Casey, D. E. (1991). Neuroleptic drug-induced extrapyramidal syndromes and tardive dyskinesia. *Schizophr. Res.* 4:109–20.

Casey, D. E. (1992a). The effect of 8-OH-DPAT on haloperidol-induced dystonia in nonhuman primates. Presented at the 31st annual meeting of the American College of Neuropsychopharmacology, San Juan, PR.

Casey, D. E. (1992b). Dopamine D_1 (SCH 23390) and D_2 (haloperidol) antagonists in drug-naive monkeys. *Psychopharmacology* 107:18–22.

Casey, D. E., & Keepers, G. A. (1988). Neuroleptic side effects: acute extrapyramidal syndromes and tardive dyskinesia. *Psychopharmacology Ser.* 5:74–93.

Ceskova, E., & Svetska, J. (1993). Double-blind comparison of risperidone and haloperidol in schizophrenic and schizoaffective psychoses. *Pharmacopsychiatry* 26:121–4.

Chakos, M. H., Mayerhoff, D. I., Loebel, A. D., Alvir, J. M., & Lieberman, J. A. (1992). Incidence and correlates of acute extrapyramidal symptoms in first episode of schizophrenia. *Psychopharmacol. Bull.* 28:81–6.

Chen, J., Paredes, W., & Gardner, E. L. (1991). Chronic treatment with clozapine selectively decreases basal dopamine release in nucleus accumbens but not in caudate-putamen as measured by in vivo brain microdialysis: further evidence for depolarization block. *Neurosci. Lett.* 122:127–31.

Chiodo, L. A., & Bunney, B. S. (1983). Typical and atypical neuroleptics: differential effects of chronic administration on the activity of A9 and A10 midbrain dopaminergic neurons. *J. Neurosci.* 3:1607–19.

Chiodo, L. A., & Bunney, B. S. (1985). Possible mechanisms by which repeated clozapine administration differentially affects and activity of two subpopulations of midbrain dopamine neurons. *J. Neurosci.* 5:2539–44.

Chipkin, R. E., Iorio, L. C., Coffin, V. L., McQuade, R. D., Berger, J. G., & Barnett, A. (1988). Pharmacological profile of SCH 39166: a dopamine D-1 selective benzonapthazepine with potential antipsychotic activity. *J. Pharmacol. Exp. Ther.* 247:1093–102.

Chouinard, G. (1990). A placebo-controlled clinical trial of remoxipride and chlorpromazine in newly admitted schizophrenic patients with acute exacerbation. *Acta Psychiatr. Scand. (Suppl. 358)* 82:111–19.

Chouinard, G., Jones, B., Remington, G., Bloom, D., Addington, D., MacEwan, G. W., Labelle, A., Beauclair, L., & Arnott, W. (1993). A Canadian multicenter placebo-controlled study of fixed doses of risperidone and haloperidol in the treatment of chronic schizophrenic patients. *J. Clin. Psychopharmacol.* 13:25–40.

Claghorn, J., Honigfeld, G., Abuzzahab, F. S., Sr., Wang, R., Steinbook, R., Tuason, V., & Klerman, G. (1987). The risks and benefits of clozapine versus chlorpromazine. *J. Clin. Psychopharmacol.* 7:377–84.

Cohen, B. M., Keck, P. E., Satlin, A., & Cole, J. O. (1991). Prevalence and severity of akathisia in patients on clozapine. *Biol. Psychiatry* 29:1215–19.

Costall, B., Fortune, D. H., Naylor, R. J., Mardsen, C. D., & Pycock, C. (1975). Serotonergic involvement with neuroleptic catalepsy. *Neuropharmacology* 14:859–68.

Costall, B., & Naylor, R. J. (1976). A comparison of the abilities of typical neuroleptic agents and of thioridazine, clozapine, sulpiride and metoclopramide to antagonize the hyperactivity induced by dopamine applied intracerebrally to areas of the extrapyramidal and mesolimbic systems. *Eur. J. Pharmacol.* 40:9–19.

Coward, D., Dixon, K., Enz, A., Shearman, G., Urwyler, S., White, T., & Karobath, M. (1989). Partial brain dopamine D_2 receptor agonists in the treatment of schizophrenia. *Psychopharmacol. Bull.* 25:393–7.

Crow, T. J., Johnstone, E. C., Deakin, J. F., & Longden, A. (1976). Dopamine and schizophrenia. *Lancet* 2:563–6.

Davidson, M., Kahn, R. S., Stern, R. G., Hirschowitz, J., Apter, S., Knott, P., & Davis, K. L. (1993). Treatment with clozapine and its effect on plasma homovanillic acid and norepinephrine concentrations in schizophrenia. *Psychiatry Res.* 46:151–63.

Delay, J., Deniker, P., & Hart, J. (1952). Traitement des états d'excitation et d'agitation par une méthode médicamenteuse dérivée de l'hibernothérapie. *Ann. Med. Psychol. (Paris)* 110:267–73.

de Leon Moral, L., & Camunas, C. (1991). Clozapine and jaw dyskinesia: a case report. *J. Clin. Psychiatry* 52:494–5.

Delini-Stula, A., Berdah-Tordjman, D., & Neumann, N. (1992). Partial benzodiazepine agonists in schizophrenia: expectations and present clinical findings. *Clin. Neuropharmacol. (Suppl. 1)* 15:405A–6A.

Duinkerke, S. J., Botter, P. A., Jansen, A. A., van Dongen, P. A., van Haaften, A. J., Boom, A. J., van Laarhoven, J. H., & Busard, H. L. (1993). Ritanserin, a selective $5\text{-HT}_{2/1C}$ antagonist, and negative symptoms in schizophrenia. A placebo-controlled double-blind trial. *Br. J. Psychiatry* 163:451–5.

Fabre, L. F. (1993). A multicenter, open, pilot trial of ICI 204,636 in hospitalized patients with acute psychotic symptomatology. *Schizophr. Res.* 9:237.

Farde, L. (1992). Selective D_1- and D_2-dopamine receptor blockade both induce akathisia in humans – a PET study with [^{11}C]SCH 23390 and [^{11}C]raclopride. *Psychopharmacology (Berlin)* 107:23–9.

Farde, L., & Nordstrom, A. L. (1992). PET analysis indicates atypical central dopamine receptor occupancy in clozapine-treated patients. *Br. J. Psychiatry (Suppl. 17)*, pp. 30–3.

Farde, L., Nordstrom, A. L., Wiesel, F. A., Pauli, S., Halldin, C., & Sedvall, G. (1992). Positron emission tomographic analysis of central D_1 and D_2 dopamine receptor occupancy in patients treated with classical neuroleptics and clozapine. Relation to extrapyramidal side effects. *Arch. Gen. Psychiatry* 49:538–44.

Farde, L., Wiesel, F. A., Nordstrom, A. L., & Sedvall, G. (1989). D_1 and D_2-dopamine receptor occupancy during treatment with conventional and atypical neuroleptics. *Psychopharmacology (Berlin)* 99:S28–31.

Fischman, L. G. (1983). Dreams, hallucinogenic drug states, and schizophrenia: a psychological and biological comparison. *Schizophr. Bull.* 9:73–94.

Fleischhacker, W. W., Roth, S. D., & Kane, J. M. (1990). The pharmacologic treatment of neuroleptic-induced akathisia. *J. Clin. Psychopharmacol.* 10:12–21.

Freedman, R., Kirch, D., Bell, J., Adler, L. E., Pecevich, M., Pachtman, E., & Denver, P. (1982). Clonidine treatment of schizophrenia: double-blind comparison to placebo and neuroleptic drugs. *Acta Psychiatr. Scand.* 65:35–45.

Friedman, A. (1978). Pizotifen (Sandomigran) used in the treatment of parkinsonian tremor (preliminary communication) (in Polish). *Neurol. Neurochir. Pol.* 12:263–7.

Friedman, L., Knutson, L., Shurell, M., & Meltzer, H. Y. (1991). Prefrontal sulcal prominence is inversely related to response to clozapine in schizophrenia. *Biol. Psychiatry* 29:865–77.

Gardner, E. L., Walker, L. S., & Paredes, W. (1993). Clozapine's functional mesolimbic selectivity is not duplicated by the addition of anticholinergic action to haloperidol – a brain stimulation study in the rat. *Psychopharmacology (Berlin)* 110:119–24.

Gelders, Y. G. (1989). Thymosthenic agents, a novel approach in the treatment of schizophrenia. *Br. J. Psychiatry* 155:33–6.

Gelders, Y., Vanden Bussche, G., Reyntjens, A., & Janssen, P. (1986). Serotonin-S2 receptor blockers in the treatment of chronic schizophrenia. *Clin. Neuropharmacol.* 9:325–7.

Gerbaldo, H., Demisch, L., Lehmann, C. O., & Bochnik, J. (1988). The effect of OPC-4392, a partial dopamine receptor agonist on negative symptoms: results of an open study. *Pharmacopsychiatry* 21:387–8.

Gerbino, L., Shopsin, B., & Collora, M. (1980). Clozapine in the treatment of tardive dyskinesia. In *Tardive Dyskinesia: Research and Treatment*, ed. W. E. Fahn, R. C. Smith, J. M. Davis, & E. F. Domino, pp. 475–89. New York: Spectrum.

Gerlach, J., & Casey, D. E. (1988). Tardive dyskinesia. *Acta Psychiatr. Scand.* 77:369–78.

Gerlach, J., & Hansen, L. (1993). Effect of chronic treatment with NNC 756, a new D-1 receptor antagonist, or raclopride, a D-2 receptor antagonist, in drug-naive *Cebus* monkeys: dystonia, dyskinesia and D-1/D-2 supersensitivity. *J. Psychopharmacol.* 7:355–64.

Goldstein, J. M., Litwin, L. C., Sutton, E. B., & Malick, J. B. (1993). Seroquel: electrophysiological profile of a potential atypical antipsychotic. *Psychopharmacology (Berlin)* 112:293–8.

Grebb, J. A., Casey, D. E., & Tamminga, C. A. (1993). A placebo-controlled trial of sertindole in schizophrenia. Presented at a meeting of the American College of Neuropsychopharmacology, Honolulu.

Greene, P., Coté, L., & Fahn, S. (1993). Treatment of drug-induced psychosis in Parkinson's disease with clozapine. *Adv. Neurol.* 60:703–6.

Gumulka, W., Kostowski, W., & Czlonkowski, A. (1973). Role of 5-HT in the action of some drugs affecting extrapyramidal system. *Pharmacology* 10:363–72.

Harnryd, C., Bjerkenstedt, L., Bjork, K., Gullberg, B., Oxenstierna, G., Sedvall, G., Wiesel, F. A., Wik, G., & Aberg-Wistedt, A. (1984). Clinical evaluation of sulpiride in schizophrenic patients – a double-blind comparison with chlorpromazine. *Acta Psychiatr. Scand. (Suppl.)* 311:7–30.

Heinrich, K., Klieser, E., Lehmann, E., Kinzler, E., & Hruschka, H. (1994). Risperidone versus clozapine in the treatment of schizophrenic patients with acute symptoms – a double blind, randomized trial. *Prog. Neuropsychopharmacol. Biol. Psychiatry* 18:129–37.

Hicks, P. B. (1990). The effect of serotonergic agents on haloperidol-induced catalepsy. *Life Sci.* 47:1609–15.

Hildebrand, J., & Delecluse, F. (1987). Effect of ritanserin, a selective serotonin-S2 antagonist, on parkinsonian rest tremor. *Curr. Ther. Res.* 41:298–300.

Hjorth, S., Carlsson, A., Wikstrom, H., Lindberg, P., Sanchez, D., Hacksell, U., Arvidsson, L. E., Svensson, U., & Nilsson, J. L. (1981). 3-PPP, a new centrally acting DA-receptor agonist with selectivity for autoreceptors. *Life Sci.* 28:1225–38.

Hommer, D. W., Zahn, T. P., Pickar, D., & van Kammen, D. P. (1984). Prazosin, a selective alpha$_1$-noradrenergic receptor antagonist, has no effect on symptoms but increases autonomic arousal in schizophrenic patients. *Psychiatry Res.* 11:193–204.

Hornykiewicz, O. (1982). Brain catecholamines in schizophrenia – a good case for noradrenaline. *Nature* 299:484–6.

Hoyberg, O. J., Fensbo, C., Remvig, J., Lingjaerde, O., Slothnielsen, M., & Salvesen, I. (1993). Risperidone versus perphenazine in the treatment of chronic schizophrenic patients with acute exacerbations. *Acta Psychiatr. Scand.* 88:395–402.

Huff, R. M., & Adams, R. N. (1980). Dopamine release in n. accumbens and striatum by clozapine: simultaneous monitoring by in vivo electrochemistry. *Neuropharmacology* 19:587–90.

Hyttel, J., Arnt, J., Costall, B., Domeney, A., Dragsted, N., Lembol, H. E., Meier, E., Naylor, R. J., Nowak, G., Sanchez, C., & Skarsfeldt, T. (1992). Pharmacologic profile of the atypical neuroleptic sertindole. *Clin. Neuropharmacol. (Suppl. 1)* 15:267A–8A.

Hyttel, J., Larsen, J. J., Christensen, A. V., & Arnt, J. (1985). Receptor-binding profiles of neuroleptics. In *Dyskinesia – Research and Treatment*, ed. D. E. Casey, T. N. Chase, A. V. Christensen, & J. Gerlach, pp. 9–18. Berlin: Springer-Verlag.

Invernizzi, R. W., Cervo, L., & Samanin, R. (1988). 8-Hydroxy-2-(di-*n*-propylamino)tetralin, a selective serotonin 1A receptor agonist, blocks haloperidol-induced catalepsy by an action on raphe nuclei medianus and dorsalis. *Neuropharmacology* 27:515–18.

Iversen, S. D. (1992). Glycine NMDA antagonists: novel antipsychotic drugs? Presented at 31st annual meeting of the American College of Neuropsychopharmacology, San Juan, PR.

Janssen, P. A., Niemegeers, C. J., Awouters, F., Schellekens, K. H., Megens,

A. A., & Meert, T. F. (1988). Pharmacology of risperidone (R-64,766), a new antipsychotic with serotonin-S2 and dopamine-D_2 antagonistic properties. *J. Pharmacol. Exp. Ther.* 244:685–93.

Javitt, D. C., & Zukin, S. R. (1990). The role of excitatory amino acids in neuropsychiatric illness. *J. Neuropsychiatry Clin. Neurosci.* 2:44–52.

Kane, J. M. (1990). Psychopharmacologic treatment of schizophrenia. In *Recent Advances in Schizophrenia*, ed. A. Kales, C. N. Stefanis, & J. Talbott, pp. 257–76. Berlin: Springer-Verlag.

Kane, J., Honigfeld, G., Singer, J., Meltzer, H., & Clozaril Collaborative Study Group (1988). Clozapine for the treatment-resistant schizophrenic: a double-blind comparison with chlorpromazine. *Arch. Gen. Psychiatry* 45:789–96.

Kane, J. M., & Lieberman, J. A. (1993). Tardive dyskinesia. In *Adverse Effects of Psychotropic Drugs*, ed. J. M. Kane & J. A. Lieberman, pp. 235–45. New York: Guilford Press.

Kane, J. M., Woerner, M. G., Pollack, S., Safferman, A. Z., & Lieberman, J. A. (1993). Does clozapine cause tardive dyskinesia? *J. Clin. Psychiatry* 54:327–30.

Kastrup, O., Gastpar, M., & Schwartz, M. (1994). Acute dystonia due to clozapine. *J. Neurol. Neurosurg. Psychiatry* 57:119.

Keller, H. H., Bartholini, G., & Pletscher, A. (1973). Increase of 3-methoxy-4-hydroxyphenylethylene glycol in rat brain by neuroleptic drugs. *Eur. J. Pharmacol.* 23:183–6.

Kohler, C., Haglund, L., Ogren, S. O., & Angeby, T. (1981). Regional blockade by neuroleptic drugs of in vivo ^{3}H-spiperone binding in the rat brain. Relation to blockade of apomorphine induced hyperactivity and stereotypies. *J. Neural Transm.* 52:163–73.

Kohler, C., Ogren, S. O., Haglund, L., & Angeby, T. (1979). Regional displacement by sulpiride of [^{3}H]spiperone binding in vivo. Biochemical and behavioural evidence for a preferential action of limbic and nigral dopamine receptors. *Neurosci. Lett.* 13:51–6.

Korsgaard, S., Noring, U., Povlsen, U. J., & Gerlach, J. (1986). Effects of citalopram, a specific serotonin uptake inhibitor, in tardive dyskinesia and parkinsonism. *Clin. Neuropharmacol.* 9:52–7.

Kostowski, W., Gumulka, W., & Czlonkowski, A. (1972). Reduced cataleptogenic effects of some neuroleptics in rats with lesioned midbrain raphe and treated with *p*-chlorophenylalanine. *Brain Res.* 48:443–6.

Krystal, J. H., Seibyl, J. P., Price, L. H., Woods, S. W., Heninger, G. R., Aghajanian, G. K., & Charney, D. S. (1993). *m*-Chlorophenylpiperazine effects in neuroleptic-free schizophrenic patients. Evidence implicating serotonergic systems in the positive symptoms of schizophrenia. *Arch. Gen. Psychiatry* 50:624–35.

Lader, M. (1988). Beta-adrenoceptor antagonists in neuropsychiatry: an update. *J. Clin. Psychiatry* 49:213–23.

Laidlaw, S. T., Snowden, J. A., & Brown, M. J. (1993). Aplastic anemia and remoxipride (letter). *Lancet* 342:1245.

Lane, R. F., & Blaha, C. D. (1987). Acute thioridazine stimulates mesolimbic but not nigrostriatal dopamine release: demonstration by in vivo electrochemistry. *Brain Res.* 408:317–20.

Lane, R. F., Blaha, C. D., & Rivet, J. M. (1988). Selective inhibition of mesolimbic dopamine release following chronic administration of clozapine: involvement of alpha$_1$-noradrenergic receptors demonsttrated by in vivo voltammetry. *Brain Res.* 460:398–401.

Lavin, M. R., & Rifkin, A. (1992). Neuroleptic-induced parkinsonism. In *Adverse Effects of Psychotropic Drugs*, ed. J. M. Kane & J. A. Lieberman, pp. 175–88. New York: Guilford Press.

Lewander, T. (1992). Differential development of therapeutic drugs for psychosis. *Clin. Neuropharmacol. (Suppl. 1)* 15:654–5.

Leysen, J. E., Gommeren, W., Eens, A., de Chaffoy de Courcelles, D., Stoof, J. C., & Janssen, P. A. (1988). Biochemical profile of risperidone, a new antipsychotic. *J. Pharmacol. Exp. Ther.* 247:661–70.

Lieberman, J., Johns, C., Pollack, S., Masiar, S., Bookstein, P., Cooper, T., Iadorola, M., & Kane, J. (1991a). Biochemical effects of clozapine in cerebrospinal fluid of patients with schizophrenia. In *Schizophrenia Research – Advances in Neuropsychiatry and Psychopharmacology*, vol. 1, ed. S. C. Schulz & C. A. Tamminga, pp. 341–9. New York: Raven Press.

Lieberman, J. A., & Safferman, A. Z. (1992). Clinical profile of clozapine: adverse reactions and agranulocytosis. *Psychiatr. Q.* 63:51–70.

Lieberman, J. A., Saltz, B. L., Johns, C. A., Pollack, S., Borenstein, M., & Kane, J. (1991b). The effects of clozapine on tardive dyskinesia. *Br. J. Psychiatry* 158:503–10.

Lindstrom, L. H. (1988). The effect of long-term treatment with clozapine in schizophrenia: a retrospective study in 96 patients treated with clozapine for up to 13 years. *Acta Psychiatr. Scand.* 77:524–9.

Lindstrom, L. H., Wieselgren, L. M., Struwe, G., Kristjansson, E., Akselson, S., Artheur, H., Andersen, T., Lindgren, S., Normon, O., Naimell, L., & Stening, G. (1990). A double-blind comparative multicentre study of remoxipride and haloperidol in schizophrenia. *Acta Psychiatr. Scand. (Suppl. 358)* 82:130–5.

Lipinski, J. F., Jr., Zubenko, G. S., Cohen, B. M., & Barreira, P. J. (1984). Propranolol in the treatment of neuroleptic-induced akathisia. *Am. J. Psychiatry* 141:412–15.

Litman, R. E., Hong, W. W., Weissman, E. M., Su, T. P., Potter, W. Z., & Pickar, D. (1993). Idazoxan, an alpha$_2$ antagonist, augments fluphenazine in schizophrenic patients: a pilot study. *J. Clin. Psychopharmacol.* 13:264–7.

Livingston, M. G. (1994). Risperidone. *Lancet* 343:457–60.

Ljungberg, T., & Ungerstedt, U. (1978). Classification of neuroleptic drugs according to their ability to inhibit apomorphine-induced locomotion and gnawing: evidence for two different mechanisms of action. *Psychopharmacology (Berlin)* 56:239–47.

McCreadie, R. G., Todd, N., Livingston, M., Eccleston, D., Watt, J. A. G., Herrington, D., Tait, D., Crocket, G., Mitchell, M. J., & Huitfeldt, B. (1990). A double-blind comparative study of remoxipride and thioridazine in the acute phase of schizophrenia. *Acta Psychiatr. Scand. (Suppl. 358)* 82:136–7.

McEvoy, J. P., Hogarty, G. E., & Steingard, S. (1991). Optimal dose of neuroleptic in acute schizophrenia. A controlled study of the neuroleptic threshold and higher haloperidol dose. *Arch. Gen. Psychiatry* 48:739–45.

McMillen, B. A., Scott, S. M., & Davanzo, E. A. (1988). Reversal of neuroleptic-induced catalepsy by novel aryl-piperazine anxiolytic drugs. *J. Pharm. Pharmacol.* 40:885–7.

Maertens de Noordhout, A., & Delwaide, P. J. (1986). Open pilot trial of ritanserin in parkinsonism. *Clin. Neuropharmacol.* 9:480–4.

Magnusson, O., Fowler, C. J., Kohler, C., & Ogren, S. O. (1986). Dopamine D$_2$ receptors and dopamine metabolism. Relationship between biochemical and behavioural effects of substituted benzamide drugs. *Neuropharmacology* 25:187–97.

Maj, J., Sarnek, J., Klimek, V., & Rawlow, A. (1976). On the anticataleptic action of cyproheptadine. *Pharmacol. Biochem. Behav.* 5:201–5.

Marder, S. R. (1992). Risperidone: clinical development: North American results. *Clin. Neuropharmacol. (Suppl. 1)* 15:92–3.

Matz, R., Rick, W., Oh, D., Thompson, H., & Gershon, S. (1974). Clozapine – a potential antipsychotic agent without extrapyramidal manifestations. *Curr. Ther. Exp. Clin. Res.* 16:687–95.

Meco, G., Marini, S., Lestingi, L., Linfante, I., Modarelli, F. T., & Agnoli, A. (1988). Controlled single-blind crossover study of ritanserin and placebo in *l*-dopa-induced dyskinesias in Parkinson's disease. *Curr. Ther. Res.* 43:262–70.

Meltzer, H. Y., Matsubara, S., & Lee, J. C. (1989). Classification of typical and atypical antipsychotic drugs on the basis of dopamine D-1, D-2 and serotonin 2 pK_i values. *J. Pharmacol. Exp. Ther.* 251:238–46.

Mendelwicz, J., de Bleeker, E., Cosyns, P., Deleu, G., Lotstra, F., Masson, A., Mertens, C., Parent, M., Peuskens, J., Suy, E., de Wilde, J., Wilmotte, J., & Norgard, J. (1990). A double-blind comparative study of remoxipride and haloperidol in schizophrenic and schizophreniform disorders. *Acta Psychiatr. Scand. (Suppl. 358)* 82:138–41.

Migler, B. M., Warawa, E. J., & Malick, J. B. (1993). Seroquel: behavioral effects in conventional and novel tests for atypical antipsychotic drug. *Psychopharmacology (Berlin)* 112:299–307.

Min, S. K., Rhee, C. S., Kim, C. E., & Kang, D. Y. (1993). Risperidone versus haloperidol in the treatment of chronic schizophrenic patients: a parallel group double-blind comparative trial. *Yonsei Med. J.* 34:179–90.

Mita, T., Hanada, S., Nishino, N., Kuno, T., Nakai, H., Yamadori, T., Mizoi, Y., & Tanaka, C. (1986). Decreased serotonin S2 and increased dopamine D_2 receptors in chronic schizophrenics. *Biol. Psychiatry* 21:1407–14.

Mueller, K. (1993). Locomotor stereotypy is produced by methylphenidate and amfonelic acid and reduced by haloperidol but not clozapine or thioridazine. *Pharmacol. Biochem. Behav.* 45:71–6.

Muller-Spahn, F. (1992). Risperidone in the treatment of chronic schizophrenic patients: an international double-blind parallel-group study versus haloperidol. The International Risperidone Research Group. *Clin. Neuropharmacol. (Suppl. 1)* 15:90–1.

Ogren, S. O., Florvall, L., Hall, H., Magnusson, O., & Angeby-Moller, K. (1990). Neuropharmacological and behavioural properties of remoxipride in the rat. *Acta Psychiatr. Scand. (Suppl. 358)* 82:21–6.

Ogren, S. O., Hall, H., Kohler, C., Magnusson, O., Lindbom, L. O., Angeby, K., & Florvall, L. (1984). Remoxipride, a new potential antipsychotic compound with selective antidopaminergic actions in the rat brain. *Eur. J. Pharmacol.* 102:459–74.

Olbrich, R., & Schanz, H. (1988). The effect of the partial dopamine agonist terguride on negative symptoms in schizophrenics. *Pharmacopsychiatry* 21:389–90.

Panteleeva, G. P., Kovskaya, M. Y., Belyaev, B. S., Minsker, E. I., Vynar, O., Ceskova, E., Svetska, J., Libiger, J., Korinkova, V., & Novotny, V. (1987). Clozapine in the treatment of schizophrenic patients: an international multicenter trial. *Clin. Ther.* 10:57–68.

Philpott, N. J., Marsh, J. C., Gordon-Smith, E. C., & Bolton, J. S. (1993). Aplastic anemia and remoxipride (letter). *Lancet* 342:1244–5.

Pickar, D., Owen, R. R., Litman, R. E., Konicki, E., Gutierrez, R., & Rapaport, M. H. (1992). Clinical and biologic response to clozapine in patients with schizophrenia. Crossover comparison with fluphenazine. *Arch. Gen. Psychiatry* 49:345–53.

Piercey, M. F., Broderick, P. A., Hoffmann, W. E., & Vogelsang, G. D. (1990). U-66444B and U-68553B, potent autoreceptor agonists at dopaminergic cell bodies and terminals. *J. Pharmacol. Exp. Ther.* 254:369–74.

Povlsen, J., Noring, U., Fog, R., & Gerlach, J. (1985). Tolerability and therapeutic effect of clozapine. A retrospective investigation of 216 patients treated with clozapine for up to 12 years. *Acta Psychiatr. Scand.* 71:176–85.

Riblet, L. A., Taylor, D. P., Eison, M. S., & Stanton, H. C. (1982). Pharmacology and neurochemistry of buspirone. *J. Clin. Psychiatry* 43:11–18.

Richardson, M. A., & Casey, D. E. (1988). Tardive dyskinesia status: stability or change? *Psychopharmacol. Bull.* 24:471–5.

Richelson, E. (1984). Neuroleptic affinities for human brain receptors and their use in predicting adverse effects. *J. Clin. Psychiatry* 45:331–6.

Rifkin, A., Doddi, S., Karajgi, B., Borenstein, M., & Wachspress, M. (1991). Dosage of haloperidol for schizophrenia. *Arch. Gen. Psychiatry* 48:166–70.

Rifkin, A., Quitkin, F., & Klein, D. F. (1975). Akinesia: a poorly recognized drug-induced extrapyramidal behavior disorder. *Arch. Gen. Psychiatry* 34:672–4.

Rosse, R. B., Theut, S. K., Banay-Schwartz, M., Leighton, M., Scarcella, E., Cohen, C. G., & Deutsch, S. I. (1989). Glycine adjuvant therapy to conventional neuroleptic treatment in schizophrenia: an open-label, pilot study. *Clin. Neuropharmacol.* 12:416–24.

Roth, B. L., Ciaranello, R. D., & Meltzer, H. Y. (1992). Binding of typical and atypical antipsychotic agents to transiently expressed 5-HT$_{1C}$ receptors. *J. Pharmacol. Exp. Ther.* 260:1361–5.

Safferman, A. Z., Kane, J. M., Aronowitz, J. S., Gordon, M. F., Pollack, S., & Lieberman, J. A. (1994). The use of clozapine in neurologic disorders. *J. Clin. Psychiatry (Suppl. B)* 55:98–101.

Safferman, A. Z., Lieberman, J. A., Pollack, S., & Kane, J. M. (1993). Akathisia and clozapine treatment. *J. Clin. Psychopharmacol.* 13:286–7.

Saller, C. F., & Salama, A. I. (1993). Seroquel: biochemical profile of a potential atypical antipsychotic. *Psychopharmacology (Berlin)* 112:285–92.

Saltz, B. L., Woerner, M. G., Kane, J. M., Lieberman, J. A., Alvir, J. M. J., Bergmann, K. J., Blank, K., Koblenzer, J., & Kahaner, K. (1991). Prospective study of tardive dyskinesia in the elderly. *J. Am. Med. Assoc.* 266: 2402–6.

Schotte, A., Janssen, P. F. M., Megens, A. A. H. P., & Leysen, J. E. (1993). Occupancy of central neurotransmitter receptors by risperidone, clozapine and haloperidol, measured ex vivo by quantitative autoradiography. *Brain Res.* 631:191–202.

Seeman, P., Lee, T., Chau-Wong, M., & Wong, K. (1976). Antipsychotic drug doses and neuroleptic/dopamine receptors. *Nature* 261:717–19.

Seibyl, J. P., Krystal, J. H., Price, L. H., Woods, S. W., D'Amico, C., Heninger, G. R., & Charney, D. S. (1991). Effects of ritanserin on the behavioral, neuroendocrine, and cardiovascular responses to meta-chlorophenylpiperazine in healthy human subjects. *Psychiatry Res.* 38:227–36.

Silver, H., & Nassar, A. (1992). Fluvoxamine improves negative symptoms in treated chronic schizophrenia: an add-on double-blind, placebo-controlled study. *Biol. Psychiatry* 31:698–704.

Skarsfeldt, T. (1988). Differential effects after repeated treatment with haloperidol, clozapine, thioridazine and tefludazine on SNC and VTA dopamine neurones in rats. *Life Sci.* 42:1037–44.

Skarsfeldt, T. (1992). Electrophysiological profile of the new atypical neuroleptic, sertindole, on midbrain dopamine neurones in rats: acute and repeated treatment. *Synapse* 10:25–33.

Skarsfeldt, T. (1993). Comparison of the effect of substituted benzamides on midbrain dopamine neurones after treatment of rats for 21 days. *Eur. J. Pharmacol.* 240:269–75.

Small, J. G., Milstein, V., Marhenke, J. D., Hall, D. D., & Kellams, J. J. (1987). Treatment outcome with clozapine in tardive dyskinesia, neuroleptic sensitivity, and treatment-resistant psychosis. *J. Clin. Psychiatry* 48:263–7.

Snyder, S. H., Greenberg, D., & Yamamura, H. I. (1974). Antischizophrenic drugs: affinity for muscarinic cholinergic receptor sites in the brain predicts extrapyramidal effects. *J. Psychiatr. Res.* 11:91–5.

Sokoloff, P., Giros, B., Martres, M. P., Bouthenet, M. L., & Schwartz, J. C. (1990). Molecular cloning and characterization of a novel dopamine receptor (D_3) as a target for neuroleptics. *Nature* 347:146–51.

Stille, G., Lauener, H., & Eichenberger, E. (1971). The pharmacology of 8-chloro-11-(4-methyl-1-piperazinyl)-5H-dibenzo(b,e)(1,4)diazepine (clozapine). *Farmaco (Pavia)* 26:603–25.

Stockmeier, C. A., DiCarlo, J. J., Zhang, Y., Thompson, P., & Meltzer, H. Y. (1993). Characterization of typical and atypical antipsychotic drugs based on in vivo occupancy of serotonin 2 and dopamine 2 receptors. *J. Pharmacol. Exp. Ther.* 266:1374–84.

Tamminga, C. A. (1994). Clozapine 1994: clozapine and tardive dyskinesia. Presented at the Garden City Hotel, Garden City, NY.

Tamminga, C. A., Cascella, N., Dixon, L., Fahouki, T., & Herting, R. L. (1990). Excitatory amino acid pharmacotherapy in schizophrenia. Presented at the 17th congress of CINP, Kyoto, Japan.

Tamminga, C. A., Cascella, N. G., Lahti, R. A., Lindberg, M., & Carlsson, A. (1992). Pharmacologic properties of (–)-3PPP (preclamol) in man. *J. Neural. Transm.* 88:165–75.

Tamminga, C., & Gerlach, J. (1987). Neuroleptics and experimental antipsychotics in schizophrenia. In *Psychopharmacology: The Third Generation in Progress*, ed. H. Y. Meltzer, pp. 1129–40. New York: Raven Press.

van Kammen, D. P., Yao, J., Gurklis, J., O'Connor, D., Nofzinger, E., & Peters, J. L. (1992). CSF noradrenergic activity and sleep EEG in clinically stable schizophrenic patients after haloperidol withdrawal. *Clin. Neuropharmacol. (Suppl. 1)* 15:325–6.

Van Putten, T. (1974). Why do schizophrenic patients refuse to take their drugs? *Arch. Gen. Psychiatry* 31:61–72.

Van Putten, T., & Marder, S. R. (1987). Behavioral toxicity of antipsychotic drugs. *J. Clin. Psychiatry (Suppl.)* 48:13–19.

Van Putten, T., Marder, S. R., & Mintz, J. (1990). A controlled dose comparison of haloperidol in newly admitted schizophrenic patients. *Arch. Gen. Psychiatry* 47:754–8.

Van Putten, T., & May, P. R. A. (1978). Akinetic depression in schizophrenia. *Arch. Gen. Psychiatry* 35:1101–17.

Van Tol, H. H. M., Bunzow, J. R., Guan, H.-C., Sunhara, R. K., Seeman, P., Niznik, H. B., & Civelli, O. (1991). Cloning of the gene for a human dopamine D_4 receptor with a high affinity for the antipsychotic clozapine. *Nature* 350:610–14.

Waddington, J. L. (1988). Therapeutic potential of selective D-1 dopamine receptor agonists and antagonists in psychiatry and neurology. *Gen. Pharmacol.* 19:55–60.

Wadenberg, M. L. (1992). Antagonism by 8-OH-DPAT, but not ritanserin, of catalepsy induced by SCH 23390 in the rat. *J. Neural Transm.* 89:49–59.

Waldmeier, P. C., & Delini-Stula, A. A. (1979). Serotonin–dopamine interactions in the nigrostriatal system. *Eur. J. Pharmacol.* 55:363–73.

Waldmeier, P. C., & Maitre, L. (1976). On the relevance of preferential increases of mesolimbic versus striatal dopamine turnover for the prediction of antipsychotic activity of psychotropic drugs. *J. Neurochem.* 27:589–97.

Weiden, P. J., Mann, J. J., Haas, G., Mattson, M., & Frances, A. (1987). Clinical nonrecognition of neuroleptic-induced movement disorders: a cautionary study. *Am. J. Psychiatry* 144:1148–53.

Westerink, B. H., & Korf, J. (1975). Influence of drugs on striatal and limbic homovanillic acid concentration in the rat brain. *Eur. J. Pharmacol.* 33:31–40.

Westerink, B. H. C., Lejeune, B., Korf, J., & Van Praag, H. M. (1977). On the significance of regional dopamine metabolism in the rat brain for the classification of centrally acting drugs. *Eur. J. Pharmacol.* 42:179–90.

White, F. J., & Wang, R. Y. (1983). Differential effects of classical and atypical antipsychotic drugs on A9 and A10 dopamine neurons. *Science* 221:1054–7.

Wiedemann, K., Benkert, O., & Holsboer, F. (1990). B-HT 920 – a novel dopamine autoreceptor agonist in the treatment of patients with schizophrenia. *Pharmacopsychiatry* 23:50–5.

Woerner, M. G., Kane, J. M., Lieberman, J. A., Alvir, J., Bergmann, K. J., Borenstein, M., Schooler, N. R., Mukherjee, S., Rotrosen, J., & Rubenstein, M. (1991). The prevalence of tardive dyskinesia. *J. Clin. Psychopharmacol.* 11:34–42.

Zivkovic, G., Guidotti, A., Revuelta, A., & Costa, E. (1975). Effect of thioridazine, clozapine and other antipsychotics in the kinetic state of tyrosine hydroxylase and on the turnover of dopamine in striatum and nucleus accumbens. *J. Pharmacol. Exp. Ther.* 194:37–46.

29

GABAergic Treatments for Tardive Dyskinesia

SHAWN L. CASSADY, M.D., GUNVANT K. THAKER,
M.D., and CAROL A. TAMMINGA, M.D.

Although the pathophysiology of tardive dyskinesia remains unknown, recent experiments have supported the possibility of a mechanism of transmission involving γ-aminobutyric acid (GABA). The earlier dopamine hypothesis of tardive dyskinesia was based on the development of dopamine receptor supersensitivity following long-term neuroleptic treatment. However, the hypothesis of dopamine receptor supersensitivity was inconsistent with certain clinical and experimental data, and adjustments to the hypothesis were made over the years. The more recent explanation is that following a cascade of neurophysiological changes upstream, there is diminished GABAergic efferent activity coming from the basal ganglia. This better fits the evidence than did the simple dopamine hypothesis. It seems, therefore, that GABA mimetics may reduce dyskinetic symptoms by enhancing GABAergic efferent activity from the basal ganglia.

Dopamine Receptor Supersensitivity Hypothesis

The dopamine receptor supersensitivity hypothesis has been widely cited as the pathophysiological mechanism in tardive dyskinesia. The supporting evidence is chiefly pharmacologic and includes findings such as the following: Dopamine agonists exacerbate dyskinesia; dopamine antagonists (e.g., haloperidol) and dopamine depleters (e.g., reserpine) ameliorate dyskinesia; withdrawal of neuroleptics, exposing supersensitive dopamine receptors, temporarily exacerbates dyskinesia. Moreover, studies have shown that cholinergic stimulation, believed to oppose dopamine in the basal ganglia, reduces some dyskinetic symptoms. Nevertheless, several clinical observations remain unexplained by the dopamine receptor supersensitivity hypothesis. For example, although it is known that neuroleptics will induce striatal dopamine receptor supersensitivity in all human brains (Mackay et al., 1982; Rupniak,

454

Jenner, & Marsden, 1985), only some patients will develop tardive dyskinesia. Also, from postmortem studies we know that the numbers of dopamine receptors in tardive dyskinesia patients are no different from those in similarly treated schizophrenics without tardive dyskinesia (Crow et al., 1982; Reidever, Jellinger, & Gabriel, 1983). Moreover, in vivo studies of patients with tardive dyskinesia and patients without tardive dyskinesia, using positron-emission tomography, have shown no differences in dopamine D_2-receptor binding (Andersson et al., 1990). Furthermore, no differences have been found between groups with and without tardive dyskinesia in terms of dopamine metabolites in cerebrospinal fluid (CSF) (Pind & Faurbye, 1970) or neuroendocrine markers in plasma (Tamminga et al., 1977). Those negative findings suggest that dopamine receptor supersensitivity may play a part, but not the operant part, in the more complex pathophysiologic process that is tardive dyskinesia.

GABAergic Modification of the Dopamine Hypothesis

Modification of the dopamine receptor supersensitivity hypothesis was needed to incorporate new findings. Clarification of the role of GABA in tardive dyskinesia allowed improvements over the previous models of the pathophysiology of tardive dyskinesia. It has been shown that GABAergic neurons of the substantia nigra reticulata (SNR) form one of the major efferent pathways from the basal ganglia, projecting to the thalamus, superior colliculus, and tegmentum (Figure 29.1), and that GABAergic projections from the striatum inhibit the SNR efferent activity (Beckstead & Frankfurter, 1982; Scheel-Krüger, 1986).

Data from several experimental animal studies support a GABAergic mechanism as part of a cascade of changes that accompany neuroleptic treatment. For example, chronic neuroleptic blockade of dopamine receptors in the neostriatum produces a reduction in striatal GABAergic efferent inhibition of the SNR, analogous to striatal lesioning (Waddington & Cross, 1978; Warzczak, Hume, & Walters, 1981). Furthermore, after long-term neuroleptic exposure, GABA receptor supersensitivity develops in the SNR, and an exaggerated response to the GABA agonist occurs in SNR efferent activity (Freed, Gillin, & Wyatt, 1980; Gale & Casu, 1981). Additional supporting animal data, including a dyskinesia-specific deficit in the GABA synthetic enzyme in monkey SNR (Gunne & Häggström, 1983), are reviewed elsewhere (Kaneda et al., 1992).

Based on this evidence, we have proposed that hypofunction in the GABAergic efferent neurons of the SNR occurs as a consequence of long-term

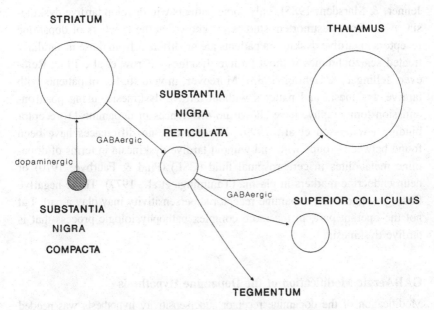

Figure 29.1. GABAergic pathways in the basal ganglia.

neuroleptic treatment and that this is the essential step in the development of tardive dyskinesia. Perhaps the neuroleptic-induced dopamine receptor super-sensitivity produces a cascade of complex neuronal changes in the basal ganglia, which in turn leads to GABA neuronal hypofunction in the SNR. Thus, reduced activity in these GABAergic projection neurons disinhibits the thalamic motor nuclei that modulate motor behavior, causing dyskinesia.

Clinical Evidence for the GABA Hypothesis

Recent clinical data provide indirect evidence for the GABA hypothesis. For instance, GABA concentrations in the CSF are reduced in schizophrenic patients with tardive dyskinesia, as compared with nondyskinetic schizo-phrenics (Thaker et al., 1987). Also, dyskinetic movements have been signifi-cantly reduced when patients with tardive dyskinesia have been treated with GABA agonists. Treatment studies will be reviewed in detail a bit later.

Neurophysiological evidence supporting GABAergic hypofunction of the SNR is also available from oculomotor studies. It appears that saccadic eye movements, ballistic eye movements mediated by the superior colliculus, which receives GABAergic efferents from the SNR, are distributed in patients

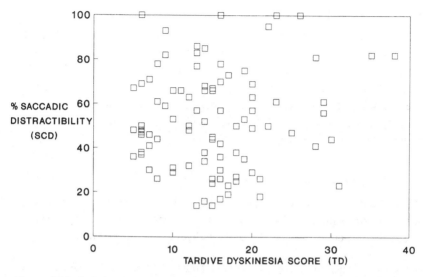

Figure 29.2. Relationship between SCD and tardive dyskinesia score; $r = .08$; mean SCD $= 52.5 \pm 22.4$; $N = 93$ dyskinetic patients.

with tardive dyskinesia. When normal saccadic eye movements occur, the GABA neuron that provides tonic inhibition to the superior colliculus neurons pauses in its firing, reducing inhibition and allowing the superior colliculus to fire and complete a saccade (Hikosaka & Wurtz, 1985). As compared with nondyskinetic schizophrenics, schizophrenic patients with tardive dyskinesia show a twofold increase in the number of inappropriate saccadic eye movements (saccadic distractibility), suggesting a deficit in GABAergic inhibitory activity to the superior colliculus from the SNR (Thaker, Nguyen, & Tamminga, 1989).

Saccadic distractibility therefore appears to mark the presence of tardive dyskinesia; however, among tardive dyskinesia patients there is no association between the severity of dyskinesia and the degree of saccadic distractibility (Figure 29.2). Furthermore, any change in dyskinesia after neuroleptic withdrawal is not associated with a corresponding change in saccadic distractibility in schizophrenics with persistent tardive dyskinesia (Cassady, Thaker, & Tamminga, 1993). Interestingly, however, there is a strong correlation between changes in saccadic distractibility and dyskinetic symptoms in response to a GABA agonist challenge (Cassady et al., 1992). This evidence supports the notion of partially shared GABAergic dysfunction in the parallel motor and oculomotor pathways in patients with tardive dyskinesia.

Clinical Trials of GABA-mimetics

Several types of GABA-mimetics are available. Our discussion will include (1) direct-acting GABA agonists, (2) GABA transaminase inhibitors, (3) weak GABA-mimetics, and (4) benzodiazepines. Although both A and B GABA receptor types have been found in the basal ganglia, it is the $GABA_A$ receptor, the one associated with the chloride ionophore and benzodiazepine receptor, that appears to be the main effector site in the therapeutic action of GABAergic treatments (Lloyd & Morselli, 1987).

$GABA_A$ Receptor Agonists

These drugs act directly on the postsynaptic $GABA_A$ receptor and have chemical structures similar to GABA itself. Three potent, direct-acting agonists are available: muscimol, progabide, and tetrahydroisoxazolopyridinol.

Muscimol. When muscimol, a potent and relatively specific $GABA_A$ agonist, was administered at 7–9 mg/day to neuroleptic-free schizophrenic patients with moderate-to-severe tardive dyskinesia (Tamminga, Crayton, & Chase, 1979), the result was a 48% reduction in the mean dyskinesia score. In some patients receiving dosages between 5 and 9 mg/day, psychotomimetic effects were noted, including intense internal preoccupation, loss of attention and orientation, and mild thought disorder. Their existing hallucinations, delusions, and paranoia, however, were not worsened.

In a more recent study, when muscimol was administered as a single 7-mg challenge dose, with a placebo control, to chronic schizophrenic patients with tardive dyskinesia who were receiving neuroleptics during the study (Cassady et al., 1992), variable effects were seen. Whereas 3 patients became significantly worse, as compared with those on the placebo treatment, another patient showed dramatic improvement. Others had intermediate responses in both directions. Although mild tremor was noted in 1 patient, no psychosis, confusion, or myoclonic twitching was observed. However, concomitant neuroleptic effects appeared to contribute to the worsening of dyskinesia in some patients, an effect not seen in the earlier study. The changes observed using the acute, single-challenge paradigm (reflecting the earliest GABA effects) may be quite different from the steady-state GABAergic effects seen in long-term treatment studies. Perhaps the presence of neuroleptics prohibited the expression of psychotic-like symptoms.

Progabide. In another study, we administered progabide, a structural analogue of GABA and a mixed $GABA_A$ and $GABA_B$ agonist, over 5 weeks at dosages starting at 300 mg daily and increasing every third day to an upper limit of 45 mg·kg^{-1}·d^{-1} (Nguyen, Thaker, & Tamminga, 1989). In addition to its known anticonvulsant actions, antidyskinetic and antidepressant effects have been reported with the use of progabide (Morselli et al., 1980; Thaker, Moran, & Tamminga, 1990a). Progabide lacks the clinical toxicity at therapeutic dosages seen with some other potent GABA-mimetics (Coquelin et al., 1985; Tamminga & Thaker, 1990). We found an average decrease in dyskinesia scores of 28%, as compared with 4% for the placebo-control subjects. No sedation or clinical side effects were seen. Thus far, 33% of our study patients have had mild increases in liver enzymes with progabide treatment, an effect that has proved to be reversible on cessation of progabide treatment, consistent with the findings in other studies (Coquelin et al., 1985; Gerbaldo et al., 1990).

In another study, progabide was given for 6 weeks to dyskinetic schizophrenics on concurrent depot neuroleptic treatment. The patients showed an overall reduction in dyskinesia scores of 43%, without significant side effects (Burner et al., 1989).

Tetrahydroisoxazolopyridinol. In a recent study, 2 young neuroleptic-free schizophrenic patients with tardive dyskinesia showed a 35% reduction in dyskinesia scores after treatment with tetrahydroisoxazolopyridinol (THIP), a direct-acting specific GABA$_A$ agonist and a bicyclic analogue of GABA. However, at dosages of 60 mg/day for 1 patient and 120 mg/day for the other, dissociative episodes occurred, as well as seizures after withdrawal (Thaker et al., 1987). In another study of elderly THIP-treated tardive dyskinesia patients on concurrent neuroleptics, no antidyskinetic effect was found at maximal dosages between 20 and 120 mg/day, although a slight worsening of parkinsonism was observed (Korsgaard et al., 1982). Also, sedation, confusion, and vomiting were prominent in that study.

GABA Transaminase Inhibitors

By inhibiting the GABA catabolic enzyme, the GABA transaminase inhibitors increase GABA concentrations. Two potent drugs available for clinical trials are vigabatrin and γ-acetylenic GABA.

Vigabatrin (γ-vinyl GABA). Vigabatrin, also a structural analogue of GABA, irreversibly inhibits GABA transaminase. It causes few side effects at effective antidyskinetic dosages and is currently used as an anticonvulsant in patients with refractory seizures (Grant & Heel, 1991). It appears that vigabatrin increases GABA concentrations in the CSF by 100% or more in a dose-dependent manner (Grove et al., 1981; Giao et al., 1987; Thaker et al., 1987). Several treatment studies have shown antidyskinetic responses to vigabatrin at maximal dosages between 2 and 8 g/day (Lambert et al., 1982; Danion et al., 1983; Korsgaard, Casey, & Gerlach, 1983; Stahl et al., 1985; Thaker et al., 1987). One negative study, which showed no overall antidyskinetic effect, and side effects of sedation, parkinsonism, and confusion, included mostly elderly patients (Giao et al., 1987).

On the other hand, a group of younger dyskinetic patients who had been withdrawn from neuroleptics showed robust antidyskinetic responses to vigabatrin at 3 g/day (Thaker et al., 1987). In fact, the 7 schizophrenic patients showed a 44% decrease in dyskinesia scores after 3 weeks of vigabatrin treatment, and there were no mental-status changes, sedation, or adverse clinical side effects.

Occasionally, confusion and worsening of psychotic symptoms have been observed with vigabatrin (Lambert et al., 1982; Danion et al., 1983; Korsgaard et al., 1983), and a withdrawal syndrome has been reported (Stahl et al., 1985). Also, increases in parkinsonian symptoms have been observed in some neuroleptic-treated patients. Individual improvements have occasionally been reported in mental status, as well as decreases in the symptoms of anergia, withdrawal, tension, and anxiety. Although a few patients have experienced exacerbation of dyskinesia with vigabatrin treatment, they have tended to be older, on concurrent neuroleptics, and experiencing concurrent dementia.

γ-Acetylenic GABA. The other potent and irreversible transaminase inhibitor, γ-acetylenic GABA, showed an overall moderate antidyskinetic effect in one study (Casey et al., 1980). However, parkinsonism was aggravated in that study's 4 oldest patients, 2 of whom also experienced worsening of dyskinesia with that treatment. Moreover, confusion and agitation were seen in another patient, although reductions in social withdrawal were noted in 2 other patients.

Weak GABA-mimetics

Baclofen and sodium valproate, early GABA-mimetic drugs, appear to have less potent GABAergic activity than the agents described earlier.

Sodium Valproate. In the late 1970s, sodium valproate, a putative GABA-mimetic, was tested in patients with tardive dyskinesia. This anticonvulsant drug raised the concentrations of GABA in the central nervous system and was thought to be an inhibitor of GABA transaminase, but its mechanism of action is unclear (Godin, Heiner, & Mark, 1969; Chapman et al., 1982). In terms of its antidyskinetic effect, mixed findings have been reported. Three controlled studies reported antidyskinetic effects of valproate at dosages between 900 and 2,700 mg/day (Linnoila, Viukari, & Hietala, 1976; Chien, Jung, & Ross-Townsend, 1978; Friis, Christensen, & Gerlach, 1983). Open studies showed similar effects (Casey & Hammerstad, 1979; Crowe, 1983). But in two studies showing no mean effect of valproate on dyskinesia, both improvement and worsening of tardive dyskinesia were observed (Gibson, 1978; Nasrallah, Dunner, & McCalley-Whitters, 1985; Fisk & York, 1987). Furthermore, when valproate alone proved ineffective, the addition of haloperidol produced an antidyskinetic effect greater than that for haloperidol alone (Nair et al., 1980).

Insufficient drug potency and inadequate durations of treatment in the various studies may have been factors that worked against any showing of an antidyskinetic effect (Crowe, 1983). Because valproate provides only weak enzymatic inhibition, higher dosages of the drug, if clinically feasible, might be more effective. Furthermore, the drug's effect is not homogeneous in all brain areas (Perry & Hansen, 1978; Ferkany, Butler, & Enna, 1979). Increased parkinsonism has been observed in a few patients.

Baclofen. Four controlled studies (Korsgaard, 1976; Gerlach, Rye, & Kristjansen, 1978; Stewart et al., 1982; Ananth et al., 1987) have shown improvements in patients with dyskinesia after treatment with baclofen, a cyclic derivative of GABA and an agonist specific to the $GABA_B$ site (Lloyd & Morselli, 1987). Also, open studies (Itil et al., 1980; Wolf et al., 1983) and case reports have shown moderations of dyskinetic and dystonic symptoms with baclofen treatment (Amsterdam & Mendels, 1979; Feder & Moore, 1980; Rosse, Allen, & Lux, 1986; Yassa & Iskander, 1988). However, three studies that examined baclofen treatment showed no antidyskinetic response (Nair et al., 1978; Simpson et al., 1978; Glazer et al., 1985). In a study in which both baclofen and haloperidol were used, significant reductions in the symptoms of tardive dyskinesia, as compared with the use of haloperidol alone, were reported (Nair et al., 1980). In those studies, mean improvements, overall, were small, and the antidyskinetic effects tended to diminish with time, suggesting tolerance, and side effects such as parkinsonism, sedation, and confusion were seen. In other studies, abrupt withdrawal of baclofen has been associated with confusion, psychosis, and worsening of symptoms (Kirubakarai, Mayfield, & Rengachary, 1984; Yassa & Iskander, 1988).

Benzodiazepines

Even before an association was demonstrated between the benzodiazepine-binding site and the $GABA_A$ receptor, benzodiazepines were used to treat involuntary movement disorders. Although benzodiazepines do not act directly on the $GABA_A$ receptor, the benzodiazepine receptor is part of the same ionophore as the $GABA_A$ receptor and facilitates the opening of the chloride channel. Numerous case reports have documented the antidyskinetic effects of diazepam (Singh, 1976; Eapen et al., 1989), alprazolam (Mehta et al., 1985; Jordan & Williams, 1990), clorazepate (Itil, Unverdi, & Mehta, 1974; Mehta, Mehta, & Mathew, 1976), and piracetam (Chaturvedi, 1987). Open treatment studies with many patients have shown success with diazepam (Jus et al., 1974) and clonazepam (O'Flanagan, 1975; Sedman, 1976). Well-controlled studies have shown the efficacy of clonazepam (Bobruff et al., 1981; Thaker et al., 1990b) and diazepam (Godwin-Austen & Clark, 1971; Singh et al., 1982), both of which produced significant antidyskinetic effects. However, two controlled trials with diazepam and alprazolam reported no positive effects (Weber et al., 1983; Csernansky et al., 1988). Finally, of 192 patients reported in the literature (Alphs & Davis, 1986; Thaker et al., 1990b), 80% experienced moderate improvements with benzodiazepine treatment (58% of cases were open and uncontrolled).

Our study of clonazepam for treatment of tardive dyskinesia showed an overall decrease in dyskinesia scores of 35% with dosages ranging from 2.0 to 4.5 mg/day (Thaker et al., 1990b). That study, with a placebo control group, monitored sedation as a study confound. Most patients were on neuroleptics. All but 1 of the 19 patients showed some antidyskinetic response, the greatest responses being seen in those with the more severe and dystonic forms of tardive dyskinesia. We found that tolerance to the antidyskinetic effects of clonazepam developed gradually over 4 months, a finding that had previously been reported (Cutler, 1981; Thaker et al., 1990b).

Unfortunately, the subcortical specificity of these moderate antidyskinetic effects is questionable because of the tendency of benzodiazepines to reduce cortical activity and produce sedation. That effect, however, was not uniformly observed in many of the reviewed studies that reported effective treatment.

Summary of GABA-mimetic Treatments

The bulk of the evidence shows that GABAergic drugs have antidyskinetic effects in the treatment of tardive dyskinesia. The potent, selectively acting compounds are more effective than the weak GABA-mimetics – the adequate dosages for many GABA-mimetics being problematic because of increased incidences of side effects occurring at or near the antidyskinetic dosages. Side effects typically seen are sedation and parkinsonism. Confusional states and organic psychoses have also been induced by the potent GABA agonists, illustrating the characteristically narrow therapeutic window. Tolerance and withdrawal reactions have been seen with many of the GABA-mimetics as well.

GABAergic treatments have not been effective in all cases of tardive dyskinesia. The particulars of neuroleptic treatment (whether or not concurrent with GABA-mimetic treatment, the use of neuroleptic-free intervals, dosage, duration of treatment) are likely to be related to the responses to GABA-mimetics. The best responses have been achieved with treatment protocols using potent GABAergic drugs in the absence of neuroleptics. Factors such as advanced age, dementia, and structural abnormalities in the brain all suggest loss of neuronal cells and appear to be associated with poor antidyskinetic responses. Furthermore, the potential for the presence of subsyndromes of tardive dyskinesia with different pathophysiologies (i.e., dystonia vs. dyskinesia, orofacial vs. truncal) may contribute to the failure to find an effective treatment agent for all cases of tardive dyskinesia.

Progabide and vigabatrin, potent agents that cause less toxicity than other GABA mimetics, may become more widely available for treating tardive dyskinesia once dosage and safety guidelines have been established. Finally, certain $GABA_A$ receptor subtypes recently identified (multiple forms of α, β, and γ subunits) appear to have neuroanatomic specificities and cell-type specificities (Fritschy et al., 1992; Wisden et al., 1992). It is expected that these findings will herald the development of GABA agonists specific to certain neurons with unique subtypes of GABA receptors. Such drugs will significantly advance the study of GABAergic mechanisms and improve treatments for patients with tardive dyskinesia.

A GABAergic Perspective on Management of Tardive Dyskinesia

Certainly the management of tardive dyskinesia should include primary prevention and consideration of pharmacologic treatments other than typical neuroleptics for treatment of psychotic patients of advanced age and those with concomitant affective syndrome and/or organic deficits. Perhaps the GABA-mimetics will be able to prevent the development of tardive dyskinesia, as suggested by animal experiments (Kaneda et al., 1992; Gao et al.,

1994), though they have yet to be tested in humans. Secondary prevention must include screening and detection of mild symptoms early in the course of tardive dyskinesia, as well as consideration of a reduction in cumulative neuroleptic dose over time. Measurement of saccadic distractibility may become a useful tool for assessment of potential GABAergic hypofunction in high-risk patients or in those for whom the diagnosis of tardive dyskinesia is questionable. Tertiary prevention must focus on alleviating the dysfunction secondary to tardive dyskinesia. In most cases, neuroleptic drugs cannot be completely withdrawn because of persistent psychotic symptoms. Even after withdrawal, and in cases where clozapine or another atypical neuroleptic has been substituted, a disabling dyskinesia may continue.

Of the currently available GABA-mimetics, we consider clonazepam to be a highly practical pharmacologic agent, given its efficacy, potency, safety, and side-effect profile. Antidyskinetic effects are seen in patients given clonazepam at dosages ranging from 2 to 4 mg/day. However, because tolerance develops over periods of 4–6 months, we advocate the use of periodic taperings and drug withdrawals. We find that giving patients a few weeks of respite without clonazepam allows them to experience the original antidyskinetic potency at the original dosages. We also usually reserve adjunctive treatment for those who suffer functional impairments (physical or psychosocial) secondary to the dyskinetic symptoms. In such patients, the potential risks from treatment are most likely outweighed by the potential benefits.

Conclusion

Our clinical studies, involving biochemical, neurophysiological, and pharmacologic data, support the idea that GABAergic dysfunction is critical in the manifestation of tardive dyskinesia. Our animal data and findings are consistent with this as well. Today, the GABA hypothesis of tardive dyskinesia, an extension of the dopamine receptor supersensitivity hypothesis, is more consistent with the accumulating evidence. As a result, the concurrence of dyskinesia and oculomotor saccadic distractibility in schizophrenics with tardive dyskinesia can be explained by parallel reductions in GABAergic inhibition at the thalamus and superior colliculus, respectively. Also, various GABA-mimetics have been tested in patients with tardive dyskinesia and have shown antidyskinetic effects. Their side effects, however, have limited the clinical use of many of these agents. Safe and potent GABAergic agents may soon become available for treatment of tardive dyskinesia. Until then, less potent and nonspecific GABA-mimetics may be clinically useful for alleviating severe dyskinetic symptoms.

References

Alphs, L. D., & Davis, J. M. (1986). Treatments for tardive dyskinesia, an overview of noncatecholaminergic/noncholinergic treatments. In *Movement Disorders*, ed. N. S. Shah & A. G. Donald, pp. 205–26. New York; Plenum Press.

Amsterdam, J. D., & Mendels, J. (1979). Treatment-resistant tardive dyskinesia: a new therapeutic approach. *Am. J. Psychiatry* 136:1197–8.

Ananth, J., Djenderedjian, A., Beshay, M., Kamal, M., Kodjian, A., & Barriga, C. (1987). Baclofen in the treatment of tardive dyskinesia. *Curr. Ther. Res.* 42:11–14.

Andersson, U., Eckernas, S. A., Hartvig, P., Ulin, J., Langstrom, B., & Häggström, J. E. (1990). Striatal binding of ^{11}C-NMSP studies with positron emission tomography in patients with persistent tardive dyskinesia: no evidence for altered dopamine D_2 receptor binding. *J. Neural. Transm.* 79:215–26.

Beckstead, R. M., & Frankfurter, A. (1982). The distribution and some morphological features of substantia nigra neurons that project to the thalamus, superior colliculus and pedunculopontine nucleus in the monkey. *Neuroscience* 7:2377–88.

Bobruff, A., Gardos, G., Tarsy, D., Rapkin, R. M., Cole, J. O., & Moore, P. (1981). Clonazepam and phenobarbital in tardive dyskinesia. *Am. J. Psychiatry* 138:189–93.

Burner, M., Giroux, C., L'Heritier, C., Garreau, M., & Morselli, P. L. (1989). Preliminary observations on the therapeutic action of progabide in tardive dyskinesia. *Brain Dysfunct.* 2:289–96.

Casey, D. E., Gerlach, J., Magelund, G., & Christensen, T. R. (1980). Gammaacetylenic GABA in tardive dyskinesia. *Arch. Gen. Psychiatry* 37:1376–9.

Casey, D. E., & Hammerstad, J. P. (1979). Sodium valproate in tardive dyskinesia. *J. Clin. Psychiatry* 40:483–5.

Cassady, S. L., Thaker, G. K., Moran, M., Birt, A., & Tamminga, C. (1992). GABA agonist-induced changes in motor, oculomotor, and attention measures correlate in schizophrenics with tardive dyskinesia. *Biol. Psychiatry* 32:192–202.

Cassady, S. L., Thaker, G. K., & Tamminga, C. A. (1993). Pharmacologic characterization of saccadic distractibility in schizophrenics with tardive dyskinesia. *Psychopharmacol. Bull.* 29:235–40.

Chapman, A., Keane, P. E., Meldrum, B. S., Simiand, J., & Vernieres, J. C. (1982). Mechanism of anticonvulsant action of valproate. *Prog. Neurobiol.* 19:315–59.

Chaturvedi, S. K. (1987). Piracetam for drug-induced dyskinesia. *J. Clin. Psychiatry* 48:255.

Chien, C., Jung, K., & Ross-Townsend, A. (1978). Efficacies of agents related to GABA, dopamine, and acetylcholine in the treatment of tardive dyskinesia. *Psychopharmacol. Bull.* 14:20–2.

Coquelin, J. P., Krall, R., Bossi, L., Musch, B., & Morselli, P. L. (1885). Drug safety profile of progabide. In *Epilepsy and GABA Receptor Agonists – Basic and Therapeutic Research*, ed. G. Bartholini, L. Bossi, K. G. Lloyd, P. L. Morselli, pp. 431–40. New York: Raven Press.

Crow, T. J., Cross, A. J., Johnstone, E. C., Owen, F., Owens, D. G. C., & Waddington, J. L. (1982). Abnormal involuntary movements in schizophrenia: Are they related to the disease process or its treatment? Are they associated with changes in dopamine receptor? *J. Clin. Psychopharmacol.* 2:336–40.

Crowe, B. M. (1983). Symptom control in tardive dyskinesia. *Br. J. Psychiatry* 143:419–25.

Csernansky, J. G., Tacke, U., Rusen, D., & Hollister, L. E. (1988). The effect of benzodiazepines on tardive dyskinesia symptoms. *J. Clin. Psychopharmacol.* 8:154–5.

Cutler, N. R. (1981). Clonazepam and tardive dyskinesia. *Am. J. Psychiatry* 138:1127.

Danion, J. M., Singer, L., Tell, G., & Schechter, P. (1983). Gamma-vinyl GABA et dyskinésies tardives: Une étude en simple insu contre placebo. *Ann. Med. Psychol. (Paris)* 142:101–10.

Eapen, V., Mukherjee, D., Chandra, P., Sinha, V., Khanna, S., & Channabasa-vanna, S. M. (1989). High-dose diazepam in neuroleptic-resistant schizophrenia with tardive dyskinesia. *J. Clin. Psychiatry* 50:309.

Feder, R., & Moore, D. C. (1980). Baclofen and tardive dyskinesia. *Am. J. Psychiatry* 137:633–4.

Ferkany, J., Butler, I., & Enna, S. (1979). Effects of drugs on rat brain, cerebrospinal fluid and blood GABA content. *J. Neurochem.* 33:29–33.

Fisk, G. G., & York, S. M. (1987). The effect of sodium valproate on tardive dyskinesia – revisited. *Br. J. Psychiatry* 150:542–6.

Freed, W. J., Gillin, J. C., & Wyatt, R. J. (1980). Anomalous behavioral response to imidazoleacetic acid, a GABA agonist, in animals treated chronically with haloperidol. *Biol. Psychiatry* 15:21–35.

Friis, T., Christensen, T. R., & Gerlach, J. (1983). Sodium valproate and biperiden in neuroleptic-induced akathisia, parkinsonism and hyperkinesia. *Acta Psychiatr. Scand.* 67:178–87.

Fritschy, J. M., Benke, D., Mertens, S., Oertel, W. H., Bachi, T., & Mohler, H. (1992). Five subtypes of A gamma-aminobutyric acid receptors identified in neurons by double and triple immunofluorescence staining with subunit-specific antibodies. *Proc. Natl. Acad. Sci. (U.S.A.)* 89:6726–30.

Gale, K., & Casu, M. (1981). Dynamic utilization of GABA in substantia nigra: regulation by dopamine and GABA in the striatum, and its clinical and behavioral implication. *Mol. Cell. Biochem.* 39:367–405.

Gao, X. M., Kakigi, T., Friedman, M. B., & Tamminga, C. A. (1994). Tiagabine inhibits haloperidol-induced oral dyskinesias in rats. *J. Neural Transm.* 95:63–69.

Gerbaldo, H., Nguyen, J. A., Thaker, G. K., Moran, M., & Tamminga, C. A. (1990). Decrease in tardive dyskinesia with progabide, a mixed GABA agonist. *Biol. Psychiatry* 27:131A.

Gerlach, J., Rye, T., & Kristjansen, P. (1978). Effect of baclofen on tardive dyskinesia. *Psychopharmacology (Berlin)* 56:145–51.

Giao, J. M., Pollak, P., Hommel, M., & Perret, J. (1987). Clinical and biochemical effects of gamma-vinyl GABA in tardive dyskinesia. *J. Neurol. Neurosurg. Psychiatry* 50:1674–8.

Gibson, A. C. (1978). Sodium valproate and tardive dyskinesia. *Br. J. Psychiatry* 133:82.

Glazer, W. M., Moore, D. C., Bowers, M. B., Bunney, B. S., & Roffman, M. (1985). The treatment of tardive dyskinesia with baclofen. *Psychopharmacology (Berlin)* 87:480–3.

Godin, Y., Heiner, L., & Mark, J. (1969). Effects of di-*n*-propylacetate, an anticonvulsant compound, on GABA metabolism. *J. Neurochem.* 16:869–73.

Godwin-Austen, R. B., & Clark, T. (1971). Persistent phenothiazine dyskinesia treated with tetrabenazine. *Br. Med. J.* 4:25–6.

Grant, S. M., & Heel, R. C. (1991). Vigabatrin. *Drugs* 41:889–926.

Grove, J., Schecter, P. J., Tell, G., Koch-Weser, J., Sjoerdsma, A., Warter, J. M., Marescaux, C., & Rumbach, L. (1981). Increased gamma-aminobutyric acid (GABA), homocarnosine and β-alanine in cerebrospinal fluid of patients treated with gamma-vinyl GABA (4-amino-hex-5-enoic acid). *Life Sci.* 28:2431–9.

Gunne, L. M., & Häggström, J. E. (1983). Reductions of nigral glutamic acid decarboxylase in rats with neuroleptic-induced oral dyskinesia. *Psychopharmacology (Berlin)* 81:191–4.

Hikosaka, O., & Wurtz, R. H. (1985). Modification of saccadic eye movements by GABA-related substances. *J. Neurophysiol.* 53:266–308.

Itil, T. M., Herkert, E., Schneider, S. J., Luhar, J., Fredrickson, J. W., & Roffman, M. (1980). Baclofen in the treatment of tardive dyskinesia: open label study. *Acta Therapeutica* 6:315–23.

Itil, T. M., Unverdi, C., & Mehta, D. (1974). Clorazepate dipotassium in tardive dyskinesia. *Am. J. Psychiatry* 131:1291.

Jordan, H. W., & Williams, B. C. (1990). Tardive dyskinesia successfully treated with alprazolam. *J. Natl. Med. Assoc.* 82:673–5.

Jus, K., Jus, A., Gautier, J., Villeneuve, A., Pires, P., Pineau, R., & Villeneuve, R. (1974). Studies on the action of certain pharmacological agents on tardive dyskinesia and on the rabbit syndrome. *Int. J. Clin. Pharmacol.* 9:138–45.

Kaneda, H., Shirakawa, O., Dale, J., Goodman, L., Bachus, S. E., & Tamminga, C. A. (1992). Co-administration of progabide inhibits haloperidol-induced oral dyskinesias in rats. *Eur. J. Pharmacol.* 212:43–49.

Kirubakarai, V., Mayfield, D., & Rengachary, S. (1984). Dyskinesia and psychosis in a patient following baclofen withdrawal. *Am. J. Psychiatry* 141:692–3.

Korsgaard, S. (1976). Baclofen (Lioresal) in the treatment of neuroleptic-induced tardive dyskinesia. *Acta Psychiatr. Scand.* 54:17–24.

Korsgaard, S., Casey, D. E., & Gerlach, J. (1983). Effect of gamma-vinyl GABA in tardive dyskinesia. *Psychiatry Res.* 8:261–9.

Korsgaard, S., Casey, D. E., Gerlach, J., Hetmar, O., Kaldan, B., & Mikkelsen, L. B. (1982). The effect of tetrahydroisoxazolopyridinol (THIP) in tardive dyskinesia. *Arch. Gen. Psychiatry* 39:1017–21.

Lambert, P. A., Cantiniaux, P., Chabannes, J. P., Tell, G. P., Schecter, P. J., & Koch-Weser, J. (1982). Essai therapeutique du gamma-vinyl GABA, un inhibiteur de la GABA-transaminase, dans les dyskinésies tardives induites par les neuroleptiques. *Encephale* 8:371–6.

Linnoila, M., Viukari, M., & Hietala, O. (1976). Effects of sodium valproate on tardive dyskinesia. *Br. J. Psychiatry* 129:114–19.

Lloyd, K. G., & Morselli, P. L. (1987). Psychopharmacology of GABAergic drugs. In *Psychopharmacology: The Third Generation*, ed. H. Meltzer, pp. 183–95. New York, Raven Press.

Mackay, A. V. P., Iverson, L. L., Rossor, M. B., Spokes, E., Bird, E., Arregui, A., Creese, I., & Snyder, S. H. (1982). Increased brain dopamine and dopamine receptors in schizophrenia. *Arch. Gen. Psychiatry* 39:991–7.

Mehta, D., Eaton, J., Burch, M., & Mehta, S. (1985). Observations in tardive dyskinesia. *J. Clin. Psychiatry* 46:73.

Mehta, D., Mehta, S., & Mathew, P. (1976). Failure of deanol in treating tardive dyskinesia. *Am. J. Psychiatry* 133:1467.

Morselli, P. L., Bossi, L., Henry, J. F., Zarifian, E., & Bartholini, G. (1980). On the therapeutic action of SL 76,002, a new GABA-mimetic agent: preliminary observations in neuropsychiatric disorders. *Brain Res. Bull.* 5:411–14.

Nair, N. P. V., Lal, S., Schwartz, G., & Thavundayil, J. X. (1980). Effect of sodium valproate and baclofen in tardive dyskinesia: clinical and neuroendocrine studies. *Adv. Biochem. Psychopharmacol.* 24:437–41.

Nair, N. P. V., Yassa, R., Ruiz-Navarro, J., & Schwartz, G. (1978). Baclofen in the treatment of tardive dyskinesia. *Am. J. Psychiatry* 135:1562.

Nasrallah, H. A., Dunner, F. J., & McCalley-Whitters, M. (1985). A placebo-controlled trial of valproate in tardive dyskinesia. *Biol. Psychiatry* 20:205–8.

Nguyen, J. A., Thaker, G. K., & Tamminga, C. A. (1989). Gamma-aminobutyric acid (GABA) pathways in tardive dyskinesia. *Psychiatr. Ann.* 19:302–9.

O'Flanagan, P. M. (1975). Clonazepam in the treatment of drug-induced dyskinesia. *Br. Med. J.* 1:269–70.

Perry, T., & Hansen, S. (1978). Biochemical effects in man and rat of three drugs which can increase brain GABA content. *J. Neurochem.* 30:679–84.

Pind, K., & Faurbye, A. (1970). Concentration of HVA and 5-HIAA in the CSF after treatment with probenecid in patients with drug-induced tardive dyskinesia. *Acta Psychiatr. Scand.* 46:323–6.

Reidever, P., Jellinger, K., & Gabriel, E. (1983). ^{3}H-spiperone binding to post-mortem putamen in paranoid and non-paranoid schizophrenics. In *Psychiatry: The State of the Art*, ed. P. Pichot, pp. 563–70. New York: Plenum Press.

Rosse, R. B., Allen, A., & Lux, W. E. (1986). Baclofen treatment in a patient with tardive dystonia. *J. Clin. Psychiatry* 47:474–5.

Rupniak, M. N., Jenner, P., & Marsden, C. D. (1985). The effect of chronic neuroleptic administration on cerebral dopamine receptor function. *Life Sci.* 32:2289–311.

Scheel-Kruger, J. (1986). Dopamine–GABA interactions: evidence that GABA transmits, modulates and mediates dopaminergic functions in the basal ganglia and the limbic system. *Acta Neurol. Scand. (Suppl.)* 73:1–54.

Sedman, G. (1976). Clonazepam in the treatment of tardive oral dyskinesia. *Br. Med. J.* 4:583.

Simpson, G. M., Lee, J. H., Shrivastava, R. K., & Branchey, M. H. (1978). Baclofen in the treatment of tardive dyskinesia and schizophrenia. *Psychopharmacol. Bull.* 14:16–18.

Singh, M. M. (1976). Diazepam in the treatment of tardive dyskinesia. *Int. Pharmacopsychiatry* 11:232–4.

Singh, M. M., Becker, R. E., Pitman, R. K., Nasrallah, H. A., Lal, H., Dufresne, R. L., Weber, S. S., & McCalley-Whitters, M. (1982). Diazepam-induced changes in tardive dyskinesia: suggestions for a new conceptual model. *Biol. Psychiatry* 17:729–42.

Stahl, S. M., Thornton, J. E., Simpson, M. L., Berger, P. A., & Napoliello, M. J. (1985). Gamma-vinyl-GABA treatment of tardive dyskinesia and other movement disorders. *Biol. Psychiatry* 20:888–93.

Stewart, R. M., Rollins, J., Beckham, B., & Roffman, M. (1982). Baclofen in tardive dyskinesia patients maintained on neuroleptics. *Clin. Neuropharmacol.* 5:365–73.

Tamminga, C. A., Crayton, J. W., & Chase, T. N. (1979). Improvement in tardive dyskinesia after muscimol therapy. *Arch. Gen. Psychiatry* 36:595–8.

Tamminga, C. A., Smith, R. C., Pandey, G., Frohman, L. A., & Davis, J. M. (1977). A neuroendocrine study of supersensitivity in tardive dyskinesia. *Arch. Gen. Psychiatry* 34:1199–203.

Tamminga, C. A., & Thaker, G. K. (1990). GABAmimetic drugs in hyperkinetic involuntary movement disorders and their effects on mental status. *Drug. Dev. Res.* 21:227–33.

Thaker, G. K., Moran, M., & Tamminga, C. A. (1990a). GABAmimetics: a new class of antidepressant agents? *Arch. Gen. Psychiatry* 47:298–8.

Thaker, G. K., Nguyen, J. A., Stauss, M. E., Jacobson, R., Kaup, B. A., & Tamminga, C. A. (1990b). Clonazepam treatment of tardive dyskinesia: a practical GABAmimetic strategy. *Am. J. Psychiatry* 147:445–51.

Thaker, G. K., Nguyen, J. A., & Tamminga, C. A. (1989). Saccadic distractibility in schizophrenic patients with tardive dyskinesia. *Arch. Gen. Psychiatry* 46:755–6.

Thaker, G. K., Tamminga, C. A., Alphs, L. D., Lafferman, J., Ferraro, T. N., & Hare, T. A. (1987). Brain gamma-aminobutyric acid abnormality in tardive dyskinesia. *Arch. Gen. Psychiatry* 44:522–9.

Waddington, J. L., & Cross, A. J. (1978). Denervation supersensitivity in the striato-nigral GABA pathway. *Nature* 276:618–20.

Warzczak, B. L., Hume, C., & Walters, J. R. (1981). Supersensitivity of substantia nigra pars reticulata neurons to GABAergic drugs after striatal lesions. *Life Sci.* 28:2411–20.

Weber, S. S., Dufresne, R. L., Becker, R. E., & Mastrati, P. (1983). Diazepam in tardive dyskinesia. *Drug Intell. Clin. Pharm.* 17:523–7.

Wisden, W., Laurie, D. J., Monyer, H., & Seeburg, P. H. (1992). The distribution of 13 GABA$_A$ receptor subunit mRNAs in the rat brain. *J. Neurosci.* 12:1040–62.

Wolf, M. E., Keener, S., Mathis, P., & Mosniam, A. D. (1983). Phenylethylamine-like properties of baclofen. *Neuropsychobiology* 9:219–22.

Yassa, R., & Iskander, H. (1988). Baclofen-induced psychosis: two cases and a review. *J. Clin. Psychiatry* 49:318–20.

30

Using Biofeedback to Train Suppression of the Oral-Lingual Movements of Tardive Dyskinesia

RONALD C. FUDGE, Ph.D., and CECILE E. SISON, Ph.D.

The involuntary movement disorder known as tardive dyskinesia typically occurs after long-term administration of neuroleptic drugs. It is most commonly manifested as oral-buccal-lingual movements that are distinct in their manifestation, often including tongue protrusion, grimacing, masticatory movements, and, at times, choreoathetoid movements of the trunk and limbs (Tarsy & Baldessarini, 1977; American Psychiatric Association, 1980; Granacher, 1981; Smith & Kane, 1982; DeVeaugh-Geiss, 1982; Wexler, 1984; Barnes, 1987; Yagi & Itoh, 1987). It is recommended that neuroleptics be withdrawn from patients with tardive dyskinesia if their clinical conditions permit. Although initially neuroleptic withdrawal may exacerbate the abnormal movements, many patients experience remission of abnormal movements after several months. But in many cases the patients' psychiatric conditions will preclude discontinuation of neuroleptics. Indeed, the dyskinesia itself may be severe enough to require neuroleptic medication. The current clinical wisdom that drugs that produce tardive dyskinesia can also suppress it, and vice versa (Jus, Jus, & Fontaine, 1979), is consistent with the dopamine-supersensitivity hypothesis. Tardive dyskinesia appears to be produced by neuroleptic medication, on the one hand, and is often treated with neuroleptic medication, on the other. This relationship of pharmacologic intervention as both cause and treatment argues for an investigation of possible nonpharmacologic treatments for tardive dyskinesia, as either alternative or adjunctive treatments for tardive dyskinesia. Nonpharmacologic interventions should have the added benefits of being low in cost and highly unlikely to exacerbate the condition.

The contents of this chapter reflect the views of the authors and in no way are to be construed as reflecting the policies of the Department of Veterans Affairs or the Franklin Delano Roosevelt Hospital.

Tardive dyskinesia is believed to be coincident with neuroleptic phar-macologic intervention. However, attentional and motor-awareness factors have reportedly been linked to the frequency, amplitude, and severity of oral-lingual-facial motor activity (Jeste & Wyatt, 1982; Kane et al., 1984). Although pervasive and distinct to an observer, the oral-lingual movements of tardive dyskinesia, in contrast to those associated with extrapyramidal symp-toms (EPSs), often occur without the patient being aware of them (Alex-opoulos, 1979).

The severity of dyskinetic movements can vary dramatically from moment to moment, and such movements are likely to increase when the patient is involved in simple motor tasks. It has been observed that when patients with oral-lingual movements are made aware of their movements, they can exer-cise limited volitional control over them.

Awareness of the occurrence of a response, as measured by the ability to discriminate that response, is an important first step in the acquisition of volitional control over that response (Brener, 1974; Roberts et al., 1984; Fudge & Adams, 1985). Because tardive dyskinesia patients apparently pos-sess some ability to control oral-lingual movements once their attention is directed to those movements, we have reasoned that the use of operant-conditioning techniques to increase that awareness might be of help in acquir-ing a measure of control over the movements. To accomplish this, we have incorporated the principles of biofeedback into a training method.

"Biofeedback" can be defined as the use of external monitoring to train people to influence their bodily processes (previously unregulated by volun-tary acts) or their physiological responses whose regulation has been inter-rupted by trauma or disease (Blanchard & Epstein, 1977). As individuals listen to a varying tone or watch the variations of a light, the variations of the tone or the light being contingent on a change in an autonomically mediated response, they can, to some extent, learn to control that response.

The work of Miller and Dworkin (1974) with operant conditioning of autonomic responses in both humans and animals, the blood-pressure studies of Shapiro, Schwartz, and Tursky (1972), and numerous other related studies seem to suggest the possibility of noninvasive treatments for certain physi-ological dysfunctions. The Health and Public Policy Committee of the Ameri-can Psychiatric Association has described the use of biofeedback for various neuromuscular disorders, noting that electromyographic (EMG) feedback has been reported to have produced positive results in many areas: spinal-cord and peripheral-nerve injuries; cerebral palsy; muscular atrophy from arthritis, or following surgery; hemiparesis caused by head injury; Huntington's chorea; tremor; Parkinson's disease; facial palsy; torsion dystonias, particularly spasmodic torticollis. Supportive of that position is a substantial literature dealing with the effective use of biofeedback in treating motor disorders such as torticollis (Brudny, Grynbaum, & Korein, 1974), stroke paralysis (Bodenhamer, Coleman, & Achterberg, 1986), hemifacial spasm (Booker, Rubow, & Coleman, 1969), and sphincter control (Mcleod, 1983).

Biofeedback

When we reviewed the behavioral literature for instances in which biofeedback techniques had been used to reduce the abnormal movements of tardive dyskinesia, our search revealed several studies that had specifically used biofeedback training to suppress the oral-lingual movements associated with tardive dyskinesia.

Albanese and Gaardner (1977) reported on 2 patients with facial tardive dyskinesia treated with EMG biofeedback training of the masseter muscle. The patients were instructed to decrease the pitch of a tone, the frequency of a "beep" sound, or the amplitude displayed on a visual gauge, all such decreases being controlled by decreases in the movement amplitude of the masseter muscle. Both patients began their training shortly after diagnosis of tardive dyskinesia. Training reduced their dyskinetic movements to negligible amounts, and both patients remained movement-free at a 3-month follow-up session. Though encouraging, the results in that study must be viewed within the context of the small number of participants and the absence of objective criteria to measure movement.

Sherman (1979) reported on 1 patient treated with EMG feedback of masseter-muscle movement. The initial use of muscle-relaxation exercises and frontalis feedback, which reduced tension headaches and self-reported anxiety, had little effect on the dyskinetic movements. However, five subsequent 20-minute sessions of biofeedback training of masseter activity, coupled with instructions to use that new muscle awareness outside of the laboratory, had reduced jaw movements completely by the fourth session. That effect was maintained at a 15-month follow-up session. The patient attributed alleviation of the dyskinetic symptoms to increased awareness of jaw movements after biofeedback training. Sherman acknowledged that no absolute measurements of masseter movements were made and that follow-up information consisted solely of the patient's self-report.

Farrar (1976) reported the treatment history of 1 patient with oral-facial dyskinesia. The patient was given a portable feedback device that provided tonal feedback for oral-facial movements. Feedback training was conducted for 2 hours each day. Although both Farrar and the patient reported a significant reduction in oral-facial movements, those results likewise must be interpreted in light of the absence of objective measurements of movement and a participant pool.

Abrams (1986) used feedback training of muscle activity and programmed instructions in deep relaxation for 8 inpatients. She noted that although the patients were able to reduce their movements during training sessions, the effects were minimal between sessions. That study is noteworthy for its objective measurements of dyskinetic movements using EMG and for its slightly larger number of participants.

Although such studies are notable for their attempts to use biofeedback training to reduce dyskinetic movements, several methodological and procedural flaws make evaluation of their findings problematic. In particular, we note the low numbers of participants. The total number of participants in all those studies was 12. In none of those studies was any attempt made to control for the effects of the experimenter or for time effects or to use nontreatment control groups to control for spontaneous recovery. Objective measurements of dyskinetic movements were lacking as well. In addition, no mention was made of attempts to standardize medication dosages, and there was no mention of the use of anticholinergic medications. Nevertheless, those studies seem to suggest a consistent positive effect of feedback training. Indeed, each reported some degree of success with biofeedback, indicating that the idea has merit. Nevertheless, questions remain regarding the efficacy, practicality, and utility of biofeedback training. To try to answer such questions and to determine for ourselves the efficacy of biofeedback in treating tardive dyskinesia, we designed a series of related studies.

Study 1

A pilot study, study 1, was conducted to develop methods for application of biofeedback in an effort to train movement suppression (Fudge et al., 1987).

Methods

Participants. Eight psychiatric inpatients at the Franklin Delano Roosevelt Department of Veterans Affairs Hospital, Montrose, New York, diagnosed as having tardive dyskinesia, with Abnormal Involuntary Movement Scale (AIMS) scores of at least 2 on two of the oral-lingual movement items, were asked to volunteer. Medication dosages were continually monitored during the study, and weekly AIMS testing was conducted to monitor dyskinetic movements.

Apparatus. Movements were assessed from EMG data on activity in the masseter, genioglossus, and frontalis muscles. EMG data were recorded using bipolar placement of 1-cm electrodes in specific locations. Lingual activity was detected from leads placed 1.5 cm apart on the ventral surface of the genioglossus muscle, starting from the symphysis menti of the mandible. Masseter activity was recorded from leads placed 1.5 cm apart on the dominant side of the masseter. Frontalis activity was recorded from leads placed 1 cm above the nasion and 1 cm from the midline. EMG signals were recorded by a Grass model 7P511 preamplifier (Grass Medical Instruments, Quincy, Massachusetts) using a 0.3-second time constant. Amplified EMG signals were integrated using Coulbourn integrators (Coulbourn Instruments, Lehigh Valley, Pennsylvania) interfaced with a Data General minicomputer (Data General Computer Corporation, Newton, Massachusetts) using a customized A/D converter. Physiological data were sampled at a rate of 1 msec per sample. All feedback and data transformations were processed by computer. The participant was seated in a reclining chair, adjusted as needed, in an air- and sound-conditioned room. To reduce extraneous noise, all instructions and feedback tones were presented through headphones.

Procedure. All participating patients were given sessions of biofeedback training, with feedback contingent on movement suppression. The length of each session was 20 minutes, with an initial 3 minutes of baseline activity, followed by 15 minutes of feedback training and another 2 minutes of baseline activity. All participants received the same training sequence. The number of sessions for the participants varied, largely as a function of their psychiatric conditions and willingness to continue the study. All participants had a minimum of 15 training sessions, with 1 patient completing 30 sessions.

All participants had electrodes placed to monitor EMG activity in the masseter, forehead, and genioglossus (tongue) muscles. The study design included a single-case format that enabled us to determine the most efficient procedures by changing the feedback contingencies and modalities. The design was an ABACA design, where condition A provided noncontingent feedback, condition B provided feedback for masseter activity, and condition C provided feedback for genioglossus activity.

Results

Our initial study indicated that biofeedback training had some efficacy for suppressing dyskinetic movements. All participants evidenced some suppression of movements following biofeedback training, with the results from the genioglossus feedback proving to be superior to those from the masseter feedback. The study also demonstrated the utility of EMG data as objective measures of movement. In other words, using EMG data we were able to quantify the suppressive effects of training. In addition, the use of the AIMS as a dependent variable proved valuable, for we were able to show that suppression was reflected in reduced AIMS scores during training. Nevertheless, although we were able to produce large-magnitude reductions of dyskinetic activity during training sessions, the effects that persisted between sessions were small.

Several confounds should be noted in this study: the small number of participants, the effects of time, and placebo and other experimenter biases that limit any extrapolation of these findings to a larger population. Indeed, behavioral and pharmacologic interventions are often seen as effective simply because of the demand characteristics (placebo effects) of the task. Moreover, because no attempt was made to monitor medication changes, and all participants were given anticholinergic medications to control dyskinetic movements, it is difficult to distinguish among medication effects, placebo effects, and training effects.

Study 2

Although we were encouraged by our findings in study 1, the aforementioned criticisms tempered our enthusiasm somewhat, prompting the design of study 2 (Fudge et al., 1991).

Methods

Participants. Twenty male inpatients at the Franklin Delano Roosevelt Department of Veterans Affairs Hospital, diagnosed as having tardive dyskinesia, were selected for the study. We administered the Brief Psychiatric Rating Scale (BPRS) (Overall & Gorham, 1962) weekly to monitor their psychiatric states during medication reductions. We also administered the AIMS, initially to verify inclusion criteria, and then weekly to monitor the severity of tardive dyskinesia. All participants with AIMS scores indicating at least mild tardive dyskinesia (rated as 2) in two of the first four AIMS areas (areas involving facial movements), or a single score of 3 (moderate) in one of those areas, were considered appropriate for inclusion. The AIMS raters were calibrated with each other at the time of the baseline rating for each participant, and at weekly intervals thereafter.

All of the patients who volunteered had histories of at least 9 months of tardive dyskinesia, with a minimum of 2 years on neuroleptic medications. Patients were excluded if they had concurrent neurological disorders or severe dental abnormalities that might mask or potentiate dyskinetic symptoms. The Mini-Mental State Examination (MMSE) (Folstein, Folstein, & McHugh, 1975) was administered at baseline. Participants with MMSE scores below 20 were considered too demented to cooperate. Participants' ages ranged from 45 to 72 years at the time of the study. Participants were randomly assigned, 10 to each of two groups (TRUE feedback or FALSE feedback).

Apparatus. The EMG signals were recorded using a Grass model 7P511 preamplifier with a 0.3-second time constant. Amplified EMG signals were integrated via Coulbourn integrators, interfaced to an IBM AT/PC computer through a Coulbourn A/D converter. Physiological data were recorded on line using the IBM AT/PC computer, with a sampling rate of 1 ms per sample. Feedback, data transformation, and data storage were all processed by computer. EMG activity was detected using 1-cm silver/silver chloride pre-jelled disposable electrodes (Vermont Medical Inc., Bellows Falls, Vermont). The participant was seated in a reclining chair, adjusted as needed, in an air- and sound-conditioned room. To reduce extraneous noise, all instructions and feedback tones were presented through headphones.

Dosage Adjustment. Prior to the biofeedback phase of the study, neuroleptic and anticholinergic medications were reduced in an attempt to find the lowest effective dosage for each participant. All participants were first shifted to a single neuroleptic. The dosage of the neuroleptic was reduced in weekly 20% decrements, with reductions titrated to BPRS scores (raters were blind as to medication status); reductions were continued until a zero dose was achieved or BPRS scores increased by 20%. After the lowest functional neuroleptic dosage was established, anticholinergic medications were reduced in similar fashion, with placebos being substituted for anticholinergics in order to keep the apparent administration of medications constant. Extrapyramidal symptoms were monitored daily. With the exception of one individual, no participant received an anticholinergic prior to feedback training. Participants were then randomly assigned to one of the two treatment groups.

Feedback Training. Participants were given 10 sessions of biofeedback training on consecutive days, each session lasting 15 minutes. The EMG activity was recorded from the genioglossus, masseter, and forehead muscles. Feedback was contingent on an increase in genioglossus activity for the TRUE feedback group, and a random presentation for the FALSE feedback group. The AIMS ratings were taken prior to feedback training and after the fifth and tenth feedback-training sessions. Ratings were also conducted at 1 week and 2 weeks after feedback training.

Results

The findings indicated that oral dyskinetic movements could be reduced through biofeedback training. Statistically significant differences were observed between the TRUE and FALSE feedback groups. Although the participants demonstrated extreme variability over training sessions, the group differences were both consistent and reliable. Training was specific to the target area (genioglossus), although notable reductions were seen in both groups for the forehead muscles. In general, both groups showed reductions in all EMG activities, with the TRUE feedback group showing significantly more suppression of oral-lingual movements than the noncontingent feedback group. The AIMS scores differed only slightly for the groups during the feedback training. The differences were so small that they were interpreted to be more the functions of artifact than of the feedback training. At 1 week and 2 weeks following training, both groups again showed AIMS scores identical with pretraining scores. These findings are graphed in Figures 30.1–30.3.

Discussion

Although our findings are somewhat more circumscribed than those from earlier reports, EMG feedback did have a suppressive effect on the oral-buccal movements of tardive dyskinesia. Moreover, because our design featured tight, double-blind placebo control, we believe that our results are due to specific training effects rather than nonspecific placebo effects. Our primary goal was to replicate the findings from previous reports using double-blind procedures, randomized assignment to treatment groups, and a sufficient number of participants to allow statistical analysis.

The failure of training effects to persist beyond the laboratory has often been noted in the biofeedback literature (Blanchard & Young, 1973). Although suppression has been shown in the laboratory, which makes for good scientific observation, clinical suppression beyond the training laboratory has been negligible. Indeed, our observation that participants showed significant variability in mastering suppression techniques during training indicates that a program of training more individualized than our quite rigorous approach might be more effective in suppression training. Additionally,

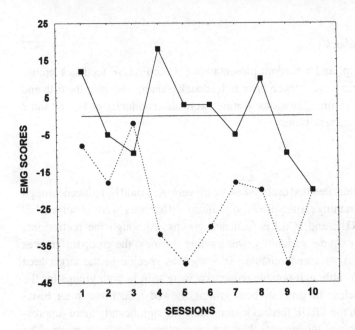

Figure 30.1. Tongue EMG scores over training sessions: squares, noncontingent feedback; circles, contingent feedback.

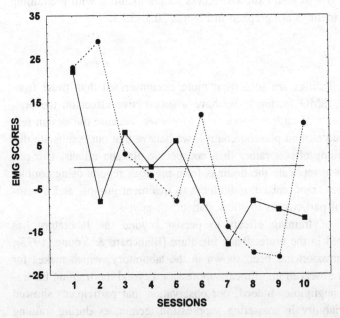

Figure 30.2. Masseter EMG scores over training sessions: squares, noncontingent feedback; circles, contingent feedback.

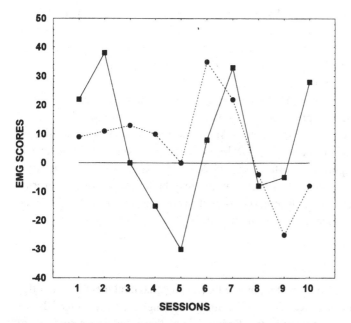

Figure 30.3. Frontalis EMG scores over training sessions: squares, noncontingent feedback; circles, contingent feedback.

individualized training might prove to be an effective approach to the problem of generalization of training effects. Also, as Taylor, Zultnick, and Hoele (1979), Jackson, Schoenfield, and Griffith (1983), and Szekely, Turner, and Jacob (1983) have shown, behavioral methods other than biofeedback may also be effective in controlling oral-lingual movements.

Ongoing Research

We have now begun looking at methods to increase training efficiency by varying feedback modalities and contingencies, instituting a more interactive program, and incorporating other behavioral methods for suppression of oral-lingual movements. In an ongoing series of studies, we are investigating combinations of feedback contingencies and sources of movement, as well as behavioral methods in vivo. We have adopted a single-case design to target several contingencies in a relatively small group of participants, for extended sessions.

All participants are started with FALSE feedback before being given TRUE feedback. We have incorporated various video presentations, different combinations of muscle groups, video feedback of facial movements, and periods of FALSE feedback. To increase generalization, all participants are allowed periods of voluntary control so that we can measure the development of self-control of movements. In addition, all participants are given a minimum of 20 sessions, at 2 sessions per week. After training, to enhance the training effects, all participants are included in either a self-monitoring/self-management group or a relaxation group.

Our findings thus far show substantial changes in EMG activity during sessions, in terms of pre- and post-feedback voluntary-control periods (within session) and weekly AIMS scores. Anecdotal reports from ward personnel indicate that during periods of TRUE feedback for several of the feedback modalities, suppressive effects are obvious. On a lesser note, we have observed that the success of such training may be a function of the severity and duration of tardive dyskinesia, as well as complex interactions of psychiatric conditions, length of hospitalization, age, and other factors.

Conclusion

In general, we have found that biofeedback and behavioral methods can offer potential adjunctive procedures for training oral-lingual suppression of dyskinetic movements. Although the findings from these and other studies are encouraging, it is nevertheless important to note the possible uses of biofeedback methods for exploring the causes of tardive dyskinesia.

We particularly note the potential uses of EMG measurements of movements. Specifically, EMG measurements can contribute to our understanding of the pathophysiological mechanisms underlying dyskinetic movements. For example, our examination of the pathology data from the BPRS and subsequent performances during feedback training indicates a nonsignificant trend. That is, in general, those participants with high BPRS scores on several of the affect-related items performed slightly better than those with lower scores. Although this observation is not statistically significant, it points to a possible relationship between affect and tardive dyskinesia in patients with schizophrenia.

Why the tongue and hands are so vulnerable to the development of dyskinetic movements is not clear. Perhaps the large representations of mouth and hand areas on the cortical motor strip provide the basis for the disorder. For example, the pathophysiological process may be one of disinhibition, with larger areas being more susceptible to release of that inhibition. We might then expect that different muscles involved in the dyskinesias (e.g., tongue, jaw, and fingers) would be excited simultaneously or with a constant time delay. EMG measurements would permit studies of the temporal patterning of abnormal involuntary movements.

Our work indicates that biofeedback training has a suppressive effect on tardive dyskinesia. Although biofeedback training by itself has not produced clinically significant suppression of tardive dyskinesia outside of the laboratory setting, we believe that this method has enormous potential for investigating the causes of tardive dyskinesia and guiding treatment strategies. More important, EMG measurements provide an objective and replicable method for assessment of patients with tardive dyskinesia. It is our belief that the use of biofeedback and objective EMG measurements of tardive dyskinesia will assist in the development of a better understanding of the causes and treatment of tardive dyskinesia.

References

Abrams, B. W. (1986). Biofeedback as an alternative form of treatment for tardive dyskinesia. Unpublished dissertation.

Albanese, H., & Gaardner, K. (1977). Biofeedback treatment of tardive dyskinesia: two case reports. *Am. J. Psychiatry* 134:1149–50.

Alexopoulos, A. (1979). Lack of complaints in schizophrenics with tardive dyskinesia. *J. Nerv. Ment. Dis.* 167:125–7.

American Psychiatric Association (1980). *Tardive Dyskinesia*. Washington, DC: American Psychiatric Association.

Barnes, T. R. E. (1987). Tardive dyskinesia. *Br. Med. J.* 296:150–1.

Blanchard, E. B., & Epstein, L. H. (1977). Clinical applications of biofeedback. In *Progress in Behavior Modification*, vol. 4, ed. M. Hersen, R. M. Eisler, & P. M. Miller, pp. 163–250. New York: Academic Press.

Blanchard, E. B., & Young, L. D. (1973). Self-control of cardiac functioning: a promise as yet unfulfilled. *Psychol. Bull.* 19:145–63.

Bodenhamer, E., Coleman, C., & Achterberg, J. (1986). Self-directed EMG training for the control of pain and spasticity in paraplegia. A case study. *Biofeedback Self Regul.* 11:199–205.

Booker, H., Rubow, R., & Coleman, P. (1969). Simplified feedback in neuromuscular retraining: an automated approach using electromyographic signals. *Arch. Phys. Med. Rehabil.* 50:621–5.

Brener, J. (1974). A general model of voluntary control applied to the phenomena of learned cardiovascular change. In *Cardiovascular Psychophysiology*, ed. P. A. Obrist, A. H. Black, J. Brener, & L. V. DiCara, pp. 365–91. New York: Plenum Press.

Brudny, J., Grynbaum, B., & Korein, J. (1974). Spasmodic torticollis: treatment by biofeedback display of EMG. *Arch. Phys. Med. Rehabil.* 55:403–8.

Casey, D. E., & Rabins, P. (1978). Tardive dyskinesia as a life-threatening illness. *Am. J. Psychiatry* 135:486–8.

DeVeaugh-Geiss, J. (1982). Epidemiology of tardive dyskinesia, part 1. In *Tardive Dyskinesia and Related Involuntary Movement Disorders*, ed. J. DeVeaugh-Geiss, pp. 33–40. Boston: John Wright.

Farrar, W. B. (1976). Using electromyographic biofeedback in treating orofacial dyskinesia. *J. Prosthet. Dent.* 35:384–7.

Folstein, M. F., Folstein, S. E., & McHugh, P. R. (1975). Mini-mental state: a practical method for grading the cognitive state of patients for the clinician. *J. Psychiatr. Res.* 12:189–98.

Fudge, R. C., & Adams, H. E. (1985). The effects of discrimination training on acquisition of voluntary control of cephalic vasomotor activity. *Psychophysiology* 22:300–6.

Fudge, R. C., Thailer, S. A., Alpert, M., & Intrator, J. (1987). The use of electromyographic feedback to reduce oral-lingual movements associated with tardive dyskinesia in elderly patients on a long-term neuroleptic regimen. Presented at the annual meeting of the Association for Advancement of Behavior Therapy, Boston.

Fudge, R. C., Thailer, S. A., Alpert, M., Intrator, J., & Sison, C. E. (1991). The effects of electromyographic feedback training on suppression of the oral-lingual movements associated with tardive dyskinesia. *Biofeedback Self Regul.* 16:117–29.

Fudge, R. C., Thailer, S., Alpert, M., Intriligator, R., & Intrator, J. (1992). Psychopathology and oral-lingual movement in tardive dyskinesia. Presented at a conference of the Society for Behavioral Medicine, New York.

Granacher, R. P., Jr. (1981). Differential diagnosis of tardive dyskinesia: an overview. *Am. J. Psychiatry* 138:1288–97.

Jackson, G. M., Schoenfield, L. I., & Griffith, A. (1983). A comparison of two behavioral treatments in decreasing the facial movement of tardive dyskinesia. *Biofeedback Self Regul.* 8:547–53.

Jeste, D. V., & Wyatt, R. J. (eds.) (1982). *Understanding and Treating Tardive Dyskinesia*. New York: Guilford Press.

Jus, A., Jus, K., & Fontaine, P. (1979). Long-term treatment of tardive dyskinesia. *J. Clin. Psychiatry* 40:72–7.

Kane, J. M., Woerner, M., Lierberman, J., & Kinon, B. (1984). Tardive dyskinesia. In *Neuropsychiatric Movement Disorders*, ed. D. V. Jeste & R. J. Wyatt. Washington, DC: American Psychiatric Press.

Mcleod, J. H. (1983). Biofeedback in the management of partial anal incontinence. *Dis. Colon Rectum* 26:244–6.

Miller, N. E., & Dworkin, B. R. (1974). Visceral learning: recent difficulties with curarized rats and significant problems for human research. In *Cardiovascular Psychophysiology*, ed. D. P. A. Obrist, A. H. Black, J. Brener, & L. V. DiCara, pp. 78–102. New York: Plenum Press.

Overall, J. E., & Gorham, D. R. (1962). The Brief Psychiatric Rating Scale. *Psychol. Rep.* 10:799–812.

Roberts, L. E., Williams, R. J., Marlin, R. G., Farrell, T., & Imiolo, D. (1984). Awareness of the response after feedback training for changes in heart rate and sudmotor laterality. *J. Exp. Psychol.* 113:225–55.

Rosenbaum, A. H., O'Connor, M. K., & Duane, D. D. (1980). Treatment of tardive dyskinesia in an agitated, depressed patient. *Psychosomatics* 41:765–6.

Shapiro, D., Schwartz, G. E., & Tursky, B. (1972). Control of diastolic blood pressure in man by feedback and reinforcement. *Psychophysiology* 9:296–304.

Sherman, R. A. (1979). Successful treatment of one case of tardive dyskinesia with electromyographic feedback from the masseter muscle. *Biofeedback Self Regul.* 4:367–70.

Smith, J. M., & Kane, J. M. (1982). Epidemiology of tardive dyskinesia: part 2. In *Tardive Dyskinesia and Related Involuntary Movement Disorders*, ed. J. DeVeaugh-Geiss, pp. 41–50. Boston: John Wright.

Szekely, B. C., Turner, S. M., & Jacob, R. G. (1983). Behavioral control of L-dopa induced dyskinesia in parkinsonism. *Biofeedback Self Regul.* 7:443–7.

Tarsy, D., & Baldessarini, R. J. (1977). The pathophysiologic basis of tardive dyskinesia. *Biol. Psychiatry* 12:431–50.

Taylor, C. B., Zultnick, S. I., & Hoele, W. (1979). The effects of behavioral procedures on tardive dyskinesia. *Behav. Ther.* 10:37–45.

Wexler, N. (1984). Huntington's disease. In *Neuropsychiatric Movement Disorders*, ed. D. V. Jeste & R. J. Wyatt. Washington, DC: American Psychiatric Press.

Yagi, G., & Itoh, H. (1987). Follow-up study of 11 patients with potentially reversible tardive dyskinesia. *Am. J. Psychiatry* 144:1496–8.

Index